D0853746

# ACCIDENT PREVENTION MANUAL for INDUSTRIAL OPERATIONS

## ADMINISTRATION and PROGRAMS

# ACCIDENT PREVENTION MANUAL for INDUSTRIAL OPERATIONS

## ADMINISTRATION and PROGRAMS

**8th Edition**

Frank E. McElroy, P.E., C.S.P.
Editor in Chief

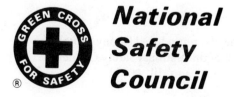

National Safety Council

**First Edition** © 1946
**Second Edition** © 1951
**Third Edition** © 1955
**Fourth Edition** © 1959
**Fifth Edition** © 1964
**Sixth Edition** © 1969
**Seventh Edition** © 1974

**Eighth Edition—in two volumes**
**Copyright © 1981 National Safety Council**
**All Rights Reserved**

International Standard Book Number: 0–87912–025–8
Library of Congress Catalog Card Number: 80–81376
Printed in the United States of America

10M0681                    Stock No. 121.41

# Occupational Safety and Health Series

The National Safety Council Occupational Safety and Health Series is dedicated to the publication of current and vital information designed to help the reader establish priorities, gather and analyze data to help identify problems, and develop methods and procedures that will eliminate or decrease the seriousness of accident problems—to mitigate injury and illness, and minimize economic loss resulting from accidents.

The principal volumes in this series are:

*Accident Prevention Manual for Industrial Operations*
  *Administration and Programs* volume
  *Engineering and Technology* volume
*Fundamentals of Industrial Hygiene*

Other hardcover books published by the Council are:

*Communications for the Safety Professional*
*Industrial Noise and Hearing Conservation*
*Motor Fleet Safety Manual*
*Supervisors Guide to Human Relations*
*Supervisors Safety Manual*

Not only are all National Safety Council books revised periodically, but new titles are introduced as the need arises. Ideas, comments, and contributions from readers are invited.

# Preface
## to the Eighth Edition

The Eighth Edition of the Accident Prevention Manual has been divided into two volumes—this one covers *Administration and Programs*; the other, *Engineering and Technology*. This is the ultimate resolution of the division that began in the Seventh Edition when chapter arrangement was improved so that those chapters encompassing management techniques were placed in the first half of the Manual and those involving the more technical duties of a safety professional were placed in the second half.

In addition to making this division, this edition does not contain those chapters that duplicate material now found in greater detail in the Council's *Fundamentals of Industrial Hygiene*. The format of the Hygiene book now matches that of the two Accident Prevention Manual volumes, so that they make an excellent three-book set—the Occupational Safety and Health Series.

However, a brief discussion of industrial hygiene methods of measurement and testing is included in Chapter 3, "Acquiring Hazard Information." Chapter 17, "Personal Protective Equipment," also duplicates some material found in *Fundamentals of Industrial Hygiene* in order to give a thorough discussion of the subject.

There were a number of reasons for dividing the content of the old Accident Prevention Manual into three volumes —one of which was the sheer bulk of all the information contained in them. Another was to physically divide the subject matter into three related books that could be consulted when the reader was faced with a specific problem in training and management, safety engineering, or industrial hygiene. This division also corresponds with the way the subjects are taught at National Safety Council and in other short courses and in college-level courses. Thus a student need not carry one big volume through three or more separate courses.

The Council hopes that this new arrangement will make this edition easier and more effective to use in preventing accidents.

This Accident Prevention Manual is not a radical venture into new fields of knowledge—it is the cumulation of facts and ideas that have become part of the safety movement's general heritage. Its goal is to organize and transmit information of value to those who toil in the vineyards of safety to prevent accidents and unwanted resultant effects—death, injury and illness, property damage, and other losses.

The term *accident* is used in its broad sense to mean that occurrence in a sequence of events that usually produces unintended injury or illness, or death, and/or property damage. This subject is discussed in greater detail in this volume. (See the Index for page references.)

## New or expanded material

This *Administration and Programs* volume picks up, updates, and expands the following chapters from the Seventh Edition—1 through 15, 18 through 23, and 45. The chapter sequence has been retained, for the most part. In addition, there are two new chapters—"The Handicapped Worker" and "Product Safety and Liability Prevention."

Specifically, here is what is new in this volume of the Eighth Edition. (Refer to the Contents page for chapter titles.)

Chapter 1, many illustrations. Chapter 2, updating of OSHA material and new description of administration, provisions, and standards of the Mine Safety and Health Act. Chapter 3, complete revision except for off-the-job portion; safety committees discussion has been reduced. Chapter 4, complete revision; many examples of inspection forms have been added. Chapter 5, minor additions. Chapter 6, update of OSHA record-keeping requirements; rearrangement of sections. Chapter 7, minimum data set

and corrective action selections are new. Chapter 8, statistics updated. Chapter 9, OSHA and MSHA training requirements included; expansion of training techniques discussion. Chapter 10, expanded. Chapter 11, extensive updating. Chapter 12, expanded. Chapter 13, minor changes. Chapter 14, major updating; videotape and CCTV is new. Chapter 15, updated and extensively revised. Chapter 16, new sections on radioactive materials and security from personal attack. Chapter 17, updating, especially respiratory equipment and safety belts and lifelines. Chapter 18, minor changes; Chapter 19, minor changes; expanded sections on neck or wrist tags for medical alert and alcohol and drug control; placement of handicapped moved to Chapter 20; Chapter 20, new. Chapter 21, portion on how to measure losses was taken out; building entrances, glazing, merchandise displays, and vertical transportation sections have been greatly expanded; crowd and panic control and swimming pools are new; product safety portion is now replaced by Chapter 22, which covers this subject in greater detail. Chapter 23, extensively revised. Chapter 24, updated; emergency and specialized information section is new.

## Contributors

National Safety Council appreciates the help and guidance of the many authorities who gave information, advice, and illustrations. Fifty-one

safety professionals and other experts contributed, as did nine professional and other associations.

Members of the Technical Publications Committee of the Industrial Division of the Council gave continuing guidance to improve this Manual.

Special thanks is given to Robert J. Firenze, president of RJF Associates, Bloomington, Ind., who prepared Chapters 3 and 4; to Richard F. Moscato, manager, Industrial Safety, International Harvester Co., World Headquarters, Chicago, who prepared Chapter 20; and to Russell E. Marhefka, director, Product Safety, National Safety Council, who prepared Chapter 22.

The following persons were on the Council staff at the time of their contribution to this volume.

I. Ahmed
G. Bombyk
A. Carpenter
R. Currie
B. Dembski
A. DiCicco
A. Hoskin
R. Hammersmith
A. Kane
R. Koziol
G. McConnell
J. Pease
A. Phillips
C. Piepho
K. Race
J. Recht ( † 1980)
P. Schmidt
J. Van Sickle
T. Worhol
D. Wu

The editor in chief of this edition, and also the previous three editions, was Frank

McElroy, a registered professional engineer and a Certified Safety Professional. Robert Pedroza ably assisted. Production help was provided by Randy Becker, Mark Cappetta, and others.

Acknowledgement is given to members of Council Staff, especially to Irvin Etter, Industrial Department manager; Roy Fisher, editor of *National Safety News*; Richard Gaw, Labor Department manager; Robert Meyer, Publications Department manager; and Frank Waszak, art director, for their assistance.

Cover design was by Jake Kasparian of the Council staff.

The information and recommendations contained in this Manual have been compiled from sources believed to be reliable and to represent the best current opinion on the subject. No warranty, guarantee, or representation is made by National Safety Council as to the absolute correctness or sufficiency of any information or statements contained in this and other publications. The National Safety Council assumes no responsibility in connection therewith. Nor can it be assumed that all acceptable safety measures are contaned in this publication, or that other or additional measures may not be required under particular or exceptional conditions or circumstances.

# Contents

# NATIONAL SAFETY COUNCIL

FOUNDED SEPTEMBER 24, 1913
INCORPORATED IN ILLINOIS OCTOBER 1, 1930
INCORPORATED BY ACT OF CONGRESS AUGUST 13, 1953

**Purposes and Powers.** Certain essential provisions of the Act of Congress which incorporated the National Safety Council are as follows:

### Objects and Purposes

"The objects and purposes of the corporation shall be --

to further, encourage; and promote methods and procedures leading to increased safety, protection, and health among employees and employers and among children in industries, on farms, in schools and colleges, in homes, on streets and highways, in recreation; and in other public and private places;

to collect, correlate, .. and disseminate educational and informative data, .. relative to safety methods and procedures;

to arouse and maintain the interest of the people of the United States, its Territories and possessions in safety and in accident prevention, and to encourage the adoption and institution of safety methods by all persons, .. and .. organizations;

to organize, establish, and conduct programs, .. for the education of all persons, .. in safety methods and procedures;

to cooperate with, enlist, and develop the cooperation of and between all persons, .. and .. organizations .. both public and private, engaged or interested in, .. any or all of the foregoing purposes .."

### Powers

"The corporation shall have power --

to establish and maintain offices for the conduct of its business, and to charter local, State, and regional safety organizations, .. in appropriate places throughout the United States, its Territories and possessions;

to charge and collect membership dues, subscription fees, and receive contributions or grants of money or property to be devoted to the carrying out of its purposes;

to choose such officers, directors, trustees, managers, agents, and employees as the business of the corporation may require.;

to adopt, amend, and alter a constitution and bylaws, ..

to organize, establish, and conduct conferences on safety and accident prevention;

to publish magazines and other publications and materials, .. consistent with its corporate purposes;

to adopt, alter, use, and display such emblems, seals, and badges as it may adopt."

### Nonpolitical Nature

"The corporation and its officers, directors, and duly appointed agents as such, shall not contribute to or otherwise support or assist any political party or candidate for office."

### No Stock or Dividends

"The corporation shall have no power to issue any shares of stock nor to declare nor pay any dividends."

### Audit and Congressional Report

The financial transactions shall be audited annually, .. by an independent certified public accountant .. A report of such audit shall be made by the corporation to the Congress not later than six months following the close of such fiscal year for which the audit is made."

### Exclusive Right to Name and Emblem

"The corporation, and its subordinate divisions and regional, state, and local chapters, shall have the sole and exclusive right to use the name, National Safety Council. The corporation shall have the exclusive and sole right to use, or to allow or refuse the use of, such emblems, seals, and badges as it may legally adopt .."

### Transfer of Assets

"The corporation may acquire the assets of the National Safety Council, Incorporated, a corporation organized under the laws of the State of Illinois, upon discharging or satisfactorily providing for the payment and discharge of all of the liability of such corporation and upon complying with all laws of the State of Illinois applicable thereto."

**Congressional and Presidential Approval.** The Act which incorporated the National Safety Council was passed during the First Session of the 83rd Congress and was designated Public Law 259. Leadership in the Congress was as follows:

| | | | |
|---|---|---|---|
| In the Senate | Bill introduced by *Arthur V. Watkins*, Senator from Utah | Approved by the Sub Committee on Federal Charges of the Judiciary Committee, *John Marshall Butler*, Chairman, Senator from Maryland | Approved by the Judiciary Committee, Chairman, *William Langer*, Senator from North Dakota | Passed by the Senate, President of the Senate, *Richard M. Nixon*, Vice President of the United States |
| In the House of Representatives | Bill introduced by *Clifford Davis*, Representative from Tennessee | Approved by the Sub Committee on Federal Charges, of the Judiciary Committee, Chairman, *John Robsion*, Representative from Kentucky | Approved by the Judiciary Committee, Chairman, *Chauncey W. Reed*, Representative from Illinois | Passed by the House, Speaker of the House, *Joseph W. Martin, Jr.*, Representative from Massachusetts |

The Act was signed by the President of the United States, Dwight D. Eisenhower, on August 13, 1953.

**Transfer of Operations to the Federal Corporation.** At the time the Act was passed granting the National Safety Council a federal charter, the Council was functioning as an Illinois corporation. This arrangement continued until _____ on which date the Council's assets, operations and organizational structure were transferred from the Illinois corporation to the federal corporation.

THE NATIONAL SAFETY COUNCIL is the only national nongovernmental, privately supported, public service organization established solely for accident prevention. In 1953, the 83rd Congress of the United States issued a Federal Charter for the Council, thus recognizing its work as an integral part of the American way of life.

# Occupational Safety

## History and Growth

# Chapter
# 1

# 1—Occupational Safety

Elimination of accidents is vital to the public interest. Accidents produce economic and social loss, impair individual and group productivity, cause inefficiency, and retard the advancement of standards of living.°

## Philosophy of Occupational Accident Prevention

There is no question that accidents are costly to industry and society. Today, failure to try to prevent injuries to employees is indefensible.

The practical and moral aspects of accident prevention are interrelated, because accidents result both in a waste of manpower and resources, and in physical and mental anguish.

In medieval days, the master craftsman tried to instruct his apprentices and journeymen to work skillfully and safely, because he could see the value of high quality and uninterrupted production, but it took the Industrial Revolution to create the conditions which led to the development of accident prevention as a specialized field.

The industrial safety philosophy developed as a result of the tremendous forces of production which were released. Without a deterrent to counter this waste of manpower and resources, the number of accidents and injuries would have challenged the imagination.

Once enlightened industrial management had accepted the responsibility for preventing accidents, the next step was workers' compensation laws. This "new" line of thinking held the employer responsible for a share of the economic loss suffered by the employee because of an accident.

It was a rather short step from this to the realization that a large proportion of accidents could be prevented and that the same industrial brain power that could produce vast quantities of goods could also be used for accident prevention. Industry soon discovered that efficient production and safety were related. From this beginning grew the safety movement as it is known today.

The progress in reducing the number of accidents and injuries in this relatively short period of time has exceeded the highest expectations of the early safety pioneers. In less than one lifetime, safety has become a vital part of industry.

Experience has shown that there is virtually no hazard or operation that cannot be overcome by practical safety measures. The future may introduce a type of unavoidable accident, but history

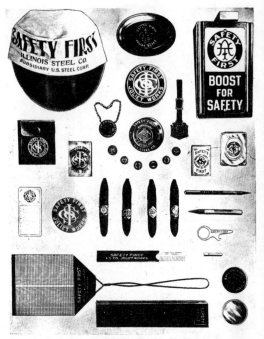

FIG. 1-1 Give the man a cigar . . . or (in summer) a fly swatter! This 1913 display used by the Joliet Works of Illinois Steel Company, the first plant to organize a safety committee, offers a variety of safety incentives: watch fobs, paper weights, cigars, and a calendar.

indicates that practically all barriers can and will be surmounted.

In summary, here are the reasons for the continuing, concerted effort to prevent accidents:

1. Needless destruction of life and health is a moral evil

2. Failure to take necessary precautions against predictable accidents involves moral responsibility for those accidents

3. Accidents severely limit efficiency and productivity

4. Accidents produce far-reaching social harm

5. The safety movement has already demonstrated that its techniques are effective in reducing accident rates and promoting efficiency

---

°Excerpt from National Safety Council policy.

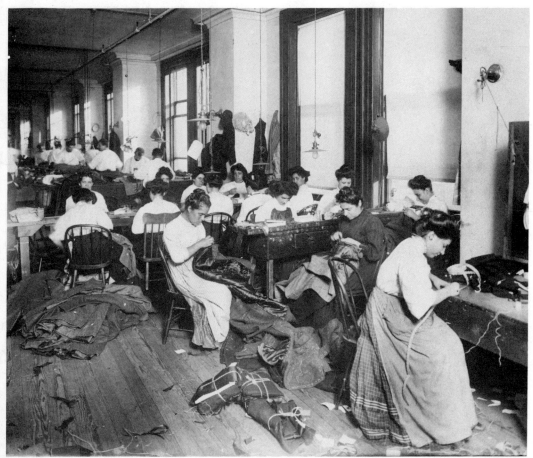

FIG. 1–2.—Old photograph shows "sweat shop" conditions that existed in the garment industry. Although factory production was far greater than the cottage industry it replaced, factories were often inferior in terms of human values, health, and safety.

*Courtesy Brown Brothers, New York, N.Y.*

6. Nothing in the available data suggests that safety professionals are near a limit in their ability to extend the moral and practical values of accident prevention.

## History of the Safety Movement

In the U.S. before the 19th Century, no industrial system existed. Families usually lived and worked on farms. No record was kept of injuries sustained by workers.

After 1800, when the effects of the Industrial Revolution were felt in the United States, factory work started.

During the last half of the 19th Century, American factories were expanding their product lines and producing at heretofore unimagined rates. While the factories were far superior in terms of production to the preceding small handicraft shops, they were often inferior in terms of human values, health, and safety.

These deficiencies were probably inevitable. The tools of mass production had to be invented and applied before anyone could begin to imagine the problems they would create, and the problems had to be known before corrective measures

**3**

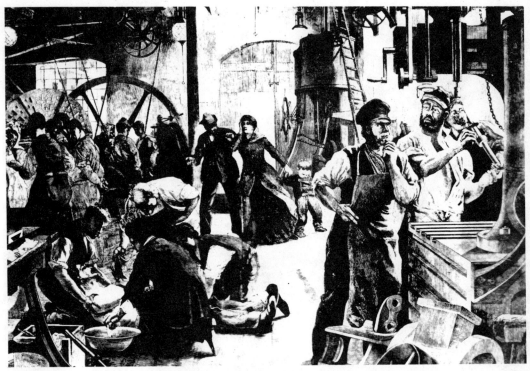

FIG. 1–3.—The accident in the machine shop—a woodcut based on a painting by John Bahr.

*Courtesy The Bettmann Archive.*

could be considered, tested, and proved. Deaths and injuries were accepted as being part of "industrial progress."

While this change in work environment was taking place, the thinking of the public, management, and the law was still reflecting the past, when the worker was an independent craftsman or a member of the family-owned shop. Common law provided the employer with a defense that gave the injured worker little chance for compensation. The three doctrines of common law that favored the employer were:

*Fellow servant rule*—Employer was not liable for injury to employee that resulted from negligence of a fellow employee.

*Contributory negligence*—Employer was not liable if the employee was injured due to his own negligence.

*Assumption of risk*—Employer was not liable because the employee took the job with full knowledge of the risks and hazards involved.

In large industrial centers, the ugly results of industrial accidents and poor occupational health conditions became more and more obvious. Voices of protest were raised. Though there were employers who denied the existence of the problem, wiser management people began to try to meet specific aspects of it.

As early as 1867, Massachusetts had begun to use factory inspectors, and ten years later that state had a law requiring the safeguarding of hazardous machinery. During 1877, Massachusetts also passed the Employer's Liability Law that made employers liable for damages when a worker was injured. However, court decisions based on common law often let the employer escape liability.

From 1898 on, there were additional efforts to make the employer financially liable for accidents. In 1911, the first effective workers' com-

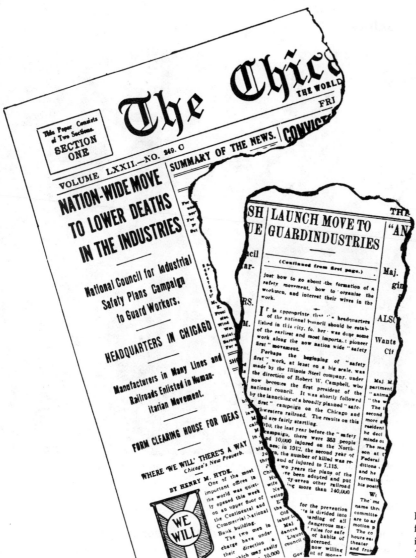

## NATION-WIDE MOVE TO LOWER DEATHS IN THE INDUSTRIES

National Council for Industrial Safety Plans Campaign to Guard Workers.

### HEADQUARTERS IN CHICAGO

Manufacturers in Many Lines and Railroads Enlisted in Humanitarian Movement.

### FORM CLEARING HOUSE FOR IDEAS

WHERE 'WE WILL' THERE'S A WAY
Chicago's New Proverb.

BY HENRY M. HYDE.

One of the most important offices in the world was quietly opened this week on an upper floor of the Continental and Commercial National Bank building.

The two men in charge here under their direction which may easily 10,000

### LAUNCH MOVE TO GUARD INDUSTRIES

(Continued from first page.)

just how to go about the formation of a safety movement, how to organize the workmen, and interest their wives in the work.

It is appropriate that the headquarters of the national council should be established in this city, fo. her: was done some of the earliest and most importa.t pioneer work along the now nation wide "safety first" movement.

Perhaps the beginning of "safety first" work, at least on a big scale, was made by the Illinois Steel company, under the direction of Robert W. Campbell, who now becomes the first president of the national council. It was shortly followed by the launching of a broadly planned "safety first" campaign on the Chicago and Northwestern railroad. The results on this road are fairly startling.

1910, the last year before the "safety campaign, there were 353 people in 10,000 injured on the North nee; in 1912, the second year of ju'a, the number of killed was re thro. and of injured to 7,115.

wo years the plans of the Chi re been adopted and put Ho ty-seven other railroad wife ing more than 140,000.

for the prevention is is divided into arding of all dangerous ma rules for safe of habits of acerned now willing nt of money.

FIG. 1–4.—Clippings from October 17, 1913, issue of *The Chicago Tribune.*

pensation act was passed in Wisconsin (some authorities give this credit to New Jersey). This was followed by similar laws in many other states.

These laws were, at first, declared invalid because of conflict with the due process of law provisions of the 14th Amendment. After the U.S. Supreme Court in 1916 declared it to be constitutional in *New York Central Railroad Co.* v. *White*, 243 U.S. 188, many states passed compulsory laws on workers' compensation.

There had also been progress on the technical side of the problem. The railroads, which, perhaps, had suffered the most adverse publicity

from accidents, adopted the air brake and the automatic coupler well before the turn of the century. Some progress was also made in such matters as safeguarding and fire prevention.

Next came the recognition that safeguarding the machine was not the total solution and that people's actions were important factors in creating accident situations.

Insurance companies began relating the cost of premiums for workers' compensation insurance to the cost of accidents. Management began to understand that there might be a relationship between successful production and safety.

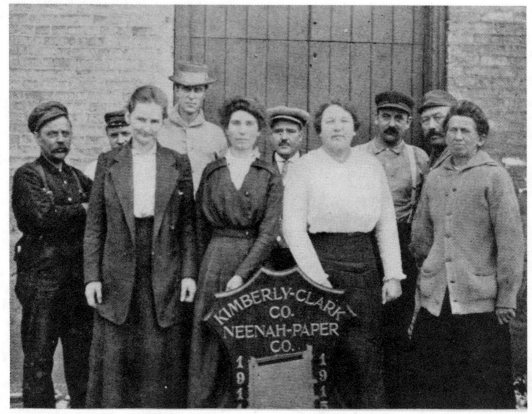

FIG. 1–5.—One of the first safety committees was formed with mill employees at Kimberly-Clark Co./Neenah Paper Co. The plaque in the foreground is dated 1915.

In the first decade of the 20th Century, two great industries, railroads and steel, began the first large-scale organized safety programs. From this period comes one of the great and historic documents of safety. In 1906, Judge Elbert Gary, president of the United States Steel Corporation, wrote:

"The United States Steel Corporation expects its subsidiary companies to make every effort practicable to prevent injury to its employees. Expenditures necessary for such purposes will be authorized. Nothing which will add to the protection of the workmen should be neglected."

The Association of Iron and Steel Electrical Engineers, organized soon after this announcement, devoted considerable attention to safety problems in its industry.

## Birth of the National Safety Council

Then, in 1911, the year in which the Wisconsin Act was passed, a request came from the Association of Iron and Steel Electrical Engineers to call a general industrial safety conference on a national scale. The result was the First Cooperative Safety Congress, which met in 1912 in Milwaukee. This gathering called for another meeting in New York the following year, and at that meeting the National Council for Industrial Safety was organized. Shortly afterward, the organization's name was changed to the National Safety Council, and its program was broadened to include all aspects of accident prevention. Yet it must be remembered that the Council was the creation of industry and that its activities have always been heavily concentrated on industrial safety.

# Attention
# Safety Committeemen!

What becomes of our safety men who have served their turn on the Safety Committee? How can they still help in the work?

There are two classes of people who have served on Safety Committees, the interested and the non-interested. The work of an active committee is always noticed. We see them when they make their monthly inspection, and later we see or hear of changes that take place—sometimes a large and sometimes just a small change. Perhaps it is a word or caution or a suggestion that guards shall not be removed without proper authority, or of a safer way to do a job, or that a cleaner room makes for better working conditions. These recommendations come to fellow employees who are working with you. While on the Committee, you are working in their interest to make their jobs more pleasant, convenient, and safe in every way. And the retired safety man is doing his share to help this work along! He knows from close acquaintance with the work just where he can help in cautioning against unsafe practices, and knows just how to approach a new man and give a friendly hint that may help a lot in that particular job, or suggest a new method to the older man so that he won't get in a rut and use old ways when there are better ways of doing things.

More important than all of these is the example that every careful workman sets for those with whom he works. The retired safety man is never retired except in name only, for his example is observed and followed by far more than he ever knows. His opportunity is to think, act, and live safety, and in this way he is doing his share to build up an organization of careful, efficient men and women.

FIG. 1–6.—A 1918 safety poster published by The National Safety Council encourages retired safety professionals to continue their safety work as a member of a safety committee.

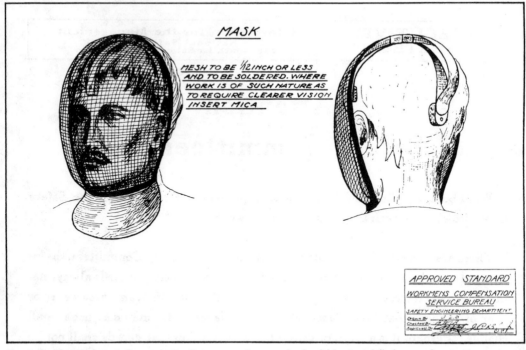

FIG. 1–7.—The Workmen's Compensation Bureau gave "approval only of the principle" of personal protective equipment and clothing. Its "Universal Safety Standard" (dated 1914) showed this mask with 1/12-inch (or less) mesh; where clear vision was required, a mica insert was allowed.

The group that met in Milwaukee and New York was composed of a few safety "professionals," some management leaders, public officials, and insurance specialists. Their one point in common was a desire to attack a problem which most people thought to be unimportant or could not be solved. Because these people were determined, the safety movement as we know it today was designed and built.

### Accident prevention discoveries

As industry developed some experience in safety, it discovered that engineering could prevent accidents, that employees could be reached through education, and that safety rules could be established and enforced. Thus the "Three E's of Safety"—Engineering, Education, and Enforcement—were developed.

There were other discoveries, too. Safety departments had often argued that savings in compensation costs and medical expenses would many times repay safety expenditures. Thought-ful business leaders soon learned that these savings were only a fraction of the financial benefits to be derived from accident prevention work. Indirect financial savings are estimated to be several times larger than the direct savings in compensation and medical bills.

### Acceleration of the drive for safety

Industrial safety received wide acceptance in the years between the two world wars. Conservation of manpower during World War II intensified the safety growth, and the federal government encouraged safety activities by its contractors. As industry expanded to meet the needs of the war effort, additional safety personnel were hastily trained to try to keep pace. The acceptance of safety as part of the industrial picture did not diminish with the end of the war. By then, the importance of safety to quality production was well established, and the small handful of dedicated people in 1912 had grown to millions.

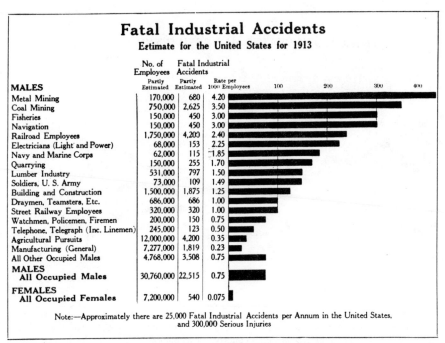

## Fatal Industrial Accidents
### Estimate for the United States for 1913

| MALES | No. of Employees Partly Estimated | Fatal Industrial Accidents Partly Estimated | Rate per 1000 Employees | | | | |
|---|---|---|---|---|---|---|---|
| | | | | 100 | 200 | 300 | 400 |
| Metal Mining | 170,000 | 680 | 4.20 | | | | |
| Coal Mining | 750,000 | 2,625 | 3.50 | | | | |
| Fisheries | 150,000 | 450 | 3.00 | | | | |
| Navigation | 150,000 | 450 | 3.00 | | | | |
| Railroad Employees | 1,750,000 | 4,200 | 2.40 | | | | |
| Electricians (Light and Power) | 68,000 | 153 | 2.25 | | | | |
| Navy and Marine Corps | 62,000 | 115 | 1.85 | | | | |
| Quarrying | 150,000 | 255 | 1.70 | | | | |
| Lumber Industry | 531,000 | 797 | 1.50 | | | | |
| Soldiers, U. S. Army | 73,000 | 109 | 1.49 | | | | |
| Building and Construction | 1,500,000 | 1,875 | 1.25 | | | | |
| Draymen, Teamsters, Etc. | 686,000 | 686 | 1.00 | | | | |
| Street Railway Employees | 320,000 | 320 | 1.00 | | | | |
| Watchmen, Policemen, Firemen | 200,000 | 150 | 0.75 | | | | |
| Telephone, Telegraph (Inc. Linemen) | 245,000 | 123 | 0.50 | | | | |
| Agricultural Pursuits | 12,000,000 | 4,200 | 0.35 | | | | |
| Manufacturing (General) | 7,277,000 | 1,819 | 0.23 | | | | |
| All Other Occupied Males | 4,768,000 | 3,508 | 0.75 | | | | |
| **MALES** All Occupied Males | 30,760,000 | 22,515 | 0.75 | | | | |
| **FEMALES** All Occupied Females | 7,200,000 | 540 | 0.075 | | | | |

Note:—Approximately there are 25,000 Fatal Industrial Accidents per Annum in the United States, and 300,000 Serious Injuries

FIG. 1–8.—Ida M. Tarbell, an American writer in the early years of this century, was present at the session of the 2nd National Safety Congress when the National Safety Council came into being. During the following year, she wrote a series of articles for *The American Magazine* telling of the "remarkable changes" that were taking place in the business world of the day. In reporting on the then-youthful safety movement, she included the chart reproduced here. (The source of the statistics is not known.)

In 1948, for example, Admiral Ben Moreell, then president of Jones and Laughlin Steel Corporation, wrote:

"Although safe and healthful working conditions can be justified on a cold dollars-and-cents basis, I prefer to justify them on the basic principle that it is the right thing to do. In discussing safety in industrial operations, I have often heard it stated that the cost of adequate health and safety measures would be prohibitive and that 'we can't afford it.'

"My answer to that is quite simple and quite direct. It is this: 'If we can't afford safety, we can't afford to be in business.'"

A discussion of current federal safety legislation follows later in this chapter under "Safety and the law."

A by-product of organized safety activity has been increased interest in safety engineering on the part of schools of higher learning. A number of schools now offer degrees and advanced courses

in this subject and are contributing to a higher standard of knowledge among professionals in the field.

The World War II labor shortage dramatically brought home to management the magnitude and seriousness of the problem of off-the-job accidents to industrial employees. The wartime theme of the National Safety Council, "Save Manpower for Warpower," focused attention on efficient and safe production. Interest in off-the-job safety has been heightened in recent years by the passage of numerous state laws on compulsory insurance which, in effect, make the employer financially responsible for all illnesses and injuries to workers, whether they originate on or off the job.

Today, an increasing number of employers are including off-the-job safety in their overall safety programs. Companies realize their operating costs and production schedules are affected as much when an employee is injured away from

## TREND OF ACCIDENTAL WORK DEATHS HAS BEEN DOWN

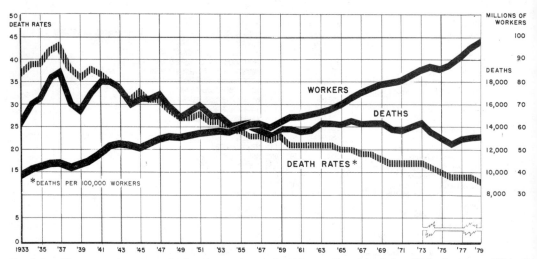

FIG. 1–9a.—The average American today has a better chance of avoiding accidental death than did the American of 30 or 40 years ago. This chart, based on figures for the entire country, shows number of deaths is down even though number of workers continues to increase.

work as when he is injured on the job. Off-the-job safety is an extension of a company's on-the-job safety program and is intended to educate the employee to follow the safe practices he uses on the job in his outside activities. Companies with sound on-the-job safety programs have found that each program complements the other.

From the earliest days of industrial safety work, it has never been possible to make a clear separation between health and accident hazards. Is dermatitis an accident or a disease? What about hernias, hearing loss, and heart trouble? Inevitably, there has been interest and activity on the part of safety professionals in many health problems that are on the borderline between diseases and accidents. Over the years, an increasingly effective organized cooperation between medical and safety professionals has developed in these areas.

### Growth

In any movement of social progress, there are many factors which must be considered in evalu-

ating the usefulness of the effort.

In evaluating the work of the safety movement, particularly, a complex set of factors must always be kept in mind.

Safety professionals, unlike designers of a new piece of machinery, cannot look philosophically upon errors and breakdowns in the experimental stage. Because they deal with human lives, human health, and immediate efficiency and productivity, safety professionals must deal with today's problems today.

On the other hand, they cannot be content to run from emergency to emergency. They must consider the long-term effects of their work—the increase of knowledge, the improvement of techniques, the development of organizational forms which will serve them well next year and for many years to come.

Since the factors are complex, no simple rating scale can indicate an answer to the question, "What has the safety movement accomplished?" In the absence of such a rating scale, an attempt to answer the question must be made by assembling several kinds of data.

Fig. 1-9b.—Since 1933, death rates per 100,000 workers were at their highest for manufacturing in 1936 and for nonmanufacturing in 1937. Since those years, both rates decreased more than 60 percent and reached their lowest levels in recent years. These lower rates resulted from deaths declining about one-third, and increased numbers of workers.

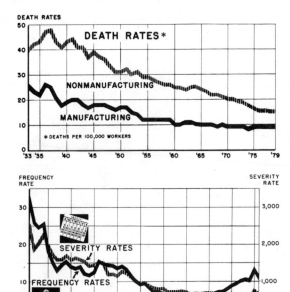

Fig. 1-9c.—The injury frequency rate of Council reporters declined rapidly to 1932, increased in World War II, then reached a record low in 1961 and increased gradually in the following decade. The severity rate followed a similar pattern.

Rates for recent years are not comparable due to significant changes in numbers of reporters, and because many employers have stopped using the ANSI Z16.1; see Chapter 6 for a discussion.

## Statistical evaluation

First, the question must be asked, "Has the safety movement, in fact, done anything in the past to prevent accidents?" To that question can be answered a clear "Yes!"

If the annual accidental death rate per 100,000 of population which held in 1912 had continued, there would have been over two million more accidental deaths than actually occurred. Since 1912, the death rate for persons of normal working age—25 to 64 years—declined more than 67 percent while the rate of all ages of the entire population declined only half that much. Medical progress accounts for some of this gain, but the larger part is certainly the product of organized safety work.

The work accident figures (Fig. 1-9a) probably understate the progress made in industrial safety, for they include a very large number of nonmanufacturing work deaths. Farm work, trades, services, and government accounted for more than half the accidental work deaths in recent years. The remaining 6900 deaths occurred in manufac-

turing, public utilities, transportation, construction, and the extractive industries (mining, quarrying, and gas and oil wells).

Overall frequency and severity rates for all industries since 1926 are not available, but figures on the experience of concerns reporting to the National Safety Council provide a dramatic summary of the progress of organized safety work in the nation—approximately a 2/3 cut in the frequency of disabling injuries through 1976.

The historical data shown in Figure 1-9c, based on the *American National Standard Method of Recording and Measuring Work Injury Experience*, ANSI Z16.1-1967 (R 1973), represent the injury experience of National Safety Council reporters and were published for the last time in the 1978 edition of *Accident Facts*. Other detailed industry data based on Z16.1, formerly shown in *Accident Facts*, have been replaced by data based on the OSHA recordkeeping requirements.

Effective with 1977 records, National Safety Council members were asked to report their occupational injury and illness records based on

**11**

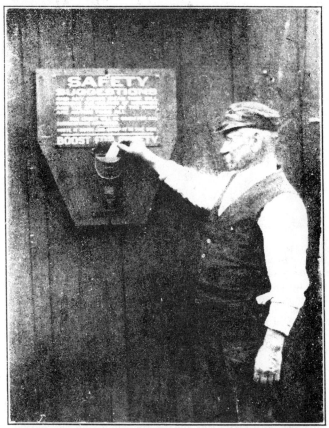

Fig. 1–10.—In 1910, U.S. Steel Corporation received 5,200 recommendations for improving the safety at 78 of its largest plants; 92 percent were accepted and put into operation. Suggestion competitions at National Cash Register Company in 1912 resulted in nearly 4000 entries and 2500 cash awards.

*Courtesy Commonwealth Steel Company.*

the OSHA Recordkeeping Requirements for the current year as well as the two prior years. Incidence rates for National Safety Council members are now kept. More details are in Chapter 6, "Accident Records and Incidence Rates."

## The dollar values

It has been estimated that the annual cost of occupational accidents in the United States exceeds $27 billion. If the 1912 accident rates had been left unchanged and if there had been no organized safety movement, this annual cost would have easily been two or three times as great.

Against such dollar savings, the relatively small expenditures for safety throughout America provide a striking contrast. Each dollar spent for safety by American industry is probably returning a clear profit of several hundred percent.

## Industry and nonwork accidents

Directly and indirectly, industry is bearing a substantial part of the burden of the cost of nonwork accidents and their prevention. The National Safety Council is the creation of industry and largely supported by it. Statewide and

# THE WANDERINGS OF CARELESS PETE
## The Electric Switchboard

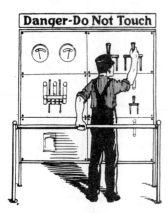

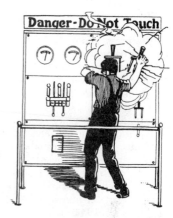

The Electric Switchboard had a certain fascination for Pete. He had no business with it but

One day he decided he'd pull one of those funny little handles just to see what would happen—

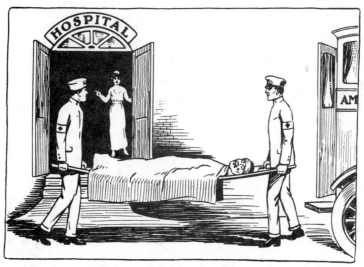

The doctor says Pete got off pretty easy. He will be around again in a few weeks, minus one eye and several weeks' wages.

—Courtesy, "The Transfer," (Milwaukee-Western Fuel Co.)

Fig. 1–11.—Employee publications, too, advanced the cause of safety.

local safety organizations play a major role in the fight against such accidents, and they, too, are largely industrial in origin and support. Thousands of safety professionals and their employers volunteer time and funds which are the mainstay of the National Safety Council's work.

Industry supports a large part of the job of informing the general public on these problems through the press, radio, and television.

The effectiveness of the nonwork accident prevention campaign is shown by the fact that, from the time records were first kept in 1921, both home and public accident death rates have declined.

If industry has been a large contributor to this successful work, it has also been a heavy beneficiary of its fruits. Disruption of labor force, worry and hardship among employees, loss of purchasing power by consumers, and heavy tax burdens for the support of hospitals and relief agencies are all results, in part, of nonwork accidents which affect industry's pocketbook.

## The safety movement's resources

Statistics measure what has been accomplished and also indicate the development of tools, methods, and knowledge which are the safety professional's capital and his resources for meeting future accident problems.

**Know-how.** A body of knowledge cannot be entirely translated into statistics, but it may be of use to note the outward signs of increased knowledge about industrial safety.

This *Accident Prevention Manual* is not a radical venture into new fields of knowledge. It is the cumulation of facts and opinions which have become a part of the safety movement's general heritage. Its purpose is to bring key points of specific, as well as general, value to safety workers.

Here are collected facts that took years to discover—years of searching and researching, of trial and error, of failure and success.

Today, an individual, whether an experienced safety professional, part-time safety administrator, or neophyte entering the field, can turn these pages and come up with better answers to a wider range of industrial safety problems than were available to the wisest and best-trained professional safety practitioner of a generation ago.

Yet this Manual contains only a fraction of the body of knowledge available to fight the never-ending war against accidents.

The volumes of National Safety Congress *Transactions* contain useful material and expert opinion on all phases of safety. In countless pamphlets and periodicals of safety organizations, government agencies, and insurance companies and in the studies and directives of individual industrial concerns is still more material. The literature of various trades and professions is likewise rich in safety information. A list of handbooks is given in Chapter 19, "Safety Engineering Tables," of the *Engineering and Technology* volume.

The National Safety Council has a very useful series of training courses, at both the beginning and advanced levels, for safety professionals. Write the Council's Safety Training Institute for details.

Finally, tremendous stores of safety information in the heads of professional safety engineers, executives, supervisors, and rank-and-file employees are made available through exchange of information in safety conferences, technical seminars, safety newsletters, and other publications.

It may be argued that, of all the achievements that the safety movement has to its credit, the greatest is the accumulation and preservation of a body of know-how which the safety professional has at his fingertips in dealing with the problems that confront him now and in the future.

**The heritage of cooperation.** The safety movement would be a far less effective force than it is if, at the outset, its members had hoarded and concealed their discoveries from their colleagues in competitive companies.

It was teamwork that created the safety activities of the Association of Iron and Steel Electrical Engineers. It was broadened teamwork which was represented at the first Milwaukee Conference and which led to the formation of the National Safety Council and other safety organizations.

Effective accident prevention requires channels of cooperation. Through the Council and other safety organizations, safety professionals found meeting places for the exchange of ideas, developed safety publications, and stimulated one another in friendly competition.

The tradition that there should be "no secrets in safety," no denial of help even to a competitor when it involves saving life, is one of the great elements of strength in the safety movement.

# Punch Press Takes Four

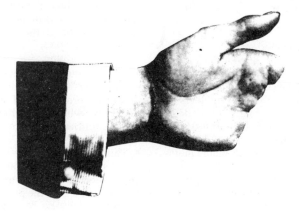

The man who lost the fingers says--"I want other fellows to know what a mistake in judgment may cost."

# Use the Guards
# Save Your Fingers

FIG. 1–12.—World War I era poster published by National Safety Council. Note "Universal Safety" emblem.

# 1—Occupational Safety

**Good will.** Like any new movement in industry, safety started with very little capital in the form of good will.

No small part of the safety professional's capital today is the prestige and good will built up for safety proposals and expenditures over the years. Where the pioneers had to battle every step of the budgetary way, safety professionals today have a far more receptive hearing from management.

**Professionalism.** Dedicated safety professionals continue to be accident prevention's most valuable asset. Their ranks have grown to the point where, in the mid-seventies, membership in the American Society of Safety Engineers is approaching 15,000. This organization, dedicated to both their interests and their professional development, has approximately one hundred chapters in the U.S. and Canada. Individual membership is worldwide.

There are many other qualified safety professionals, in addition to the ASSE members, who, together with thousands of specialists and technicians, carry out a limited scope of activities within the field, and numerous individuals who devote less than 50 percent of their time to safety functions.

In 1968, the ASSE was instrumental in forming a new organization, the Board of Certified Safety Professionals. Its purpose is to provide a means of giving professional status to qualified safety people by certification after meeting strict educational and experience requirements and passing an examination. Several thousand safety professionals have been certified, since the BCSP was formed.

Both the ASSE and the BCSP are described in Chapter 24, "Sources of Help," in this volume.

**Advancement of knowledge.** There has always been an orderly development of knowledge, which, when applied with sufficient skill and judgment, has produced significant reductions in many types of accidents and accidental injuries and occupational illnesses. However, the tremendous increase in scientific knowledge and technological advancement since the close of World War II has added to the complexities of safety work.

The approach has oscillated between one that emphasizes environmental control or engineering, and one that emphasizes human factors.

From this, several important trends in the pattern of the safety professional's development have emerged. All are discussed in detail in subsequent chapters of this volume.

• First, increasing emphasis toward analyzing the loss potential of the activity with which the safety professional is concerned. Such analysis will require greater ability (a) to predict where and how loss- and injury-producing events will occur and (b) to find the means of preventing such events.

• Second, increased development of factual, unbiased, and objective information about loss-producing problems and accident causation, so that those who have ultimate decision-making responsibilities can make sound decisions.

• Third, increasing use of the safety professional's help in developing safe products. The application of the principles of accident causation and control to the product is becoming more important because of the increase in product liability cases, the sudden emphasis in law of the entire field of negligent design, and the obvious impact a safer product would have on the overall safety of the environment.

To identify and evaluate the magnitude of the safety problem, the safety professional must be concerned with all facets of the problem—personal and environmental, transient and permanent—to determine the causes of accidents or the existence of loss-producing conditions, practices, or materials. From the information he collects and analyzes, he proposes alternate solutions, together with recommendations based upon his specialized knowledge and experience, to those who have ultimate decision-making responsibilities.

Therefore, future application of this knowledge in all aspects of our civilization—whether to industry, to transportation, at home, or in recreation—makes it imperative that those in this field be trained to utilize scientific principles and methods to achieve adequate results. Of prime importance will be the knowledge, skill, and ability to integrate machines, equipment, and environments with man and his capabilities.

The safety professional in performing these functions will draw upon specialized knowledge in both the physical and social sciences. He will apply the principles of measurement and analysis to evaluate safety performance. He will be required to have fundamental knowledge of statistics, mathematics, physics, chemistry, and engineering.

He will use knowledge in the field of behavior, motivation, and communications. Knowledge of management principles as well as the theory of business and government organization will also be required. His specialized knowledge must include a thorough understanding of the causative factors contributing to accident occurrence as well as methods and procedures designed to control such events.

The safety professional will also need diversified education and training, if he is to meet the challenges of the future. The population explosion, the problems of urban areas and future transportation systems, as well as the increasing complexities of man's everyday life, will create many problems and stretch the safety professional's creativity to its maximum, if he is to successfully provide the knowledge and leadership to conserve life, health, and property.

Training of the safety professional of the future can no longer be the "on-the-job," one-on-one type, only. It must contemplate specialized undergraduate level training, leading to a bachelor's degree or higher degree.

Training courses, such as those conducted by the National Safety Council, have and will continue to serve a very useful purpose for a large number of individuals who begin performing safety functions and must receive initial training or advanced training in certain specialized areas.

Approximately 200 four-year colleges and universities currently offer courses in safety, and several dozen offer a bachelor's degree or higher in safety. An increasing number of two-year, community colleges are offering associate degrees or certificates for courses designed for the safety technician or part-time administrator. Governmental agencies and ASSE are also actively promoting and conducting such professional development programs.

This is the creative challenge of tomorrow—not only improved performance on the job, but also professionalizing and perpetuating this field of endeavor.

## Summary of achievements

The safety movement has helped save many thousands of lives. It is saving industry and its employees billions of dollars a year.

It faces the future with great resources for eliminating accidents—resources in know-how, teamwork, good will, and trained and dedicated safety workers.

It has, therefore, done much to meet the double challenge presented to it: to deal with accidents now and to build soundly for the long-range attack upon accidents in the future.

### Safety Today

The answer to the question, "What has the safety movement accomplished?" is in purely positive terms—accomplishments, advances, achievements. The answer to the question, "How does the safety movement stand today?" demands a look at what is wrong, as well as what is right, with the present situation. The answer can be found in an appraisal of how the safety movement stands in relation to how it ought to stand. The first point to be considered is simple and grim:

- Accidents still bleed this country of more than 100 thousand lives a year, cause more than 10 million disabling injuries, and account for a total financial loss of more than $70 billion.

- Work accidents destroy more than 13,000 lives a year, about half these deaths occurring in what is normally considered industry. Work accidents injure more than 2 million persons annually and cost more than $27 billion.

In recent years, the ratio of off-the-job deaths to on-the-job deaths was about 3 to 1 and more than half of the injuries suffered by employees occurred off the job.

In terms of time loss, all injuries to workers, both on and off the job, caused a loss of about 45 million man-days of work directly and 200 million man-days indirectly.

Within the industrial community, there are very large variations in accident rates from industry to industry and from company to company.

Trade, service, and manufacturing are, on the average, low-accident businesses. Transportation, agriculture, construction, and the extractive industries are high-accident fields. These low and high rankings hold for both deaths and injuries. The communications industry has accidental death rates substantially below the national average and has the lowest injury rates.

How much the variation from one industry to

another reflects unavoidable differences in hazards and how much it reflects other factors, such as accident prevention activity or government regulation, has not been fully determined. Certainly, the mining industry, for example, has had a maximum amount of regulation and assistance from government, yet its rate remains high.

In construction and logging operations, the high rates may be due in part to the fact that the typical operation is small, or that it moves from place to place.

## Large and small establishments

It is generally assumed that small companies with, say, fewer than 100 employees have proportionately more work injuries than large corporations. However, since many small companies have not been accurately recording and reporting their experience, it is difficult to establish any valid ratio comparing work injury experience. However, it is safe to say that companies, large or small, that ignore systematic safety effort will, in the main, have more than their share of work accidents and injuries.

The seriousness of the small-enterprise problem has been widely recognized for many years, and the National Safety Council has devoted much effort to meeting it. Some promising steps have been taken to increase small-establishment participation in the organized safety movement, principally through the establishment of liaison between the National Safety Council and the trade associations representing many small companies.

Certain aspects of the small-company problem can be stated with assurance:

1. The small establishment may not need or cannot employ specialized safety personnel to deal with the accident problem.

2. The number of accidents in a significant amount of time or the financial position of many small concerns makes it difficult to convince them that spending the money necessary for proper equipment, layout, guarding, and other elements is important.

3. Managers of small operations are harried by a host of problems in all fields. Seldom do they have the expertise or can they find time for proper study of accidents and their causes.

4. In small units, statistical measures of performance are unreliable, so that it is difficult to

produce clear-cut evidence as to the cost of accidents versus the effectiveness of accident prevention work. In other words, a small operation may have, by luck, a good or bad accident record over a few years, whether or not its safety program is sound.

These are obstacles to progress—real and serious ones. They are not, of course, excuses for failure to try to prevent accidents. The trade association approach offers some real hope for improvement on a group basis.

## Labor-management cooperation

From its inception, one of the prime goals of organized labor has been the safety of its members. Many of today's international unions were organized originally to deal with extremely hazardous situations in the workplace, and have a sincere desire to work together with management on methods to prevent occupational injury.

In 1949, the National Safety Council issued a policy statement declaring the common interest of labor and management in accident prevention. Even before this date, representatives of leading labor organizations served as members of the Council's governing boards. At a number of National Safety Congresses, reports were made by labor and management people on specific examples of local and company-wide cooperation between unions and corporations. In 1955, a Labor Department and a Labor Conference (now known as Labor Division) were formally established to function within the organizational framework of the National Safety Council.

Labor has been represented at the various presidential and gubernatorial industrial safety conferences, and was instrumental in promoting legislation such as the Occupational Safety and Health Act of 1970 (OSHAct), described in the next chapter.

Some unions have independently done extensive safety work and have published printed matter and released films which are real contributions to the safety movement.

Through the auspices of the National Safety Council, the Labor Division and the Industrial Division, along with other affected divisions, frequently have cooperated in preparing Council positions on matters pertaining to standards action, oversight testimony, publicity releases, and other areas which bear on occupational safety and health. As a result of these joint committees,

Council positions are being recognized as more representative of all elements of society, allowing them to have even greater impact on administrative agencies and legislative bodies.

It is the hope of the great majority of farsighted safety professionals in both labor and management that every opportunity for cooperation will continue to be pressed to the fullest extent.

Through a program begun in January of 1978 with a symposium of leaders from government, industry, and organized labor, the National Safety Council has begun an extensive program (with the cooperation of these three elements of our society) for determining causal factors of injuries. Realizing that most data in the past have only given us the numbers of types of injuries, the focus of this program is to change investigatory and reporting methods, as well as to provide an information exchange bank of the factors that have actually caused injury or occupational illness.

### Research and standards

Statistical data on industrial accidents have been compiled by the National Safety Council for more than 50 years. Analyses computed annually and published in industry rate pamphlets and *Accident Facts* have proven of utmost importance in evaluating leading accident causes.

Some industries through their trade associations have recorded accident rates for almost 60 years. In most instances, even the divisions of an industry can establish their positions with regard to number and types of accidents and can determine their experience in comparison with national averages.

There are a large number of standards relating to safety. Continuing research has been necessary over the years to keep these standards in line with current industrial development and the development of new products and materials.

Special research projects, such as those making studies of walkway surfaces and safety belts, can be and have been financed by private sources and coordinated by the National Safety Council. Since the Council is not an approval agency, results of these projects are given as a summary of findings with no attempt to set minimum standards.

### Safety and the law

The early legal action in industrial safety took the form of laws to regulate and investigate. The

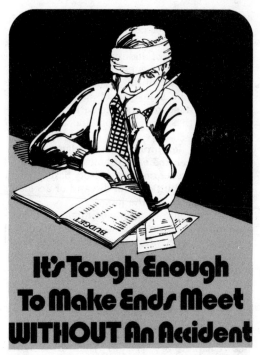

It's Tough Enough To Make Ends Meet WITHOUT An Accident

FIG. 1–13.—Modern posters produced by the National Safety Council combine eye appeal and an easily understood message.

next phase was largely concerned with workers' compensation payments.

The following years have seen a gradual growth in regulation of industry on safety matters by federal, state, and local governments. The Walsh-Healey Act, which deals with companies having supply contracts with the federal government, is an example of such regulation.

In certain industries—notably mining and transportation—federal government regulation and inspection have been extensive. The Construction Safety Act, which was passed in 1969, deals with the particular problems of that industry.

In 1970, the Williams-Steiger Occupational Safety and Health Act was passed and, for the first time, the United States had a *national* safety law. Every business, with one or more employees, which is affected by interstate commerce is covered by the law. Safety in this country has taken on a new direction and meaning as a result of the Occupational Safety and Health Act. More details are in Chapter 2, "Federal Legislation."

Today industry accepts almost without exception the idea of financial responsibility for work injuries. Not all of industry, however, is convinced of the effectiveness of government regulation of safety procedures. Several states, with the cooperation of management and labor, have developed standards and regulations that have been effective in reducing the number of accidents.

A recent development in the laws of some states has been the establishment of health and accident insurance on a compulsory basis to cover employee disabilities from diseases or accidents which originate off the job.

This compulsory insurance might be considered either a drastic extension of the principle of workers' compensation or an extension of social security legislation. It differs from workers' compensation in that it puts a financial burden upon management for diseases and accidents which are products of conditions beyond its control.

Whatever the theory, the result of these laws is to give the employer a direct financial stake in dealing with the off-the-job accident problem. See Chapter 3, "Hazard Control Program Organization."

## Safety and occupational health

Even though medical and safety cooperation in accident prevention started back in the earliest days of the safety movement, interest in safety on the part of the medical profession is increasing. Part of this interest is the result of concern with occupational disease, noise, radiation, and other problems beyond the former concepts of occupational accident prevention.

Safety is, of course, the beneficiary of many medical advancements—notably prevention of industrial diseases and infections.

Industry's growing concern with problems of ionizing radiation has brought the physicist into partnership with medical and safety professionals.

Knowledge in the field of industrial hygiene has been greatly extended in a number of areas.

The utilization by industry of the physically handicapped has led progressive companies to adjust their policies on preemployment physical examinations, to make sure that they are screening out only the unfit and not those with defects that do not rule out useful work under proper conditions and limits.

For more details, refer to the Council's *Fundamentals of Industrial Hygiene*, part of the Occupational Safety and Health Series.

## Psychology and "accident proneness"

The safety professional who is thoughtfully looking for ways to improve his work encounters a great deal of challenging information in modern psychological writing—and also a great deal of careless and misleading generalizations.

Concern about the so-called "accident-prone" individual in industry is as old as the safety movement. Statistical information suggests existence of such individuals, though clear and sharp data proving this point are remarkably hard to come by. Too many alleged "proofs" turn out to be statistically deceptive, or based on inadequate samples, or the result of highly subjective diagnoses.

The elusiveness of statistical proof of the existence of accident-prone individuals suggests to some thoughtful safety professionals that accident proneness may be a passing phase in the individual rather than a permanent characteristic.

Realistically, objective analysis might disclose some supervisory deficiency or procedural weakness which may aggravate the hazard of certain operations or performance of individuals or groups of workers.

The same observation applies to psychological tests used as screening devices for new employees. Spectacular claims have been made from time to time for the effectiveness of such tests in predicting accident proneness, but none has established itself to the general satisfaction of the safety profession.

The work of psychologists like Dunbar and the Menningers has aroused great interest among safety professionals. However, great contributions to the practical day-to-day fight against accidents have not yet been made by psychologists—or have not been recognized if they have been made.

Refer to the discussions in Chapters 9 and 11.

## Summary

The present situation in the field of industrial safety is one of progress and improvement, largely through the continued application of techniques and knowledge slowly and painfully acquired through the years.

There appears to be no limit to the progress

possible through the application of the universally accepted safety techniques of education, engineering, and enforcement.

Yet large and serious problems remain unsolved. A number of industries still have high accident rates. There are still far too many instances where management and labor are not working together or have different goals for the safety program.

The resources of the safety movement are great and strong—an impressive body of knowledge, a corps of able professional safety people, a high level of prestige, and strong organizations for cooperation and exchange of information.

## Current Problems

Some problems of the safety movement are directly related to traditional strengths and weaknesses. Some of these problems are social and political in nature. Still others are essentially organizational.

### Technology and public interest

There is no reason for the safety professional to view the public's interest in product safety, a better environment, and general technological trends with alarm. Emphasis upon automation and more refined instrumentation will probably continue. New specific problems will arise, but they will be of a type that well-established methods of safety engineering are competent to solve.

The use of new materials and techniques—particularly radioactive materials and lasers—is likely to present more serious difficulties to the safety professional. However, even here, there is considerable experience.

### Political problems

On the political side remains the timeworn problem of industry–government relations. The difficult task of the serious safety professional is to objectively advise his management regarding legislation and what may be considered government interference in safety matters and still, at the same time, encourage good people in public service to work to improve safety standards.

If safety people simply fight government "on principle," they will lose their objectivity and professional stature, and this will probably only heighten the pressure from other quarters for stiff and inflexible regulation.

### Organizational problems

On the national scale, a wide variety of organizations are attacking specific aspects of the safety problem. The National Safety Council is, of course, the giant in the field—a strong, constructive, and nonpolitical, noncommercial giant. It has repeatedly sought and often achieved cooperative division of labor between itself and other organizations in the safety field.

One of the guiding principles of the Council has been that there was work enough and credit enough for all.

It remains to be seen whether the best organizational forms have been found for participation by all businesses in safety work. Safety professionals should be ready to consider new ideas and new forms.

### A look to the future

The future is, as it always has been, most uncertain. Problems large and small, predictable and unpredictable, can be expected to crowd upon the safety professional.

Some of these problems will call for reapplication of established safety techniques. Others will call for radical departures and the creation of new methods and new organizational forms.

To be able to discriminate between the two situations will, perhaps, be the safety professional's greatest test.

## References

American Engineering Council. *Safety and Production.* New York, Harper & Brothers Publishers, 1928.

American Insurance Association, Accident Prevention Department, 85 John St., New York, N.Y. *Handbook of Industrial Safety Standards.* 10th rev., 1962.

Andrews, E. W. "The Pioneers of 1912." *National Safety News,* 66:24-25,. 64-65 (July 1952).

Beyer, David Stewart. *Industrial Accident Prevention,* 3rd ed. Boston and New York, Houghton Mifflin Co., 1928.

# 1—Occupational Safety

Blake, Roland P., editor. *Industrial Safety*, 3rd ed. Englewood Cliffs, N.J., Prentice-Hall, Inc., 1963.

Campbell, R. W. "The National Safety Movement." *Proceedings of the Second Safety Congress of the National Council for Industrial Safety*, pp. 188-192, 1913.

DeBlois, Lewis A. *Industrial Safety Organization for Executive and Engineer*. New York City, McGraw-Hill Book Company, 1926.

DeReamer, Russell. *Modern Safety and Health Technology*. New York, John Wiley and Sons, Inc., 1980.

Eastman, Crystal. *Work Accidents and the Law*. New York, Charities Publication Committee, 1910. Reprint. New York, Arno Press, 1969.

Grimaldi, John V., and Rollin H. Simonds. *Safety Management*, 3rd ed. Homewood, Ill., Richard D. Irwin, rev. 1975.

Heinrich, H. W. *Industrial Accident Prevention*, 4th ed. New York, McGraw-Hill Book Company, 1959.

Heinrich, H. W., Petersen, Dan, and Roos, Nester. *Industrial Accident Prevention*, 5th ed. New York, McGraw-Hill Book Co., 1980.

Holbrook, Steward H. *Let Them Live*. New York, The Macmillan Co., 1939.

Menninger, K. A. *Man Against Himself*. New York, Harcourt, Brace and World, Inc., 1956.

National Safety Council, 444 North Michigan Ave., Chicago, Ill. 60611.
*Accident Facts*. Issued annually.
"Golden Anniversary Issue." *National Safety News*, 87:5 (May 1963).
*National Safety News*. Issued monthly.
*Proceedings of the First Co-Operative Safety Congress*, 1912.
*Proceedings of the National Safety Congress*. Issued annually from 1914-1925.
*Proceedings of the Second Safety Congress of the National Council for Industrial Safety*. 1913.

Schaefer, Vernon G. *Safety Supervision*. New York, N.Y., McGraw-Hill Book Company, 1941.

Schulzinger, Morris S. "Accident Syndrome—A Clinical Approach." *Archives of Industrial Health*, 11:66-71, 1955. Chicago, Ill., American Medical Assn.

Schwedtman, Ferd., and James A. Emery. *Accident Prevention and Relief*. New York, National Association of Manufacturers in the United States of America, 1911.

# Federal Legislation

## Chapter
## 2

## 2—Federal Legislation

The two major pieces of federal legislation having an impact on occupational safety and health passed by the Congress in the last decade are the Occupational Safety and Health Act of 1970 and the Federal Mine Safety and Health Act of 1977. Although other federal legislation affecting occupational safety and health to a lesser degree remain on the books, this chapter will focus on the Occupational Safety and Health Act and the Federal Mine Safety and Health Act.

# PART I
# The Occupational Safety and Health Act

A new national policy was established on December 29, 1970, when President Richard M. Nixon signed into law the Occupational Safety and Health Act of 1970 (Public Law No. 91-596).* The Congress of the United States declared that the purpose of this piece of legislation is "to assure so far as possible every working man and woman in the Nation safe and healthful working conditions and to preserve our human resources."

The OSHAct took effect April 28, 1971. It was coauthored by Senator Harrison A. Williams (Dem.-N.J.) and the late Congressman William Steiger (Rep.-Wis.) and hence is sometimes designated as the Williams-Steiger Act. The Act is regarded by many as landmark legislation since it goes beyond the present workplace and considers the working environment of the future as related to health hazards.

The information provided in Part I of this chapter focuses on federal OSHA programs. State OSHA programs may differ from the federal program in certain areas. However, unless specifically instructed to the contrary, the recommendations in this chapter can be followed whether the jurisdiction rests at the federal or state level.

### Legislative History

Historically, the enactment of safety and health laws has been left to the states. Prior to the 1960's only a few federal laws (such as the Walsh-Healey Public Contracts Act and the Longshoremen's and Harbor Workers' Compensation Act) directed any attention to occupational safety and health. The decade of the sixties, however, saw significant congressional action in this arena. A number of pieces of legislation passed by the Congress during the sixties, including the Service Contract Act of 1965, the National Foundation on Arts and Humanities Act, the Federal Metal and Nonmetallic Mine Safety Act, the Federal Coal Mine Health and Safety Act and the Contract Workers and Safety Standards Act (Con-struction Safety Act), directed attention to occupational safety and health.

Each of these federal laws was applicable to a limited number of employers. These laws were directed at those who had obtained federal contracts or they zeroed-in on a specific industry. Even collectively, all the federal safety legislation passed prior to 1970 was not applicable to the majority of employers or employees. Until 1970, congressional action related to occupational safety and health was, at best, sporadic, covering only specific sets of employers and employees with little attempt for an omnibus coverage that is a part of the OSHAct.

Proponents of more significant federal presence in occupational safety and health, mostly represented by organized labor, based their position primarily on the following:

• With few exceptions, the states failed to meet their obligation in regard to occupational safety and health. Only a few of the states had safety and health legislation that was considered reasonable or adequate. Many states legislated safety and health only in specific industries. In general, states had inadequate safety and health standards, inadequate enforcement procedures, inadequate staff with respect to quality and quantity, and inadequate budgets.

• In the late 1960's, approximately 14,300 employees were being killed annually on or in connection with their job and more than 2.2 million employees suffered a disabling injury each year as a result of work-related accidents. The injury/death toll was considered by most to be much too high and therefore not acceptable.

• The nation's work injury rates in most indus-

---

*29 U.S.C. §§651-678.

tries were increasing throughout the decade of the sixties. Since the trend was in the wrong direction, proponents of federal presence felt that federal legislation would assist in reversing this trend.

The act evolved amid a stormy atmosphere in both houses of Congress. Highly controversial issues were involved. Such issues were responsible for sharply drawn lines between political parties and between the business community and organized labor. After three years of political hassle, numerous compromises were made; this ultimately enabled the passage of the OSHAct of 1970 by both houses of Congress.

## Administration

Administration and enforcement of the OSHAct are vested primarily with the Secretary of Labor and the Occupational Safety and Health Review Commission (discussed later). With respect to the enforcement function, the Secretary of Labor performs the investigation and prosecution aspects of the enforcement process and the Review Commission performs the adjudication portion of the enforcement process.

Research and related functions and certain educational functions are vested in the Secretary of Health, Education, and Welfare (now known as the Secretary of Health and Human Services) and are, for the most part, carried out by the National Institute for Occupational Safety and Health established within the Department of Health and Human Services (DHHS). Compiling injury and illness statistical data is handled by the Bureau of Labor Statistics, U.S. Department of Labor.

To assist the Secretary of Labor, the Act authorizes the appointment of an Assistant Secretary of Labor for Occupational Safety and Health. This position is filled by Presidential appointment with the advice and consent of the Senate. The Assistant Secretary is the chief of the Occupational Safety and Health Administration (OSHA) established within the Department of Labor (DOL). The Assistant Secretary acts on behalf of the Secretary of Labor. For the purpose of this chapter, OSHA is also synonymous with the term Secretary or Assistant Secretary of Labor.

The primary functions of the four major governmental units assigned to carry out the provisions of the Act are described in this section on administration.

## Occupational Safety and Health Administration

The Occupational Safety and Health Administration (OSHA) came into existence officially on April 28, 1971, the date the Williams–Steiger Occupational Safety and Health Act became effective. This agency was created by the Department of Labor to discharge the Department's responsibilities assigned by the Act.

**Major areas of authority.** The Act grants OSHA the authority, among other things, (a) to promulgate, modify, and revoke safety and health standards; (b) to conduct inspections and investigations and to issue citations, including proposed penalties; (c) to require employers to keep records of safety and health data; (d) to petition the courts to restrain imminent danger situations; and (e) to approve or reject state plans for programs under the Act.

The Act also authorizes OSHA (a) to provide training and education to employers and employees; (b) to consult with employers, employees, and organizations regarding prevention of injuries and illnesses; (c) to grant funds to the states for identification of program needs and plan development, experiments, demonstrations, administration and operation of programs; and (d) to develop and maintain a statistics program for occupational safety and health.

**Major duties delegated.** In establishing the Occupational Safety and Health Administration, the Secretary of Labor delegated to the Assistant Secretary for Occupational Safety and Health the authority and responsibility for safety and health programs and activities of the Department of Labor, including responsibilities derived from:

1. Occupational Safety and Health Act of 1970

2. Walsh-Healey Public Contracts Act of 1936, as amended

3. Service Contract Act of 1965

4. Public Law 91-54 of 1969 (construction safety amendments)

5. Public Law 85-742 of 1958 (maritime safety amendments)

6. National Foundation on the Arts and Humanities Act of 1965

7. Longshoremen's and Harbor Workers' Compensation Act (Title 33, Chapter 18, §§901, 904, *U.S. Code*; Act of March 4, 1927, Chapter 509, 44 Stat. 1424)

8. Federal safety program under Title 5 U.S. Code §7902

Similarly, the Commissioner of the Bureau of Labor Statistics was delegated the authority and given the responsibility for developing and maintaining an effective program for collection, compilation, and analysis of occupational safety and health statistics, providing grants to the states to assist in developing and administering programs in such statistics, and coordinating functions with the Assistant Secretary for Occupational Safety and Health.

The Solicitor of Labor is assigned responsibility for providing legal advice and assistance to the Secretary and all officers of the Department in the administration of statutes and Executive Orders relating to occupational safety and health. In enforcing the Act's requirements, the Solicitor of Labor also has the responsibility for representing the Secretary in litigation before the Occupational Safety and Health Review Commission, and, subject to the control and direction of the Attorney General, before the federal courts.

To assist in carrying out its responsibilities, OSHA has established ten regional offices in the cities of Boston, New York, Philadelphia, Atlanta, Chicago, Dallas, Kansas City, Denver, San Francisco, and Seattle. (See *Directory of Federal Agencies.*) The primary mission of the regional office chief, known as the Regional Administrator, is to supervise, coordinate, evaluate, and execute all programs of OSHA in the region. Assisting the Regional Administrator are Assistant Regional Administrators for (*a*) training, education, consultation, and federal agency programs, (*b*) technical support, and (*c*) state and federal operations.

Area offices have been established within each region, each headed by an Area Director. The mission of the Area Director is to carry out the compliance program of OSHA within designated geographic areas. The area office staff carries out its activities under the general supervision of the Area Director with guidance of the Regional Administrator, using policy instructions received from the national headquarters. The real action for implementing the enforcement portion of the OSHAct is carried out by the area offices in those

states that do not have an approved state plan. The area office monitors state activities in those states that have a state plan. (See Federal–State Relationships, pages 45 and 46.)

## Occupational Safety and Health Review Commission

The Occupational Safety and Health Review Commission (OSHRC) is a quasi-judicial board of three members appointed by the President and confirmed by the Senate. The Commission is an independent agency of the Executive Branch of the U.S. Government and is not a part of the Department of Labor. The principal function of the Commission is to adjudicate cases resulting from an enforcement action initiated against an employer by OSHA when any such action is contested by the employer or by his employees or their representatives.

The Commission's actions are limited to contested cases. In such cases, OSHA notifies the Commission of the contested cases and the Commission hears all appeals on actions taken by OSHA concerning citations, proposed penalties, and abatement periods, and determines the appropriateness of such actions. When necessary, the Commission may conduct its own investigation and may affirm, modify, or vacate OSHA's findings.

There are two levels of adjudication within the Commission: (*a*) the administrative law judge, and (*b*) the three-member Commission. All cases not resolved on informal proceedings are heard and decided by one of the Commission's administrative law judges. The judge's decision can be changed by a majority vote of the Commission if one of the members, within 30 days of the judge's decision, directs that the judge's decision be reviewed by the Commission members. The Commission is the final administrative authority to rule on a particular case, but its findings and orders can be subject to further review by the courts. (For further information, see Contested Cases later in this chapter.)

The headquarters of the OSHRC is located at 1825 K Street, NW., Washington, D.C. 20006.

## National Institute for Occupational Safety and Health

The National Institute for Occupational Safety and Health (NIOSH) was established within the HEW (currently known as the Department of Health and Human Services) under the provisions of the OSHAct. Administratively, NIOSH is located in DHHS's Center for Disease Control. NIOSH is the principal federal agency engaged in research, education, and training related to occupational safety and health.

The primary functions of NIOSH are to (a) develop and establish recommended occupational safety and health standards, (b) conduct research experiments and demonstrations related to occupational safety and health, and (c) conduct education programs to provide an adequate supply of qualified personnel to carry out the purposes of the OSHAct.

**Research and related functions.** Under the OSHAct, NIOSH has the responsibility for conducting research for new occupational safety and health standards. NIOSH develops criteria for the establishment of such standards. Such criteria are transmitted to OSHA which has the responsibility for the final setting, promulgation, and enforcement of the standards.

The OSHAct also requires NIOSH to publish an annual listing of all known toxic substances and the concentrations at which such toxicity is known to occur. While the entry of a substance on the list does not mean that it is to be avoided, it does mean that the listed substance has a documented potential of being hazardous if misused and, therefore, care must be exercised to control the substance. Conversely, the absence of a substance from the list does not necessarily mean that a substance is nontoxic. Some hazardous substances may not qualify to be listed because the dose that causes the toxic effect is not known.

**Education and training.** NIOSH also has the responsibility to conduct (a) education and training programs which are aimed at providing an adequate supply of qualified personnel to carry out the purpose of the Act and (b) informational programs on the importance and proper use of adequate safety and health equipment. The long-term approach to an adequate supply of training personnel in occupational safety and health is found in the colleges and universities and other institutions in the private sector. NIOSH encourages such institutions, by contracts and grants, to expand their curricula in occupational medicine, occupational health nursing, industrial hygiene, and occupational safety engineering.

**Employer and employee services.** Of principal interest to individual employers and employees are the technical services offered by NIOSH. The five main services that are provided upon request to NIOSH's Division of Technical Services, Cincinnati, Ohio 45226, are:

1. Hazard evaluation—Provides on-site evaluations of potentially toxic substances used or found on the job.

2. Technical information—Provides technical information concerning health or safety conditions at workplaces, such as the possible hazards of working with specific solvents, and when to use protective equipment.

3. Accident prevention—Provides technical assistance for controlling on-the-job injuries including the evaluation of special problems and recommendations for corrective action.

4. Industrial hygiene—Provides technical assistance in the areas of engineering and industrial hygiene, including the evaluation of special health-related problems in the workplace and recommendations for control measures.

5. Medical service—Provides assistance in solving occupational medical and nursing problems in the workplace including the assessment of existing medically related needs and the development of recommended means for meeting such needs.

NIOSH approves coal mine dust personal sampler units, gas detector tube units, and respiratory protective devices including self-contained breathing apparatus, gas masks, supplied-air respirators, chemical-cartridge respirators, and dust, fume, and mist respirators. NIOSH also has a certification program for sound level meters.

NIOSH representatives, although not authorized to enforce the OSHAct, are authorized to make inspections and to question employers and employees in order to carry out those duties assigned to the DHHS under the Act.

## Bureau of Labor Statistics

The responsibility for conducting statistical surveys and establishing methods used to acquire injury and illness data is placed in the Bureau of Labor Statistics (BLS). Questions regarding recordkeeping requirements and reporting procedures can be directed to any of the OSHA regional or area offices or the BLS regional offices.

# 2—Federal Legislation

## Advisory committees

The Act established a 12–member National Advisory Committee on Occupational Safety and Health (NACOSH) to advise, consult with, and make recommendations to the Secretaries of Labor and Health and Human Services (HHS) with respect to the administration of the Act. Eight members are designated by the Secretary of Labor and four by the Secretary of HHS. Members include representatives from management, labor, occupational safety and health professions, and the public.

The Act also authorizes the appointment of 15-member advisory committees to assist OSHA in the development of standards. The Standards Advisory Committees on Construction Safety and Health and on Cutaneous Hazards are the two currently in place.

## Major Provisions of the OSHAct

### Coverage

Except for specific exclusions, the Act is applicable to every employer who has one or more employees and who is engaged in a business affecting commerce. The law applies to all 50 states, the District of Columbia, Puerto Rico, and all U.S. possessions.

Specifically *excluded* from coverage are all federal, state, and local government employees. There are, however, special provisions in the Act for federal employees and potential coverage for state and local government employees. The Act requires each federal agency head to establish and maintain an occupational safety and health program consistent with the standards promulgated by the Secretary of Labor. Executive Orders setting requirements for federal programs have been issued, the last (up to the time this chapter was written) being Executive Order 12196 issued February 26, 1980.

Employees of states and political subdivisions of the states are excluded from the federal OSHAct. However, states with approved state plans are required to provide coverage for these public employees. Public employees in states that do not have approved plans are not covered by the OSHAct in any manner.

The OSHAct is also not applicable to those operations where a federal agency (and state agencies acting under the Atomic Energy Act of 1954), other than the Department of Labor, has statutory authority to prescribe or enforce standards or regulations affecting occupational safety or health and is performing that function. An example of this exclusion is specific issues covered by Department of Transportation regulations in the railroad industry.

Also excluded from the OSHAct are operators and miners covered by the Federal Mine Safety and Health Act of 1977 (see Part II of this chapter) which is applicable to mines of all types; coal and noncoal, surface and underground.

Curiously, inspection restrictions can vary from year to year, depending on the whims of Congress at the time it considers appropriations for the Department of Labor. In its yearly appropriation bills since 1977, Congress has placed restrictions on OSHA enforcement. For example, items exempt from inspection in fiscal year (FY) 1980 include:

• Farmers with ten or fewer employees on the day of inspection and the 12 months preceding the day of inspection

• Any work activity in any recreational, hunting, fishing or shooting area

• Employers with ten or fewer employees in industries with three-digit Standard Industrial Classification injury/illness rates of less than seven per 100 employees

The exemption is inapplicable to situations involving, among others, employee complaints, imminent danger, health hazards, accidents resulting in a fatality or hospitalization involving five or more employees, or discrimination complaints.

OSHA clarified its interpretation of coverage with respect to certain employees by issuing a regulation.° It has been declared that churches and religious organizations, with respect to their religious activities, are not regarded as employers. Likewise, persons who in their own residences employ others to perform domestic household tasks are not regarded as employers. Further, any person engaged in agriculture who is a member of the immediate family of the farmer is not regarded as an employee and hence is not covered by the Act.

---

°The regulation clarifying policy regarding "Coverage of Employees Under the Williams–Steiger Occupational Safety and Health Act of 1970" is contained in *Code of Federal Regulations* (C.F.R.), Title 29, Chapter XVII, Part 1975.

## Employer and employee duties

Each employer covered by the Act:

1. Has the general duty to furnish each of his employees employment and places of employment which are free from recognized hazards that are causing or likely to cause death or serious physical harm (this is commonly known as the "general duty clause")

2. Has the specific duty of complying with safety and health standards promulgated under the Act

Each employee, in turn, has the duty to comply with the safety and health standards and all rules, regulations, and orders which are applicable to his own actions and conduct on the job.

For employers, the general duty provision is used only where there are no specific standards applicable to a particular hazard involved. A hazard is "recognized" if it is a condition that is generally recognized as a hazard in the particular industry in which it occurs and is detectable (a) by means of the human senses, or (b) there are accepted tests known in the industry to determine its existence which should make its presence known to the employer. An example of a "recognized hazard" in the latter category is excessive concentration of a toxic substance in the work area atmosphere, even though such concentration could only be detected through use of measuring devices.

During the course of an inspection a compliance safety and health officer is concerned primarily with determining whether the employer is complying with the promulgated safety and health standards. However, he will also direct attention to determining whether the employer is complying with the general duty clause.

The law provides for sanctions against the employer in the form of citations and civil and criminal penalties if the employer fails to comply with his two duties. However, there is no provision for government sanctions against an employee for failure to comply with the employee's duty. While some may view the latter as unjust, significantly, it was not one of the controversial issues in the formative stages of the Act.

Both management and organized labor have long agreed that safety and health on the job is a management responsibility. The business community generally did not want the law structured to provide for government sanctions against an erring employee because there are measures which management can invoke against an employee who obstructs the employer's efforts to provide a safe workplace.

While the law expressly places upon each employee the obligation to comply with the standards, final responsibility for compliance with the requirements of the Act remains with the employer. Employers thus should take all necessary action to assure employee compliance with the promulgated standards and establish within their safety system a means whereby they become aware of situations where employees are not complying with applicable standards.

## Employer rights

An employer has the right to:

• Seek advice and off-site consultation as needed by writing, calling, or visiting the nearest OSHA office

• Request and receive proper identification of the OSHA compliance officer prior to inspection

• Be advised by the compliance safety and health officer (CSHO) of the reason for an inspection

• Have an opening and closing conference with the CSHO

• File a Notice of Contest with the OSHA area director within 15 working days of receipt of a notice of citation and proposed penalty

• Apply to OSHA for a temporary variance from a standard if unable to comply because of the unavailability of materials, equipment, or personnel needed to make necessary changes within the required time

• Take an active role in developing safety and health standards through participation in OSHA Standards Advisory Committees, through nationally recognized standards-setting organizations, and through evidence and views presented in writing or at hearings

• Avail himself, if a small business employer, of long-term loans through the Small Business Administration to help bring the establishment into compliance, either before or after an OSHA inspection

• Be assured of the confidentially of any trade secrets observed by an OSHA compliance officer.

## 2—Federal Legislation

### On-Site Consultation

Congress has authorized, and OSHA now provides through a state agency or private contractors free on-site consultation service for employers in every state. These consultants help employers identify hazardous conditions and determine corrective measures.

The service is available upon employer request. Priority is given to smaller businesses, which are generally less able to afford private sector consultation, and emphasis is placed on highly hazardous jobs.

The consultative visit consists of an opening conference, a walk-through of the company's facility, a closing conference and a written summary of findings. During the walk-through, the employer is told which OSHA standards are applicable and what they mean. The employer is told of any apparent violations of those standards and, where possible, is given suggestions on how to reduce or eliminate the hazard.

Because employers, not employees, are subject to legal sanctions of the OSHA standards, the employer controls the extent of participation by employees or their representatives in the visit. However, the consultant must be allowed to confer with individual employees during the walk-through in order to identify and judge the nature and extent of hazards.

### Employee rights

Although the employee has the legal duty to comply with all the standards and regulations issued under the OSHAct, there are many employee rights that are also incorporated in the Act. Since these rights may affect labor relations as well as labor negotiations, employers as well as employees should be aware of the employee rights contained in the Act. Employee rights fall into three main areas and are related to (a) standards, (b) access to information, and (c) enforcement.

With respect to standards:

1. Employees may request OSHA to begin proceedings for adoption of a new standard or to amend or revoke an existing one.

2. Employees may submit written data or comments on proposed standards and may appear as an interested party at any hearing held by OSHA.

3. Employees may file written objections to a proposed federal standard and/or appeal the final decision of OSHA.

4. Employees must be informed when an employer applies for a variance of a promulgated standard.

5. Employees must be afforded the opportunity to participate in a variance hearing as an interested party and have the right to appeal OSHA's final decision.

With respect to access to information:

1. Employees have the right to information from the employer regarding employee protections and obligations under the Act and to review appropriate OSHA standards, rules, regulations, and requirements that the employer should have available at the workplace.

2. Affected employees have a right to information from the employer regarding the toxic effects, conditions of exposure, and precautions for safe use of all hazardous materials in the establishment by means of labeling or other forms of warning where such information is prescribed by a standard.

3. If employees are exposed to harmful materials in excess of levels set by the standards, the affected employees must be so informed by the employer and the employer must also inform the employees thus exposed what corrective action is being taken.

4. If a compliance safety and health officer determines that an alleged imminent danger exists, he must inform the affected employees of the danger and that he is recommending that relief be sought by court action if the imminence of such danger is not eliminated.

5. Upon request, employees must be given access to records of their history of exposure to toxic materials or harmful physical agents that are required to be monitored or measured and recorded.

6. If a standard requires monitoring or measuring hazardous materials or harmful physical agents, employees must be given the opportunity to observe such monitoring or measuring.

7. Employees have the right of access to (a) the list of toxic materials published by NIOSH, (b)

criteria developed by NIOSH describing the effects of toxic materials or harmful physical agents, and (c) industrywide studies conducted by NIOSH regarding the effects of chronic, low-level exposure to hazardous materials.

8. On written request to NIOSH, employees have the right to obtain the determination of whether or not a substance found or used in the establishment is harmful.

9. Upon request, the employees should be allowed to review the Log and Summary of Occupational Injuries (OSHA No. 200) at a reasonable time and in a reasonable manner.

**With respect to enforcement:**

1. Employees have the right to confer in private with the compliance officer and to respond to questions from the compliance officer, in connection with an inspection of an establishment.

2. An authorized employee representative must be given an opportunity to accompany the compliance officer during an inspection for the purpose of aiding such inspection. (This is commonly known as the "walk-around" provision.) Also, an authorized employee has the right to participate in the opening and closing conferences during the inspection.

3. An employee has the right to make a written request to OSHA for a special inspection if the employee believes a violation of a standard threatens physical harm, and the employee has the right to request OSHA to keep his identity confidential.

4. If an employee believes any violation of the Act exists, he has the right to notify OSHA or a compliance officer in writing of the alleged violation, either before or during an inspection of the establishment.

5. If a request is made for a special inspection and it is denied by OSHA, the employee must be notified in writing by OSHA, together with the reasons, that the complaint was not valid. The employee has the right to object to such a decision and may request a hearing by OSHA.

6. If a written complaint concerning an alleged violation is submitted to OSHA and the compliance officer responding to the complaint

fails to cite the employer for the alleged violation, OSHA must furnish the employee or his authorized representative a written statement setting forth the reasons for its final disposition.

7. If OSHA cites an employer for a violation, employees have the right to review a copy of the citation which must be posted by the employer at or near the place where the violation occurred.

8. Employees have the right to appear as an interested party or to be called as a witness in a contested enforcement matter before the Occupational Safety and Health Review Commission.

9. If OSHA arbitrarily or capriciously fails to seek relief to counteract an imminent danger and an employee is injured as a result, that employee has the right to bring action against OSHA for relief as may be appropriate.

10. An employee has the right to file a complaint to OSHA within 30 days if he believes he has been discriminated against because he asserted his rights under the Act.

11. An employee has the right to contest the abatement period fixed in the citation issued to his employer by notifying the OSHA Area Director that issued the citation within 15 working days of the issuance of the citation.

## The OSHA poster

The OSHA poster (OSHA 2203, see Fig. 2–1) must be prominently displayed in a conspicuous place in the workplace where notices to employees are customarily posted. The poster informs employees of their rights and responsibilities under the Act.

## Occupational safety and health standards

The Act authorizes OSHA to promulgate, modify, or revoke occupational safety and health standards.° OSHA is responsible for promulgating legally enforceable standards which may require conditions, or the adoption or use of

---

°The rules of procedure for promulgating, modifying or revoking standards are codified in the *Code of Federal Regulations* (C.F.R.), Title 29, Chapter XVII, Part 1911.

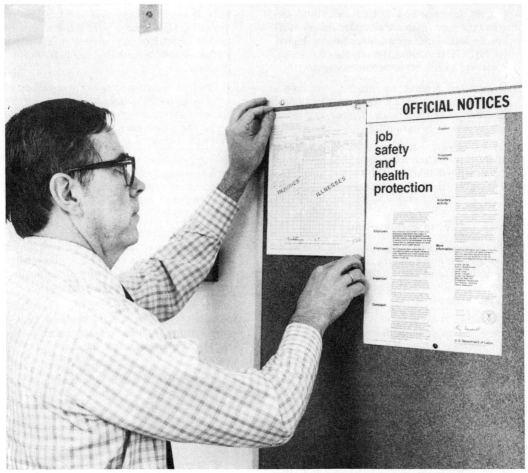

Fig. 2–1.—OSHA poster (OSHA 2203), "Safety and Health Protection on the Job," must be posted conspicuously at every plant, job site, or other establishment. At left is the annual Log and Summary of Occupational Injuries and Illnesses, OSHA Form 200, that must be posted by February 1 of the following year and remain in place until March 1.

practices, means, methods, or processes that are reasonably necessary and appropriate to protect employees on the job. It is the employer's responsibility to become familiar with the standards applicable to their establishments and to make sure that employees have and use personal protective equipment required for safety. In addition, employers are responsible for complying with the Act's general duty clause.

In order to get the initial set of standards in place without undue delay, the Act authorized OSHA to promulgate any existing federal standard or any national consensus standard without regard to the usual rulemaking procedures prior to April 28, 1973. The initial set of standards, Part 1910, appeared in the *Federal Register* of May 29, 1971. Subscriptions to the *Federal Register* are obtained through the Government Printing Office, Washington, D.C. 20402.

Standards° contained in Part 1910 are applica-

---

°The Occupational Safety and Health Standards, Title 29, C.F.R., Chapter XVII, Parts 1910, 1926, and 1915–1918 are available at all OSHA regional and area offices.

ble to general industry. Those contained in Part 1926 are applicable to construction. Standards applicable to ship repairing, shipbuilding, shipbreaking, and long-shoring are contained in Parts 1915 through 1918 respectively. Because standards cannot remain static due to use of new equipment, methods, and materials, all are subject to updating via modification.

OSHA standards incorporate by reference other standards adopted by standards-producing organizations. Standards incorporated by reference in OSHA standards in whole or in part as of June 30, 1980, include, but are not limited to, standards adopted by the following standards-producing organizations:

American Conference of Governmental Industrial Hygienists
American National Standards Institute
American Petroleum Institute
American Society of Agricultural Engineers
American Society of Mechanical Engineers
American Society for Testing and Materials
American Welding Society
Compressed Gas Association
Crane Manufacturers Association of America, Inc.
Institute of Makers of Explosives
National Electrical Manufacturers Association
National Fire Protection Association
National Plant Food Institute
National Institute for Occupational Safety and Health
Society of Automotive Engineers
The Fertilizer Institute
Underwriters Laboratories Inc.
U.S. Department of Commerce
U.S. Public Health Service

OSHA has the authority to promulgate emergency temporary standards where it is found that employees are exposed to grave danger. Emergency temporary standards can take effect immediately upon publication in the *Federal Register*. Such standards will remain in effect until superseded by a standard promulgated under the procedures prescribed by the Act. The law requires OSHA to promulgate a permanent standard no later than six months after publication of the emergency temporary standard.

Any person adversely affected by any standard issued by OSHA has the right to challenge its validity by petitioning the U.S. Court of Appeals

within 60 days after its promulgation.

**Input from the private sector.** Occupational safety and health standards promulgated by OSHA will never cover every conceivable hazardous condition that could exist in any workplace. Nevertheless, new standards and modification of existing standards are of significant interest to employers and employees alike. Industry organizations as well as individuals and employee organizations should express their views by responding to (*a*) OSHA's advance notice of proposed rulemaking, which usually calls for information upon which to base proposed standards, and (*b*) OSHA's proposed standards, since it is within the private sector that most of the expertise and the technical competence lies. To do less means that industry and employees are willing to let the standards development process rest in the hands of OSHA.

Sources used by OSHA for the revision of existing occupational safety and health standards or the development of new standards are standards advisory committees appointed by the Secretary of Labor and NIOSH criteria documents.

In order to promulgate, revise, or modify a standard, OSHA must first publish in the *Federal Register* a notice of any proposed rule that will adopt, modify, or revoke any standard and invite interested persons to submit their views on the proposed rule. The notice will include the terms of the new standard and will provide an interval of at least 30 days from the date of publication and usually 60 days or more for interested persons to respond. Interested persons may file objections to the rule and are entitled to a hearing on their objections if they request a hearing be held. However, objections must specify the parts of the proposed rule to which they object and the grounds for such objection. If a hearing is requested, OSHA must hold one. Based on (*a*) the need for control of an exposure to an occupational injury or illness, and (*b*) the reasonableness, effectiveness and feasibility of the control measures required, OSHA may issue a rule promulgating an additional standard or modify or revoke an existing standard.

## Recordkeeping requirements

Most employers covered by the Act are required to maintain in each establishment records of recordable occupational injuries and

## 2—Federal Legislation

illnesses.° Such records consist of:

• A log and summary of occupational injuries and illnesses, OSHA Form 200

• A supplementary record of each occupational injury or illness, OSHA Form 101

• An annual summary of occupational injuries and illnesses—OSHA Form 200 to be used in preparing the summary. The annual summary must be posted by February 1 of the following year and remain posted until March 1. (See Fig. 2-1.)

For details concerning recording and reporting occupational injuries and illnesses, see Chapter 6.

OSHA Forms 200 and 101 are available at all Bureau of Labor Statistics (BLS) regional offices and OSHA area and regional offices. If your state has an OSHA approved plan, be sure to check for any additional recordkeeping requirements.

In an effort to relieve small businesses from recordkeeping requirements, OSHA has ruled that an employer who had no more than ten employees at any time during the calendar year immediately preceeding the current calendar year, need not comply with the recordkeeping requirements. However, if an employer, regardless of size, has been notified in writing by the Bureau of Labor Statistics that he has been selected to participate in the statistical survey of occupational injuries and illnesses, then he will be required to maintain the log and summary and to make reports for the period of time specified in the notice. Further, no employer is relieved of his obligation to report to the nearest OSHA area office any fatalities or multiple hospitalization accidents.

### Reporting requirements

Within 48 hours after the occurrence of an accident which is fatal to one or more employees or which results in the hospitalization of five or more employees, the employer must report the accident either orally or in writing to the nearest area director of OSHA. In states with approved state plans, the report must be made to the state agency which has the enforcement responsibilities for occupational safety and health. If an oral report is made, it shall always be followed with a confirming letter written the same day. The report must relate to the circumstances of the accident, the number of fatalities, and the extent of any injuries.

### Variances from standards

There will be some occasions when, for various reasons, standards cannot be met. In other cases, the protection already afforded by an employer to employees is equal to or superior to the protection that would be granted if the standard were followed strictly to the letter. The Act provides an avenue of relief from these situations by empowering OSHA to grant variances°° from the standards, providing the granting of such variances would not degrade the purpose of the Act.

There are two types of variances—temporary and permanent. An employer may apply for an order granting a temporary variance provided he establishes that (a) he cannot comply with the applicable standard because of unavailability of personnel or equipment or time to construct or alter facilities; (b) he is taking all available steps to protect his employees against exposure covered by the standard; and (c) his program will effect compliance with the standard as soon as possible.

Employer applications for an order for a temporary variance must contain at least the following:

1. Name and address of the applicant

2. Address(es) of the place(s) of employment involved

3. Identification of the standard from which the applicant seeks a variance

4. A representation by the applicant that he is unable to comply with the standard and a detailed statement of reasons therefor

5. A statement of the steps the applicant has taken and will take, with dates, to protect employees against the hazard covered by the standard

6. A statement of when the applicant expects to

---

°Regulations pertaining to recording and reporting injuries and illnesses are codified in Title 29, C.F.R., Chapter XVII, Part 1904.

°°The detailed "Rules of Practice for Variances, Limitations, Variations, Tolerances, and Exemptions" are codified in Title 29, C.F.R., Chapter XVII, Part 1905.

be able to comply with the standard and what steps he has taken, with dates, to come into compliance with the standard

7. A certification that he has informed his employees of the application. A description of how employees have been informed is to be included in the certification. Information to employees must also inform them of their right to petition for a hearing

An employer may also apply for a permanent variance from a standard. A variance order can be granted if OSHA determines that an employer has demonstrated by a preponderance of evidence that he will provide a place of employment as safe and healthful as that which would prevail if he complied with the standard.

Employer applications for an order for a permanent variance must contain at least the following:

1. Name and address of the applicant

2. Address(es) of the place(s) of employment involved

3. A description of the countermeasures used or proposed to be used by the applicant

4. A statement showing how such countermeasures would provide a place of employment which is as safe and healthful as that required by the standard for which the variance is sought

5. Certification that he has informed his employees of the application

6. Any request for a hearing

7. A description of how employees were informed of the application and of their right to petition for a hearing

An employer may request an interim order permitting either kind of variance until his formal application can be acted upon. Again, the request for an interim order must contain statements of fact or arguments why such interim order should be granted. If a request for an interim order is denied, the applicant will be notified promptly and informed of the reasons for the decision. If the order is granted, all concerned parties will be informed and the terms of the order will be published in the *Federal Register*. In such cases, the employer must inform the affected employees regarding the interim order in the same manner

used to inform them of the variance application.

Upon filing an application for a variance, OSHA will publish a notice of such filing in the *Federal Register* and invite written data, views, and arguments regarding the application. Those affected by the petition may request a hearing. After review of all the facts, including those presented during the hearing, OSHA publishes its decision regarding the application in the *Federal Register*.

## Workplace inspection

Prior to the U.S. Supreme Court's decision on the controversial Barlow case,° the Department of Labor's Compliance Safety and Health Officers (CSHO) could enter, at any reasonable time and without delay, any establishment covered by the OSHAct to inspect the premises and all its facilities.°° However, the Barlow decision requires the OSHA compliance officer to present a search warrant if the employer demands that he do so. OSHA's entitlement to a warrant does not depend on demonstrating probable cause to believe that conditions on the premises violate the OSHA regulations, but merely that reasonable legislative or administrative standards for conducting an inspection are satisfied. As a general rule, it is not advisable for the employer to refuse entry to a CSHO without a search warrant, since such action normally would result in only delaying an inspection a day or two, the time necessary for OSHA to obtain a search warrant. Since the Barlow decision, OSHA has had to obtain a warrant in about 2.5 percent of the inspections.

The OSHAct authorizes an employer representative as well as an authorized employee representative to accompany the CSHO during the official inspection of the premises and all its facilities. Employee representatives also have the right to participate in both the opening and closing conferences.

Usually the authorized employee representative is the union steward or the chairman of the employee safety committee. Occasionally there

---

°Marshall v. Barlow's Inc., 436 U.S. 307 (1978).

°°The regulations governing enforcement procedures, including inspections, citations, and proposed penalties, are codified in Title 29, C.F.R., Chapter XVII, Part 1903.

may be no authorized employee representative, especially in those establishments that are nonunion shops. In the absence of an employee representative, the CSHO will confer with employees whom he picks at random.

An employer should not refuse to compensate employees for the time spent participating in an inspection tour and for related activities such as participating in the opening and closing conferences. A 1977 amendment to OSHA regulations provided that a denial of pay for the time spent assisting compliance personnel amounts to discrimination, but this may be revoked.

**Inspection priorities.** OSHA has established priorities for assignment of manpower and resources. The priorities are as follows:

1. Investigation of imminent dangers. Allegations of an imminent danger situation will ordinarily trigger an inspection within 24 hours of notification.

2. Catastrophic and fatal. Accidents will be investigated if they include any one of the following:

   One or more fatality

   Five or more employees hospitalized for more than 24 hours

   Significant publicity

   Issuance of specific instructions for investigations in connection with a national office special program.

3. Investigations of employee complaints. Highest priority is given those complaints that allege an imminent danger situation. Complaints alleging a "serious" situation are given high priority. If time and resources allow, the CSHO will normally inspect the entire workplace rather than limit the inspection to the condition alleged in the complaint.

4. Programmed high-hazard inspections. Industries are selected for inspection based on the death, injury, and illness incidence rates, employee exposure to toxic substances, etc.

5. Reinspections. Establishments cited for alleged serious violations normally are reinspected to determine whether the hazards have been abated.

**General inspection procedures.** The primary responsibility of the CSHO, who is under the supervision of the OSHA area director, is to conduct an effective inspection to determine if employers and employees are in compliance with the requirements of the standards, rules, and regulations promulgated under the OSHAct. OSHA inspections are almost always conducted without prior notice.

To enter an establishment, the CSHO will present his credentials to a guard, receptionist, or other person acting in such a capacity. Employers should always insist on seeing and checking the CSHO's credentials carefully before allowing the individual to enter their establishment for the purpose of an inspection (see Fig. 2–2). Anyone who tries to collect a penalty or promotes the sale of a product or service is not a CSHO.

The CSHO will usually ask to meet an appropriate employer representative. It is recommended that employers furnish written instructions to the security, receptionist, and other affected personnel regarding the right of entry, treatment, who should be notified, and to whom and where the CSHO should be directed so that undue delay can be avoided.

**Opening conference.** The CSHO will conduct a joint opening conference with employer and employee representatives. Where it is not practical to hold a joint conference, separate conferences are to be held for employer representatives. If there is no employee representative, then a joint conference is not necessary. In those instances where separate conferences are held, a written summary of each conference is to be made and the summary made available on request to employer and employee representatives.

Since the CSHO will want to talk with the safety personnel, such personnel should participate in the opening conference. The employer representative who accompanies the CSHO during the inspection should also participate in the opening conference.

At the opening conference, the CSHO will:

1. Inform the employer that the purpose of his visit is to make an investigation to ascertain if the establishment, procedures, operations, and equipment are in compliance with the requirements of the OSHAct.

2. Give the employer copies of the Act, standards, regulations, and promotional materials, as necessary.

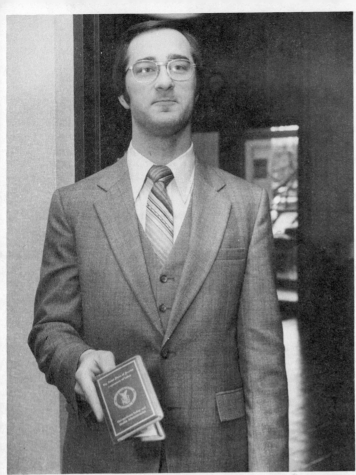

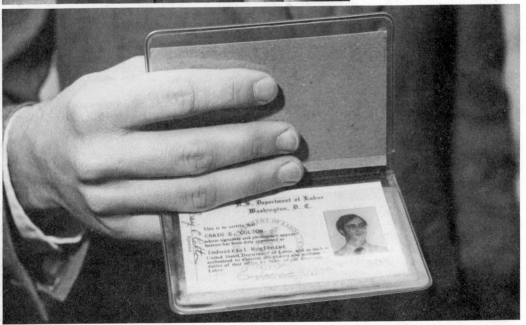

FIG. 2–2.—Bona-fide OSHA compliance officers are equipped with official identification as shown here. The credentials are signed by the current or former Assistant Secretary of Labor for Occupational Safety and Health. If in doubt about the validity of the credentials, it is recommended that the employer contact the nearest OSHA area office and determine whether or not the area office has scheduled an inspection at the establishment in question and verify the serial number on the credentials.

3. Outline in general terms:

   The scope of the inspection

   The records he wants to review

   His obligation to confer with employees

   The physical inspection of the workplace

   The closing conference

4. If applicable, furnish a copy of the complaint(s).

5. Answer questions those in attendance might have.

In the opening conference, the employer representative should determine which areas of the establishment the CSHO wishes to inspect. If the inspection includes areas of the plant in which trade secrets are maintained, the employer representative should orally request *confidential treatment* of all information obtained from such areas and follow up with a trade secret letter to the CSHO requesting him to keep information identified in the letter strictly confidential by not discussing any of it or providing copies to any person not authorized by law to receive the information without prior written consent of the employer.

During the course of the opening conference, the CSHO may request to review company records. The CSHO is authorized to review only the records required to be maintained by the OSHAct, regulations and standards. In general, these records include the "Log and Summary of Occupational Injuries and Illnesses" (OSHA Form 200) and the "Supplemental Record of Occupational Injuries and Illnesses" (OSHA Form 101). Such records should be made readily available to him the officer.

The CSHO may want to obtain information regarding the safety and health program that the employer now has in operation so that he can evaluate such a program. Naturally, a comprehensive safety and health program that shows evidence of effective performance in accident prevention will be impressive to all concerned.

The CSHO will also ascertain from the employer whether employees of another employer (for example, a contracting employer for maintenance or remodeling) are working in or on the establishment. If so, the CSHO will afford the authorized representative of those employees a reasonable opportunity to accompany him during the inspection of the workplaces where they are working.

During the conference, the CSHO will explain the employee representative's rights and ask for the authorized employee representative. Generally the employee representative will be an employee of the establishment inspected. However, if, in the judgment of the CSHO, good cause has been shown that accompaniment of a third party (such as an industrial hygienist or safety consultant) who is not an employee of the employer (but is, indeed, an authorized employee representative) is reasonably necessary to conduct an effective and thorough inspection, such a third party may accompany the CSHO during the inspection. The final decision will rest with the CSHO.

The employer is not permitted to designate the employee representative. Employee representatives may change as the inspection process moves from department to department. The CSHO may deny the right of accompaniment to any person whose conduct interferes with a full and orderly inspection. If there is no authorized employee representative, the CSHO will consult with a reasonable number of employees concerning matters of safety and health in the workplace during the course of the inspection.

*Inspection of facilities.* The CSHO will normally take the time necessary to inspect all of the operations in the establishment. The inspections have as their primary objective the enforcement of the occupational safety and health standards as well as the enforcement of other promulgated regulations such as the posting of the OSHA poster (Fig. 2–1).

The CSHO will have the necessary instruments for checking certain items, such as noise levels, certain air contaminants and toxic substances, grounding, and the like. During the course of inspection, the CSHO will note any apparent violation of the standards and will normally record any apparent violation, including its location, and any comments that he has regarding the violation. He will do the same for any apparent violation of the general-duty clause. The notes will serve as the basis of information for the area director when issuing citations or proposed penalties. For these reasons, the employer representative should ascertain any apparent violations from the CSHO during the actual inspection of the facilities. The employer representative should make notes identical to the CSHO's during the actual inspection so that he will have precisely the same information that the CSHO has.

It should be noted that the CSHO is only required to record apparent violations and is not required to present a solution or method of correcting, minimizing, or eliminating the violation. OSHA, however, will respond to requests for technical information concerned with complying with given standards. In such cases, the employer is urged to contact the regional or area office.

If, during the course of an inspection, the CSHO receives a complaint from an employee regarding a condition which is alleged to be in violation of an applicable standard, the CSHO, even though the complaint is brought to him via an informal process, will normally inspect for the alleged violation.

In the course of his normal inspection, the CSHO may make some preliminary judgments with respect to environmental conditions affecting occupational health. In such cases, he will generally use direct-reading instruments. Should this occur, and if proper instrumentation is available, it would be prudent for the employer to have qualified personnel at the establishment make duplicate tests in the same area at the same time under the same conditions. In addition, the employer representative should again take careful notes on the CSHO's methods as well as the results. If the inspection indicates a need for further investigation by an industrial hygienist, the CSHO will notify the Area Director who may assign a qualified industrial hygienist to investigate further. If a laboratory analysis is required, samples are sent to OSHA's laboratory in Salt Lake City and the results will be reported back to the Area Director.

*Closing conference.* Upon completion of the inspection, the CSHO will hold a joint closing conference with employee representatives and representatives of the employer. If a joint conference is not possible, a separate conference will be held. Again, the employer's safety personnel should be present at the closing conference. It is at this time that the CSHO will advise the employer and employee representatives of all conditions and practices which may constitute a safety or health violation. He should also indicate the applicable section or sections of the standards that may have been violated.

The CSHO will normally advise that citations may be issued for alleged violations and that

penalties may be proposed for each violation. Administratively, the authority for issuing citations and proposed penalties rests with the Area Director or his representative.

The employer will also be informed that the citations will fix a reasonable time for abatement of the violations alleged. The CSHO will attempt to obtain from the employer an estimate of the time he feels would be required to abate the alleged violation, and then he will take such estimate into consideration when recommending a time for abatement. Although the employer is not required to do so, it might be advantageous to give the officer copies of any correspondence or orders concerning equipment to achieve compliance since it may help to establish a reasonable abatement period and may reduce the proposed penalty by demonstrating good faith.

The CSHO should also explain the appeal procedures with respect to any citation or any notice of a proposed penalty.

*Informal post-inspection conferences.* Issues raised by inspections, citations, proposed penalties, or notice of intent to contest may be discussed at the request of an affected employer, employee, or employee representative at an informal conference held by the Assistant Regional Director. Whenever an informal conference is requested by either the employer or employee representatives, both parties shall be afforded the opportunity to participate fully.

**Followup inspections.** Followup inspections will always be made for those situations involving imminent danger or where citations have been issued for serious, repeated or willful violations. Followup inspections for all other cases will be conducted at the discretion of the Area Director.

The followup inspection is intended to be limited to verifying compliance of those conditions which were alleged to be in violation. The followup inspection is conducted with all of the usual formality of the original inspection, including the opening and closing conferences, and the walk-around rights of the employer and employee representative.

## Violations

In addition to the general-duty clause, the occupational safety and health standards promulgated under the OSHAct are used as a basis for determining alleged violations. There are four types of violations: imminent danger, serious, nonserious, and de minimis (very minor).

**Imminent danger.** The OSHAct defines imminent danger as "Any condition or practice in any place of employment which is such that a danger exists which could reasonably be expected to cause death or serious physical harm immediately or before the imminence of such danger can be eliminated through the enforcement procedures otherwise provided by this Act." Therefore, for conditions or practices to constitute an imminent danger situation, it must be determined that there is a reasonable certainty that immediately or within a short period of time such conditions or practices could result in death or serious physical harm.

"Serious physical harm" includes the permanent loss or reduction in efficiency of a part of the body, or inhibition of a part of the body's internal system such that life is shortened or physical or mental efficiency is reduced.

Normally a health hazard would not constitute an imminent danger except in *extreme* situations, such as the presence of potentially lethal concentrations of airborne toxic substances that are an immediate threat to the life or health of employees.

If, during the course of inspection, the CSHO deems that the existing set of conditions appears to constitute an imminent danger situation, he will immediately advise the employer or his representative that such a danger exists and will attempt to have the danger corrected immediately through voluntary compliance. Further, if any employees appear to be in imminent danger, they will be informed of the danger and the employer will be requested to remove them from the area of imminent danger.

An employer will be deemed to have abated the imminent danger if he eliminates the imminence of the danger by (a) removing employees from the danger area and assuring the CSHO that employees will not return until the hazardous condition has been eliminated or (b) eliminating the conditions or practices which constitute the imminent danger. Normally abatement is achieved in these two ways. When the employer voluntarily eliminates the danger, no imminent danger procedure is instituted and no Notice of Imminent Danger is issued. However, citations and proposed penalties are, nonetheless, issued.

If the employer refuses to voluntarily abate the alleged imminent danger, the CSHO will inform the affected employees of the danger involved and will inform the employer as well as the affected employees that he will recommend to the Area Director a civil action (in the form of a court order) for appropriate relief (*e.g.*, to shut down the operation). In such cases the CSHO will personally post the imminent danger notice at or near the area in which the exposed employees are working. The federal CSHO has no authority to order the closing down of an operation or to direct employees to leave the area of imminent danger or the workplace.

In such cases, the Area Director normally will request the Regional Solicitor to obtain an injunction permanently restraining the employer's practices. In order to protect the employees until the hearing on the injunction, a temporary restraining order, issued without notice to the employer and effective for up to five days, may be issued. The Act vests jurisdiction in the U.S. district courts to restrain any condition or work practice in imminent danger situations.

**Serious violation.** A serious violation is one where a substantial *probability* of death or serious physical harm could result, and that the employer knew, or should have known, of the hazard.

OSHA's *Field Operations Manual* (Chapter VIII) sets forth four steps for the CSHO to follow to determine whether a violation is serious or other than serious.

1. Determine the type of accident or health hazards that the standard is designed to prevent. (Example: a guard designed to prevent an operator's hand from coming in contact with the circular blade of a table saw.)

2. Determine what type of injury could be reasonably expected to result from the hazard. (In the example stated above, it could be reasonably predicted that contact between the operator's hand and the saw blade could result in the amputation of a finger or fingers, laceration of fingers or of an entire hand, or amputation of a hand.)

3. Determine whether the injury noted in Step 2 is likely to cause death or serious physical injury which involves the loss of use of part of the body or substantial reduction of efficiency of a part of the body. (In the example stated, a

deep laceration of the fingers or hand could result in substantial reduction in the efficiency of that limb.)

4. Determine that the employer knew of the violative condition which means that the employer had actual knowledge or could have known of the hazardous conditions if he had exercised reasonable diligence.

It is obvious that the CSHO must make an evaluation that death or serious physical harm could result from a condition which is an alleged violation.

Note that the emphasis in deciding whether or not a condition represents a serious violation is based on the *seriousness* or *severity* of a potential injury that could arise out of the potential accident, rather than on the *probability* that the accident will occur as a result of the violation. In many cases, the decision in determining whether a violation is serious or not will require professional judgment.

The *Industrial Hygiene Field Operations Manual* is used as a guide for handling health inspections and citations. (See Chapter 24, "Governmental Regulations," of *Fundamentals of Industrial Hygiene*, 2nd ed.)

**Other than serious violation.** An other than serious violation is one that has a direct relationship to job safety and health, but probably would not cause death or serious physical harm. For example, a violation of housekeeping standards that might result in a tripping accident would be classified as a nonserious violation since the probable consequence of such a condition would be strains or contusions which are not classified as serious physical harm.

**De minimis violations.** De minimis° violations are those that have no immediate or direct relationship to safety or health.

**Special types.** There are two other special types of violations: a willful violation, and a repeated violation.

• A willful violation exists where evidence shows that:

1. The employer committed an intentional and knowing violation of the Act and knows that such action constitutes a violation.

2. Even though the employer was not con-

sciously violating the Act, he was aware that a hazardous condition existed and made no reasonable effort to eliminate the condition.

• A repeated violation is where a second citation is issued for a violation of a given standard or the same condition which violates the general-duty clause. A repeated violation differs from a failure to abate in that repeated violations exist where the employer has abated an earlier violation, and upon later inspection, is found to have violated the same standard.

## Citations

When an investigation or inspection reveals a condition that is alleged to be in violation of the standards or general-duty clause, the employer may be issued a written citation which will describe the specific nature of the alleged violation, the standard allegedly violated and will fix a time for abatement. *Each citation*, or copy thereof, *must be prominently posted by the employer at or near the place where the alleged violation occurred.* All citations will be issued by the Area Director or his designee and will be sent to the employer by certified mail.

A "Citation for Serious Violation" will be prepared to cover those violations which fall into the "serious category." This type of violation *must* be assessed a monetary penalty.

A citation is used for other than serious violations which *may* or *may not* carry a monetary penalty. A citation may be issued to the employer for employee actions which violate the safety and health standards.

A notice, in lieu of a citation, is issued for de minimus violations which have no direct relationship to safety and health. Unlike the citation, the employer is not required to post this notice.

If an inspection has been initiated as a result of an employee complaint, the employee or authorized employee representative may request an informal review of any decision not to issue a citation.

Employees may not contest citations, amendments to citations, penalties, or lack of penalties. They may contest the time for abatement of a

---

°"De minimis" is short for the legal maxim, *De minimis non curat lex,* "The law does not concern itself with trifles."

hazardous condition specified in a citation. They also may contest an employer's Petition for Modification of Abatement (PMA), which requests an extension of the abatement period. Employees must contest the PMA within 10 working days of its posting or within 10 working days after an authorized employee representative has received a copy.

Within 15 working days of the employer's receipt of the citation, an employee may submit a written objection to OSHA. The OSHA area director forwards the objection to the Occupational Safety and Health Review Commission, which operates independently of OSHA.

Employees may request an informal conference with OSHA to discuss any issues raised by an inspection, citation, notice of proposed penalty, or employer's notice of intention to contest.

**Petition for modification of abatement.** Upon receiving a citation, the employer must correct the cited hazard by the prescribed date. However, factors beyond the employer's reasonable control may prevent the completion of corrections by that date. In such a situation, the employer who has made a good faith effort to comply may file for a Petition for Modification of Abatement date.

The written petition should specify all steps taken to achieve compliance, the additional time needed to achieve complete compliance, the reasons such additional time is needed, all temporary steps being taken to safeguard employees against the cited hazard during the intervening period, that a copy of the PMA was posted in a conspicuous place or near each place where a violation occurred, and that the employee representative (if there is one) received a copy of the petition.

## Penalties

In proposing civil penalties for citations, a distinction is made between serious violations and all other violations. There is no requirement that a penalty be proposed when a violation is not a serious one, but a penalty *must* be proposed for a serious violation. In either case the maximum penalty that may be proposed is $1000. In case of willful or repeated violations, a civil penalty of up to $10,000 may be proposed. Criminal penalties may be imposed on any employer who, among other things, willfully violates a standard and that violation causes death to any employee. There are no penalties for de minimis violations.

Penalties may be proposed for an alleged violation even though the employer immediately abates or initiates steps to abate the alleged violation. However, actions to abate should be favorably considered when determining the amount of adjustment applied for "good faith."

The information that follows describes the system that OSHA uses to arrive at its proposed penalties. Since it is unlikely that most employers comply with all of the promulgated standards, the employer can use a similar strategy to establish his own priorities for voluntary compliance with the standards.

**Other than serious violations.** For other than serious violations, the penalty may range from 0 to $1000 for each violation. An "unadjusted penalty" is based on the gravity of the alleged violation. Three factors are used to determine gravity and all factors require professional judgment.

1. The *severity* of injury or illness most likely to result. The severity factors are rated as follows:

   "A"—For conditions in which the injury would require first aid treatment or less, such as minor cuts, bruises or splinters

   "B"—For conditions in which the injury would require treatment by a doctor, such as sutures or setting broken bones in a finger

   "C"—For conditions in which the injury would require hospitalization for 24 hours or more.

2. The *probability* or likelihood that an injury or illness would result from the alleged violation. Consideration is given to the extent that such a condition has already resulted in injury or illness and the number of employees exposed to the substandard condition. The probability is rated as follows:

   "A"—If the likelihood is low

   "B"—If the likelihood is moderate

   "C"—If the likelihood is high

3. The *extent* to which the standard is violated. Here there are two factors involved—(a) standards pertaining to the workplace and (b) standards pertaining to employee procedures. The rating scheme for standards pertaining to

the workplace is as follows:

"A"—If any isolated violations are observed; that is, no more than 15 percent of the units covered by the standards are in violation.

"B"—If from 15 to 50 percent of the affected units are in violation.

"C"—If over 50 percent of such units are in violation.

With respect to standards pertaining to employee procedures, the rating system is as follows:

"A"—If the violation occurs occasionally

"B"—If the violation occurs frequently

"C"—If the violation occurs regularly

It is obvious from these measurement schemes that an "A" rating is the least severe and that the "C" rating is the most severe. These ratings are averaged to determine the final rating. (An "X" rating is used when the employer clearly demonstrates a blatant disregard for the violation in question.) Each final letter rating has been assigned the following dollar ranges for the purpose of establishing an "unadjusted penalty."

"A" = none

"B" = $100 to $200

"C" = $201 to $500

"X" = $501 to $1000

**Penalty reductions.** The "unadjusted penalty" may then be adjusted downward up to 50 percent depending on the employer's "good faith," size of business, and history of previous violations. A reduction of up to 20 percent may be given for "good faith." Evidence of good faith includes awareness of the OSHAct and any overt indications of the employer's desire to comply with the Act. A reduction of up to 10 percent may be given for business size measured in terms of the number of employees employed by the employer. A reduction of up to 20 percent may be given for a favorable history regarding previous violations. Normally, such history is based on the employer's past experience under the OSHAct. However, in certain cases, the employer's past history under other federal or applicable state safety and health statutes may be considered. The penalty adjustment factors are applied to the "unadjusted penalty" to determine the "adjusted penalty."

The "adjusted penalty" is further reduced by 50 percent (the abatement credit) if the employer corrects the violation within the abatement period specified in the citation. This reduction is made at the time the proposed penalty is calculated to determine the proposed penalty to be assessed for each violation.

**Serious violations.** The law requires that any employer who has received a citation for a serious violation must be assessed a proposed civil penalty of up to $1000 for each such violation. Due to the severity of a serious violation, the amount of the proposed penalty for each cited serious violation is usually calculated from a base of $1000 (the unadjusted penalty), which is the maximum penalty allowed. The unadjusted penalty may then be adjusted downward by up to 50 percent, depending on the employer's good faith, size of business, and history of violations, just as in the case of other than serious violations. However, the additional 50 percent "abatement credit" applicable to other than serious violations is *not* applicable to serious violations.

**Imminent danger.** Penalties may be proposed in cases of imminent danger even though the employer immediately eliminates the imminence of such danger or initiates steps to abate such danger. If the danger is abated, the situation can be reduced in gravity to the "serious" category, and some to the "nonserious" category—all dependent on what was done to remove the imminence and how much of the hazard is removed.

**Proposed penalties.** Once the proposed penalties have been calculated, each is listed in the "Citation and Notification of Penalty" (OSHA-2 Form), which is used to officially inform the employer of violations found during the inspection and penalties proposed for those violations. This is sent to the employer by certified mail. An information copy is sent to an employee representative or the employee organization.

**Notice of failure to correct.** The Act provides that any employer who fails to correct an uncontested violation within the abatement period may be assessed a proposed penalty of up to $1000 for each day that the violation continues after the expiration of the abatement period. This penalty provision can be applied when a followup inspection discloses that the employer has not abated a violation for which a citation has been issued and the citation and proposed penalty have become final.

**Time for payment of penalties.** When a citation and/or proposed penalty is uncontested, the payment is due after the lapse of 15 working days following receipt of the citation. When a citation and/or penalty are contested, the payment (if any) is not due until the final order of the Occupational Safety and Health Review Commission or the appropriate Circuit Court of Appeals is issued.

### Contested Cases

An employer has the right to contest an OSHA action if he feels that such action is not justified. The employer may contest a citation, a proposed penalty, a notice of failure to correct a violation, the time allotted for abatement of an alleged violation, or any combination of these.° An employee or authorized employee representative may contest only the time allotted for an abatement of an alleged violation.

Prior to going through the formality of initiating a contest, employers should request an informal hearing with the Area Director or the Assistant Regional Director. Many times such informal sessions will resolve the questions and the issues; therefore, the formal contested case proceedings can be avoided.

If the informal conference fails to resolve the dispute between OSHA and the employer and the latter elects to contest the case, it must be remembered that affected employees or the authorized employee representative are automatically deemed to be parties to the proceeding. In contesting an OSHA action, the employer must comply with the following which are applicable to the specific case:

1. Notify the Area Office which initiated action that he is contesting. *This must be done within 15 working days from receipt of OSHA's notice of proposed penalty;* it must be sent by certified mail. If the employer does not contest within 15 working days after receipt of the notice of proposed penalty, the citation and proposed assessment of penalties are deemed to be a final order of the Occupational Safety and Health Review Commission and are not subject to review by any court or agency and the alleged violation must be corrected within the abatement period specified in the citation.

2. If any of the employees working on the site of the alleged violation are union members, a copy of the notice of contest must be served upon their union.

3. If employees who work on the site are not represented by a union, a copy of the notice of contest must either be posted at a place where the employees will see it or be served upon them personally.

4. The notice of contest must also contain a listing of the names and addresses of those parties who have been personally served a notice and, if such notice is posted, the addresses of the place the notice was posted.

5. If the employees at the site of the alleged violation are not represented by a union and have not been personally served with a copy of the notice to contest, posted copies must specifically advise the unrepresented employees that they may be prohibited from asserting their status as parties to the case if they fail to properly identify themselves to the Commission or the Hearing Examiner prior to the commencement of the hearing or at the beginning of the hearing.

6. There is no specific form for the notice of contest. However, such notice should clearly identify what is being contested— the citation, the proposed penalty, the notice of failure to correct a violation, or the time allowed for abatement—for each alleged violation or combination of alleged violations.

If the employer contests an alleged violation in good faith, and not solely for delay or variance of penalties, the abatement period does not begin until the entry of the final order by the Review Commission.

When a notice of contest is received by an Area Director from an employer or from an employee or an authorized employee representative, he will file with the Review Commission the

---

°The regulations concerning the rules of procedure for contested cases adopted by the Occupational Safety and Health Review Commission are codified in Title 29, C.F.R., Chapter XX, Part 2200.

notice of contest and all contested citations, notice of proposed penalties, or notice of failure to abate.

Upon receipt of the notice of contest from the Area Director, the Commission will assign the case a docket number. Ultimately, an Administrative Law Judge (ALJ) will be assigned to the case and will conduct a hearing at a location reasonably convenient to those concerned. OSHA presents its case and is subject to cross examination by other parties. The party contesting then presents his case and is also subject to a cross examination by other parties. Affected employees or an authorized employee representative may participate in the hearings. The decision by the ALJ will be based *only* on what is in the record. Therefore, if statements are unchallenged, the statements will be assumed to be fact.

Upon completion of the hearings, the ALJ will submit the record and his report to the Review Commission. If no Commissioner orders a review of a ALJ's recommendation, such recommendation will stand as the Review Commission's decision. If any Commissioner orders a review of the case, the Commission itself must render a decision to affirm, modify, or vacate the judge's recommendation. The Commission's orders become final 15 days after issuance, unless stayed by a court order.

Any person adversely affected or aggrieved by an order of the Commission may obtain a review of such order in the U.S. Court of Appeals if sought within 60 days of the order's issuance.

## Small Business Loans

The Act enables economic assistance for small businesses. It amends the Small Business Act to provide for financial assistance to small firms for changes that will be necessary to comply with the standards promulgated under the OSHAct or standards promulgated by a state under a state plan. Before approving any such financial assistance, the Small Business Administration (SBA) must first determine that the small firm is likely to suffer substantial economic injury without such assistance.

An employer can make an application for a loan under one of two procedures: (*a*) before he has been inspected in order to come into compliance, or (*b*) after he has been inspected to correct alleged violations.

When an employer has not been inspected and requests a loan to bring his establishment into compliance before it is inspected, he must submit to the SBA:

A statement of the conditions to be corrected

A reference to the OSHA standards that require correction

A statement of his financial condition that necessitates applying for a loan

The employer should submit this information to the nearest SBA field office along with any background material. The SBA will then refer the application to the appropriate OSHA Regional Office, Office of Technical Support. The OSHA Regional Office will review the application and advise SBA whether the employer is required to correct the described conditions in order to come into compliance and whether his proposed use of funds will accomplish the needed corrections. Direct contact with the applicant will be initiated by OSHA only after clearance with the SBA.

If the employer is making an application after an inspection to correct alleged violations, the procedure is the same as before inspection, except that the applicant also must furnish SBA a copy of the OSHA citation(s). SBA then refers the application to the OSHA Area Office that conducted the inspection. That office will notify SBA whether the proposed use of loan funds will adequately correct cited violations.

Forms for loan applications may be obtained from any SBA field office. In some instances, private lending institutions will be able to provide the form for SBA/bank participation loans.

## Federal–State Relationships

The OSHAct encourages the states to assume the fullest responsibility for the administration and enforcement of their own occupational safety and health laws. Any state may assume responsibility for the development and enforcement of occupational safety and health standards relating to any occupational safety and health issue covered by a standard promulgated under the OSHAct. However, in order to assume this responsibility, such state must submit a state plan° to OSHA for approval. If such a plan

---

°The regulations pertaining to state plans for the development and enforcement of state standards are codified in C.F.R., Title 29, Chapter XVII, Part 1902.

satisfies designated conditions and criteria, OSHA must approve the plan.

The basic criteria for approval of state plans is that the plan must be "at least as effective as" the federal program. There was no congressional intent to require the state programs to be a "mirror image" of the federal program. Congress believed rules for developing state plans should be flexible to allow consideration of local problems, conditions, and resources.

The Act provides for funding the implementation of the state program, up to half the costs.

A state plan must include any occupational safety and health "issue" (industrial, occupational, or hazard group) for which a corresponding federal standard has been promulgated. A state plan cannot be less stringent, but it may include subjects not covered in the federal standards. However, state plans that do not include those issues covered by the federal program, in effect, surrender such issues to OSHA. For example, a state plan may cover all industry except construction. If such is the case, the state surrenders its jurisdiction for safety and health programs in construction operations to OSHA and it is then OSHA's obligation to enforce the federal standards for those operations not covered by the state plan.

Following approval of a state plan, OSHA will continue to exercise its enforcement authority until it determines on the basis of actual operations that the state plan is indeed being satisfactorily carried out. If the implementation of the state plan is satisfactory during the first three years after the plan's approval, then the federal standards and federal enforcement of such standards under the OSHAct can become inapplicable with respect to issues covered under the plan. This means that for the interim period of dual jurisdiction, employers must comply with the state standards as well as the federal standards.

While the state agencies administering the state plan are vitally concerned with its success, this is not always the case with the members of the state legislature. The state legislature must appropriate not only an adequate budget, but in many cases must pass legislation that will ultimately enable the state agency to carry out all the functions incorporated in the state plan. Should the state agency responsible fail to fully implement the state plan and the state's performance falls short of the mark of being "at least as effective as" the federal program, OSHA has the right and the obligation to withdraw its approval of the state plan and once again reassume full jurisdiction in that state.

## What Does It All Mean?

Congressional action in the form of the OSHAct is only a limited step in achieving the full purpose of the Act. Getting it to work with reasonable efficiency is the second and more difficult task. Achieving the *purpose* will depend on the willingness and cooperation of all concerned–employees and organized labor as well as business and industry.

There is no doubt that the Act has given new visibility to the whole realm of occupational safety and health. Since there are many employee rights incorporated in the OSHAct, it has given the employees a significant part of the action related to occupational safety and health matters. It has moved the laggards from "little or no safety" to "some safety," but not to "optimum safety." It has raised occupational safety and health to a higher priority in business management. It has given new status and responsibility to the occupational safety and health professional. Management is now relying more heavily on the safety profession for advice. And, it has given a new status to nationally recognized consensus standards-producing organizations.

New impetus is given to the field of occupational health, a much more difficult discipline with which to work when compared to occupational safety. Much more needs to be done to determine what kind of exposures are indeed hazardous to humans and under what conditions. Further, much more needs to be done to determine what countermeasures are not only adequate, but also reasonable and feasible to eliminate or minimize exposures to occupational health hazards. There exists a great need for much more research and data in occupational health to achieve optimum occupational safety and health programming.

The OSHAct has encouraged greater training for professionals in occupational safety and health. New curricula and university programs leading to various degrees in safety and health have been inaugurated by several universities and more are yet to come.

The OSHAct added new impetus to the product safety discipline. Until the passage of the Consumer Product Safety Act, the OSHAct was the most significant piece of legislation affecting product safety ever passed by the Congress. Designers and manufacturers of equipment now used by industry have a moral (but not legal) obligation to design, deliver, and install such equipment in accordance with the applicable standards.

The OSHAct, as well as the Occupational Safety and Health Administration, is not without limitations. Mere compliance with the requirements of the Act will not achieve optimum safety and health in terms of cost, benefits, and human values. All concerned must recognize that occupational safety and health cannot be handed to the employer or to the employee by legislative enactment or administrative decree. At best, state or federal occupational safety and health standards can cover only those things that are enforceable—namely control over physical conditions and environment.

As a matter of hard reality, enforcement standards simply do not adequately relate to the man in the man–machine–environment system. Important elements of a complete safety program, such as (a) establishment of work procedures to limit risk, (b) supervisory training, (c) job instruction training for employees, (d) job safety analysis, and (e) human factors engineering, to name a few, have not, for the most part, been included in the standards promulgated under the OSHAct—nor do the standards relate to employee attitudes, morale, or teamwork.

For the most part, the occupational safety and health standards promulgated under the OSHAct are minimal criteria and represent a floor rather than a goal to achieve. Thus, to rely on mere compliance with the occupational safety and health standards is to invite disaster since the residual risk after compliance remains unacceptable. Effective accident prevention and control of occupational health hazards must go beyond the OSHAct.

A violation of a standard is only symptomatic of something wrong with the management safety system. Only complete occupational safety and health programming as described elsewhere in this Manual will achieve a level of risk that is acceptable to employers as well as employees. The *real objective* and the purpose of the OSHAct is better occupational safety and health performance and not more compliance with a promulgated set of standards.

# PART II
# The Federal Mine Safety and Health Act

On November 9, 1977, President Carter signed into law the Federal Mine Safety and Health Act of 1977, Public Law 95-164. The Act became effective March 9, 1978.

The Federal Mine Safety and Health Act of 1977 (subsequently referred to as the Mine Act) is intended to ensure, so far as possible, safe and healthful working conditions for miners, it is applicable to operators of all types of mines, both coal and noncoal and both surface and underground. The Mine Act states that mine operators are responsible for the prevention of conditions or practices unsafe and unhealthful in mines, which endanger the safety and health of miners.

Mine operators are required to comply with the safety and health standards promulgated and enforced by the Mine Safety and Health Administration (MSHA), an agency within the Department of Labor. Like OSHA, MSHA may issue citations and propose penalties for violations. Unlike the OSHAct, miners (employees) are sub-ject to government sanctions for violations of standards relating to smoking. Similarly, employers and other supervisory personnel may be personally liable for violations as the operator's agent.

## Legislative History

Historically, the Bureau of Mines within the Department of the Interior administered the mine safety and health laws. Before the Congress passed the Mine Act, mine operators were governed by two separate laws, the Federal Coal Mine Health and Safety Act of 1969 and the Federal Metal and Nonmetallic Mine Safety Act of 1966.

Because the Bureau of Mines was also charged with promoting mine production, critics charged that this responsibility produced an inherent conflict of interest with respect to enforcement of safety and health laws. The establishment of the Mine Enforcement Safety Administration

(MESA) in 1973 within the Interior Department failed to reduce the criticism. Congress looked for alternative solutions, including the transfer of mine safety and health to the OSHAct. Congress finally settled on a solution by adopting the Federal Mine Safety and Health Act of 1977 which repealed the Federal Coal Mine Health and Safety Act of 1969 and the Federal Metal and Nonmetallic Mine Safety Act of 1966.

## Administration

The administration and enforcement of the Federal Mine Safety and Health Act are vested primarily with the Secretary of Labor and the Federal Mine Safety and Health Review Commission. The agency that administers the investigation and prosecution aspects of the enforcement process is the Mine Safety and Health Administration. The Federal Mine Safety and Health Review Commission,° an independent agency created by the Act, reviews contested MSHA enforcement actions.

The Mine Act separates *health* research and *safety* research. Miner *health* research and standards development is the responsibility of the National Institute for Occupational Safety and Health (NIOSH), located in the Department of Health and Human Services. The Department of the Interior is responsible for mine *safety* research and mine inspector training.

## Mine Safety and Health Administration

The Mine Safety and Health Administration, located within the Department of Labor, administers and enforces the Mine Act. MSHA is headed by an Assistant Secretary of Labor for Mine Safety and Health and is appointed by the President with the advice and consent of the Senate. The Assistant Secretary acts on behalf of the Secretary of Labor. For the purposes of this chapter, MSHA is also synonymous with the term Secretary or Assistant Secretary of Labor.

MSHA is authorized to adopt procedural rules and regulations to carry out the provisions of the Act. The agency also has the responsibility and authority to perform the following:

Promulgate, revoke or modify safety and health standards

Conduct mine safety and health inspections

Issue citations and propose penalties for violations

Issue orders for miners to be withdrawn from all or part of the mine

Grant variances

Seek judicial enforcement of its orders

Assisting the Assistant Secretary in carrying out the provisions of the Act is, among others, (a) an Administrator for Coal Mine Safety and Health and (b) an Administrator for Metal and Nonmetal Mine Safety and Health. Each administrator is responsible for a Division of Safety and a Division of Health.

## Federal Mine Safety and Health Review Commission

The five-member Federal Mine Safety and Health Review Commission serves as the administrative adjudication body. The Review Commission is completely independent from the Department of Labor. The commission has the authority to assess all civil penalties provided in the act. It reviews contested citations, notices of proposed penalties, withdrawal orders, and employee discrimination complaints. The Commission is appointed by the President for six-year terms with the advice and consent of the Senate. The first commissioners took office for staggered terms of two, four and six years.

The Commission appoints Administrative Law Judges (ALJ's) to conduct hearings on behalf of the Commission. The decision of an ALJ becomes a final decision of the Commission 40 days after its issuance unless the Commission directs a review.

## National Institute for Occupational Safety and Health

The functions carried out under the Mine Act by the National Institute for Occupational Safety and Health (NIOSH), Department of Health and Human Services (DHHS), include the following:

Miner health research

Recommending standards to MSHA for adoption

Conducting health hazard evaluations at a mine upon request

---

°Headquarters located at 1730 K Street, NW., Washington, D.C. 20006; (202) 653-5633.

To carry out its responsibilities, NIOSH is given authority to enter workplaces for the purpose of gathering information for research and for making health hazard evaluations. NIOSH also has the authority to provide medical examinations for miners at government expense for research purposes, to develop recordkeeping regulations relating to toxic exposure, and to require mine operators to make additional reports from time to time.

NIOSH also has the responsibility for reviewing toxic materials or harmful physical agents which are used or found in mines and to determine whether such substances are potentially toxic at the concentrations found. Further, NIOSH must thereafter review the toxicity of new substances brought to its attention. NIOSH is also required to submit criteria documents on toxic substances to assist MSHA in setting its standards.

## Department of the Interior

The Mine Act assigns the responsibility for mine safety research and the training of mine inspectors, operators, and miners to the Department of the Interior. Mine safety and health inspectors and technical support personnel of MSHA are trained by the DOI's National Mine Health and Safety Academy located in Beckley, West Virginia. The DOI is also authorized to conduct education and training programs for operators and miners in safety and health matters.

## Major Provisions of the Mine Act

### Coverage

The Mine Act covers all mines that affect commerce. The Act defines "mines" as all underground or surface areas from which minerals are extracted and all surface facilities used in preparing or processing the minerals. Structures, equipment, and facilities including roads, dams, impoundments, and tailing ponds used in connection with mining and milling activities are also included.

OSHA and MSHA established an interagency agreement° which, among other things, delineates certain areas of authority and provides for coordination between OSHA and MSHA in all areas of mutual interest. In case of jurisdictional disputes between OSHA/MSHA, the Secretary of Labor is authorized to assign enforcement responsibilities to one of the agencies.

### Advisory committees

The Act requires the Secretary of the Interior to appoint an Advisory Committee on Mine Safety Research.

The Secretary of HHS is required to appoint an Advisory Committee on Mine Health Research.

The Secretary of Labor or the Secretary of HHS may appoint other advisory committees as deemed appropriate to advise in carrying out the provisions of the Act.

### Miners' rights

The Act affords miners (employees) a number of rights, including the following:

• Miners may request in writing an inspection if they believe a violation of a standard or an imminent danger situation exists in the mine. Similarly, written notification of alleged violations or imminent danger situations may be given to an inspector before or during an inspection.

• An authorized representative of miners must be given the opportunity to accompany the inspector during the inspection process. Also, miners have the right to participate in post-inspection conferences held by the mine inspector at the mine.

• At least one representative of the miners who accompanies the inspector during the inspection must be paid at his regular rate of pay for the time spent accompanying the inspector.

• Miners are entitled to observe monitoring and examine monitoring records when the standards require monitoring exposure to toxic materials or harmful physical agents.

• Miners, including former miners, must be provided access to records relating to their own exposures.

• Operators must notify miners who are exposed to toxic substances in concentrations which exceed prescribed limits of exposure. Further, those miners must be informed of the corrective action being taken.

---

°Published at 44 FR 22827, April 17, 1979.

• Miners given new work assignments for medical reasons because of exposure to hazardous substances must be paid at their regular rate if the related standard so provides.

• Miners who are not working because of a withdrawal order are entitled to be compensated subject to certain limits.

• Miners or their authorized representatives may contest the issuance, modification, or termination of any order issued by MSHA or the time period set for abatement.

• Miners adversely affected or aggrieved by an order of the Review Commission may obtain judicial review.

• Miners may file a complaint with the Review Commission concerning compensation for not working arising out of a withdrawal order or for acts of employee discrimination.

• Miners, through their authorized representative, may petition for a variance from mine safety or health standards.

• MSHA is required to send to the miners' authorized representative copies of proposed safety or health standards. In addition, the mine operator must provide a copy of such standards on its office bulletin board.

• To keep miners informed, mine operators are required to post copies of orders, citations, notices, and decisions issued by MSHA or the Review Commission.

• Miners are entitled to receive training for their specific jobs and must be given refresher training annually and are entitled to normal compensation while being trained. When a miner leaves the operator's employ, he is entitled to copies of his training certificates.

• Operators may not discriminate against miners or representatives of miners.

• Miners suffering from black lung disease are entitled to extensive black lung benefits.

### Duties

Mine operators are required to comply with the safety and health standards and other rules promulgated under the Act and are subject to sanctions for failing to comply. Similarly, every miner is required to comply with the safety and health standards promulgated under the Act. However, no sanctions are imposed against miners except for willful violation of safety standards relating to smoking or to the carrying of smoking materials, matches, or lighters.

### Miner training

Mine operators are required to have a safety and health training program approved by MSHA which provides the following:

• At least 40 hours of instruction for new underground miners. The training must include the statutory rights of miners and their representatives under the Act, use of the self-rescue device and use of respiratory devices, hazard recognition, escapeways, walk-around training, emergency procedures, basic ventilation, basic roof control, electrical hazards, first aid, and the health and safety aspects of the task assignment.

• Twenty-four hours of instruction for new surface miners. The training must include all of the items for underground miners just listed, except escapeways, basic ventilation, and basic roof control, none of which are essential to surface mining.

• At least 8 hours of refresher training for all miners on an annual basis.

The Mine Act requires that the training must be conducted during normal working hours and that the miners must be paid at their normal rate during the training period. Regulations concerning training and retraining of miners are codified at Title 30, CFR, Part 48. (See Chapter 9.)

### Mine Safety and Health Standards

The Mine Act authorizes MSHA to promulgate, modify, or revoke mine safety and health standards.

To get the initial set of standards in place without delay under the Mine Act, the safety and health standards under the Coal Mine Health and Safety Act of 1969 were adopted under the Mine Act. These standards are codified in Title 30 CFR, Parts 70, 71, 74, 75, 77, and 90.

Similarly, the Mine Act adopted the mandatory standards that prevailed under the Metal and Nonmetallic Mine Safety Act of 1966. Later, many of the advisory standards were adopted as mandatory standards under the Mine Act. All of the noncoal standards are codified in Title 30 CFR, Parts 55, 56, and 57.°

If MSHA should determine that a standard is needed, it may propose a standard or seek assistance from an advisory committee. The proposed standard must be published in the *Federal Register* and a time period of at least 30 days must be established for public comment. MSHA may hold public hearings if objections are made to a proposed standard. Upon adoption by MSHA, the standard must be published in the *Federal Register*. The new standard becomes effective upon publication or at a date specified.

## Judicial review

Any person adversely affected by any standard issued by MSHA has the right to challenge the validity of the standard by petitioning in the U.S. Court of Appeals within 60 days after promulgation of the standard. The filing of such a petition does not stay enforcement of the standard, but the Court may order a stay before conducting a hearing on the petition. Objections that were not raised during rulemaking will not be considered by the Court, unless good cause is shown for the failure to have raised an objection.

## Input from the private sector

Mine safety and health standards, promulgated by MSHA, can never cover every conceivable hazardous condition that could exist in mines. Nevertheless, new standards, modification or revocation of existing standards are of significant interest to mine operators and miners alike. Mining operator organizations, miner organizations as well as individuals should express their views in the rulemaking process by responding to MSHA's proposed standards since it is within the private sector that most of the expertise and the technical competence lies. To do less means that mining operators and miners are willing to let the standards development process be done by MSHA.

## Emergency temporary standards

MSHA has the authority to publish emergency temporary standards if it deems that immediate action must be taken to protect miners "exposed to grave danger" from toxic substances or physically harmful agents. The emergency temporary standard is effective immediately upon publication in the *Federal Register* and remains in effect until superseded by a permanent standard promulgated under the normal rulemaking procedures. MSHA is required to promulgate a permanent standard within nine months after publication of an emergency temporary standard.

## Variances

Upon petition by an operator or a representative of miners, MSHA may modify the application of any mandatory *safety* standard. The Act does not allow for variances of *health* standards.

A petition may be granted if MSHA deems that an alternative method of compliance will achieve the same measure of protection for miners as the standard would provide or that the standard in question will result in less safety to miners.

A variance petition should be filed with the Assistant Secretary of Labor for Mine Safety and Health. If the mining operator submits a petition, a copy must be served on the miners' representative. Similarly, if the miners' representative petitions for a variance, a copy must be served on the mine operator. The petition must include the name and address of the petitioner and the mailing address and identification, and name or number of the affected mine. It must also identify the standard, describe the desired modification, and state and basis for the request.

MSHA will publish a notice of the petition in the *Federal Register*. The notice will contain information contained in the petition. Interested parties have 30 days to comment. MSHA then will conduct an investigation on the merits of the petition and the appropriate Administrator issues a proposed decision. The proposed decision becomes final 30 days after service unless a hearing request is filed within that time.

## Accident, injury, illness reporting

For the purpose of reporting accidents, injuries and illnesses under the Mine Act, the term "accident" includes:

---

°A list of all of the standards promulgated under authority of the Mine Act are listed in References, at the end of this chapter.

A fatality at a mine

An injury which has the potential to cause death

Entrapment for more than 30 minutes

An unplanned ignition or explosion of gas or dust

An unplanned fire not extinguished within 30 minutes of its discovery

An unplanned ignition or explosion of a blasting agent or an explosive

Roof fall in active workings where roof bolts are in use or a roof fall that impairs ventilation or impedes passage

Coal or rock outbursts that disrupt mining activities for more than one hour

Conditions requiring emergency action or evacuation

Damage to hoisting equipment in a shaft or slope that endangers an individual or interferes with use of equipment for more than 30 minutes

An event at the mine that causes a fatality or bodily injury to an individual not at the mine at the time of occurrence

"Occupational injury" means an injury that results in death, loss of consciousness, administration of medical treatment, temporary assignment to other duties, transfer to another job, or inability to perform all duties on any day after the injury.

"Occupational illness" is an illness or disease that may have resulted from work at a mine or for which a compensation award is made.

All mine operators are required to *immediately* report accidents (as defined earlier) to the nearest MSHA district or subdistrict office. Similarly, operators must investigate and submit to MSHA, upon request, an investigation report on accidents and occupational injuries. The investigation report must include:

The date and hour of occurrence

The date the investigation began

The names of the individuals participating in the investigation

A description of the site

An explanation of the accident or injury

The name, occupation, and experience of any miner involved

If appropriate, a sketch, including dimensions

A description of actions taken to prevent a similar occurrence

Identification of the accident report submitted.

All mine operators must submit to MSHA within 10 days of occurrence a report of each accident, occupational injury or illness on Form No. 7000-1. A separate form is to be prepared for each miner affected.

Accident investigation reports as well as the injury/illness reports filed by means of Form 7000-1 must be retained for five years at the mine office closest to the mine in which the accident/injury/illness occurs.

### Inspection and investigation procedures

Inspections of a mine are conducted by MSHA to determine if an imminent danger exists in the mine and if the mine operator is complying with the safety and health standards and with citations, orders, or decisions issued. Mine inspectors from MSHA or representatives of NIOSH have the right to enter any mine to make an inspection or an investigation. Although a representative of NIOSH has the authority to enter mines, he has no enforcement authority. The Mine Act's provision for warrantless inspection has been held valid.

As in OSHA, the advance notice of inspection for the purpose of ascertaining compliance is prohibited. However, NIOSH may give advance notice of inspections for research and other purposes.

**Frequency.** All underground mines are to be inspected by MSHA in their entirety at least four times a year. Surface mines are to be inspected at least two times a year. Spot inspections must be conducted by MSHA based on the number of cubic feet of methane or other explosive gases liberated during a 24 hour period. The Act authorizes MSHA to develop guidelines for additional inspections based on other criteria.

**Miner complaints.** A miners' authorized representative, or a miner if there is no authorized representative, may request in writing an immediate inspection by MSHA, if there is reasonable grounds to believe that a violation of a standard or an imminent danger situation exists. MSHA will normally conduct a special inspection soon after receiving the complaint of an alleged violation or imminent danger situation. If MSHA determines that a violation does not exist, it must notify the complaintant in writing.

Similarly, before or during an inspection, the miners' authorized representative, or a miner if there is no authorized representative, may notify the inspector in writing of any alleged violation or imminent danger situation believed to exist in the mine.

**Health hazard evaluations.** Upon written request of an operator or authorized representative of miners, NIOSH is authorized to enter a mine to determine whether any toxic substance, physical agent or equipment found or used in the mine is potentially hazardous. A copy of the evaluation will be submitted to both the operator and the miners' representative.

**The inspection procedure.** An MSHA inspector will normally begin the inspection at the mine office. He will inform the mine operator why he is there and will state what records he wants to examine. His review of the records will likely focus on the preshift or on-shift examination record. Such records help the inspector determine where he should concentrate his efforts during the inspection.

An operator's representative and a representative authorized by the miners must be given the opportunity to accompany the MSHA inspector during the inspection. Similarly, each must be given the opportunity to participate in the post-inspection conference. One miner representative (who is an employee of the operator) must be paid his regular wage for the time spent accompanying the inspector.

If the inspector observes a condition that he believes is a violation of the standards, a citation must be issued. If, in the opinion of the mine inspector, an imminent danger condition exists, then the inspector must issue a withdrawal order.

After completing the inspection, the inspector will hold a close-out conference with the representatives of the mine operator and the miners to discuss his findings. Occasionally, in the interests of all concerned, a separate closing conference may be held with the mine operator and another with the miners' representative.

## Withdrawal orders

MSHA has the authority under specified conditions, to issue orders to an operator requiring the operator to withdraw the miners from all or part of a mine. Miners idled by such an order are entitled to receive compensation at their regular rate of pay for specified periods of time. All miners in the affected area must be withdrawn except those necessary to eliminate the hazard, public officials whose duty requires their presence in the area, representatives of the miners qualified to make mine examinations, and consultants.

If an imminent danger is found to exist during an inspection, MSHA is required to order the withdrawal of all persons from the affected area except those referred to in Section 104 of the Act until the danger no longer exists. The order must describe the conditions or practices which cause and constitute the imminent danger and the area affected. The withdrawal order does not preclude issuance of a citation and proposed penalty.

There are other situations in which MSHA may issue a withdrawal order such as the following:

• If, during a follow-up inspection, MSHA finds that a mine operator has failed to abate a violation for which a citation has been issued and there is no valid reason to extend the abatement period, MSHA must issue a withdrawal order until the violation is abated.

• If a mine operator fails to abate a respirable dust violation for which a citation has been issued and the abatement period has expired, MSHA must either extend the abatement period or issue a withdrawal order.

• If two violations constituting "unwarrantable failures" to comply with the standards are found during the same inspection, or if the second unwarrantable violation is found within 90 days of the first, a withdrawal order must be issued. An unwarrantable failure violation (second within 90 days) is a situation of such a nature that the operator knew or should have known that a violation existed and failed to take corrective action.

• A miner may be ordered to be withdrawn from a mine if he has not received the safety training required by the Act. Miners withdrawn for this reason are protected by the Act from discharge or loss of pay.

# 2—Federal Legislation

Except for withdrawal orders issued for respirable dust violations and imminent danger situations, an operator or a miner may file a written request for a temporary stay of the order with the Review Commission. Also, temporary relief may be requested from any modification or termination of a withdrawal order. The Review Commission may grant a stay of a withdrawal order if the granting of such relief would not adversely affect the safety and health of miners.

Both operators and miners, or their representatives may contest an imminent danger withdrawal order by filing with the Review Commission an application for review of the order within 30 days of its receipt, or within 30 days of any modification or termination of such an order if the modification or termination is being contested.

## Citations

If an MSHA inspector or his supervisors believe that the mine operator is in violation of any standard, rule, order, or regulation promulgated under the Mine Act, a citation must be issued to the operator with "reasonable promptness." A citation may be issued at the site of the alleged violation. In any case, a citation for all alleged violations will be issued before the inspector leaves the mine property, unless mitigating circumstances exist.

Citations must be in writing, describe the nature of the violation, and include a reference to the provision of the Mine Act, standard, rule, regulation, or order allegedly violated. The citation, based on the inspector's opinion, will establish a reasonable time period for abatement.

The Act requires that the citations be posted on the mine's bulletin board. Copies are sent to the miners' representative, to the state agency charged with administering mine safety and health laws, and to those designated by the operator as having responsibility for safety and health in the mine.

## Penalties

A civil penalty of not more than $10,000 must be assessed for each violation of the Act. Penalties up to $1000 per day may be assessed for each day the operator fails to correct a violation for which a citation has been issued. A fine of $25,000 and/or one year imprisonment may be assessed for a willful violation of a standard. A penalty of up to $250 per occurrence may be assessed miners having willfully violated a standard relating to smoking or the carrying of smoking materials, matches or lighters.

After the alleged violation has been abated or a final action has been taken to terminate the citation, MSHA's assessment office will conduct an initial review in which a proposed penalty is established. In determining the amount of the penalty, MSHA considers six criteria:

1. The operator's history of previous violations
2. The size of the operator's business
3. Whether or not the operator is negligent
4. The effect of the operator's ability to continue in business
5. The gravity of the violation
6. The demonstrated good faith in attempting to achieve rapid compliance after notification of the alleged violation.

Proposed penalty assessments are assigned a range of penalty points for each of the above criterion. The total points are then converted into a dollar penalty. The mine operator or a miners' representative may request, within 10 days of receipt of a proposed penalty, an informal conference if either or both wishes to dispute the proposed penalty. If the informal conference fails to resolve the issues, either may contest the proposed penalty within 30 days from receipt of the proposed penalty.

## Contested Cases

Operators and miners (or miners' representatives) have 30 calendar days from the receipt to contest a citation, a withdrawal order, or a proposed penalty. The notice of contest must be filed with the Assistant Secretary of Labor for Mine Safety and Health at the MSHA headquarters located at 4015 Wilson Boulevard, Arlington, Va. 22203, by registered or certified mail. A copy of the notice of contest must be sent to the representative of the miners.

If a mine operator fails to notify MSHA within the 30 day period and no notice is filed by any miner or miners' representative, then the citation and/or the proposed penalty is deemed a final order of the Federal Mine Safety and Health Review Commission and is not subject to review by any court or agency. However, it should be understood that the citation and the penalty have separate 30 day periods within which they may be contested. For instance, if a mine operator fails to contest the citation, all is not lost. When the proposed penalty is received at some later date, the mining operator has 30 days within which to contest that penalty. In addition, if the penalty is contested, the citation may be reopened for negotiation at the same time.

A citation may be contested before the operator receives a notice of proposed penalty, even if the alleged violation has been abated. A notice of contest consists of a statement of what is being contested and the relief sought. A copy of the order or citation being contested must accompany the notice of contest.

Upon receiving the notice of contest, MSHA immediately notifies the Review Commission and a docket number and an Administrative Law Judge (ALJ) are assigned to the case. The Review Commission will provide an opportunity for a hearing via the ALJ. The ALJ may hold an informal conference with all parties involved to clarify and settle the issues. If the issues are not resolved, then a formal hearing conducted by the ALJ will take place.

Mine operators, miners or representatives of miners, and applicants for employment may be parties to the Review Commission proceedings. Miners or their representatives may become parties by filing a written notice with the Executive

Director of the Review Commission prior to the hearing.

The Review Commission's ALJ's are authorized, among other things, to administer oaths, issue subpoenas, receive evidence, take depositions, conduct hearings, hold settlement conferences, and render decisions. The decision will include findings of facts, conclusions of law, and an order. A copy of the decision will be issued to each of the parties involved and to each of the Commissioners. Any person aggrieved by the decision of the ALJ may, within 30 days of issuance of an order or decision, file a petition for a discretionary review by the Review Commission.

The Review Commission on its own motion and with the affirmative vote of two members may direct review of an ALJ's decision within 30 days of issuance only if the decision may be contrary to law or to Commission policy or if a novel question of policy has been presented.

Any person adversely affected by a decision of the Review Commission, including MSHA, may appeal to the U.S. Court of Appeals within 30 days of issuance. The court may affirm, modify or set aside the Commission's decision in whole or in part.

## DIRECTORY OF FEDERAL AGENCIES

### The Occupational Safety and Health Act

**National headquarters**

*OSHA*

Occupational Safety and Health Administration, U.S. Department of Labor, Department of Labor Building, 200 Constitution Avenue, NW., Washington, D.C. 20210

*NIOSH*

National Institute for Occupational Safety and Health, U.S. Department of Health and Human Services, Parklawn Building, 5600 Fishers Lane, Rockville, Md. 20857

*BLS*

Bureau of Labor Statistics, U.S. Department of Labor, 200 Constitution Avenue, NW., Washington, D.C. 20210

*OSHRC*

Occupational Safety and Health Review Commission, 1825 K Street, NW., Washington, D.C. 20006

**OSHA regional offices**

*Region I* (Connecticut, Maine, Massachusetts, New Hampshire, Rhode Island, Vermont)
16–18 North Street, 1 Dock Square, Boston, Mass. 02109

*Region II* (New York, New Jersey, Puerto Rico)
1515 Broadway (1 Astor Plaza), New York, N.Y. 10036

*Region III* (Delaware, District of Columbia, Maryland, Pennsylvania, Virginia, West Virginia)
Gateway Building, 3535 Market Street, Philadelphia, Pa. 19104

## 2—Federal Legislation

*Region IV* (Alabama, Florida, Georgia, Kentucky, Mississippi, North Carolina, South Carolina, Tennessee)
1375 Peachtree Street, NE.,
Atlanta, Ga. 30309

*Region V* (Illinois, Indiana, Michigan, Minnesota, Ohio, Wisconsin)
J.C. Kluczynski Federal Building,
230 South Dearborn Street,
Chicago, Ill. 60604

*Region VI* (Arkansas, Louisiana, New Mexico, Oklahoma, Texas)
555 Griffin Square Building,
Dallas, Texas 75202

*Region VII* (Iowa, Kansas, Missouri, Nebraska)
Old Federal Office Building,
911 Walnut Street, Kansas City, Mo. 64106

*Region VIII* (Colorado, Montana, North Dakota, South Dakota, Utah, Wyoming)
Federal Building, 1961 Stout Street,
Denver, Colo. 80294

*Region IX* (Arizona, California, Hawaii, Nevada, Guam, American Samoa, Trust Territory of the Pacific Islands)
Federal Building, 450 Golden Gate Avenue,
San Francisco, Calif. 94102

*Region X* (Alaska, Idaho, Oregon, Washington)
Federal Office Building, 909 First Avenue,
Seattle, Wash. 98174

### The Mine Safety and Health Act

Mine Safety and Health Administration, U.S. Department of Labor, 4015 Wilson Boulevard, Arlington, Va. 22203

National Institute for Occupational Safety and Health, U.S. Department of Health and Human Services, Parklawn Building, 5600 Fishers Lane, Rockville, Md. 20857

National Mine Health and Safety Academy, P.O. Box 1166, Beckley, W.Va. 25801

Federal Mine Safety and Health Review Commission, 1730 K Street, NW., Washington, D.C. 20006

### The 'Federal Register' and the 'Code of Federal Regulations'

The safety specialist and the industrial hygienist should be familiar with two U.S. Government publications, *The Federal Register (FR)* and *The Code of Federal Regulations (CFR)*. Both documents, published by the Office of *The Federal Register*, National Archives and Records Service, General Services Administration, are available on subscription basis from the Superintendent of Documents, U.S. Government Printing Office, Washington, D.C. 20402.

*The Federal Register*, published daily Monday through Friday, provides a system for making publicly available regulations and legal notices issued by all federal agencies. In general, an agency will issue a regulation as a proposal in *FR*, followed by a comment period, then will finally promulgate or finally adopt the regulation in *FR*. Reference to material published in *FR* is usually in the format A *FR* B, whereby A is the volume number, *FR* indicates *Federal Register*, and B is the page number. For example, 43 *FR* 58946, indicates volume 43, page 58946.

The *Code of Federal Regulations*, published annually in paperback volumes, is a compilation of the general and permanent rules and regulations that have been previously released in *FR*.

The *CFR* is divided into 50 different titles, representing broad subject areas of federal regulations, for example, Title 29—"Labor;" Title 40—"Protection of Environment;" Title 49—"Transportation," etc. Each title is divided into chapters (usually bearing the name of the issuing agency), and then further divided into parts and subparts covering specific regulatory areas. Reference is usually in the format 40 *CFR* 250.XX, meaning Title 40 *CFR* Part 250 (Hazardous Waste Guidelines and Regulations), or 49 CFR 172.XX, (Hazardous Materials Table and Hazardous Materials Communications Regulations). The "XX" refers to the number of the specific regulatory paragraph.

The *Code of Federal Regulations* is kept up to date by the individual issues of The *Federal Register*. These two publications must be used together to determine the latest version of any given rule or regulation.

Source: J. T. Baker Chemical Co.

## References

Bureau of National Affairs, Inc., 1231 25th Street, NW., Washington, D.C. 20037. *Occupational Safety and Health Reporter.*

Commerce Clearing House, Inc., 4025 West Peterson Avenue, Chicago, Ill. 60646. *Employment Safety and Health Guide.*

National Institute for Occupational Safety and Health, 5600 Fishers Lane, Rockville, Md. 20857.
"The Advisor" (newsletter).
"Occupational Safety and Health Directory."

National Safety Council, 444 North Michigan Avenue, Chicago, Ill. 60611.
*National Safety News* (magazine)
"OSHA Up-to-Date" (newsletter).
*OSHA Standards Handbook for Business and Industry* (self-evaluation checklist).

Superintendent of Documents, U.S. Government Printing Office, Washington, D.C. 20402.
*Annual List of Toxic Substances.*
*Directory of Federal Agencies.*
*Federal Register.*
*Field Operations Manual.*
*Industrial Hygiene Field Operations Manual.*
Occupational Safety and Health Act of 1970 (P.L. 91-596).
*Occupational Safety and Health Regulations,* Title 29, *Code of Federal Regulations* (C.F.R.)
    Part 11—Department of Labor, National Environmental Policy Act (NEPA) Compliance Procedures.
    Part 1901—Procedures for State Agreements.
    Part 1902—State Plans for the Development and Enforcement of State Standards.
    Part 1903—Inspections, Citations and Proposed Penalties.
    Part 1904—Recording and Reporting Occupational Injuries and Illnesses.
    Part 1905—Rules of Practice for Variances, Limitations, Variations, Tolerances, and Exemptions.
    Part 1906—Administration Witnesses and Documents in Private Litigation.
    Part 1907—Accreditation of Testing Laboratories.
    Part 1908—On-Site Consultation Agreements.
    Part 1910—Occupational Safety and Health Standards.
    Part 1911—Rules of Procedure for Promulgating, Modifying, or Revoking Occupational Safety or Health Standards.
    Part 1912—Advisory Committees on Standards.
    Part 1912a—National Advisory Committee on Occupational Safety and Health.
    Part 1913.10—OSHA Access to Employee Medical Records.
    Part 1915—Safety and Health Regulations for Ship Repairing.
    Part 1916—Safety and Health Regulations for Shipbuilding.
    Part 1917—Safety and Health Regulations for Shipbreaking.
    Part 1918—Safety and Health Regulations for Longshoring.
    Part 1926—Safety and Health Regulations for Construction.
    Part 1950—Development and Planning Grants for Occupational Safety and Health
    Part 1951—Procedures for 23(g) Grants to State Agencies
    Part 1952—Approved State Plans for Enforcement of State Standards
    Part 1953—Changes to State Plans for the Development and Enforcement of State Standards
    Part 1954—Procedures for the Evaluation and Monitoring of Approved State Plans
    Part 1955—Procedures for Withdrawal of State Plan Approval
    Part 1956—Safety and Health Provisions for Public Employees in Non-approved Plan States
    Part 1960—Safety and Health Provisions for Federal Employees
    Part 1975—Coverage of Employees under the Williams-Steiger Occupational Safety and Health Act of 1970

# 2—Federal Legislation

Part 1977—Discrimination Against Employees Exercising Rights Under the Williams-Steiger Occupational Safety and Health Act of 1970
Part 1990—Identification, Classification and Regulation of Potential Occupational Carcinogens
Part 2200—Review Commission Rules of Procedure
Part 2201—Regulations Implementing the Freedom of Information Act
Part 2202—Standards of Ethics and Conduct of Occupational Safety and Health Review Commission Employees
Part 29-12—Coverage of Persons Receiving Occupation or Job Training Under Department of Labor Who Are Not Employees of Contractors

Federal Mine Safety and Health Act of 1977 (P.L. 95-164)

*Mine Safety and Health Regulations and Standards*
29 CFR Part 2700—Federal Mine Safety and Health Review Commission, Rules of Procedure
30 CFR Part 11—Certification of Vinyl Chloride Respiratory Protective Devices
Part 40—Representatives of Miners at Mines
Part 41—Notification of Legal Identity of Mine Operators
Part 43—Procedures for Processing Hazardous Condition Complaints
Part 44—Procedures for Processing Petitions for Modification of Safety Standards
Part 45—Independent Contractors
Part 48—Training and Retraining of Miners
Part 49—Mine Rescue Teams
Part 50—Notification, Investigation, Reports and Records of Accidents, Injuries, Illnesses, Employment, and Coal Production in Mines
Part 55—Health and Safety Standards: Metal and Nonmetallic Open Pit Mines
Part 56—Health and Safety Standards: Sand, Gravel and Crushed Stone Operations
Part 57—Health and Safety Standards: Metal and Nonmetallic Underground Mines
Part 70—Mandatory Health Standards: Underground Coal Mines
Part 71—Mandatory Health Standards: Surface Work Areas of Underground Coal Mines and Surface Coal Mines
Part 74—Coal Mine Dust Personal Sampler Units
Part 75—Mandatory Safety Standards: Underground Coal Mines
Part 77—Mandatory Safety Standards: Surface Coal Mines and Surface Work Areas of Underground Coal Mines
Part 90—Procedure for Transfer of Miners with Evidence of Pneumoconiosis
Part 100—Civil Penalties for Violation of the Federal Mine Safety and Health Act of 1977
42 CFR Part 37—Specifications for Medical Examinations of Underground Coal Miners
Part 85—Requests for Health Hazard Evaluations
Part 85a—NIOSH Policy on Workplace Investigations

# Hazard Control Program Organization

# Chapter
# 3

# 3—Hazard Control Program Organization

To be effective, a hazard control program must be planned and be logical. Unlike Topsy, it can't "just grow." Program objectives and safety policies need to be established. Responsibility for the hazard control program needs to be determined. Specific processes to identify and control hazards need to be performed; these will be discussed later in this chapter. But first, those who are to design and participate in the hazard control program need to understand the nature of hazards, their effects on the work process, the basic causes of accidents, and ways that they can be controlled.

## Accidents and Hazard Control

### Definition of hazards

Hazards are a major cause of accidents. A workable definition of *hazard* is any existing or potential condition in the workplace which, by itself or by interacting with other variables, can result in the unwanted effects of deaths, injuries, property damage, and other losses (Firenze, 1978).

This definition carries with it two significant points.

• First, a condition does not have to exist at the moment to be classified as a hazard. When the total hazard situation is being evaluated, *potentially* hazardous conditions must be considered.

• Secondly, hazards may result not from independent failure of workplace components but from one workplace component acting upon or influencing another. For instance, if gasoline or another highly flammable substance comes in contact with sulfuric acid, the reaction created by the two substances produces both toxic vapors and sufficient heat for combustion.

Hazards are generally grouped in two broad categories: those dealing with safety (i.e., injuries) and those dealing with health (i.e., illnesses). Hazards that involve only property damage must also be considered.

### Effect of hazards on the work process

In a well-balanced operation, workers, equipment, and materials interact within the work environment to produce a product or perform a service. When operations go smoothly and time is used efficiently and effectively, production is at its highest.

What happens when an accident interrupts an operation? Does it carry a price tag? An accident increases the time needed to complete the job, reduces the efficiency and effectiveness of the operation, and raises production costs. If the accident results in injury, materials waste, equipment damage, or other property loss, there is a further increase in operational and hidden costs and a decrease in effectiveness.

### Controlling hazards: a team effort

Traditionally, management personnel have relied only on their safety and production people to locate, evaluate, and prescribe methods of controlling hazardous situations. However, the more that is learned about hazard and loss control, the more evident it becomes that the job is too large for any individual or small group to do by itself. Accident and hazard reduction requires a team effort by employees and management.

Here is how several departments can work together.

• The engineering departments can design facilities free of uncontrolled hazards and provide technical services to other departments to aid in hazard identification and analysis. They must be sure that designs comply with federal, state or provincial, and local laws and standards.

• Manufacturing can reduce hazards through such efforts as effective tool design, changes in processes, job hazard analysis and control, and coordinating and scheduling production.

• Quality control can test and inspect all materials and finished products and conduct studies to determine whether alternate design, material, and methods of manufacture could improve quality and safety of the product and the safety of the employees who make the product.

• Purchasing departments can make sure that materials and equipment which enter the workplace meet established safety and health standards, that adequate protective devices are an integral part of equipment, and that information about safety and health hazards associated with substances and materials used in the workplace is disseminated to line management and workers.

• Maintenance can perform construction and installation work in conformance with good engineering practices, comply with acceptable safety and health criteria, and provide planned preven-

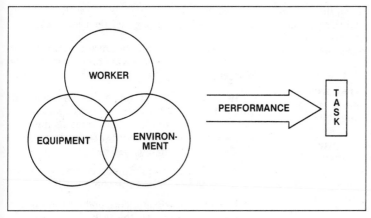

FIG. 3–1.—A system approach to hazard control recognizes the interaction between worker, equipment, and environment in the performance of the work task.

tive maintenance on electrical systems, machinery, and other equipment to prevent abnormal deterioration, loss of service, or safety and health hazards.

• Industrial relations often administer many programs directly related to health and safety.

Input can also come from the joint safety and health committee (discussed later in this chapter).

### Hazard control and management

In order to coordinate these departmental efforts, a program of hazard control is necessary as part of the management process (Windsor, 1979). Such a program provides hazard control with such management tools as programs, procedures, audits, and evaluations. Sometimes hazard control programs, in their rush to be competitive and innovative, to deal with increasingly complex employee relations issues and government involvement, and to address the *technical* aspects of the programs, neglect the *basics*. A program of hazard control assures that the old standbys will also be addressed. These basics include sound operating and design procedures, operator training, inspection and test programs, and communicating essential information about hazards and their control.

A hazard control program coordinates shared responsibility among departments. For example, if one department makes a product and another distributes it, they share responsibility for hazard control. The producer knows the nature of the process, its known and suspected hazards, and

FIG. 3–2.—An accident causes the work system to break down. It intervenes between the worker, equipment, and environment and the task to be performed.

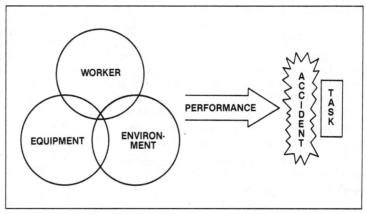

their control. The producer and the distributor are responsible for making sure that this information does not end with the production department but is available to the purchaser or the next unit in the manufacturing process.

Coordination is also important when manufacturing responsibility is transferred from one department to another (as when a pilot program becomes a full-blown manufacturing unit). When a process is phased out, coordination is also necessary to assure that experienced personnel with knowledge of the hazards involved are retained throughout the phase-out and that appropriate hazard control activities are carried out until the process is fully terminated.

## Worker/equipment/environment system

Those involved in establishing effective hazard control programs must understand the interrelationships between the worker/equipment/ environment system. Chapter 10, "Human Factors Engineering," will examine the system in greater detail. This chapter will touch on the elements of the system as depicted in Fig. 3–1. As Fig. 3–2 illustrates, an accident intervenes between the system and the task to be accomplished.

**Worker.** In any worker/equipment/environment system, the worker performs three basic functions:

Sensing

Information processing

Controlling.

• As a *sensor*, the worker serves to monitor or gather information.

• As an *information processor*, the worker uses the information collected to make a decision about the relevance or appropriateness of various courses of action.

• The third function, *control*, flows from the first two. Once information is collected and processed, the worker keeps the situation within acceptable limits or takes the necessary action to bring the system back into an acceptable (i.e., safe) range.

Evaluating an accident in the light of these three functions can pinpoint the cause(s).

Did the error occur while the worker was gathering information as a *sensor*? Was the worker able to gather information accurately (e.g., no glare, adequate illumination)?

Did the error occur as a result of faulty information *processing* and decision making?

Did the error occur because an appropriate *control* option was not available or because the worker took inappropriate action?

In order for the system to move toward its production objectives, the employee must carry out his role effectively and avoid taking unnecessary risks. To do this, he must be made aware of the following (Firenze, 1978):

1. The necessary requirements of the task and the steps he will take to accomplish it

2. His own knowledge, skill, and limitations and how they relate to the task

3. What will be gained if he attempts the task and succeeds

4. What will result if he attempts the task and fails, and

5. What will be lost if he does not attempt to accomplish the task at all.

**Equipment.** The second component in the system is equipment, which must be properly designed, maintained, and used. From a hazard control standpoint, questions should be raised about the shape of tools, their size and thickness, the weight of equipment, operator comfort, and the strength required to use or operate tools, equipment, and machinery. Such questions relate to the interaction between worker and equipment. Other equipment variables important in hazard recognition include speed of operation and mechanical hazards. (Olishifski, 1979.)

**Environment.** Special consideration must be given to those environmental factors that might detract from the comfort, health, and safety of the worker. Emphasis should be placed on such factors as:

1. Layout (whether the worker has sufficient room while performing his assigned task)

2. Maintenance and housekeeping

3. Adequate illumination (poorly lit areas increase not only eyestrain but also the chance of making mistakes and having accidents)

4. Temperature, humidity, noise, vibration, and ventilation of toxic materials.

Interpersonal relations are another factor within the system which play an important role in operational effectiveness. The task performed by one worker is related to tasks performed by others. Special consideration must be given to coordinating information, materials, and human effort. (Hannaford, 1976.)

## Accident Causes and Their Control

Accidents are caused. Close examination of each accident situation shows that it can be attributed, directly or indirectly, to one or more of the following (Firenze, 1978):

1. Oversight or omissions or malfunction of the management system (as related to the three following items). (Refer to discussion later in this chapter.)

2. Situational work factors (for example, facilities, tools, equipment, and materials)

3. Human factor (either the worker or another person)

4. Environmental factors (such as noise, vibration, temperature extremes, illumination)

If the management system is adequate and properly interfaces with the worker, the equipment, and the environment, then the likelihood of accidents occuring in the workplace is greatly reduced.

## Human factors

The human factor is the person who, by his commission (what he does) or by his omission (what he fails to do), causes an accident. Both workers and management may cause an accident by their commission, for example, when a worker sharpens a wood gouge on a grinder without resting the tool on the grinder's rest. He may contribute to the cause of an accident by an act of omission when he fails to wipe an oil spot from the floor. Each of these actions is generally described as an unsafe act—a human action that departs from hazard control or job procedures or practices to which the person has been trained or otherwise informed, or which causes unnecessary exposure of a person to a hazard or hazards.

Very often an unsafe act is a deviation from the standard job procedures, such as:

1. Using equipment without authority

2. Operating equipment at an unsafe speed or in any other improper way

3. Removing safety devices (such as guards) or rendering them inoperative, and

4. Using defective tools.

Unsafe acts can be a deviation from a standard or written job procedure, safety rules or regulations, instructions, or job safety analysis. The real question is, "Why the deviation?" The unsafe act could occur because, among other contributing factors, one or more of the following situations existed. Note the countermeasure(s), given in parentheses after the cause, that alter the safety or management system. This is where the emphasis should be placed in a hazard control program. (The following are examples of both management and employee unsafe acts or omissions.)

1. There was no standard or otherwise well-known job procedure. (Countermeasure: Perform a job safety analysis [JSA] and develop a good procedure through job instruction training [JIT].)

2. The employee did not know the standard job procedure. (Countermeasure: Train in the correct procedure and/or its applicability.)

3. Employee knew, but did not follow, the standard job procedure. (Countermeasure: Consider an employee performance evaluation. Test the validity of the procedure and/or motivation.)

4. Employee knew and followed the procedure. (Countermeasure: Change a wrong job procedure.)

5. Procedure encouraged risk-taking incentive, such as incentive piecework. (Countermeasure: Change incorrect job design or procedures.)

6. Employee changed job procedure or equipment. (Countermeasure: Change method so that it cannot be bypassed.)

7. Employee did not follow correct procedure because of pressure of work or supervisor's influence. (Countermeasure: Counsel employee and supervisor; consider change in work procedures or job requirements.)

8. The individual characteristics of the employee, which may involve a handicap,

made him unable or unwilling to follow the correct procedures. (Countermeasure: Counsel employee; consider change in work procedures or job requirements. Also consider training.)

Whenever a worker is directly involved in an accident, it often seems that his actions are automatically called "unsafe." A great many accidents are the result of someone deviating from the standard job procedures, doing something that he is *not* supposed to do, or failing to do something that he *is* supposed to do. In other situations, the worker becomes the target for criticism when, although he was directly involved in the accident, other factors forced him into this involvement. The following example will illustrate this point (Firenze, 1981).

Suppose a newly hired worker, after receiving what was thought to be sufficient instruction on the use of a table saw guard, is required to make a particular cut which cannot be made with the guard in proper position. In this case the required task causes the worker to remove the guard temporarily so that the cut can be made. While removing the guard, his hand slips off the wrench and is cut on the saw blade. Obviously the worker was instrumental in the accident situation, and consequently many people would view what he did as an unsafe act. A closer analysis of the situation reveals, however, that the primary cause factor cannot be placed solely on his shoulders.

In this instance, a failure in the management system contributed to the accident. First of all, those in charge of purchasing the particular guard should have done so with a better knowledge of its capabilities, limitations, and compatibility with process requirements. Second, the new worker should have been instructed in the use of the guard, as well as how to maintain and remove it when necessary. Most importantly, a contingency plan should have provided protection if and when the saw would have to be used without adequate safeguarding.

Differentiating between worker error and supervisory error is a very important first step in hazard control. Other ways to reduce human error are (a) for supervisors and workers to know the correct methods and procedures to accomplish given tasks; (b) for workers to demonstrate a skill proficiency before using a particular piece of equipment; (c) for higher management and supervisors to consider the relationship between worker performance and physical characteristics and fitness; (d) for the entire organization to give high and continuous regard to potentially dangerous situations and the corrective action necessary to avoid accidents; and (e) for supervisors to provide proper direction, training, and surveillance. The supervisor must be aware of the worker's level of skill with each piece of equipment and process and adjust the supervision of each worker accordingly. When the supervisor lets it be known that he will accept nothing less than safe work practices and as safe a workplace as possible, he shapes the workers' attitudes and actions.

## Situational factors

Situational factors are another major cause of accidents. These factors are those operations, tools, equipment, facilities and/or materials that contribute to accident situations. Examples are unguarded, poorly maintained, and defective equipment; ungrounded equipment which can cause shock; equipment without adequate warning signals; poorly arranged equipment, buildings, and layouts which create congestion hazards; and equipment located in positions which can expose more people to a potential hazard than is necessary.

Some causes of situational problems are:

1. Defects in design (for example, a container for use with flammable materials, constructed from lightweight metal and without adequate venting devices, or lack of a guard on a power press);

2. Poor, substandard construction (for example, a ladder built with defective lumber or with a variation in the space of its rungs);

3. Improper storage of hazardous materials (for example, oxygen and acetylene cylinders stored in an unstable manner and ready to topple over with the slightest impact); and

4. Inadequate planning, layout, and design (for example, a welding station located near combustible materials or placed where many workers without eye protection are exposed to the intense light of the welding arc).

An example of a situational problem occurred in a light industrial manufacturing plant where maintenance workers found themselves periodically replacing a bearing on an expensive machine. Something had to be done to save downtime, labor, and the cost of the bearing. The industrial engineering and maintenance departments jointly devised a solution. They placed on the machine a system which fed oil at set intervals to the bearing, keeping it lubricated. It was no longer necessary to replace the bearing frequently.

But new hazards had been created. When oil was fed onto the bearing, it ran onto the floor in an aisle adjacent to the machine. Workers could have slipped on the oil spot and sustained serious injuries. Fork lifts were driven over the oil. With oil on the rubber wheels, the fork lift driver might not have been able to stop the vehicle.

Had the maintenance and industrial engineering organizations been thinking of accident causes, they could have avoided situational hazards by correcting their design. As an interim action, they might have collected the oil by placing a pan under the motor where the bearing was housed. This would "buy time." A tube could be installed to return the oil to the system, thus saving the oil as well as eliminating the hazard.

## Environmental factors

The third factor in accident causation is the environmental one, the way in which the workplace directly or indirectly can cause or contribute to accident situations. Environmental factors fall into three broad categories: physical, chemical, and biological.

**Physical category.** Noise, vibration, radiation, illumination, and temperature extremes are examples of factors that have the capacity directly or indirectly to influence or cause accidents and/or illnesses. If operations on a machine lathe, for example, produce high noise levels that can damage the worker's hearing, his communications with others may be impaired. Thus, workers may be unable to warn one another of a hazard in time to avoid an accident.

**Chemical category.** Under this category are classified toxic fumes, vapors, mists, smokes, and dusts. In addition to causing illnesses, these elements often impair a worker's skill, reactions, judgment, or concentration. For example, a worker who has been exposed to the narcotic effect of some solvent vapors may experience an alteration of his judgment and move his hand too close to the cutting blade of a milling machine.

**Biological category.** Biological factors are those which are capable of making a person ill from contact with bacteria, viruses, and other micro-organisms or from contact with fungi or parasites (for example, boils and inflammations caused by staphylococci and streptococci; grain itch caused by parasites).

## Sources of situational and environmental hazards

Situational and environmental hazards enter the workplace from many sources: purchasing agents; those responsible for tool, equipment, and machinery placement and for providing adequate machine guards; and those responsible for maintaining shop equipment, machinery, and tools.

Employee contribution to situational and environmentally caused hazards could include disregarding safety rules and regulations by making safety devices inoperative, by using equipment and tools incorrectly, by using defective tools rather than taking the time to secure serviceable ones, by failing to use exhaust fans when required, and by using toxic substances in unventilated areas or without proper protection.

Purchasing agents can be instrumental in causing situational and environmental hazards if they give little consideration to hazards. Purchasing agents may acquire tools, equipment, and machinery without adequate guards and other safety devices, especially if such items can be obtained at a bargain. Sometimes toxic and hazardous materials are purchased when less toxic and hazardous materials could be substituted. Sometimes purchasing agents fail to acquire from the vendor and to disseminate to those in charge of the particular process the necessary warning and control information. However, in many companies, the purchasing agent is controlled as to what he buys by engineering, safety, and government standards and regulations.

Those involved in layout, design, and placement of equipment and machinery must also consider adequate safeguarding and safety devices or equipment; otherwise, they contribute to hazardous situations in the workplace. Examples are:

1. Placing equipment and machinery with reciprocating parts where workers can be crushed between the equipment and substantial objects

2. Installing electrical control switches on machinery in such a manner that the operator

must be exposed to the hazards of cutting tools, blades, etc., in order to start and stop the equipment

3. Installing on equipment and machinery guards that interfere with work operations

4. Locating work stations with high hazard potential where they expose workers unnecessarily (for example, placing a welding station in the middle of a floor area instead of locating it in a corner or along a wall where better control over the welding arc light is possible).

Those responsible for maintenance, both management and employees among others, sometimes cause hazards in the workplace. Examples are:

1. Improperly identifying high and low pressure steamlines, compressed air and sanitary lines;

2. Not detecting or replacing worn or damaged machine and equipment parts (e.g., abrasive wheels on power grinders);

3. Failing to adjust and lubricate equipment and machinery on a scheduled basis;

4. Failing to inspect and replace worn hoisting and lifting equipment;

5. Failing to replace worn and frayed belts on equipment;

6. Over-oiling motor bearings, resulting in oil being thrown onto the insulation of electrical wiring and onto the floor, perhaps damaging the bearings;

7. Failing to replace guards; and

8. Failing to tag and/or lock out unsafe equipment.

More details are included in this chapter under the sideheading, Responsibility for the hazard control program.

## Need for a balanced approach

Prior to the development of the concept of hazard control, accidents were viewed as chance occurrences or "acts of God," a view still held by some today. A variation of this point of view is that accidents are an inherent consequence of production. Such approaches accept accidents as inevitable and yield no information about causation. Control strategies are limited to mitigating

the consequences of the occurrence.

In the early days of hazard control, accident prevention activities focused on the human element. Findings indicated that a small proportion of workers accounted for a significant percentage of accidents. From these findings came the "accident proneness" theory of causation. Control strategies were devised to reduce human error through training, education, motivation, communication, and other forms of behavior modification. During World War II, industrial psychology aimed at matching employees to particular jobs, and personnel screening and selection were seen as ways to prevent accidents. The weakness of accident proneness and other behavioral models is that, while useful for understanding human behavior, they do not consider the interaction between the worker and the other parts of the system. (See the discussion in Chapters 9 and 11.)

The 1950's and 1960's saw the emphasis change to engineering and control programs aimed at the machine and/or equipment. With the implementation of the OSHAct in 1970, emphasis was placed on preventing accidents through control of the work environment and the elements of the workplace. Specification standards and compliance rules and regulations were spelled out.

## Management oversight and omission

The emphasis of many organizations over the last few decades have taken into account *system defects*, which result from management oversight or omission, or malfunction of the management system. A balanced approach to hazard control looks at each component of the system and includes such weaknesses as inadequate training and education, improper assignment of responsibility, unsuitable equipment, or badly budgeted funds. Because managers are the people responsible for the design of systems, system defects can occur because of management errors.

## Examining accident causation

There are two basic approaches to examining how accidents are caused, "after-the-fact" and "before-the-fact."

**"After-the-fact."** The "after-the-fact" approach relies on examining accidents that already have occurred in order to determine cause and develop corrective measures. Evaluation of past performance uses information derived from acci-

## TYPICAL LIST OF INCIDENTS

An "incident" is any observable human activity sufficiently complete in itself to permit references and predictions to be made about the person performing the act.

1. Adjusting and gauging (calipering) work while the machine is in operation.
2. Cleaning a machine or removing a part while the machine is in motion.
3. Using air hose to remove metal chips from table or work (a brush or other tool should be used for this purpose, except on recessed jigs).
4. Using compressed air to blow dust or dirt off of clothing or out of hair.
5. Using excessive pressure on air hose.
6. Operating machine tools (turning machines, knurling and grinding machines, drill presses, milling machines, boring machines, etc.) without proper eye protection (including side shields).
7. Not wearing safety glasses in a designated eye-hazard area.
8. Failing to use protective clothing or equipment (face shield, face mask, ear plugs, safety hat, cup goggles, etc.).
9. Failure to wear proper gloves or other hand protection when handling rough or sharp-edged material.
10. Wearing gloves, ties, rings, long sleeves, or loose clothing around machine tools.
11. Wearing gloves while grinding, polishing, or buffing.
12. Handling hot objects with unprotected hands.
13. No work rest or poorly adjusted work rest on grinder (1/8 in. maximum clearance).
14. Grinding without the glass eye-shield in place.
15. Making safety devices inoperative (removing guards, tampering with adjustment of guard, "beating" or "cheating" the guard, failing to report defects).
16. Using an ungrounded (or uninsulated) portable electric hand tool.
17. Improperly designed safety guard (for example, a wide opening on a barrier guard which will allow the fingers to reach the cutting edge).

FIG. 3–3.

dent and inspection reports and insurance audits. This approach too often is used only after there has been an accident that results in injury or damage, or system ineffectiveness. Furthermore, accident frequency and severity rates do not answer the crucial questions *what, why,* and *when.*

**"Before-the-fact."** "Before-the-fact" methods rely on inspecting and systematically identifying and evaluating the nature of undesired events in a system. One such method is known as the "critical incident technique."

• *Critical incident technique.* The critical incident technique can assist in the identification of causes of potential accidents before a loss occurs. In order to obtain a representative sample of workers exposed to various hazards, persons are selected from various departments of the plant. An interviewer questions a number of persons who have performed particular jobs within certain environments. He asks them to describe existing hazards and unsafe conditions that have come to their attention. Fig. 3–3 lists typical incidents described. Incidents are then classified into hazard categories, and problem areas are identified.

The technique measures safety performance and identifies practices or conditions that need to be corrected. Inquiry can be made into the management systems that should have prevented the occurrence of unsafe acts or the existence of unsafe conditions. The technique can lead to improvements in hazard control program management.

The procedure needs to be repeated because the worker/equipment/environment system is not static. Repeating the technique with a new sample of workers can reveal new problem areas and measure the effectiveness of the accident prevention program.

• *Safety sampling*, also called behavior or activity sampling, is another technique that uses the expertise of those within the organization to inspect, identify, and evaluate hazards (Pollina, 1962). This method relies on personnel—usually management or safety staff members—who are familiar with operations and well trained in recognizing unsafe practices. While making rounds of the plant or establishment, they record on a safety sampling sheet both the number and type of safety defects they observe. A code number can be used to designate specific unsafe conditions (for example, hands in dies, failure to wear eye protection and protective clothing, failure to lock out source of power while working on machinery, crossing over belt conveyors, working under suspended loads, improper use of tools, transporting unbanded steel).

Observations must be made at different times of the day, on a planned or random basis in the actual work setting, and throughout the various parts of the plant. In a short time the observations can be easily converted to a simple report which shows in sharp relief what specific unsafe conditions exist in what areas and what supervisors and foremen need help in enforcing good work practices. The information is unbiased and therefore irrefutable. What has been recorded is what has been observed. Like the umpire in a baseball game, the observer "calls 'em as he sees 'em."

## Principles of Hazard Control

*Hazard control* can be defined as the function which is directed toward recognizing, evaluating, and eliminating (or at least reducing) the destructive effects of hazards emanating from human errors and from the situational and environmental aspects of the workplace (Firenze, 1978). Its primary function is to locate, assess, and set effective preventive and corrective measures for those elements detrimental to operational efficiency and effectiveness.

The process exists on three levels:

1. National (laws, regulations, exposure limits, codes, standards of governmental, industrial, and trade bodies);

2. Organizational (management of hazard control program; safety committees); and

3. Component (worker/equipment/environment).

Hazard control can be thought of as a *failure-oriented* method. In the first place, there are fewer failures than successes. Second, it is easier to agree on what constitutes failure than on what is success. Failure is the inability of a system (or a part of a system) to perform as required under specified conditions for a specific length of time. The causes of failures often can be determined by answering a series of questions. What can fail? How can it fail? How frequently can it fail? What are the effects of failure? What is the importance of the effects? The manner in which a system (or portion of a system) can exhibit failure is commonly known as the *mode of failure*.

The opposite of failure is not necessarily total success—that error-free performance which is an ideal state, not a reality—but the *minimum acceptable* success. That is the point where processes are accomplished with a tolerable number of losses and interruptions, keeping efficiency and effectiveness of the operation within acceptable limits of control.

Management builds into each of its production systems lower and upper limits of control. Each of these interfacing subsystems—maintenance, quality control, production control, personnel, purchasing, to name a few—is designed to move the system within acceptable limits toward its objective. This concept of keeping operations within acceptable limits gives substance and credibility to the process of hazard control. In addition to familiarizing management with the full consequences of system failures, hazard control can pinpoint hazards *before* failures occur. The anticipatory character of hazard control increases productivity.

## Processes of Hazard Control

An effective hazard control program has six essential processes (Firenze, 1978):

1. Hazard identification and evaluation

2. Ranking hazards by risk

3. Management decision making

4. Establishing preventive and corrective measures

5. Monitoring, and

6. Evaluating program effectiveness.

Let's discuss each in turn.

### Hazard identification and evaluation

The first process in a comprehensive hazard control program is to identify and evaluate hazards located in the workplace. These hazards are associated with machinery, equipment, tools, operations, and the physical plant.

There are many ways to acquire information about hazards associated with the workplace. A good place to begin is with those who are familiar with plant operations and the hazards associated with them. See Chapter 24, "Sources of Help," for a description of many organizations that can be of help. The critical incident technique (described on the previous two pages) is useful for obtaining information from workers and supervisors. Insurance company loss control representatives know those hazards that have caused damage, injuries, and fatalities. In addition to the National Safety Council, such associations as the American Society of Safety Engineers (ASSE), American Industrial Hygiene Association (AIHA), and the American Conference of Governmental Industrial Hygienists (ACGIH) have information about safety and health experience. Manufacturers of equipment, tools, and machinery used in the plant offer information about the hazards associated with their products, as can suppliers of materials and substances. Labor representatives and business agents may offer a perspective on hazards

overlooked by others. Safety and health personnel in organizations doing similar work can be of inestimable value.

A second place to look would be old inspection reports, either internal (by a safety and health committee or company management and specialists) or external (by local, state or provincial, or federal enforcement agencies). OSHA can supply information that may be helpful in describing violations uncovered in similar operations and in outlining compliance regulations. See Chapter 2, "Federal Legislation," for descriptions of state agencies and private concerns that give on-site inspection and consultation services under OSHA and NIOSH.

Hazard information also can be obtained from accident reports. Information concerning how a particular injury, illness, or fatality occurred often will reveal hazards which require control. Close review of accident reports filed in the past three to five years also will identify the individuals and specific operations involved, the department or section of a plant where the accident occurred, the extent of supervision, and possibly deficiencies in knowledge and skill on the part of the injured. OSHA incident rates also are useful. Although they are historical and reflect what has happened, not the current status of safety performance, they provide, from a large sample, data that reflects what actually has occurred in the workplace.

Other sources which can be valuable are described in other chapters, in the data sheets of the National Safety Council, in the specifications for particular equipment and machines which are published by the American National Standards Institute (ANSI), UL, ASTM, and NFPA, and in the information about work activities, facilities, and equipment which is distributed by the National Institute for Occupational Safety and Health (NIOSH).

Hazard analysis is another avenue available for acquiring meaningful hazard information and a thorough knowledge of the demands of a particular task. Analysis probes operational and management systems to uncover hazards that (*a*) may have been overlooked in the layout of the plant or the building and in the design of machinery, equipment, and processes; (*b*) may have developed after production started; or (*c*) may exist because original procedures and tasks were modified.

The greatest benefit of hazard analysis is that it

| HAZARD CONSEQUENCE CATEGORY | EXPLANATION |
|---|---|
| I. Catastrophic Hazard | Imminent danger exists. The hazard is capable of causing death, possible multiple deaths, widespread occupational illnesses, and loss of facilities. |
| II. Critical Hazard | The hazard can result in severe injury, serious illness, and property and equipment damage. |
| III. Marginal Hazard | The hazard can cause injury, illness, and equipment damage, but the injury, illness, and equipment damage would not be serious. |
| IV. Negligible Hazard | The hazard will not result in a serious injury or illness. Damage beyond a minor first aid case is extremely remote. |

FIG. 3-4.—Relative consequences of various hazard categories.

### HAZARD PROBABILITY CATEGORY
### (Qualitative Estimate)

A. Probable. Likely to occur immediately or within a short period of time.

B. Reasonably Probable. Probably will occur in time.

C. Remote. May occur in time.

D. Extremely Remote. Unlikely to occur.

FIG. 3-5.—Qualitative probability estimate for use in decision making.

forces those conducting the analysis to view each operation as part of a system. In so doing, each step in the operation is assessed while consideration is paid to the relationship between steps and the interaction between workers and equipment, materials, the environment, and other workers. Other benefits of hazard analysis include (a) identifying hazardous conditions and potential accidents; (b) providing information with which effective control measures can be established; (c) determining the level of knowledge and skill as well as the physical requirements that workers need to execute specific shop tasks; and (d) discovering and eliminating unsafe procedures, techniques, motions, positions, and actions.

The topic of hazard analysis—its underlying philosophy, the basic steps to be taken, and its ultimate use as a safety, health, and decision-making tool—will be treated in Chapters 4 and 5.

### Ranking hazards by risk (consequence and probability)

The second process in hazard control is to rank hazards by risk. Such ranking takes into account both the consequence (the severity) and the probability (the frequency). This second process is necessary so that hazards can be addressed according to the principle of "worst first." Ranking provides a consistent guide for corrective action, specifying which hazardous conditions warrant immediate action, which have secondary priority, and which can be addressed in the future.

The classification scheme outlined in Fig. 3-4 is suggested for rating hazards by consequence.

Once hazards have been ranked according to their potential destructive consequences, the next step is to estimate the probability of the hazard resulting in an accident situation. Quantitative data for ranking hazard probability are desirable, but almost certainly they will not be available for each potential hazard being assessed. Whatever quantitative data exist should be part of the risk-rating formula used to estimate probability. Qualitative data—estimates based on experience—are a necessary supplement to quantitative data. Fig. 3–5 shows how probability estimates should be made.

When the hazards have been ranked according to both criteria, it is easy to determine where action is mandated. A hazard rated "I-A", for example, demands corrective action before a hazard with a rating of "I-D".

## Management decision making

The third process involves providing management with full and accurate information, including all alternatives at its disposal, so that it can make intelligent, informed decisions concerning hazard control. Such alternatives will include recommendations for training and education, the need for better methods and procedures, equipment repair or replacement, environmental controls, and—in rare cases where modification cannot suffice—recommendations for redesign. Information must be presented to management in a form that makes clear what actions are required to improve conditions. The person who reports hazard information must do so in a way that promotes, rather than hinders, action.

Once those in the position to make decisions receive hazard reports, they normally have three alternatives:

1. They can choose to take no action.

2. They can modify the workplace and/or its components.

3. They can redesign the workplace or its components.

• When management chooses to take no positive steps to correct hazards uncovered in the workplace, it usually is for one of three reasons:

a. It feels that it cannot take the required action. Immediate constraints—be they financial, crucial production schedules, or limitations of personnel—loom larger than the risks involved in taking no action.

b. It is presented with limited alternatives. For example, it may receive only the best and most costly solutions with no less-than-totally-suc-cessful alternatives to choose from.

c. It does not agree that a hazard exists. However, the situation may require additional consultation and study to resolve any problem.

• When management chooses to modify the system, it does so with the idea that its operation is generally acceptable but that, with the reported deficiencies corrected, performance will be improved. Examples of modification alternatives are the acquisition of machine guards, personal protective equipment, or ground-fault circuit interrupters to prevent electrical shock; a change in training or education; a change in preventive maintenance; isolating hazardous materials and processes; replacing hazardous materials and processes with non- or at least less-hazardous ones; and purchasing new tools.

• Although redesign is not a popular alternative, it is sometimes necessary. When redesign is selected, management must be aware of certain problems. Redesign usually involves substantial cash outlay and inconvenience. For example, assume that the air quality in a plant is found to be below acceptable standards. The only way to correct this situation is to completely redesign and install the plant's general ventilation system. The cost and inconvenience are obvious.

Another problem is the distinct possibility that the new design may contain hazards of its own. For this reason, whenever redesign is offered as an alternative, those making such a recommendation must establish and execute a plan to detect problems in both their design and early stages so that they can be eliminated or reduced.

One way to expedite decision making regarding actions for hazard control is to present findings in such a manner that management can clearly understand the nature of the hazards, their location, their importance, the necessary corrective action, and the estimated cost.

Fig. 3–6 shows a record of occupational and safety health deficiencies. It illustrates one approach for recording and displaying hazard information for decision making. It indicates the hazard ranking, the specific location and nature of the hazard, and what costs are likely to be incurred. Furthermore, it tells what specific corrective action is recommended. At a glance, it makes clear if the corrective action has been taken and what was the actual cost.

## RECORD OF OCCUPATIONAL SAFETY AND HEALTH DEFICIENCIES

Location _____ Shipping

Inspector _____ Pete Varga

| Deficiency No. | Date Recorded | Description of Hazardous Condition | Specific Location | Identification of Acceptable Standard | Hazard Rating | | Corrective Action | Estimated Cost of Correction | Date Deficiency Corrected | Resources Used for Correction |
|---|---|---|---|---|---|---|---|---|---|---|
| | | | | | Conse-quence | Proba-bility | | | | |
| S – 1 | 12/11/80 | Ungrounded Tools and Equipment | Throughout Shop | OSHA; Subpart S National Electrical Code, Article 250; 4S | I | A | Provide receptacles with the 3-prong outlet.<br><br>Test each to make certain it is grounded.<br><br>Make sure that all tools (other than double-insulated) have a grounding plug. | $5,000 | 1/9/80 | $4,900 |

FIG. 3-6.—One approach to recording and displaying hazard information for decision making.

*Developed by RJF Associates, Inc.*

## Establishing preventive and corrective measures

After hazards have been identified and evaluated and information for informed decisions has been provided, the next process involves the actual installation of control measures.

Controls are of two kinds: administrative (i.e., through personnel, management, monitoring, limiting worker exposure, measuring performance, training and education, housekeeping and maintenance, purchasing) and engineering (i.e., isolation of source, lockout procedures, design, process or procedural changes, monitoring and warning equipment, chemical or material substitution).

Before installation of controls takes place, it is essential that those involved in safety and health activities understand how hazards are controlled. Fig. 3–7 illustrates the three major areas where

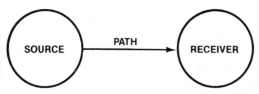

FIG. 3–7.—Three major areas where hazards can be controlled—the contaminant source, the path it travels, and the employee's work pattern and use of personal protective equipment.

hazardous conditions can be either eliminated or controlled.

• The first and perhaps best control alternative is to attack a hazard at its source. One method is to substitute a less harmful agent for the one causing the problem. For example, if a certain solvent is highly toxic and flammable, the first step is to determine whether the hazardous substance can be exchanged for one that is nontoxic, nonflammable, and still capable of doing the job. If a nonhazardous substance that meets these criteria is not available, then a less toxic, less flammable substance can be used and additional safeguards employed.

• The second alternative is to control the hazard along its path. This can be done by erecting a barricade between the hazard and the worker. Examples of such engineering controls are (a) machine guards, which prevent a worker's hands

from making contact with the table saw blade; (b) protective curtains, which prevent eye contact with welding arc flashes; and (c) a local exhaust system, which removes toxic vapors from the breathing zone of the workers.

• The third alternative is to direct control efforts at the receiver, the worker. Removing the worker from exposure to the hazard can be accomplished by (a) employing automated or remote control options (for example, automatic feeding devices on planers, shapers); (b) providing a system of worker rotation or rescheduling some operations to times when there are few workers in the plant; or (c) providing personal protective equipment when all options have been exhausted and it is determined that the hazard does not lend itself to correction through substitution or engineering redesign.

Protective equipment may be selected for use in two instances: when there is no immediately feasible way to control the hazard by more effective means, and when it is employed as a temporary measure, while more effective solutions are being installed. There are, however, major shortcomings associated with the use of personal protective equipment:

1. Nothing has been done to eliminate or reduce the hazard.

2. If the protective equipment (such as gloves or an eye shield) fails for any reason, the worker is exposed to the full destructive effects of the hazard.

3. The protective equipment may be cumbersome and interfere with the worker's ability to perform a task, thus compounding the problem.

Chapters 5 and 17, "Removing the Hazard from the Job" and "Personal Protective Equipment," will treat these subjects more fully.

## Monitoring

The fifth process in the hazard control program deals with the monitoring of activities in order to locate new hazards and assess the effectiveness of existing controls. Monitoring includes inspection, industrial hygiene testing, and medical surveillance. These subjects will be dealt with in Chapter 4, "Acquiring Hazard Information."

Monitoring is necessary (a) to provide assurance that hazard controls are working properly;

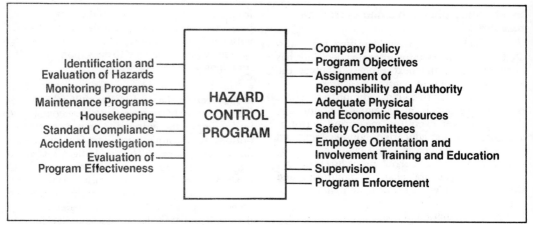

Fig. 3–8.—Major components of a hazard control program.

*Developed by RJF Associates, Inc.*

(*b*) to make sure that modifications have not so altered the workplace that hazard controls can no longer function adequately; and (*c*) to discover hazards that are new or previously undetected.

### Evaluating program effectiveness

The final process in hazard control is to evaluate the effectiveness of the safety and health program. Evaluation involves answering the following questions. How much is being spent to locate and control hazards in the plant? What benefits are being received, for example, reduction of injuries, workers' compensation cases, and damage losses? What impact are the benefits having on improving operational efficiency and effectiveness?

Evaluation examines the program to see whether it has accomplished its objectives (effectiveness evaluation) and whether they have been achieved in accordance with the program plan (administrative evaluation, including such factors as schedule and budget).

Evaluation must be adapted to (*a*) the time, money, and kinds of equipment and personnel available for the evaluation; (*b*) the number and quality of data sources; (*c*) the particular operation; and (*d*) the needs of the evaluators.

Among the criteria which may assist management in determining the effectiveness of its safety and health program effort are the number and severity of injuries to workers compared with work hours; the cost of medical care; material

damage costs; facility damage costs; equipment and tool damage or replacement costs; and the number of days lost from accidents.

One of the indicators of the effectiveness of a hazard control program is the experience rating given a company by the insurance carrier responsible for paying workers' compensation. Experience rating is a comparison of the actual losses of an individual (company) risk with the losses that would be expected from a risk of such size and classification. Experience rating determines whether the individual risk is better or worse than the average and to what extent the premium should be modified to reflect this variation. Experience modification is determined in accordance with the Experience Rating Plan (ERP) formula, which has been approved by the insurance commissioner and is used in all states except California, Delaware, New Jersey, and Pennsylvania. Loss frequency is penalized more heavily than loss severity because it is assumed that the insured can control the small loss more easily than the less frequent, severe loss.

### Organizing an Occupational Safety and Health Program

The purposes of a hazard control program organization are to assist management in developing and operating a program designed to protect workers, prevent and control accidents, and increase effectiveness of operations. Fig. 3–8 illustrates the major organizational components of a hazard and loss control program.

## Establishing program objectives

Critical to the design and organization of a safety and health program is the establishment of objectives and policy to guide the program's development. If the organization has a joint safety and health committee, it could be the logical body to set objectives. It is assumed that those recommending objectives for adoption by management would involve employee representatives, supervisors, upper management, and safety professionals (safety directors, managers, supervisors, and administrators; industrial hygiene technicians and professionals; and fire protection engineers).

Among the program objectives should be:

1. Gaining and maintaining support for the program at all levels of the organization

2. Motivating, educating, and training those involved in the program to recognize and correct or report hazards located in the workplace

3. Engineering hazard control into the design of machines, tools, and facilities

4. Providing a program of inspection and maintenance for machinery, equipment, tools, and facilities

5. Incorporating hazard control into training and educational techniques and methods, and

6. Complying with established safety and health standards.

## Establishing organizational policy

Once the objectives have been formulated, the second step is for management to adopt a formal policy. A written policy statement, over the signature of the chief administrator of the organization, should be made available to all personnel. It should state the purpose behind the hazard control program and require the active participation of all those involved in the program's operation. The policy statement also should reflect:

1. The importance that management places on the health and well-being of employees

2. Management's commitment to occupational safety and health

3. The emphasis the company places on efficient

operations, with a minimum of accidents and losses

4. The intention of integrating hazard control into all operations, including compliance with applicable standards

5. The necessity for active leadership, direct participation, and enthusiastic support of the entire organization.

The policy of the Bell System is probably the shortest statement, but it drives home the point that:

NO JOB IS SO IMPORTANT AND NO SERVICE IS SO URGENT—THAT WE CANNOT TAKE TIME TO PERFORM OUR WORK SAFELY.

The National Safety Council publishes a 12-page Industrial Data Sheet, "Management Safety Policies," No. 585, that covers this subject more fully.

After a safety policy has been established, it should be publicized so that each employee becomes familiar with it, particularly how it applies directly to him. Meetings, letters, pamphlets, bulletin boards: these are ways to publicize the statement. It should also be posted in management offices to serve as a constant reminder of management's commitment and responsibility.

## Responsibility for the hazard control program

Responsibility for the hazard control program can be established at the following levels: board of directors, chief executive officers, managers and administrators; department heads, supervisors, foremen, and employee representatives; purchasing agents; housekeeping and maintenance personnel; employees; safety personnel; (staff) medical personnel; and safety and health committees.

**Management and administration.** Before any hazard control program gets underway, it must receive full support and commitment from top management and administration. The president, board members, directors, and other management personnel have the responsibility for the hazard control program by furnishing the motivation to get the program started and to oversee its operations. Responsibility involves the continuing obligation to ascertain that an effective safety and health program is in operation. Top management must initiate discussions with personnel during preplanning meetings and periodically review the performance of its hazard control program. Such discussions will deal with program progress, specific needs, and a review of company procedures and alternatives for handling emergencies in the event an accident occurs.

Specifically, responsibility at this level appears in the form of setting objectives and policy and supporting safety personnel in their requests for necessary information, facilities, tools, and equipment to conduct an effective hazard control program and establish a safe and healthy work environment. Management must realize that it is not fulfilling its organization's potential efficiency and effectiveness until it brings its operations at least into compliance with federal and state or provincial safety and health standards, whether or not these standards are mandatory.

In order for any hazard control program to succeed, it is necessary for management and administration to delegate the necessary prerogatives to those at various levels in the organization. Although management cannot delegate to others its responsibility for employee safety and health, it can assign to others responsibility for certain parts of the hazard control program. But when responsibilities are delegated, so too must be the authority to carry them out. While authority always must start with those in the highest administrative levels, it eventually must be delegated to other responsible people at lower levels in order to achieve desired results. If safety professionals, safety committees, department heads, supervisors, foremen, and employee representatives are to conduct a vigorous and thorough hazard control program, if they are to accept and assert the authority delegated to them when circumstances warrant it, they must be fully confident that they have administrative support.

Management must understand that, although it can assert authority, it may find resistance to this authority unless it has enlisted support from the earliest stages of the program. If supervisors, employees, and their representatives are not aware of the reasons for and the benefits of a thoroughgoing hazard control program, they may resist any changes in their methods of operation and instruction and may do as little as possible to assist the overall program effort.

Management must insist that safety and health information is an integral part of training, methods, materials, and operations. It must guarantee a system where hazard control is considered an important part of equipment purchase and process design, operation, preventive maintenance, and layout and design. It must make sure that effective fire prevention and protection controls exist. Management also has the responsibility to be certain that subcontractors, at the time of negotiating the contract, are fully informed of applicable standards. Management must see that subcontractors comply fully with company and other applicable safety regulations.

Administrators are required to safeguard employees' health by seeing to it that the work environment is adequately controlled. They must be aware of those operations that produce airborne fumes, mists, smokes, vapors, dusts, noise, and vibration that have the capacity to cause impaired health or discomfort among their workers. Administrators must be aware that occupational illnesses that begin in the workplace environment may eventually take their toll during the years to come, even after a worker retires. To protect the future of its employees, management must maintain a constant industrial hygiene monitoring system.

Management must provide meaningful criteria to measure the success of the hazard control program and to provide information upon which to base future decisions. It must decide what the hazard control program should give in terms of reduced accidents, injuries, illnesses, and their associated losses.

There are many concrete ways that management can show evidence of its commitment to safety: attending safety meetings, reviewing and acting upon accident reports, reviewing safety records through conferences with department heads and joint employee/management committees, and by setting a good example.

**Department heads, supervisors, foremen, and employee representatives.** Department heads, supervisors, foremen, and stewards and other employee representatives are in strategic positions within the organization. Their leadership and influence should assure that safety and health standards are enforced and upheld in each individual area and that standards and enforcement are uniform throughout the workplace.

What are some responsibilities of department heads? They make certain that materials, equipment, and machines slated for distribution to the areas under their jurisdiction are hazard-free or that adequate control measures have been provided. They make certain that equipment, tools, and machinery are being used as designed and are properly maintained. They keep abreast of accident and injury trends occurring in their areas and take proper corrective action to reverse these trends. They investigate all accidents occurring within their jurisdiction. They should see to it that all hazard control rules, regulations, and procedures are enforced in their departments. They require that a hazard analysis be conducted for certain operations, particularly those that they regard as dangerous, either from past accident history or from their perception of accident potential. They require that hazard recognition and control information be included in instruction, training, and demonstration sessions for both supervisors and employees. They actively participate in and support the safety and health committee and follow up on its recommendations.

Supervisors, foremen, and employee representatives carry great influence. With their support, top management can be assured of an effective safety and health program. Supervisors have a moral and professional responsibility to safeguard, educate, and train those who have been placed under their direction. Thus, they are generally responsible for creating a safe and healthy work setting and for integrating hazard recognition and control into all aspects of work activities. By their careful monitoring, they can prevent accidents.

For all practical purposes supervisors, foremen, and employee representatives are the eyes and ears of the workplace control system. On a day-to-day basis, they must be aware of what is happening in their respective areas, who is doing it, how various tasks are being performed, and under what conditions. As they monitor their areas, they must prevent accidents from occurring. If, despite their vigilance, they see that a danger is imminent, they must be prepared to intervene in the operation and take immediate corrective action.

What are chief among the safety and health responsibilities of supervisors? They train and educate workers in methods and techniques which are free from hazards. They should be certain that employees understand the properties and hazards of the material stored, handled, or used by them. They make sure that employees observe necessary precautions, including proper

guards and safe work practices. They furnish employees with the proper personal protective equipment, instruct them in its proper use, and make certain that it is worn.

Supervisors demonstrate an active interest in and comply with hazard control policy and safety and health regulations. They actively participate in and support the safety and health committees. They supervise and evaluate worker performance, with consideration given to safe behavior and work methods. They should first try to convince employees of the need for safe performance, and then, unpleasant though it may be, they should administer appropriate corrective action when health and safety rules are violated. Corrections for the violation of rules demand tact and good judgment. Enforcement should be viewed as education rather than discipline. However, if a supervisor feels that a worker is deliberately disobeying rules and/or through unsafe acts endangering his life and the lives of others, then prompt and firm action is called for. Laxity in the enforcement of safety rules undercuts the entire safety and health program and allows accidents to happen.

Supervisors monitor their area on a daily basis for human, situational, and environmental factors capable of causing accidents. They should make sure that meticulous housekeeping practices are developed and used at all times. They should correct hazards detected in their monitoring or report such hazards to the persons who can take corrective action. They should investigate all accidents occurring within their areas to determine causes.

Foremen and employee representatives share much of the responsibility for safety and health with upper management. Their job is to inspect, detect, and correct. What are specific responsibilities of foremen and representatives? They should encourage fellow workers to comply with the organization's safety and health regulations. They detect safety violations and hazardous machinery, tools, equipment, and other implements. They take corrective action when possible and report to the supervisor the hazard and the corrective action taken or still required. They participate in accident investigations. They represent the interest of the workers on the safety and health committee.

Practical training aids for employee representatives, foremen, and supervisors do exist. The Council's *Supervisors Safety Manual* and accompanying "Home Study Course," also available through the National Safety Council, have been widely accepted by industry.

**Purchasing agents.** Those responsible for purchasing items for the organizations are in a key position to help reduce hazards associated with operations. The purchasing department has much latitude in selecting machinery, tools, equipment, and materials used in the organization. In maintaining standards of quality, efficiency, and price, the purchasing department must make certain that safety has received adequate attention in designing, manufacturing, and shipping items.

Depending upon the company organization, other departments—such as safety, engineering, quality control, maintenance, industrial hygiene, and medical—should indicate to the purchasing department what equipment and materials meet with their approval. The purchasing department is responsible for soliciting such guidance and direction.

Chapter 5, "Removing the Hazard from the Job," will outline specific guidelines for cooperation between purchasing and safety departments. Three points, however, need to be emphasized here.

• First, the purchasing agent must make certain that all items comply with federal and state or provincial regulations and with local ordinances. A statement to this effect must be part of the purchase order. Purchasing agents also will be guided by (a) codes and standards of the American National Safety Institute (ANSI), Canadian Standards Association (CSA), and other standards and specifications groups; (b) products approved or listed by such agencies as Underwriters Laboratories Inc. and the National Fire Protection Association; and (c) recommendations by such agencies as the National Safety Council, insurance carriers or associations, the Factory Mutual System in its *Factory Mutual Handbook of Industrial Loss Prevention* and *Loss Prevention Data*, and trade or industrial organizations. (See Chapter 24, "Sources of Help".)

• Second, the purchasing agent must make certain that tools, equipment, materials, and machinery are purchased and shipped with adequate regard for safety. This requirement applies even to such ordinary items as boxes, cleaning rags, paint, and common hand tools. It is essential when purchasing personal protective equipment and

larger items, especially machines. Sometimes the cost of an adequately guarded machine seems out of proportion to that of an unguarded machine to which makeshift guards can be added after installation. But experience has proven repeatedly that the best time to eliminate or minimize a hazard is in the design stage. Safeguards that are integral parts of a machine are the most efficient and durable.

• Third, the purchasing agent must be cost-conscious, realizing that every accident has both direct and indirect costs. He will understand that the organization cannot afford "bargains" which later result in accident losses and occupational disease.

**Housekeeping and preventive maintenance.** Housekeeping and preventive maintenance can be regarded as two sides of the same coin. No hazard control program can succeed if housekeeping and maintenance are not seen as integral parts.

• *Good housekeeping* reduces accidents, improves morale, and increases efficiency and effectiveness. Most people appreciate a clean and orderly workplace, and can accomplish their tasks without interference and interruption.

An industrial organization, by its very nature, contains tools that must be kept clean. In its operation, it uses flammable substances and materials that require special storage and removal. It generates dust, scrap metal filings and chips, waste liquids, and scrap lumber which must be disposed of.

Housekeeping is a continuous process involving both workers and custodial personnel. A good housekeeping program incorporates the housekeeping function into all processes, operations, and tasks performed in the workplace. The ultimate goal is for each worker to see housekeeping as an integral part of performance, not as a supplement to the job to be done.

When the workplace is clean and orderly and housekeeping becomes a standard part of operations, less time and effort will be spent keeping it clean, making needless repairs, and replacing equipment, fixtures, and the like. When the worker can concentrate on his required tasks without excess scrap material, tools, and equipment interfering with his work, he can operate more efficiently and create a product of higher quality. Time will be used for work, not searching for tools, materials, or parts. When a plant is clean and orderly as well as safe, employee morale is heightened.

When everything has an assigned place, there is less chance that materials and tools will be taken from the plant or misplaced. In a few moments, the foreman or supervisor can determine what is missing before quitting time. Different colors of paint can be applied to tools to identify the department to which they belong. Tool racks or holders should be painted a contrasting color as a reminder to workers to return the tools to their proper places. The space directly behind each tool stored on a rack should be painted or outlined in color to call attention to a missing tool.

Money is saved and efficiency is increased when workers treat materials with the care they deserve by minimizing spillage and scrap, by saving pieces of material for use in future projects, and by returning even small quantities of parts to their storage area. When aisle and floor space is uncluttered, movement within the plant is easier and safer, and machinery and equipment can be cleaned and maintained. When the plant has adequate work space and when oil, grease, water, and dust are removed from floors and machinery, workers are less likely to slip, trip, fall, or inadvertently come into contact with dangerous parts of machinery.

When a workplace is kept free from accumulations of combustible materials which may burn upon ignition or, in the case of certain material relationships, spontaneously ignite without the aid of an external source of ignition, the chances of fires are minimized. Furthermore, an orderly plant permits easy exit by keeping exits and aisles leading to exits free from obstructions. A neat and orderly workplace also makes it easier to locate and obtain fire emergency and extinguishment equipment.

• *Preventive maintenance* may be defined as orderly, uniform, continuous and scheduled action to prevent breakdown and prolong the useful life of equipment and buildings. Preventive maintenance must be understood as a shared responsibility. Workers caring for tools and equipment accomplish specific maintenance tasks. Other maintenance duties (such as oiling, tightening guards, adjusting tool rests, and replacing wheels) are routinely performed by workers.

Some advantages to be gained from preventive maintenance include safer working conditions, decreased "down time" of equipment because of breakdown, and increased life of the equipment.

Satisfactory production depends on having buildings, equipment, machinery, portable tools, safety devices, and the like in operating condition and maintained in such a manner that production activities will not be interrupted while repairs are being made or equipment replaced.

Preventive maintenance prolongs the life of the equipment by ensuring its proper use. When tools are kept dressed or sharpened and in satisfactory condition, the right tool will be used for the job. When safe and properly maintained tools are issued, workers have an added incentive to give the tools better care. When repairs are made so that equipment is not inoperative for long periods of time, workers do not need to improvise by using a piece of equipment for a purpose for which it was not intended. Sound and efficient maintenance management anticipates machine and equipment deterioration and sets up overhaul procedures designed to correct defects as soon as they develop. Such a repair and overhaul system obviously requires close integration of maintenance with inspection.

Preventive maintenance has four main components:

1. Scheduling and performing periodic maintenance functions

2. Keeping records of service and repairs

3. Repairing and replacing equipment and equipment parts, and

4. Providing spare parts control.

Maintenance schedules can be set up on either a time or use basis, whichever comes first. Factors to be considered include:

The age of the machine

The number of hours per day the machine is used

Past experience

The manufacturer's recommendations.

Manufacturer's specifications provide standards which need to be maintained for safe and economical use of the machine. These specifications give maintenance personnel definite guidelines to follow. Examples of various activities which need to be scheduled include lubricating each piece of equipment; replacing belts, pulleys, fans, and other parts; and checking and adjusting brakes.

Two kinds of records need to be kept. The first is a maintenance service schedule for each piece of equipment in the establishment. Such a schedule indicates the date the equipment was purchased or placed in operation, its cost (if known), the place in which it is used, each part to be serviced, the kind of service required, the frequency of service, and the one assigned to do the servicing. Each piece of equipment also requires a repair record, which includes an itemized list of parts replaced or repaired and the name of the person who did the work.

In addition to scheduled adjustments and replacements, maintenance personnel must repair malfunctioning or broken equipment in accordance with manufacturer's specifications. Sometimes equipment must be sent back to the manufacturer or his representative for repair. Maintenance personnel should be aware of their limitations and recognize that their experience and expertise are not sufficient for all repairs. Those assigned repair responsibilities require special safety training. Many of the jobs to be performed include testing or working on equipment with guards and safety devices removed. Therefore, a statement of necessary precautions should accompany the repair directive.

Maintenance personnel (along with others) have a responsibility to tag and lock out defective equipment, or tag if the equipment (like a ladder) cannot be locked out.

Another element of the total preventive maintenance program is the survey of spare parts requirements. In order to keep needed repair parts on hand, it is necessary to review periodically material required for repair orders and the delivery schedule of such parts. If maintenance personnel keep purchasing agents informed of their anticipated stock needs, lengthy "down time" while waiting for parts to arrive will be prevented.

The difference between a mediocre maintenance program and a superior one is that the first is aimed at maintaining facilities, the second at improving them. If conditions are good, a mediocre program will keep them that way but will not make them better; if conditions are not good, a mediocre program will not improve them. Preventive maintenance, on the other hand, is a program of mutual support which creates safe

conditions, eliminates costly delays and breakdowns, and prolongs equipment life.

**Employees.** Employees make the safety and health program succeed. Well-trained and educated employees are the greatest deterrent to damage, injuries, and health in the plant or establishment.

What are specific ways that the hazard control program can be rooted in employee involvement and concern? Employees can observe safety and health rules and regulations and work according to standard procedures and practices. They can recognize and report to the foreman or supervisor hazardous conditions or unsafe work practices in the plant. They can develop and practice good habits of hygiene and housekeeping. They can use protective and safety equipment, tools, and machinery properly. They can report all injuries or exposure to harmful agents as soon as possible. Employee can help develop safe work procedures and make suggestions for improving work procedures.

What shapes an employee's attitude toward safety? From the day an employee goes to work, whether or not the firm has a formal training program, the employee starts to form his attitude. Substantial if subtle influence is exerted on him by the attitudes he sees in upper management, supervisors, foremen, and his fellow workers. If they regard safety as integral to effective operation, a mark of skill and good sense, if they participate actively and cooperatively in the safety program, if employees are recognized for having good safety records, then the employee will regard safety as something important, not as window-dressing or a gimmick to which lip service is paid periodically.

Introduction to the safety program should come on the employee's first day on the job. A three-pronged approach is suggested (Kane, 1979):

1. Coverage of general company policy and rules; discussion of various benefit programs (for example, hospitalization, pension plan, holidays, sick leave). The personnel department usually is responsible for giving such information immediately after the new employee is added to the payroll.

2. Discussion of general safety rules and the safety program. This part of the program should be the responsibility of a safety profes-

## COMPANY SAFETY RULES

*All Employees Will Abide By The Following Rules:*

1. Report unsafe conditions to your immediate supervisor.

2. Promptly report all injuries to your immediate supervisor.

3. Wear hard hats on the jobsite at all times.

4. Use eye and face protection where there is danger from flying objects or particles, such as when grinding, chipping, burning and welding, etc.

5. Dress properly. Wear appropriate work clothes, gloves, and shoes or boots. Loose clothing and jewelry should not be worn.

6. Never operate any machine unless all guards and safety devices are in place and in proper operating condition.

7. Keep all tools in safe working condition. Never use defective tools or equipment. Report any defective tools or equipment to immediate supervisor promptly.

8. Properly care for and be responsible for all personal protective equipment.

9. Be alert and keep out from under overhead loads.

10. Do not operate machinery if you are not authorized to do so.

11. Do not leave materials in aisles, walkways, stairways, roads or other points of egress.

12. Practice good housekeeping at all times.

13. Do not stand or sit on sides of moving equipment.

14. The use of, or being under the influence of, intoxicating beverages or illegal drugs while on the job is prohibited.

15. All posted safety rules must be obeyed and must not be removed except by management's authorization.

16. Comply at all times with all known federal, state and local safety laws as well as employer regulations and policies.

17. Horseplay causes accidents and will not be tolerated.

Violations of any of these rules may be cause for immediate disciplinary action.

Fig. 3-9.

*Developed by the Construction Advancement Foundation SAFE Committee.*

sional. The company's safety handbook should be given to the new employee, and the company's safety policy statement should be explained. The "why" aspect of general safety rules should be explored with the employee, who is more likely to follow rules when he understands the reasons for them.

3. Explanation of specific safety rules that are applicable in the new employee's department.

At this point the supervisor's role overlaps with that of the safety professional. The supervisor can show how some hazards have been eliminated while others, which could not be designed out of the operation, are guarded against. This discussion provides an opportunity to talk about safe work practices and emergency procedures as well as to show how personal protective equipment can further reduce the effects of the hazard. The employee's responsibilities for safety and health also must be stressed. These responsibilities include reporting all accidents (whether or not they result in injuries), checking equipment and tools before use, and operating equipment only with proper authorization and prior instruction.

Fig. 3-9 lists the company safety rules developed by the Construction Advancement Foundation SAFE Committee and distributed to construction employees in Indiana.

### Professionals in hazard control

The roles of various professionals in the hazard control program are described in National Safety Council's *Fundamentals of Industrial Hygiene*, 2nd ed.: Chapter 25, "The Industrial Hygienist"; Chapter 26, "The Safety Professional"; Chapter 27, "The Occupational Physician"; and Chapter 28, "The Occupational Health Nurse." The following discussion, therefore, describes only briefly the responsibilities of the safety professional, the industrial hygienist, and (staff) medical personnel.

**Safety professionals (hazard control specialists).** To assure the continuity of the safety program, top management usually places the administration of the program in the hands of a safety director or manager of safety. The number of full-time safety professionals is increasing as the nature of their duties is better understood.

To effectively administer a safety program requires considerable training and/or many years of experience. A safety program has many facets: occupational health, product safety, machine design, plant layout, security, damage control, fire prevention. Safety as a profession combines engineering, management, preventive medicine, industrial hygiene, and organizational psychology. It requires knowledge of system safety analysis, job safety analysis, job instruction training, human factors engineering, biomechanics, and product safety. The professional must have thorough knowledge of his organization's equipment, facilities, manufacturing process, and workers' compensation. He must be able to communicate and work with all types of people. He must be able to see both management and employee viewpoints, and also be a good trainer himself. A list of tasks performed by occupational safety professionals is included in the Board of Certified Safety

Professionals, "Curricula Development and Examination Study Guidelines," Technical Report No. 1. (See References.)

The passage of the Occupational Safety and Health Act of 1970 requires that certain safety standards be met and maintained. Generally, organizations with moderate or high hazards and/or employing 500 or more persons need a full-time safety professional. The nature of the operation may indicate the need for a full-time professional, regardless of the number of people employed.

The growing number of safety professionals is reflected in the growing membership of the American Society of Safety Engineers (ASSE), which is now approaching 15,000. This organization has approximately one hundred chapters in the U.S. and Canada.

In 1968 the ASSE was instrumental in forming a new organization, the Board of Certified Safety Professionals (BCSP). Its purpose is to provide professional status by certification to qualified safety people who meet strict educational and experience requirements and pass an examination. Several thousand safety professionals have been certified since the BCSP was formed. (Details of both organizations are given in Chapter 24, "Sources of Help.")

The safety professional—whether called a safety engineer, safety director, hazard control specialist, loss control manager, or some other title—normally functions as a specialist on the management level. The hazard control program should enjoy the same position as other established activities of the organization, such as sales, production, engineering, or research. Its budget reflects top management's commitment to the safety and health of its employees and includes the safety professional's salary, the salary of staff to help him, travel allowance, cost of safety equipment, cost of training and continuing education, and other related items. Safety professionals must define needs of their program and, according to priorities, make short- and long-range (three to five years) budget projections. With such projections in hand, they are able to present their needs to those with fiscal responsibility and stand a better chance of acquiring what they need to make their programs function.

Fig. 3-10 is the ASSE's description of the functions of the safety professional. (He does not necessarily need to do all of them all the time, however.)

# THE SCOPE OF THE PROFESSIONAL SAFETY POSITION

A safety professional brings together those elements of the various disciplines necessary to identify and evaluate the magnitude of the safety problem. He is concerned with all facets of the problem, personal and environmental, transient and permanent, to determine the causes of accidents or the existence of loss producing conditions, practices or materials.

Based upon the information he has collected and analyzed, he proposes alternate solutions, together with recommendations based upon his specialized knowledge and experience, to those who have ultimate decision-making responsibilities.

The functions of the position are described as they may be applied in principle to the safety professional in any activity.

The safety professional in performing these functions will draw upon specialized knowledge in both the physicial and social sciences. He will apply the principles of measurement and analysis to evaluate safety performance. He will be required to have fundamental knowledge of statistics, mathematics, physics, chemistry, as well as the fundamentals of the engineering disciplines.

He will utilize knowledge in the fields of behavior, motivation, and communications. Knowledge of management principles as well as the theory of business and government organization will also be required. His specialized knowledge must include a thorough understanding of the causative factors contributing to accident occurrence as well as methods and procedures designed to control such events.

The safety professional of the future will need a unique and diversified type of education and training if he is to meet the challenges of the future. The population explosion, the problems of urban areas, future transportation systems, as well as the increasing complexities of man's every day life will create many problems and extend the safety professional's creativity to its maximum if he is to successfully provide the knowledge and leadership to conserve life, health, and property.

## Functions of the Professional Safety Position

The major functions of the safety professional are contained within four basic areas. However, application of all or some of the functions listed below will depend upon the nature and scope of the existing accident problems, and the type of activitiy with which he is concerned.

The major areas are:

A. Identification and appraisal of accident and loss producing conditions and practices and evaluation of the severity of the accident problem.

B. Development of accident prevention and loss control methods, procedures, and programs.

C. Communication of accident and loss control information to those directly involved.

D. Measurement and evaluation of the effectiveness of the accident and loss control system and the modifications needed to achieve optimum results.

### A. Identification and Appraisal of Accident and Loss Producing Conditions and Practices and Evaluation of the Severity of the Accident Problem

These functions involve:

1. The development of methods of identifying hazards and evaluating the loss producing potential of a given system, operation or process by:
   a. Advanced detailed studies of hazards of planned and proposed facilities, operations and products.
   b. Hazard analysis of existing facilities, operations and products.

2. The preparation and interpretation of analyses of the total economic loss resulting from the accident and losses under consideration.

3. The review of the entire system in detail to define likely modes of failure, including human error and their effects on the safety of the system.

   a. The identification of errors involving incomplete decision making, faulty judgment, administrative miscalculation and poor practices.

FIG. 3–10.

*(Continued on next page.)*

   b. The designation of potential weaknesses found in existing policies, directives, objectives, or practices.

4. The review of reports of injuries, property damage, occupational diseases or public liability accidents and the compilation, analysis, and interpretation of relevant causative factor information.
   a. The establishment of a classification system that will make it possible to identify significant causative factors and determine needs.
   b. The establishment of a system to ensure the completeness and validity of the reported information.
   c. The conduct of thorough investigation of those accidents where specialized knowledge and skill are required.

5. The provision of advice and counsel concerning compliance with applicable laws, codes, regulations, and standards.

6. The conduct of research studies of technical safety problems.

7. The determination of the need of surveys and appraisals by related specialists such as medical, health physicists, industrial hygienists, fire protection engineers, and psychologists to identify conditions affecting the health and safety of individuals.

8. The systematic study of the various elements of the environment to assure that tasks and exposures of the individual are within his psychological and physiological limitations and capacities.

## B. Development of Accident Prevention and Loss Control Methods, Procedures, and Programs

In carrying out this function, the safety professional:

1. Uses his specialized knowledge of accident causation and control to prescribe an integrated accident and loss control system designed to:

   a. Eliminate causative factors associated with the accident problem, preferably before an accident occurs.

   b. Where it is not possible to eliminate the hazard, devise mechanisms to reduce the degree of hazard.

   c. Reduce the severity of the results of an accident by prescribing specialized equipment designed to reduce the severity of an injury should an accident occur.

2. Establishes methods to demonstrate the relationship of safety performance to the primary function of the entire operation or any of its components.

3. Develops policies, codes, safety standards, and procedures that become part of the operational policies of the organization.

4. Incorporates essential safety and health requirements in all purchasing and contracting specifications.

5. As a professional safety consultant for personnel engaged in planning, design, development, and installation of various parts of the system, advises and consults on the necessary modification to ensure consideration of all potential hazards.

6. Coordinates the results of job analysis to assist in proper selection and placement of personnel, whose capabilities and/or limitations are suited to the operation involved.

7. Consults concerning product safety, including the intended and potential uses of the product as well as its material and construction, through the establishment of general requirements for the application of safety principles throughout planning, design, development, fabrication and test of various products, to achieve maximum product safety.

8. Systematically reviews technological developments and equipment to keep up to date on the devices and techniques designed to eliminate or minimize hazards, and determine whether these developments and techniques have any applications to the activities with which he is concerned.

## C. Communication of Accident and Loss Control Information to those Directly Involved

In carrying out this function the safety professional:

1. Compiles, analyzes, and interprets accident statistical data nd prepares reports designed to communicate this information to those personnel concerned.

2. Communicates recommended controls, procedures, or programs designed to eliminate or minimize hazard potential, to the appropriate person or persons.

3. Through appropriate communication media, persuades those who have ultimate decision making responsibilities to adopt and utilize those controls which the preponderance of evidence indicates are best suited to achieve the desired results.

4. Directs or assists in the development of specialized education and training materials and in the conduct of specialized training programs for those who have operational responsiblity.

5. Provides advice and counsel on the type and channels of communications to insure the timely and efficient transmission of useable accident prevention information to those concerned.

## D. Measurement and Evaluation of the Effectiveness of the Accident and Loss Control System and the Needed Modifications To Achieve Optimum Results

1. Establishes measurement techniques such as costs statistics, work sampling or other appropriate means, for obtaining periodic and systematic evaluation of the effectiveness of the control system.

2. Develops methods that will evaluate the costs of the control system in terms of the effectiveness of each part of the system and its contribution to accident and loss reduction.

3. Provides feedback information concerning the effectiveness of the control measures to those with ultimate responsibility, with the recommended adjustments or changes as indicated by the analyses.

FIG. 3–10.—(Concluded)

*This is taken from a brochure prepared by the American Society of Safety Engineers and is reprinted through the courtesy of the Society.*

In general, the safety professional advises and guides management, supervisors, foremen, employees, and such departments as purchasing, engineering, and personnel on all matters pertaining to safety. He formulates, administers, and constantly monitors, evaluates, and improves the accident prevention program.

The safety professional usually investigates serious accidents personally or through his staff. He reviews supervisors' accident reports and checks corrective actions taken to eliminate accident causes. He makes necessary reports to management and maintains the accident report system, including files. He recommends safety provisions in (a) plans and specifications for new building construction, (b) repair or remodeling of existing structures, (c) safety equipment, (d) designs of new equipment, (e) processes, operations, and materials. He provides (or cooperates with the training supervisor to provide) safety training and education for employees. He and his staff also take continuing education and attend professional meetings like the National Safety Congress.

Further, the safety professional makes certain that federal, state or provincial, and local laws, ordinances, orders, and regulations relating to safety and health are complied with and that standards, whether mandatory or recommended, are met. He is responsible for preparing the necessary reports (for example, OSHA Forms 100 and 102) for management. On jobs involving subcontractors, the safety professional informs each subcontractor of his hazard control responsibilities; this is often spelled out in the contract. (See the discussion in the *Engineering and Technology* volume, Chapter 2, "Construction and Maintenance of Plant Facilities.")

He supervises disaster control, fire prevention and firefighting activities where they are not responsibilities of other departments. He stimulates and maintains employee interest in and commitment to safety.

It is not uncommon to find that the safety professional has been given the authority to order immediate changes on fast-moving and rapidly changing operations or in cases where delayed action could endanger lives (as in construction, demolition, or emergency work, fumigation, and some phases of manufacture of explosives, chemicals, or dangerous substances). Where the safety professional exercises this authority, he does so with discretion, realizing that he is accountable to management for errors in judgment but that errors on the side of caution are more easily justified than unnecessary risk-taking.

# 3—Hazard Control Program Organization

**Industrial hygienists.** The industrial hygienist is trained to recognize, evaluate, and control health hazards—particularly chemical, physical, and biological agents—that exist in the workplace and have injurious effects on workers. Specialists work in such fields as toxicology, epidemiology, chemistry, ergonomics, acoustics, ventilation engineering, and statistics.

The American Board of Industrial Hygiene (ABIH) examines and certifies persons in industrial hygiene. Many certified industrial hygienists are also certified safety professionals. Physicians, nurses, and safety professionals can move part or all of the way into industrial hygiene functions.

What are the specific responsibilities of the industrial hygienist in the hazard control program? He recognizes and identifies those chemical, physical, and biological agents that may adversely affect the physical and mental health and well-being of the worker. He measures and documents levels of environmental exposure to specific hazardous agents. He evaluates the significance of exposures and their relationship to occupationally and environmentally induced diseases. He establishes appropriate controls and monitors their effectiveness. He recommends to management how to correct unhealthy (or potentially unhealthy) conditions.

**(Staff) medical personnel.** Occupational health services vary greatly from one organization to another, depending on number of employees, nature of the operation, and the commitment of the employer. One plant may include a full-time physician, nurses, and technicians, with treatment rooms and a dispensary. Another may have only the required first aid kit and an adequately trained person to render first aid and cardiopulmonary resuscitation (CPR). The small plant has special need for persons thoroughly trained in first aid and CPR to take care of the employees on all shifts throughout each working day. Sometimes small companies and plants in the same locality share the services of a qualified physician on either a part- or full-time basis.

How much responsibility a part- or full-time nurse assumes generally depends on the availability of a licensed physician. It is not unusual for an occupational nurse to be solely and completely responsible for the occupational safety and health program with medical direction from a physician who rarely visits the workplace.

The American Association of Occupational Health Nurses in 1977 defined occupational health nursing as "the application of nursing principles in conserving the health of workers in all occupations. It involves prevention, recognition, and treatment of illness and injury, and requires special skills and knowledge in the fields of health, education, and counseling, environmental health, rehabilitation, and human relations." In addition to being responsible for health care, the occupational nurse may on occasion monitor the workplace, perform industrial hygiene sampling, act as a consultant on sanitary standards, and be responsible for health education.

Chapter 19, "Occupational Health Services," deals specifically with the duties of the industrial physician, nurse, and first aid attendants. Regardless of size, health programs share common goals: to maintain the health of the work force, to prevent or control diseases and accidents, and to prevent or at least reduce disability and resulting lost time.

Staff medical personnel are a vital part of the total health and safety program. Their most obvious contribution is to provide emergency medical care for employees who are injured or become ill on the job. An outgrowth of this responsibility is to provide followup treatment of employees suffering from occupational disease or injuries. For many, periodic examinations are required by OSHA regulations. A further outgrowth is medical personnel's promotion of health education programs for employees and their families. Assisting with problems of alcohol and drug abuse; keeping immunizations up to date; promoting mental health, weight control, and regular exercise: these are only some ways that medical personnel can encourage the health and well-being of employees.

Medical personnel foster a healthful environment by occasional tours of the workplace. Such tours also familiarize medical personnel with the materials and processes used and procedures performed by the employees under their care.

Another way that medical personnel are important to the health and safety organization is in the placement of employees. Proper placement matches the worker to the demands of the job. Often a preplacement examination gives the medical staff an opportunity to recommend where a prospective worker is to be assigned. This placement should take into consideration the physical capacity and mental ability of the employee so that he subjects neither himself nor others to unnecessary safety and health risks.

## Safety and Health Committees

Safety and health committees can be invaluable to the hazard control program, providing the active participation and cooperation of many key people in the organization. They also can be neither productive nor effective. The difference between success and failure lies with the original purpose of the committee, its staffing and structure, and the support it receives while carrying out its responsibilities.

A safety and health committee is a group that aids and advises both management and employees on matters of safety and health pertaining to plant or company operations. In addition, it performs essential monitoring, educational, investigative, and evaluative tasks.

Committees may represent various constituencies or levels within the organization. Another division is based on function: management or workplace committees. The joint safety and health committee is discussed here.

The OSHAct in Section 2 (b)(13) clearly contemplates the possibility of joint safety and health initiatives as a supplementary approach to more effectively accomplishing OSHA's objectives. Joint committees have considerable potential for reducing injuries and illnesses, thus leaving OSHA free to target enforcement according to the worst-first principle (Tofany, 1980).

The joint committee concept stresses cooperation and a commitment to safety as a shared responsibility. Employees can become actively involved in and make positive contributions to the company's safety and health program. Their ideas can be translated into actions. The committee serves as a forum for discussing changes in regulations, programs, or processes and potential new hazards. Employees can communicate problems to management openly and face to face. Information and suggestions can flow both ways. The knowledge and experience of many persons combine to accomplish the objectives of creating a safe workplace and reducing accidents. With many minds addressing a problem simultaneously, with so much "thinking power" concentrating on an issue, effective solutions often are produced in a give-and-take atmosphere. Because they facilitate communication and cooperation,

joint committees usually result in higher morale as well.

Even though a joint committee represents both employees and management, analyses and recommendations of the committee—whether they pertain to policy or practice—should be reviewed and confirmed by those with expertise when they relate to specialized areas (for example, electrical safety, exposure levels).

Labor/management cooperation was discussed in Chapter 1, "Occupational Safety: History and Growth." Committee organization and operation are covered in the Council publication "You Are the Safety and Health Committee."

## Off-the-Job Safety Programs

There is a certain amount of confusion as to what off-the-job (OTJ) safety really includes. Essentially, off-the-job safety involves employees, and is a term used by employers to designate that part of their safety program directed to the employee when he is not at work.

The principal aim of off-the-job safety is to get an employee to follow the same safe practices in his outside activities as he uses on the job. Experience indicates, however, that many individuals tend to leave their safety training at the work place when they go home. Therefore, off-the-job safety should not be a separate program, but rather an extension of a company's on-the-job safety program.

One of the basic reasons for a company to become involved in off-the-job safety is manpower. While companies now have a legal responsibility to prevent injuries on the job, they have a moral responsibility to try to prevent injuries away from the job. All injuries are a waste of a valuable resource—people. Injuries and fatalities happen to people who call on customers, make a product, service equipment, keep the books, and do many other jobs involved in running a business.

The other reason for an off-the-job safety program is cost. Operating costs and production schedules are affected as much when employees are injured away from work as when they are injured on the job. (These costs are discussed in detail in Chapter 7, "Accident Investigation, Analysis, and Costs.")

Although accidents occur off the job, a large part of the cost is borne by employers. Some cost is paid directly in the form of wages to absent

# 3—Hazard Control Program Organization

## OTJ Cost Categories

### 1. Direct

Wages paid to injured workers while off the job.

### 2. Indirect (disabling)

a. Wage cost due to decreased output of injured worker after he returns to work.

b. Personnel cost of hiring replacement workers.

c. Wage cost of supervisors for time spent in training replacement workers.

d. Wage cost due to lower output of replacement workers during break-in period.

e. Products, materials, tools, etc., spoiled by replacement workers during break-in period.

f. Wage cost of time lost by other workers who were delayed getting started because injured worker was a member of a team, his output was needed, or other workers discussed the accident.

g. Wages paid during time spent by non-injured workers for visiting the injured, attending funerals.

### 3. Indirect (nondisabling)

This cost arises in connection with the following (many workers will lose some hours from work even though they do not lose a full day at any one time).

a. Wages paid during time lost by workers for doctor or dispensary visits.

b. Wage cost due to decreased output of worker because of his injury.

c. Wage cost of other workers who may be slowed down, either because the injured worker was slow, temporarily absent, or needed help of other workers.

d. Spoilage of product or materials due to less efficient work because of the injury.

### 4. Insurance

Each company can determine its own insurance cost covering off-the-job accidents. Generally this will be included in some form of health and accident coverage, and the insurance company will be able to state that portion of the premium which is for the accident portion of the policy. While this cost is not as flexible as others listed above, most policies do provide for some form of credit for improved experience.

*Note.* Every one of these costs will not arise in connection with every off-the-job accident, but each is a potential cost, and during a period of time, many or all of them will arise whether actually identified or not.

Fig. 3–11.

---

workers and the cost of hiring and training replacement workers. Some of the cost is hidden. For example, a skilled tool maker, or a sales person injured off the job may not be replaced immediately. Their absences may result in lost sales, late deliveries, and loss of customers.

Some of the cost is hidden even deeper, although it is still very real. As accidents in a community increase, so do insurance costs, taxes, and welfare contributions. Probably no company is fully aware of all the costs that result from off-the-job accidents, and the impact they have on operations and profits. Enough experience has been accumulated, however, to develop a simplified plan for estimating such costs (see Fig. 3–11).

There is nothing special about techniques for promoting off-the-job safety. The same principles and techniques used to put across safety on the job are employed. From a safety standpoint, operating power tools at home is the same as operating the same equipment at work; driving the family car is the same as driving a company vehicle.

A company *does* have to depend more on education and persuasion to get its message across, because once an employee leaves his office, plant, or job site he is on his own and the supervision factor is no longer available. An employee must realize that accidents do not always happen to other people.

As with any other program—whether it be attendance, quality control, waste reduction—management support and guidance is essential. Once management has been shown the seriousness of the problem (through experience and cost records), there should be little problem in obtaining support.

The approach to off-the-job safety should not be negative—"Don't do this" or "Don't participate in that activity"—but positive. That is done by pointing out that any activity can be performed safely if the employee only thinks through the activity first, finds out what hazards are involved, takes instruction if needed, and uses the correct procedure and equipment.

An important element of off-the-job safety programming is to keep the activities seasonal. Generally, employees are more receptive to subjects when they coincide with their normal routine. Examples are: water safety in summer, and home fires in the winter. Of course some subjects, safety belts, falls, poison prevention, to name a few, can be used any time.

Take advantage of national programs, if possible. Activities such as Fire Prevention Week, Poison Prevention Week, and Safe Boating Week get a great deal of national publicity and can be used as a springboard for an activity.

Another important element in off-the-job safety programming is the help available in the community. That is particularly true for recreational activities. Local gun clubs, powerboat squadrons, the Red Cross, YMCA, health, police and fire departments, to name a few, have proven to be of valuable assistance in promoting off-the-job safety. Most of those organizations have materials that can be distributed; some have speakers and films available for company meetings. All can serve as sources of ideas for activities.

A company does not necessarily need actually to conduct activities itself to have an effective off-the-job safety effort. One important way to promote off-the-job safety is to encourage employees to take advantage of swimming and life saving classes, safe boating courses, safe hunting classes, Driver Improvement Courses, Occupant Restraint Programs, first aid courses, and others available in the community.

The same methods used to sell safety on the job can also be used to sell safety off the job—meetings, a company magazine, bulletin board notices, video tapes, films, displays, and posters. (See Chapter 12, "Maintaining Interest in Safety.")

While some companies conduct elaborate open houses, safety fairs, and other large programs that have good results, others obtain equally good results with rather simple activities. Many companies work off-the-job safety activities right into their regular plant safety programs. One company, for example, selected the month of May to cover lifting and material handling. In-plant problems were covered in departmental meetings and notices. It was also pointed out that plant safety principales and practices for safe lifting of heavy objects could be used at home, while moving furniture and doing other spring housecleaning chores.

There are three benefits a company can realize from expanding its safety program to include off-the-job safety. The first is a reduction in lost production time and operating costs from both on- and off-the-job injuries. Second, companies have found that efforts in off-the-job safety have produced an increased interest by employees in their on-the-job safety program. The third benefit, often overlooked, is that of better public relations.

The aim of safety education, namely changing the employee's attitude, is especially true of off-the-job safety. No asset is more important to a company than its employees. They should be protected not only during working hours, but also be given every incentive to also be safe *off* the job.

## References

Board of Certified Safety Professionals of the Americas, 501 S. Sixth St., Champaign, Ill. 61820. "Curricula Development and Examination Study Guidelines," Tech. Report No. 1.

Construction Advancement Foundation, Hammond, Ind. *Safety Manual.*

Factory Mutual Engineering Corp., Norwood, Mass. 02062.
*Handbook of Industrial Loss Prevention.*
*Loss Prevention Data.*

Firenze, Robert J. *Guide to Occupational Safety and Health Management.* Dubuque, Ia., Kendall/Hunt Publishing Co., 1973.

# 3—Hazard Control Program Organization

————. *The Process of Hazard Control.* Dubuque, Ia., Kendall/Hunt Publishing Co., 1978.

————. *Safety and Health in Industrial/Vocational Education.* Cincinnati, Ohio, National Institute for Occupational Safety and Health, 1981.

Hannaford, Earle S. *Supervisors Guide to Human Relations,* 2nd ed. Chicago, Ill., National Safety Council, 1976.

Johnson, William G. *MORT Safety Assurance Systems.* New York, N.Y., Marcel Dekker, Inc., 1980.

Kane, Alex. "Safety Begins the First Day on the Job," *National Safety News,* January 1979, p. 53.

Manuele, Fred A. "How Effective Is Your Hazard Control Program?" *National Safety News,* February 1980, pp. 53-58.

Maryland, State of, Department of Labor and Industry, Safety Engineering and Education Division. "Safety Program Safety Committee Manual," 1967.

National Association of Suggestion Systems, 435 N. Michigan Ave., Chicago, Ill. 60611.
*Performance Magazine* (6 times a year).
"Suggestion Newsletter" (6 times a year).

National Safety Council, 444 N. Michigan Ave., Chicago, Ill. 60611.
*Communications for the Safety Professional.*
Industrial Data Sheets
*Management Safety Policies,* No. 585.
*Off-the-Job Safety,* No. 601.
*Safety Committees,* No. 631.
*Supervisors Safety Manual.*
"You Are the Safety and Health Committee."

Olishifski, Julian B., ed. *Fundamentals of Industrial Hygiene,* 2nd ed. Chicago, Ill., National Safety Council, 1979.

Peters, George A. "Systematic Safety," *National Safety News,* September 1975, pp. 83–90.

Pollina, Vincent. "Safety Sampling," *Journal of the American Society of Safety Engineers,* August 1962, pp. 19-22.

Tainter, Sarah A., and Monro, Kate M. *The Secretary's Handbook.* New York, The Macmillan Co.

Tofany, Vincent L. Remarks at Oversight Hearings on the Occupational Safety and Health Act of 1970, U.S. Senate Committee on Labor and Human Resources, March 28, 1980.

U.S. Department of Human Resources, National Institute for Occupational Safety and Health, Division of Technical Services, Cincinnati, Ohio 45226. *Self-Evaluation of Occupational Safety and Health Programs,* Publication 78-187, 1978.

U.S. Department of Labor, Bureau of Labor Standards. *Safety Organization,* Bulletin 285, 1967.

U.S. Department of Labor, Occupational Safety and Health Administration. *Organizing a Safety Committee,* OSHA 2231, June 1975.

Windsor, Donald G. "Process Hazards Management," a speech given before the Chemical Section, National Safety Congress, October 17, 1979.

# Acquiring Hazard Information

# Chapter
# 4

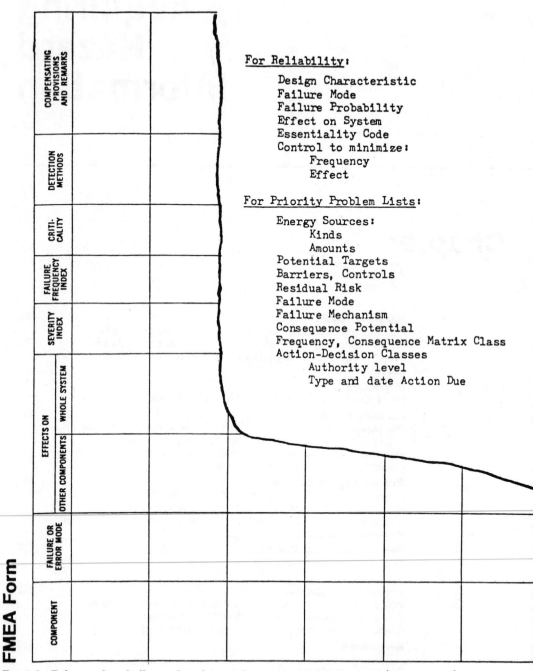

For Reliability:

Design Characteristic
Failure Mode
Failure Probability
Effect on System
Essentiality Code
Control to minimize:
Frequency
Effect

For Priority Problem Lists:

Energy Sources:
Kinds
Amounts
Potential Targets
Barriers, Controls
Residual Risk
Failure Mode
Failure Mechanism
Consequence Potential
Frequency, Consequence Matrix Class
Action-Decision Classes
Authority level
Type and date Action Due

FIG. 4-1.—Failure mode and effect analysis form used at Aerojet Nuclear Company (Johnson, 1980.)

Before hazards can be controlled, they must be discovered. Monitoring is an effective means of acquiring hazard information. *Monitoring* can be defined as a set of observation and data collection methods to detect and measure deviations from plans and procedures in current operations (Johnson, 1980).

Monitoring is important to ascertain (*a*) that controls are functioning as intended; (*b*) that workplace modifications have not altered conditions so that controls no longer function effectively; and (*c*) that new problems have not crept into the workplace since the most recent controls were introduced (Firenze, 1978).

Monitoring can involve four functions: hazard analysis, inspection, measurement, and accident investigation. Including all four functions means that monitoring is performed *before* the operation begins, *during* the life cycle of the operation, and *after* the system has broken down. A systems approach to hazard control will use each of these methods. The remainder of this chapter tells how.

## Hazard Analysis

Data from hazard analysis can be thought of as being the baseline for future monitoring activities. Before the workplace can be inspected to assure that environmental and physical factors fall within safe ranges, the hazards inherent in the system must be discovered. Hazard analysis has proven itself an excellent tool to identify and evaluate hazards.

The idea of analyzing a problem or situation to extract data for decision making is not new. Good workers and their supervisors are always—though sometimes unconsciously—making assessments which guide their actions. Written analyses carry the process one step further. They provide the means to document hazard information.

### Philosophy behind hazard analyses

Written analyses can form the basis for more thorough inspections. They can communicate data about hazards and risk potential to those in command positions. They can educate those in the line and staff organizations who must know the consequences of hazards which exist within their operations and the purpose and logic behind established control measures. Management may require formal, written analysis for each critical operation. By doing so, it not only gathers information for immediate use, but it also reaps

benefits over the long run. Once important hazard data are committed to paper, they become part of the technical information base of the organization. These documents show the employer's concern for locating hazards and establishing corrective measures prior to any accident that may happen.

Traditionally, when systems have been analyzed to determine failures that detracted from their effectiveness, they were analyzed during their operational phase. Hazard analytical techniques applied during this phase of a system's life cycle returned substantial dividends by reducing both accident and overall system losses.

But during the last decade, a shift has taken place. Hazard control specialists no longer concentrate solely on operations. Instead, they are looking at the conceptual and design stages of the systems for which they are responsible. They are using analytical methods and techniques *before accidents happen*, to identify and judge the nature and effects of hazards associated with their systems. This widened assessment, in many instances, has altered significantly the direction of hazard control efforts. When potential failures can be located prior to the production or on-stream process stage of a system's life cycle, specialists can cut costs and avoid damage, injuries, and death. Systems engineering was initially concerned with increasing effectiveness, not profits. Properly applied, however, it can point out profitable solutions to many of top management's most perplexing operational problems.

### What is hazard analysis?

*Hazard analysis* is an orderly process used to acquire specific information (hazard and failure data) pertinent to a given system. (Firenze, 1978.) A popular adage holds that "most things work out right for the *wrong* reasons." By providing data for informed management decisions, hazard analysis helps things work out right for the *right* reasons. The method forces those conducting the analysis to ask the right questions, and it also helps to answer those questions. By locating those hazards that are the most probable and/or have the severest consequences, hazard analyses produce information essential in establishing effective control measures. Analytic techniques assist the investigator in deciding what facts to seek, determining probable causes and contributing factors, and arranging results so that they are orderly and clear.

| Operational Step | Equipment and Materials | Potential Hazardous Condition | Potential Human Error | Potential Accident | Accident Probability Estimate 1 | 2 | 3 | Effect | Haz. Cl. | Applicable Standard |
|---|---|---|---|---|---|---|---|---|---|---|
| Installing a conduit in a trench | Backhoe, Conduit, Sling, Bulldozer, Compactor, Spoil pile | Workman exposure to unstable trench walls | Failure to achieve proper trench wall sloping | Cave in of trench walls | x | | | Death or injury | III | OSHA P1 |
| | | | Incorrect determination or evaluation of soils at the site | | | x | | | II | P-1 1926.651(h) |
| | | | Failure to recognize the effects of surcharges | Earth sliding into the trench | | | x | Permanent damage to workman's circulatory system | III | 1926.651(e) .651(o) .651(q) |
| | | | Failure to recognize the effects of vibration | | | | x | | III | .651(k) .651(e) |
| | | | Failure to recognize previous excavations | | | | x | | III | 1926.652(e) |
| | | | Failure to recognize a change in soils | | | x | | | II | P-1 |
| | Backhoe, Conduit, Sling, Bulldozer, Compactor, Spoil pile | exposure to Workman unstable trench walls | Failure to recognize a water problem | Cave in of trench walls | x | | | Death or injury | III | .651(d) (e) (f) (h) (p) |
| | | | Altered design without subsequent change in side sloping | Earth sliding into the trench | | | x | Permanent damage to workman's circulatory system | II | P-1 .651(e) .652(b) |
| | | Workman exposed to falling objects in trench | Failure to keep all excavated materials and equipment well back from the edge of the trench | | | x | | | III | .651(i1) (i2) |

What are some uses to which hazard analysis can be put?

1. It can uncover hazards that may have been overlooked in the original design, mock up, or setup of a particular process, operation, or task.

2. It can locate hazards that may have developed after a particular process, operation, or task was instituted.

3. It can determine the essential factors in and requirements for specific job processes, operations, and tasks. It can indicate what qualifications are prerequisites to perform work safely and productively.

4. It can indicate the need for modifying processes, operations, and tasks.

5. It can identify situational hazards in facilities, equipment, tools, materials, and operational events (for example, unsafe conditions).

6. It can identify human factors responsible for accident situations (for example, deviations from standard procedures).

7. It can identify exposure factors that contribute to injury and illness (such as contact with hazardous substances, materials, or physical agents).

8. It can identify physical factors that contribute to accident situations (noise, vibration, insufficient illumination, to name a few).

9. It can determine appropriate monitoring methods and maintenance standards needed for safety.

## Formal methods of hazard analysis

Formal hazard analytical methods can be divided into two broad categories: inductive and deductive.

Inductive method. The inductive analytical method uses observable data to predict what can happen. It postulates how the component parts of a system will contribute to the success or failure of the system as a whole. Inductive analysis considers a systems operation from the standpoint of its components, their failure in a particular operating condition, and the effect of that failure on the system.

The inductive method forms the basis for such analyses as failure mode and effect analysis (FMEA) and construction hazard analysis (CHA).

In Failure Mode and Effect Analysis, the failure or malfunction of each component is considered, including the mode of failure. The effects of the hazard(s) that led to the failure are traced through the system, and the ultimate effect on the task performance is evaluated. However, because only one failure is considered at a time, some possibilities may be overlooked. Fig. 4–1 illustrates the FMEA format used at Aerojet Nuclear Co., Idaho Falls, Idaho. Fig.4–2 illustrates the CHA format used in construction.

Once the inductive analysis is completed and the critical failures that require further investigation are detected, then the fault tree analysis will facilitate an inspection.

Chapter 5, "Removing the Hazard from the Job," discusses job safety analysis (JSA), an analysis using the inductive method. That chapter indicates the basic steps to be taken and the uses to which a job safety analysis can be put.

Deductive method. If inductive analysis tells us *what* can happen, deductive analysis tells us *how*. It postulates the failure of the entire system and then identifies how the components could contribute to the failure.

Deductive methods use a combined-events analysis, often in the form of trees. The positive tree calls for stating the requirements for success; see Fig. 4–3. Positive trees are less commonly used than fault trees because they easily become a list of "you shoulds" and sound preachy and moralizing.

Fault trees are reverse images of positive trees and show ways troubles can occur. An undesired event is selected. All the possible happenings that can contribute to the event are diagrammed in the form of a tree. The branches of the tree are continued until independent events are reached. Probabilities are determined for the independent events.

The fault tree requires rigorous, thorough analysis; all known sources of failure must be listed. The fault tree is a graphic model of the various parallel and sequential combinations of system component faults that may result in a single, selected system fault. Fig. 4–3 illustrates three types of analytical trees.

Analytical trees have three advantages:

1. They accomplish rigorous, thorough analysis

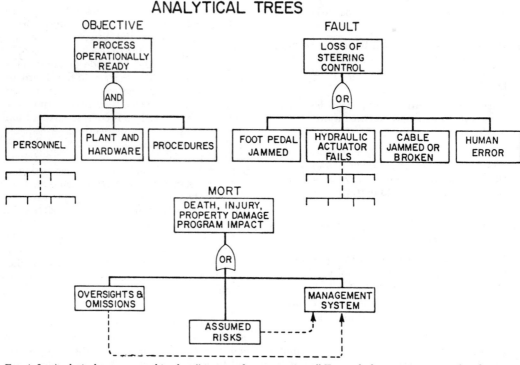

FIG. 4–3.—Analytical trees are nothing but "structured common sense." Trees of of two major types—the *objective or positive trees*, which emphasize what must be done if a job is to be done properly, and the *fault trees*, which are based upon a specific failure and emphasize those things that can go wrong to produce the failure. A fault tree structured for one job can be generalized to cover a wide variety of jobs. The MORT diagram describes the ideal safety program in an orderly, logical manner; it is based on three basic "branches"—(a) a branch that deals with specific oversights and omissions at the work site, (b) a branch that deals with the management system that establishes policies and makes the system go, and finally (c) an assumed risk branch that visually recognizes that no activity is completely risk-free and that risk-management functions must exist in any well-managed organization. (Nertney, 1977.) (Used with permission.)

without wordiness. Using known data, the analyst can identify the single and multiple causes capable of inducing the undesired event.

2. They make the analytical process visible, allowing for the rapid transfer of hazard data from person to person, group to group, with few possibilities for miscommunication during the transfer.

3. They can be used as investigative tools. By reasoning backwards from the accident (the undesired event), the investigator may be able to reconstruct the system and pinpoint those elements that were responsible for the undesired event.

**Cost-effectiveness.** The cost-effectiveness method can be used as part of either the inductive or deductive approach. The cost of system changes made to increase safety is compared with the decreased costs of fewer serious failures or with the increased efficiency of the system. Cost-effectiveness frequently is used to decide among several systems, each of which can perform the same task.

**Choosing which method to use.** To decide what hazard analytical approach is best for a given situation, the hazard control specialist will want to answer five questions:

1. What is the quantity and quality of information desired?

| System Safety Method or Concept | Scaled-Down Version | Comments |
|---|---|---|
| Hazard Analysis and Risk Projection | 1. Think like an insurance agent—try to reduce hazards to consequences.<br>2. Use insurance companies. "How much would you charge to insure us?" | Safety people too often try to communicate with line managers in terms of "hazards" rather than reducing the hazards to risks and consequences. |
| Biomechanics | Looking at the job from the worker's point of view in terms of physical characteristics. | For example, does the vehicle cab "fit" small men and women? Can the largest person, the smallest person, the person with the shortest reach, etc. operate the equipment effectively—or have the designers given us another "average-man" design? Can the job be done on the hottest and coldest days? Are the people going to be completely exhausted half way through the job, etc.? |
| Human Factors | 1. Simple step-by-step walk-through of the work<br>2. Misuse analysis<br>3. Select equipment that is easy to operate *and* matches existing equipment in operational logic. | Most of the fancy human factors analyses have shown that a simple walk-through will indicate many very obvious booby traps for the workers in terms of job steps that are hard to do or things that invite the people to do it wrong or to misuse equipment. |
| Job Information Systems<br><br>Formal Change Analysis Methods | 1. Do job-site surveillance and monitoring in an orderly manner.<br>2. Pay attention to what the *workers* say.<br>3. Be sensitive to *any changes* in people, hardware, or plans. | "Following one's nose" can too easily lead to oversights and failure to "pick up" on changes. Studies have shown that in a series of six accidents, workers had reported all major contributing factors in questionnaire-type studies performed prior to the accident. Another analysis indicated two typewritten pages of changes which contributed directly to five major accidents. |
| Formal Work-Flow Charting for Safety Reasons | 1. Formal work-flow charting to get the job done properly<br>2. Job Safety Analysis | 1. Experience is indicating that the benefits of formal use of work and project flow-charting go far beyond safety benefits. This is particularly true in avoiding foul-ups between different working groups.<br>2. Use of step-by-step job safety analysis at worker and first-line supervisor level has been adopted by a number of large business-managed tax-paying industrial firms as a cost-effective, efficient method for producing on-the-job safety. |

Fig. 4–4—Areas in which system safety methods and ideas can, with a little adaptation, be applied in ordinary occupational-type work. (Nertney, 1977.) (Used with permission.)

2. What information already is available?

3. What is the cost of setting up and conducting analyses?

4. How much time is available before decisions must be made and action taken?

5. How many people are available to assist in the hazard analysis, and what are their qualifications?

Conducting a hazard analysis can be expensive. It is important to determine what information is needed and how important it is before hazard analysis technique is chosen.

It is beyond the scope of this Manual to go into detail regarding other applications of system safety. (See Johnson, 1980.) A few other areas in which large-project system safety methods and ideas can, with a little adaptation, be scaled down to apply in ordinary industrial-type work are indicated in Fig. 4–4. (Nertney, 1977.)

## Who should participate in hazard analysis?

A hazard analysis, to be fully effective and reliable, should represent as many different viewpoints as possible. Each person who is familiar with a process or operation has acquired insights concerning problems, faults, and situations which can cause accidents. These insights need to be recorded along with those of the initiator of · hazard analysis, who usually will be the safety professional. Input from workers and employee representatives may be extremely valuable at this stage.

## What processes, operations, and tasks need to be analyzed?

Many processes, operations, and tasks in the establishment or plant are good candidates for hazard analysis because they have the potential to cause accidents. However, in this instance as in most others, some are more equal than others. In determining which processes, operations, and tasks receive priority, those making the decisions should take the following into consideration:

1. *Frequency of accidents.* An operation or task that has repeated accidents associated with its performance is a good candidate for analysis, especially if different employees have the same kind of accident while performing the same operation or task.

2. *Potential for injury.* Some processes and operations may have a low accident frequency but a high potential for major injury (e.g., tasks on the grinder conducted without the use of a tool rest or tongue guard).

3. *Severity of injury.* A particular process, operation, or task may have a history of serious injuries and be a worthy candidate for analysis, even if the frequency of such injuries is low.

4. *New or altered equipment, processes, and operations.* As a general rule, whenever a new process, operation, or task is created or an old one altered (e.g., because of machinery or equipment changes), a hazard analysis should be conducted. For maximum benefit the hazard analysis should be done while the process or operation is in the planning stages. No equipment should be put into regular operation until it has been checked for hazards, its operation studied, any necessary additional safeguards installed, and safety instructions or procedures developed. Adhering to such a procedure ensures that employees can be trained in hazard controlled safe operations and serious injuries and exposures avoided.

5. *Excessive material waste or damage to equipment.* Processes or operations that produce excessive material waste and/or damage to tools and equipment are candidates for hazard analysis. The same problems which are causing the waste or damage may be the ones which, given the right situation, could cause injuries.

Eventually all jobs should be covered.

## Inspection

Hazard analysis is a process that can take place during the planning, design, and operational phases of the system. Inspection can be defined as that monitoring function conducted in an organization to locate and report existing and potential hazards which have the capacity to cause accidents in the workplace (Firenze, 1978). Inspection works because it is an essential part of hazard control. It is a vital managerial tool, not a gimmick.

### Philosophy behind inspection

Inspection can be viewed negatively or positively:

• Fault-finding, with the emphasis on criticism, or

• Fact-finding, with the emphasis on locating potential hazards that can adversely affect safety and health.

The second viewpoint makes the most sense. To be effective, this viewpoint depends on three things: (a) yardsticks adequate for measuring a particular situation, (b) comparison of what is with what ought to be, and (c) corrective steps being taken to achieve desired performance. (Firenze, 1978.) Failure to analyze inspection reports for *causes* of defects ultimately means the failure of the monitoring function. Corrective action may fix the specific item but fail to fix the system.

What are the purposes of inspection? Its primary purpose is to detect potential hazards so that they can be corrected *before* an accident occurs. Inspection can determine those conditions which need to be corrected or improved to bring operations up to acceptable standards, both from safety and operational standpoints. Secondary purposes are to improve operations and thus increase efficiency, effectiveness, and profitability.

While management ultimately has the responsibility for inspecting the workplace, authority for carrying out the actual inspecting process extends throughout the organization. Obviously supervisors, foremen, and employees fulfill an inspection function, but so do departments as diverse as engineeering, purchasing, quality control, personnel, maintenance, and health care.

## Types of inspection

Inspection can be classified as one of two types—either continuous or at intervals.

**Continuous, ongoing inspection** is conducted by employees, foremen, supervisors, and maintenance personnel alike as part of their job responsibilities. Continuous inspection involves noting an apparent or potential hazardous condition or unsafe act and either correcting it immediately or making a report to initiate corrective action. Continuous inspection of personal protective equipment is especially important.

Supervisors continuously make sure that tools, machines, and equipment are properly maintained and safe to use and that safety precautions are being observed. Toolroom employees regu-

larly inspect all hand tools to make sure that they are in safe condition. Foremen are often responsible for continuously monitoring the workplace and seeing that equipment is safe and that employees are observing safe practices. When foremen or supervisors inspect machines at the beginning of a shift to see if they are ready to operate, a safety inspection must be part of the operation.

Continuous inspection is one ultimate goal of a good safety and health program. It means that each individual is vigilant, alert to any condition that has accident potential, and willing to take the initiative necessary for corrective action.

Continuous inspection is sometimes called "informal" because it does not conform to a set schedule, plan, or checklist. Critics argue that continuous inspection is erratic and superficial, that it does not get into out-of-the-way places, and that it misses things. The truth is that both kinds of inspections are necessary. They complement one another.

The supervisor's greatest advantage in continuous inspection—his familiarity with the employees, equipment, machines, and environment—can also be a disadvantage. Just as an old newspaper left on a table in time becomes part of the decor, a hazard can become so "familiar" that it is no longer noticed. The supervisor's blind spot is particularly likely to occur with housekeeping and unsafe acts. Poor housekeeping conditions may not be noticed because the change is gradual and the effect is cumulative. A similar phenomenon may occur with such unsafe acts as employees smoking in prohibited areas or failing to wash thoroughly before taking a break for eating or smoking.

No matter how conscientious the supervisor is, he cannot be objective. Inspections of his own area reflect personal and vested interest, knowledge and understanding of the production problems involved in the area, and concern for the employees. A planned periodic inspection of his area by another supervisor can be used as an audit of his efforts. Furthermore, the supervisor who inspects another area may return to his own section with renewed vision. Having looked at the trees day in and day out, he needs occasionally to take the long view and see the forest.

Though this section will be devoted primarily to discussing planned inspections continuous inspections should be regarded as a cooperative, not a competitive, activity.

# 4—Acquiring Hazard Information

**Planned inspection at intervals** is what most people think of as "real" safety and health inspection. It is deliberate, thorough, and systematic by design. In many cases specific items or conditions are examined. An established procedure is followed and a checklist may be used. Planned inspection is of three types: periodic, intermittent, and general.

• *Periodic inspection* includes those inspections scheduled to be made at regular intervals. Such inspections may be of the entire plant, a specific area, a specific operation, or a specific type of equipment. They may take place weekly, monthly, semi-annually, annually, or at other suitable intervals. Items such as safety guard mountings, scaffolds, elevator wire ropes (cables), two-hand controls, and fire extinguishers, and other items that are relied on for safety, require frequent inspection. The greater the accident severity potential, the more often the item should be inspected.

Periodic inspections can be of several different types:

1. Inspections by the safety professional, industrial hygienist, and joint safety and health committees.

2. Inspections for preventing accidents and damage or breakdowns (checking mechanical functioning, lubricating, and the like), performed by electricians, mechanics, and maintenance personnel. Sometimes these persons are asked to serve as roving inspectors.

3. Inspections by specially trained certified or licensed inspectors, often from outside the organization (for example, inspection of boilers, elevators, unfired pressure vessels, cranes, power presses, fire extinguishing equipment).

4. Inspections done by outside investigators to determine compliance with government regulations.

The advantage of periodic inspection is that it covers a specific area and allows detection of unsafe conditions in time to provide effective countermeasures. The staff or safety committee that periodically inspects a certain area is familiar with operations and procedures and therefore quick to recognize deviations. A disadvantage of periodic inspection is that deviations from accepted practices are rarely discovered because employees are usually aware of the presence of inspectors.

• *Intermittent* inspections are those made at irregular intervals. Sometimes the need for an inspection is indicated by accident tabulations and analysis. If a particular department or location shows an unusual number of accidents or if certain types of injuries occur with greater frequency, then an inspection is called for. When construction or remodeling is going on within or around a facility, an unscheduled inspection may be needed to find and correct unsafe conditions before an accident occurs. The same is true when new equipment is installed or when new processes are instituted or old ones modified.

Another form of intermittent inspection is that made by the industrial hygienist when a health hazard is suspected or present in the environment. This monitoring of the workplace is covered in detail in Measurement and Testing, later in this chapter. It usually involves:

Sampling the air for the presence of toxic vapors, fumes, gases, and particulates

Testing of materials for toxic properties

Testing of ventilation and exhaust systems for proper operation.

• *A general inspection* is a planned inspection of places which do not receive periodic inspection. A general inspection covers those areas where "no one ever visits" and "where no one ever gets hurt." It includes parking lots, sidewalks, fencing, and similar outlying regions.

Many out-of-the-way hazards are located overhead, where they are difficult to spot. Overhead inspections frequently disclose the need for repairs to skylights, windows, cranes, roofs, and other installations that affect the safety of both the employees and the physical plant. Overhead devices may require adjustment, cleaning, oiling, and repairing.

Inspections of overhead areas are necessary to determine that all reasonable safeguards are provided and safe practices observed. Inspectors must be certain that persons performing overhead jobs are provided with suitable staging, safety belts, and lifelines. They must apply this safety directive to themselves during the inspection. They must look for loose tools, bolts, pipe lines, shafting, pieces of lumber, windows, electrical fixtures, and other objects that may fall from building structures, cranes, roofs, and similar overhead locations.

Safety conditions change after dark, when the only illumination is artificial. Therefore, when an organization has more than one shift, it is important that inspections also be performed at night to make sure that adequate illumination is provided and that the lighting system is maintained in a satisfactory condition. The safety professional should make this inspection, aided by a photometer and camera, where necessary.

Even when there are no regular night shifts, some employees—maintenance personnel, firefighters, and night watchmen—are required to work after dark. The safety professional occasionally needs to check on the conditions in which they work.

General inspections are usually required before reopening a plant after a long shutdown.

## Planning for Inspection

A safety and health inspection program requires:

1. Sound knowledge of the plant

2. Knowledge of relevant standards, regulations, and codes

3. Systematic inspection steps

4. A method of reporting, evaluating, and using the data.

An effective program begins with analysis and planning. If inspections are casual, shallow, and slipshod, the results will reflect the method. Before instituting an inspection program, the answer to five questions is necessary:

1. What items need to be inspected?

2. What aspects of each item need to be examined?

3. What conditions need to be inspected?

4. How often must items be inspected?

5. Who will conduct the inspection?

## The hazard control inspection inventory

To determine what factors affect the inspection, a hazard control inspection inventory can be conducted. Such an inventory is the foundation upon which a program of planned inspection is based. It resembles a planned preventive mainte-nance system and yields many of the same benefits.

The entire facility—yards, building, equipment, machinery, vehicles—should be divided into areas of responsibility. Once these areas have been determined, they should be listed in an orderly fashion. A color-coded map of the facility or floor plan might possibly be developed. It may be desirable to divide large areas or departments into smaller areas that can be assigned to each first-line supervisor and/or the hazard control department's inspector.

## What items need to be inspected?

Once specific areas of responsibility have been determined, an inventory should be made of those items that can become unsafe or cause accidents. These would include:[*]

1. Environmental factors (illumination, dusts, gases, sprays, vapors, fumes, noise).

2. Hazardous supplies and materials (explosives, flammables, acids, caustics, toxic materials or by-products).

3. Production and related equipment (mills, shapers, presses, borers, lathes).

4. Power source equipment (steam and gas engines, electrical motors).

5. Electrical equipment (switches, fuses, breakers, outlets, cables, extension and fixture cords, grounds, connectors, connections).

6. Handtools (wrenches, screwdrivers, hammers, power tools).

7. Personal protective equipment (hard hats, safety glasses, safety shoes, respirators).

8. Personal service and first aid facilities (drinking fountains, wash basins, soap dispensers, safety showers, eyewash fountains, first aid supplies, stretchers).

9. Fire protection and extinguishing equipment (alarms, water tanks, sprinklers, standpipes, extinguishers, hydrants, hoses).

10. Walkways and roadways (ramps, docks, sidewalks, walkways, aisles, vehicle ways).

11. Elevators, electric stairways, and manlifts (controls, wire ropes, safety devices).

---

[*]Adapted from *Facility Inspection* (see References).

# 4—Acquiring Hazard Information

## List of Possible Problems To Be Inspected

| | | | | |
|---|---|---|---|---|
| Acids | Closets | Fork lifts | Piping | Shapers |
| Aisles | Connectors | Fumes | Pits | Shelves |
| Alarms | Containers | Gas cylinders | Platforms | Sirens |
| Atmosphere | Controls | Gas engines | Power tools | Slings |
| Automobiles | Conveyors | Gases | Presses | Solvents |
| Barrels | Cranes | Hand tools | Racks | Sprays |
| Bins | Crossing lights | Hard hats | Railroad cars | Sprinkler systems |
| Blinker lights | Cutters | Hoists | Ramps | Stairs |
| Boilers | Docks | Horns and signals | Raw materials | Steam engines |
| Borers | Doors | Hoses | Respirators | Sumps |
| Buggies | Dusts | Hydrants | Roads | Switches |
| Buildings | Electric motors | Ladders | Roofs | Tanks |
| Cabinets | Elevators | Lathes | Ropes | Trucks |
| Cables | Explosives | Lights | Safety devices | Vats |
| Carboys | Extinguishers | Mills | Safety shoes | Walkways |
| Catwalks | Eye protection | Mists | Scaffolds | Walls |
| Caustics | Flammables | Motorized carts | Shafts | Warning devices |
| Chemicals | Floors | | | |

FIG. 4–5.

Adapted from Principles and Practices of Occupational Safety and Health, Student Manual, *Booklet Three, U.S. Department of Labor, OSHA 2215.*

12. Working surfaces (ladders, scaffolds, catwalks, platforms, sling chairs).

13. Material handling equipment (cranes, dollies, conveyors, hoists, fork lifts, chains, ropes, slings).

14. Transportation equipment (automobiles, railroad cars, trucks, front-end loaders, helicopters, motorized carts and buggies).

15. Warning and signaling devices (sirens, crossing and blinker lights, klaxons, warning signs).

16. Containers (scrap bins, disposal receptacles, carboys, barrels, drums, gas cylinders, solvent cans).

17. Storage facilities and areas both indoor and outdoor (bins, racks, lockers, cabinets, shelves, tanks, closets).

18. Structural openings (windows, doors, stairways, sumps, shafts, pits, floor openings).

19. Buildings and structures (floors, roofs, walls, fencing).

20. Miscellaneous—any items that do not fit in preceding categories.

Sources of information on items to be inspected are many. Maintenance employees know what problems can cause damage or shutdowns. The workers in the area are qualified to point to causes of injury, illness, damage, delays, or bottlenecks. Medical personnel in the organization can list problems that cause job-related illnesses and injuries. Manufacturers' manuals often specify maintenance schedules and procedures and safe work methods.

Gathering the information about standards, regulations, and codes is a necessary first step in determining what items need to be inspected. A great deal of work already has been done for the safety inspector. Each March the *National Safety News* publishes a list of occupational safety and health standards and references. This guide is arranged according to the various subparts of OSHAct's rules and regulations. It also lists related standards, checklists, and data sheets published by the American National Standards Institute (ANSI), the National Fire Protection Association (NFPA), Underwriters Laboratories Inc., the National Bureau of Standards, the

## 29 CFR 1910
## OCCUPATIONAL SAFETY AND HEALTH STANDARDS

### Subparts

D — Walking-Working Surfaces
E — Means of Egress
F — Powered Platforms, Manlifts, and Vehicle-Mounted Work Platforms
G — Occupational Health and Environmental Control
H — Hazardous Materials
I — Personal Protective Equipment
J — General Environmental Controls
K — Medical and First Aid
L — Fire Protection

M — Compressed Gas and Compressed Air Equipment
N — Materials Handling and Storage
O — Machinery and Machine Guarding
P — Hand and Portable Powered Tools and Other Hand-Held Equipment
Q — Welding, Cutting, and Brazing
R — Special Industries
S — Electrical
T — Commercial Diving Operations
Z — Toxic and Hazardous Substances

## 29 CFR 1926
## STANDARDS FOR THE CONSTRUCTION INDUSTRY

### Subparts

C — General Safety and Health Provisions
D — Occupational Health and Environmental Controls
E — Personal Protective and Life Saving Equipment
F — Fire Protection and Prevention
G — Signs, Signals, and Barricades
H — Materials Handling, Storage, Use and Disposal
I — Tools—Hand and Power
J — Welding and Cutting
K — Electrical
L — Ladders and Scaffolding
M — Floors and Wall Openings and Stairways

N — Cranes, Derricks, Hoists, Elevators, and Conveyors
O — Motor Vehicles, Mechanized Equipment, and Marine Operations
P — Excavations, Trenching, and Shoring
Q — Concrete, Concrete Forms, and Shoring
R — Steel Erection
S — Tunnels and Shafts, Caissons, Cofferdams, and Compressed Air
T — Demolition
U — Blasting and Use of Explosives
V — Power Transmission and Distribution
W — Rollover Protection Structures; Overhead Projection

FIG. 4-6.

National Safety Council, and other sources of similar information. Using this annual bibliography can save the safety officer much time and effort.

Building codes, building inspection books, guides to building and plant maintenance: these also will be useful references. Publications of the National Fire Protection Association will be helpful in making certain that fire hazards are being effectively controlled. Sometimes insurance company surveys contain checklists to determine the condition of buildings. Research and reference material is contained in subsequent chapters of this Manual. Other publications of the National Safety Council, such as *Accident Facts*, may prove useful.

State or provincial and federal governments also publish accident statistics. The Walsh-Healey Public Contracts Act (41 CFR 50) gives safety and health standards for federal supply contracts. In one of its publications OSHA gave examples of possible problems that can be found in the work area. These are cited in Fig. 4-5. The *Federal Register* and the *Code of Federal Regulations*, Title 29, parts 1900-1950, gives OSHA regulations. Fig. 4-6 shows the special subjects addressed by the subparts of 29 CFR 1910 (General Industry) and the subparts of 29 CFR 1926 (Construction). It is important to remember, however, that usually federal and state or provincial laws, codes, and regulations set up minimum requirements only. To comply with company policy and secure maximum safety, it frequently is necessary to exceed these requirements. OSHA publications indicate not only what standards are required but also what violations are most frequent. These same sources are helpful in the next step—determining critical factors to be inspected.

### What aspects of each item need to be examined?

Particular attention should be paid to the parts most likely to cause the greatest problems when they become unsafe. These parts are most likely to develop unsafe or unhealthy conditions because of stress, wear, impact, vibration, heat, corrosion, chemical reaction, and misuse. Safety devices, guards, controls, work or wearpoint components, electrical and mechanical components, and fire hazards would become unsafe first. For a particular machine, critical parts would include the point of operation, moving parts, and accessories (flywheels, gears, shafts, pulleys, key ways, belts, couplings, sprockets, chains, controls, lighting, brakes, exhaust systems). Also to be checked would be feeding, oiling, adjusting, maintenance, grounding, how attached, work space, and location.

The most critical parts of an item are not always obvious. When the security of a heavy load depends on a cotter pin being in place, then that pin is a critical part. *Poor Richard's Almanac* is relevant to today's hazard control efforts: "A little neglect may breed great mischief..."

### What conditions need to be inspected?

The unsafe conditions for each part to be inspected should be described specifically and clearly. A checklist question that reads "Is ... safe?" is meaningless because it does not define what makes an item unsafe. The unsafe conditions for each item to be inspected must not only be listed but also described. Usually, conditions to look for can be indicated by such words as *jagged, exposed, broken, frayed, leaking, rusted, corroded, missing, vibrating, loose,* or *slipping.* Sometimes exact figures are needed; for example, the maximum pressure in a boiler.

Guidelines for safety and health inspections

have been developed by OSHA and are included in its publication, *Safety and Health Inspections for an Effective Safety and Health Program* (U.S. Department of Labor, February 1977). The 75-page guideline shows how specific subparts of the General Industry Standards can be simplified and ordered to help in the monitoring process. The Center for Disease Control, U.S. Department of Health, has devised a suggested checklist for the safety evaluation of shop and laboratory areas. The work sheet is referenced to the OSHA "General Industry Standards."

The National Safety Council also has an extensive checklist in its *OSHA Standards Handbook for Business and Industry.*

Many different types of checklists are available for use in monitoring, varying in length from thousands of items to only a few. Each type has its place. Generally, the longer checklists refer to OSHA standards. These are useful in determining which standards or regulations apply to individual situations. Once the relevant applicable standards are identified, a checklist can be tailored to organizational needs and uses and computerized for action and followup.

Checklists serve as reminders of what to look for and as records of what has been covered. They give inspections direction. They allow on-the-spot recording of all findings and comments before they are forgotten. In case an inspection is interrupted, checklists provide a record of what has and what has not been inspected. Without checklists, inspectors may miss things that they should see or be unsure, after inspecting an area, that they have covered everything.

Good checklists also help in followup. Of course merely running through a checklist does little to locate or correct problems. If the inspector simply checks off the items on the list, he is checking the list, not conducting a safety inspection. The checklist must be used as an aid to the inspection process, not as an end in itself. A hazard observed during inspection must be recorded, even though it may not be part of the checklist.

Refer to the following portfolio of checklists.

*(Text continues on page 117.)*

The following 12 pages comprise a portfolio of various companies' inspection checklists. The first nine are used with computer followup on inspection results, actions to be taken, and corrections made.

| Mechanical Inspection | | | | | |
|---|---|---|---|---|---|

**Mechanical Inspection**

Acct. No. 26023-61
Ord. No. 759223
Dept. No. 862

Koch Dry Ovens and
Paint Booth Make Up
Air Blowers

Inspec's. Name: _____
Inspec. Date: _____

Inspect For: Security, Condition, Operation,
Vibration, Belt Tension, Safety

To Be Inspected-
Jan-Mar-May-Jul-Sep-Nov

Dept. 862

| Mach. No. | Bearings | Belts and Pulleys | Belt Guards | Lube & Lube Lines O.K. | Inspector's Comments | Mach. No. | Bearings | Belts and Pulleys | Belt Guards | Lube & Lube Lines O.K. | Inspector's Comments |
|---|---|---|---|---|---|---|---|---|---|---|---|
| | Sub Assembly Paint System on Mezzanine - North to South | | | | | | Combine Finish Paint Syst. - Dry Ovens and Paint Booth Make Up Air Units | | | | |
| | | | | | | | Bldg. - "V1" South to North | | | | |
| 7227 | | | | | | | | | | | |
| 7226 | | | | | | 7251 | | | | | |
| 7186 | | | | | | 7252 | | | | | |
| 7187 | | | | | | | | | | | |
| 7188 | | | | | | 7259 | | | | | |
| 7225 | | | | | | 7260 | | | | | |
| 7189 | | | | | | 7261 | | | | | |
| | Paint Booth Make Up Air Bldg. - "V" Roof - East Side | | | | | 7262 | | | | | |
| 6790 | | | | | | 7297 | | | | | |
| 6791 | | | | | | 7298 | | | | | |
| 7219 | | | | | | 7300 | | | | | |
| 7221 | | | | | | | Touch Up Paint Dry Oven (3-Ovens) Bldg. - "V2" North East Corner | | | | |
| 7220 | | | | | | 6390 | | | | | |
| 7218 | | | | | | | | | | | |
| | Work in Process Paint System on Mezzanine - North to South | | | | | | | | | | |
| 6760 | | | | | | | | | | | |
| 6758 | | | | | | | | | | | |
| 6795 | | | | | | | | | | | |
| 6796 | | | | | | | | | | | |

**MECHANICAL INSPECTION**

**FLOOR CONVEYORS**

Acct. No. 90059-67
Ord. No. 759225
Dept. No. 862

Monthly Inspection

Inspecting Dept. - 862

Inspection Date

Inspector's Name: _____

SUPERVISOR'S NAME: _____

Inspect for: Security – Safety
Operation – Condition

If item is O.K. use ☑ mark. If work is needed use W and explain. If inspector completes repair, use R and explain.

Column headings:

- Remarks
- Proper Function, Hydrostatic Drive Unit w/Hyd. Motor – Oil Level.
- Check Chain, Tracks or Channel Guides for Wear, "Makeup," Mechanism for
- Check Roller and Wear - Check Guides and Alignment
- Check Roller or Chain - Main Rollers and Return Chain Guides - Worn
- Check Hyd. Hoist Cylinders and Tubing, Hoses and parts
- Check Hyd. Hoist Cylinders, Leaks, Worn
- Check Conveyor Chain for Operation, Wear, Adequate Lube, System for Operation, Wear,
- Check Security Auto Lube Systems for proper Function
- Check Shafts, Mech., Overload Device and Sprockets, "Makeups," bearings & Lube
- Check Chain Drives and Sprockets for Alignment and Tension – Replace as Necessary
- Check Chain, "Makeups," & Lube for Alignment and
- Check Belts and Pulleys for Alignment
- Check Drive Couplings for Operation.
- Check 2 Gear Reduction Boxes for Lubrication.
- Security & Noise Tension

| Machine Number and Name of Conveyor |
| --- |
| 9160 – East (N. Pit) Assembly Line Conveyor |
| 6951 – Hydraulic Hoist System |
| 9160 South Pit |
| 9159 – West (N. Pit) Assembly Line Conveyor |
| 6949 – Hydraulic Hoist System |
| 9159 South Pit |
| 7313 – Combine Paint Conveyor – S. Pit |
| 7313 – Combine Paint Conveyor – N. Pit |

106

**66**  HOIST INSPECTION — FACTORY

Fed.Reg.-1910.179
Acct. No. - 90059-79 Sheet 1 of 7
Ord. No. - 759230
Dept. Chrg. - 862

Insp. Dept. - 862

Insp. Frequency - Monthly

Check off ✓ if O.K. Mark W for work needed and explain. Mark R for items repaired and explain.

V1,V2,V4, & R-BLDGS
Building - R-7   Floor - 1

MONTHLY INSPECTIONS          Yearly Jan.

Inspection categories (column headings):
Controls or Hand Chain. Operation. · Identification - Safety Chain or Cable (Strain) · Upper and Lower Limits - Condition & Security · Operation & Safety Cbl.-Condition & Security · Hoist and Lower Cable - Safety Cable · Brake (function & Sound) of Hoist · Chain Bucket & Chute & Holds Load · Load Chain Sprockets (or Cable Drum) & Lube Chain or Cable · Upper Sprockets (or Collector-Trolley-Track-Collector-Coil) Cord-Air Hose · Fd. Rail Hanger & Lower Hoist Hanger & Guides · All Hardware & Comments (Hoist-Track-Anchors-Bridge · Operator's Comments (Hoist-Trolley-Track-Bridge · Hook Crack Check (Magnaflux-Die Check) · REMARKS · Supervisor's Approval · Inspector's Signature · Date

| Hoist Location Bay or Post Numbers | Mfg.& Type Hoist | Size Hoist | Mach. No. |
|---|---|---|---|
| 93860 | CM ELEC | ½ TON | 4990 |
| 93860 | CM ELEC | ½ TON | |
| 93862 | IR AIR | 500# | |
| 94502 | THOR BAL | | |
| 94502 | IR AIR | 2000# | |
| ON GIB CRANE 94502 | IR AIR | 300# | |
| 94502 | IR AIR | ½ TON | |
| 94502 | IR AIR | 1000# | |
| 94502 | CP BAL | | |
| 94500 | IR AIR | 300# | |
| 94510 | CM ELEC | ½ TON | |

107

**Monthly Mechan. Inspec. (862)  (43)**

**V-BUILDING – HYD. TRACK DROP SECTIONS**

Inspect For: Security – Safety / Operation – Cleanliness

Sheet 1 of 1

INSPEC'S. SIG: _____
SUPERVISOR SIG: _____
ACCT. NO. 90059-67
ORDER NO. 75922.5
DEPT. NO. 862

DATE _____

**2-Hyd. Syst's.–Ea.**

If Item is O.K. Use ☑ Mark. If work is needed use Ⓦ and explain. If inspector completes work, use Ⓡ and explain.

ITEM NUMBER: 1 2 3 4 5 6 7 8 9 10 11 12 13

Item descriptions:
1. DROP SECTION HANGERS
2. DROP SECTION AND STRUCTURAL MEMBERS
3. DROP SECTION WELDS AND BOLTED JOINTS
4. STOPS – TELESCOPIC CYLINDER GUIDES WITH ROLLERS
   STOP SECTION TRACK ACTUATORS – HARDWARE – GUIDES
   HYDRAULIC CONNECTING CYLINDER – CONNECTING PINS & COTTER PINS
5. HYDRAULIC SWITCHOVER VALVE
   UP/DOWN CONTROL SWITCH WITH CORD
   180-GAL. OIL TANK WITH GAGE
   BREATHER – OIL (ENOUGH OIL?)
   HYDRAULIC FILTER CHANGE (NEED FILTER WITH GAGE?)
   15 HP ELEC. MOTOR & GAGE – AIR
   HYD. OIL PUMP & COUPLING
   ALL HOSES – CONNECT & GAGE & HOSE CLAMPS

| Location Post No's. | Machine Number | AREA OF USAGE | INSPECTOR'S COMMENTS |
|---|---|---|---|
| G-13 | 9161 | BODY (LOAD CONVEY.) | 1-Hyd. Syst. |
| F-16 | 9162 | BODY (LINE) | |
| C-16 | 9164 | BODY (LINE) | 1-Hyd. Syst. |
| D-13 | 9163 | BODY (LOAD CONVEY) | |

Loca. No's. / Mach. No.

INSPECTOR'S COMMENTS

**8818 - 3-TON HEMAG STACKER CRANE - WIP STORAGE BUILDING V-5**

ACCT. NO. - 90059-79
ORD. NO. - 759228
DEPT. CHG. 862

MECHANICAL INSPECTION

INSPECTING DEPARTMENT 862

INSPECTOR'S SIGNATURE

SUPERVISOR'S SIGNATURE

INSPECTION DATE

ITEM NUMBER column headings:
- Security - Condition & Adjustment
- Brake - Condition & Adjustment
- Alignment - Operation
- Open Gearing - Bearings & Seals
- Gear Box lube levels
- All Bolts - Rivets & Seals

| | Component |
|---|---|
| A | Bridge |
| B | Trolley |
| C | Bridge Drive - Slow Motor (2) |
| D | Bridge Drive - Fast Motor (2) |
| E | Trolley Drive Motor |
| F | Rotation Motor |
| G | Hoist Drive - Slow Motor |
| H | Hoist Drive - Fast Motor |
| I | Bridge Drive - Slow Gear Box (2) |
| J | Bridge Drive - Fast Gear Box (2) |
| K | Trolley Drive - Gear Box |
| L | Rotation - Gear Box |
| M | Hoist Drive - Slow Gear Box |
| N | Hoist Drive - Fast Gear Box |
| | **LIFTING CARRIAGE AND CAB** |
| O | Fork Adjusting Motor |
| P | Fork Adjusting Gear Box |
| Q | Fork Adjusting Chains & Sprockt |
| R | Fork Rails & Forks |
| S | Lift Carriage & Guide Rollers |
| T | Cab & Door, Windows, Mirror |
| U | Cab, Carriage & Guide Roller |
| V | Cab, Stool & Fire Extinguisher |
| W | Lift Carriage - Catching Device |
| X | Rescu - Escape Device |
| Y | All Safety Guards |

Numbered inspection items (1–29):
1. Gear Box Gearing
2. Bridge bumpers
3. Trolley Bumpers
4. All Travel Bumpers
5. Travel Wheels & Bearings
6. Travel Rail Rails & Splices
7. Travel Rail hold Downs & Welds
8. Travel Rail Sweeps
9. Rotation Ring Gear & Pinion
10. Rotation Ball Bearing
11. All safety Bearing
12. Service Walks & Safety Rails
13. Upper - Hoist Safety Rails
14. Return Sheave - Hoist Guards
15. Hoist Sheave Pivots
16. Hoist Cable Return Sheave
17. Lower Cable - Hoist Drum & Cable Sheave
18. Hoist Cable Dead Anchors
19. Hoist Cable Return Sheave
20. Governor & Cable Dead End
21. Governor Cable Overload Device
22. Governor Cable Sheaves (2)
23. Vertical mast and Rails (2)
24. Mounting bolts (Vertical Mast)
25–29. 6000 lbs. - Load Cap. Check

**INSPECTION NOTE**

IN ALL INSPECTIONS CHECK FOR: CONDITION, SECURITY, ALIGNMENT, OPERATION, CLEANLINESS.

IF ITEM TO BE INSPECTED IS OKAY PLACE A [✓] MARK IN THE PROPER BOX. IF ITEM IS NOT OKAY PLACE A "W" IN THE BOX INDICATING "WORK REQUIRED". THEN LIST WORK REQUIRED IN THE SPACE PROVIDED BELOW.

COMMENTS FOR WORK REQUIRED

ITEM #

| MECHANICAL INSPECTION ㉝ | Inspector's Name: | | | | | | | Dept. 862 |
|---|---|---|---|---|---|---|---|---|

**"HEATER-VENTILATOR BLOWERS"**

INSPECTIONS TO BE MADE
FEB  −  APR  −  JUN
AUG  −  OCT  −  DEC

Bldgs. "V" and "V2"
Roof
Acct. No. 26845-79
Ord. No. 759224
Dept. No. 862

Date of Inspection
To Be Inspected -
Feb-Apr-Jun-Aug-Oct-Dec

Start Inspection at Southwest
Corner of "V" Bldg. Roof. Check
Off if Item is "OK". Make Remarks
For Needed Repairs.

| Heater - Ventilator Number | Bearings Check - OK | Lube - OK -Lube Lines O.K. | Belts in Good Condition - | Belt Tension - OK | Pulleys in Good Condition - | Pulleys Secure | Belt Guards "In Place" and Secure | All Filters in Good Condition and Clean | Inspector's Remarks |
|---|---|---|---|---|---|---|---|---|---|
| 6640 | | | | | | | | | |
| 6641 | | | | | | | | | |
| 6643 | | | | | | | | | |
| 6642 | | | | | | | | | |
| 6644 | | | | | | | | | |
| 6645 | | | | | | | | | |
| 6646 | | | | | | | | | |
| 6650 | | | | | | | | | |
| 6649 | | | | | | | | | |
| 6648 | | | | | | | | | |
| 6647 | | | | | | | | | |
| 6651 | | | | | | | | | |
| 6652 | | | | | | | | | |
| 6653 | | | | | | | | | |
| 6657 | | | | | | | | | |
| 6656 | | | | | | | | | |
| 6655 | | | | | | | | | |
| 6654 | | | | | | | | | |
| 6658 | | | | | | | | | |
| 6659 | | | | | | | | | |
| 6660 | | | | | | | | | |
| 6664 | | | | | | | | | |
| 6663 | | | | | | | | | |
| 6662 | | | | | | | | | |
| 6661 | | | | | | | | | |
| 6665 | | | | | | | | | |
| 6666 | | | | | | | | | |
| 6667 | | | | | | | | | |
| 6378 | | | | | | | | | |
| 6379 | | | | | | | | | |
| 6380 | | | | | | | | | |

| EXHAUST BLOWERS & AIR CONDI. HEAT EXCHANGER & DOOR SEAL BLOWERS |
|---|

3-Month Inspection
Feb-May-Aug-Nov

Inspector's Name _____  Inspection Date _____

Acct. No. 26023 -79  Ord. No. 759223  Dept. No. -862

| Blower Machine Number | Check for Excessive Vibration | Chk. Belts and Pulleys for Ten. & Align. & Condi. | All Safety Shields are in Place and Secure |
|---|---|---|---|
| "V" Bldg. Roof E. Side | | | |
| 7426-Air Condi.Heat Exchanger | | | |
| 7429-Air Condi.Heat Exchanger | | | |
| Sub.Assemb.Paint & Wash Ovens Mezzanine - North to South | | | |
| 7228 | | | |
| 7178 | | | |
| 7179 | | | |
| 7181 | | | |
| 7180 | | | |
| 7183 | | | |
| 7182 | | | |
| 7185 | | | |
| 7224 | | | |
| 7223 | | | |
| 7187 | | | |
| 7190 | | | |
| Flow Coat Booth | | | |
| 7192 | | | |
| 7193 | | | |
| 7194 | | | |
| 7195 | | | |
| 7196 | | | |
| 7197 | | | |
| Spray Paint Booth | | | |
| 7205 | | | |
| 7206 | | | |
| 7208 | | | |
| 7207 | | | |
| 7212 | | | |
| 7213 | | | |
| 7215 | | | |
| 7214 | | | |

| Blower Machine Number | Check for Excessive Vibration | Chk. Belts & Pulleys for Ten. & Align. & Condi. | All Safety Shields are in Place and Secure |
|---|---|---|---|
| W.I.P. Paint Dip | | | |
| 5765 | | | |
| 6767 | | | |
| 6766 | | | |
| 6764 | | | |
| W.I.P. Paint Spray | | | |
| 6784 | | | |
| 6785 | | | |
| 6786 | | | |
| 6787 | | | |
| 6763 | | | |
| W.I.P. Wash Dry Off | | | |
| 6761 | | | |
| 6760 | | | |
| 6759 | | | |
| 6757 | | | |
| W.I.P. Paint Dry | | | |
| 6793 | | | |
| 6794 | | | |
| 6798 | | | |
| 6797 | | | |
| W.I.P. Wash Booth | | | |
| 6755 | | | |
| 6754 | | | |
| 6753 | | | |
| Comb. Finish Paint | | | |
| 7241 | | | |
| 7242 | | | |
| 7243 | | | |
| 7249 | | | |
| Wash Dry Off | | | |
| 7250 | | | |
| 7253 | | | |

| Blower Machine Number | Check for Excessive Vibration | Same as Other | Same |
|---|---|---|---|
| Wash Cool Down | | | |
| 7255 | | | |
| 7256 | | | |
| 7257 | | | |
| Combine Paint | | | |
| 7268 | | | |
| 7269 | | | |
| 7270 | | | |
| 7271 | | | |
| 7272 | | | |
| 7263 | | | |
| 7264 | | | |
| 7265 | | | |
| 7266 | | | |
| 7267 | | | |
| Combine Flash Off | | | |
| 7292 | | | |
| 7293 | | | |
| Combine Paint Dry | | | |
| 7295 | | | |
| 7296 | | | |
| 7299 | | | |
| 7301 | | | |
| Combine Cool Down | | | |
| 7303 | | | |
| 7304 | | | |
| 7305 | | | |
| 7310 | | | |
| 7312 | | | |
| 7306 | | | |
| 7311 | | | |
| Spray & Dry - N.E. Corner-"V2" | | | |

# 4—Acquiring Hazard Information

<table>
<tr><td colspan="2">㊴    AIR COMPRESSOR INSPECTION<br>TIRE ROOM  DEPT. 945</td><td colspan="3">ACCT. NO. 26021-67<br>SHOP ORD. 759226<br>DEPT. 945</td><td colspan="2">DATE: _____<br>INSPECTOR: _____<br>SUPERVISOR: _____</td></tr>
</table>

MECHANICAL - ㊶

IF ITEM IS O.K. USE ✔ MARK. IF WORK IS NEEDED USE ☐W☐ AND EXPLAIN. IF INSPECTOR COMPLETES REPAIR USE ☐R☐ & EXPLAIN

| ITEM NO. | PART TO BE INSPECTED | | CHECK OFF 7694 | CHECK OFF 7840 | | | |
|---|---|---|---|---|---|---|---|
| | | | 1stWK | 2ndWk | 3rdWk | 4thWk | 5thWk |
| 1. | CHECK CRANKCASE OIL LEVEL (ANDEROL-500 OIL) | 7694 | | | | | |
| | | 7840 | | | | | |
| 2. | CHANGE CRANKCASE OIL (ANDEROL-500 OIL) (JAN-MAR-MAY-JUL-SEP-NOV) | | | | | | |
| 3. | CHECK CONDITION OF COMPRESSOR AND AIR RECEIVER | | | | | | |
| 4. | | | | | | | |
| | | | 1stWk | 2ndWk | 3rdWk | 4thWk | 5thWk |
| 5. | CHECK CONDITION OF AIR RECEIVER CONDENSATE TRAP. DRAIN AS NECESSARY | 7694 | | | | | |
| | | 7840 | | | | | |
| 6. | CLEAN OR REPLACE INTAKE AIR FILTER (JAN-JUL) | | | | | | |
| 7. | DISASSEMBLE COMPRESSOR VALVES. CLEAN OR REPLACE ALL PARTS AS NECESSARY - PER INSTRUCTIONS ON PAGE 25 OF I.R. INSTRUCTION FORM NO. 1050-H (JAN-JUL) | | | | | | |
| 8. | CHK. CONDITION OF DRIVE BELTS. REPLACE AS NECESSARY. CHECK TENSION. | | | | | | |
| 9. | CHK. CONDITION, SECURITY, SOUND-ELEC. MOTOR (LUBE-JAN G-1 GREASE) | | | | | | |
| 10. | CLEAN COMPRESSOR & RECEIVER WITH AIR JET (JAN-JUL) (EXTERNAL SURFACE OF CYLINDERS & INTERCOOLER TUBES) | | | | | | |

TORQUE CHECK ALL CAP SCREWS

| ITEM NO. | LOCATION OF CAP SCREWS (JAN-JUL) | QUANT. SCREW | TORQUE | CHECK OFF 7694 | CHECK OFF 7840 |
|---|---|---|---|---|---|
| 11. | CONSTANT SPEED UNLOADERS | | | | |
| 12. | AIR HEADS | | | | |
| 13. | CYLINDER BOLTS | | | | |
| 14. | SHAFT END COVER | | | | |
| 15. | CRANKCASE COVER PAN | | | | |
| 16. | DISCHARGE AIR MANIFOLD | | | | |
| 17. | | | | | |
| 18. | | | | | |
| 19. | | | | | |
| 20. | | | | | |

| ITEM NO. | POST ITEM NUMBER AND LIST MAINTENANCE TO BE DONE |
|---|---|
| | |
| | |
| | |
| | |
| | |

| | | |
|---|---|---|
| **(44.)** GRAIN TANK TRACK DROP SECTION "V" BUILDING | | Inspect For: Security-Safety-Operation-Condition |
| INSPECTION DEPT. - (862) | ACCT. NO. - 90059-**67** ORD. NO. - **759225** DEPT. NO. - **862** | If Item is O.K. use [✓] mark. If work is needed use [W] and explain. If inspector completes repair, use [R] and explain. |

DATE _____

INSPECTOR'S SIGNATURE _____

SUPERVISOR'S SIGNATURE _____

Inspector is to perform lubrications listed in each box at the time indicated.

| ITEM NO. | ITEM FOR INSPECTION | CHECK OFF LOCATION COL. F-19 9190 W. Line | COL. C-19 9191 E. Line | INSPECTOR'S COMMENTS |
|---|---|---|---|---|
| 1. | Drop Section Structural Members and Bolted & Welded Joints | | | |
| 2. | (4) Trolley End Trucks and (2) Drop Section Main Track | | | |
| 3. | Power and Free Drop Track Section with Hardware - Stops - Stop Actuators - Guides - Upper Stops - Carrier Release | | | |
| 4 | (4) Hoisting Cables and (2-Each) Connecting Points and Hardware | | | |
| 5. | Hoist Shaft - (2) Cable Drums - (4) Pillow Block Bearings. Grease Lube: Jan-Apr-July-Oct Use "G-1" Grease | | | |
| 6. | Hoist Shaft Worm Gear Reducer - (3) Drive Couplings - Hydraulic Motor Check Oil level - MONTHLY - Use "0-52" Change Oil in OCTOBER | | | |
| 7. | Hoist Shaft Cam Switch - Drive Sprockets & Chain Hand Oil - MONTHLY - "0-31" | | | |
| 8. | (4) Outboard - Hoist Cable Pulleys Grease - MONTHLY "G-14" | | | |
| 9. | Slack Cable Limit Switch | | | |
| 10. | Hydraulic Drive Unit-Check Oil Level-MONTHLY-Change Oil - OCTOBER "0-30" | | | |
| 11. | Horizontal Drive - (2) Drive Wheels-(6) Bearings - Drive Gear Box - Drive Motor. Grease Bearings-January&July "G-1" Chk.Gear Box Oil Level Monthly Change Oil - OCTOBER "0-48" *Oil* | | | |
| 12. | Electric Control Station with Strain Chain | | | |
| 13. | Power Cable Festoon | | | |
| | | | | |
| | | | | |
| | | | | |
| | | | | |

**113**

# 4—Acquiring Hazard Information

BUTLER MANUFACTURING COMPANY
WEEKLY INSPECTION OF FIRE PROTECTIVE EQUIPMENT
Kansas City Plant

Instructions: Fill out this blank while making inspection. Do not report a valve open unless you personally have inspected and tested it. Every valve controlling sprinklers or water supplies to sprinklers should be listed. When the blank is filled out, it should be sent to the Safety Department.

| Valve No. | AREA CONTROLLED | Location | Open | Shut | Sealed | Pressure |
|---|---|---|---|---|---|---|
| 1 | Entire West System | Bldg. 57 | | | | |
| 2 | Bldg. 43-43B | Bldg. 57 | | | | |
| 3 | Valves 4-5-6-7-8-9-10-11 | Bldg. 43 | | | | PIV |
| 4 | East End Bldg. 2-2B | Bldg. 2 | | | | |
| 5 | Center 2-2B, Paint Line | Bldg. 2 | | | | |
| 6 | West End Bldg. 2 | Bldg. 2 | | | | |
| 7 | Valves 8-9-10-11 | Bldg. 2 | | | | PIV |
| 8 | Valves 9-10-11 | Bldg. 62 | | | | |
| 9 | Bldg. 3 | Bldg. 62 | | | | |
| 10 | Bldg. 62-62B-6A-5C-5 | Bldg. 62 | | | | |
| 11 | Bldg. 4-4A-5-5A-5C | Bldg. 62 | | | | |
| 12 | Paint Booth P34KC | Bldg. 1 | | | | |
| 13** | Oven | Bldg. 1 | | | | |
| 14 | Paint Booth P57KC | Bldg. 1 | | | | |
| 15 | Paint Booth P58KC | Bldg. 1 | | | | |
| 16 | Paint Booth P59KC | Bldg. 1 | | | | |
| 17 | Paint Booth P56KC | Bldg. 1 | | | | |
| 18 | Locker Room Offices | Bldg. 67 | | | | |
| 19 | Laboratory Paint Room | Bldg. 58A | | | | |
| 20 | Paint Shop Bldg. 23 | Bldg. 23 | | | | |
| 21 | Bldg. 65 | Bldg. 65 | | | | |
| 22 | Paint Booth P49KC | Bldg. 63 | | | | |
| 23 | Paint Booth P710G | Bldg. 63 | | | | |
| 24 | Bldg. 17 | Bldg. 17 | | | | |
| 25 | Bldgs. 53-63 | Bldg. 17 | | | | |
| 26* | Bldg. 57 | Bldg. 57 | | | | |
| 27 | Bldg. 17A Offices | Bldg. 15 | | | | |
| 28 | Bldg. 17A Balcony | Bldg. 15 | | | | |
| 29 | Entire East System | 12th St. | | | | PIV |
| 30* | Bldg. 52 | Driveway | | | | PIV |
| 31* | Bldg. 46 | Driveway | | | | PIV |
| 32 | Valves 21-22-23-24-25 | Driveway | | | | PIV |
| | | | | | | |
| | | | | | | |
| | | | | | | |
| | | | | | | |
| | | | | | | |

SPRINKLER VALVES

\* Controls Dry System
\*\*Manually Operated, always shut

GENERAL CONDITIONS

HYDRANTS: In good condition? _____

Clear? _____ Remarks _____

_____

AUTOMATIC SPRINKLERS: Any heads missing? _____ Disconnected? _____

Obstructed by high-piled stock? _____

Any rooms not sufficiently heated

to prevent freezing? _____ How

many extra heads available? _____

SPRINKLER ALARMS: Tested? _____ In

good condition? _____ Do not test

hydraulic alarms when temperatures

are below freezing.

EXTINGUISHERS, SMALL HOSE: In good

condition? _____

FIRE DOORS: All inspected? _____

In good order? _____

HOUSEKEEPING: Good throughout? _____

Combustible waste removed before

night? _____

REMARKS on other matters relating to

fire hazard: _____

_____

_____

Date _____ Signed _____

*Courtesy Butler Manufacturing Company.*

114

# PITTSBURGH ROLLS CORPORATION
## CRANE INSPECTION REPORT

Crane No............................Type.......................... Capacity................................

### RUNWAY AND CONDUCTORS

Track Alignment.....................Spread.......................... Fastenings ...............................
Line Conductors....................................Conductor Supports...............................

### TRUCKS AND MAIN COLLECTORS

Truck Wheels, Flat Spots?.....................Flanges..........................End Play..........................
Axle Bearings..............................Lubrication ..........................
Truck Drive Bearings......................Lubrication.................. Gears ...............................
Gear Screws......................Pinion..........................Key.................. Collectors ...............................

### GIRDERS AND DRIVE

Drive Shaft....................Couplings...................Bearings.................. Lubrication ...............................
Foot Brake Shaft...................Couplings...................Bearings.................. Lubrication ...............................
Bridge Brake Case......................Adjustment.......................... Lubrication ...............................
Walkway.............................. Railing ........................ Ladder ...............................
Bridge Motor Support.......................Shaft Extension........................ Couplings ...............................
Bridge Drive Gear Case.......................Gears.............. Lubrication ...............................

### MOTORS

| Location | Armature | Commutator | Brushes | Brush Holders | Bearings | Lubrication |
|---|---|---|---|---|---|---|
| Bridge | | | | | | |
| Hoist | | | | | | |
| Aux. Hoist | | | | | | |
| Trolley | | | | | | |

### CONTROLLERS

| | Brushes | Brush Holders | Contacts | Wiring | Springs | Resistance |
|---|---|---|---|---|---|---|
| Bridge | | | | | | |
| Hoist | | | | | | |
| Aux. Hoist | | | | | | |
| Trolley | | | | | | |

Trolley Wheels....................Trolley Wheel Bearings.......................... Lubrication ...............................
Trolley Gear Case..............Case Support..............Gears.............. Lubrication ...............................
Hoist Gear Case..............Main Gear Train............Comp. Train..........Lubrication...............................
Mech. Brake.............Drift..............Elec. Brake............ Adjustment ..........Lubrication...............................
Drum................Cable or Chain.......................Cable Pin.................Limit Switch...............................
Limit Switch Adjustment...................Hook............. Sheaves ............Lubrication...............................
Trolley Conductors...................Trolley Collectors.....................Cage Roof....................Door...............................
Windows.................Foot Brake Treadle.......................Cont. Levers....................Load Test...............................
Bell or Signal...............................................................................................................
Inspected by............................................................ Date...............................

KEY WORDS—G=Good; F=Fair; W=Worn; A=Need Attention;
C=Need Cleaning; T=Too Tight

*Courtesy Pittsburgh Rolls Corporation.*

## 4—Acquiring Hazard Information

## STATIONARY SCAFFOLD SAFETY CHECK LIST

PROJECT: _____

ADDRESS: _____

CONTRACTOR: _____

DATE OF INSPECTION: _____  INSPECTOR:_____

| | Yes | No | Action/Comments |
|---|---|---|---|
| 1. Are scaffold components and planking in safe condition for use and is plank graded for scaffold use? | | | |
| 2. Is the frame spacing and sill size capable of carrying intended loadings? | | | |
| 3. Have competent persons been in charge of erection? | | | |
| 4. Are sills properly placed and adequate size? | | | |
| 5. Have screw jacks been used to level and plumb scaffold instead of unstable objects such as concrete blocks, loose bricks, etc.? | | | |
| 6. Are base plates and/or screw jacks in firm contact with sills and frame? | | | |
| 7. Is scaffold level and plumb? | | | |
| 8. Are all scaffold legs braced with braces properly attached? | | | |
| 9. Is guard railing in place on all open sides and ends above 10′ (4′ in height if less than 45″) | | | |
| 10. Has proper access been provided? | | | |
| 11. Has overhead protection or wire screening been provided where necessary? | | | |
| 12. Has scaffold been tied to structure at least every 30′ in length and 26′ in height? | | | |
| 13. Have free standing towers been guyed or tied every 26′ in height? | | | |
| 14. Have brackets and accessories been properly placed: Brackets? | | | |
| Putlogs? | | | |
| Tube and Clamp? | | | |
| All nuts and bolts tightened? | | | |
| 15. Is scaffold free of makeshift devices or ladders to increase height? | | | |
| 16. Are working level platforms fully planked between guard rails? | | | |
| 17. Does plank have minimum 12″ overlap and extend 6″ beyond supports? | | | |
| 18. Are toeboards installed properly? | | | |
| 19. Have hazardous conditions been provided for: Power lines? | | | |
| Wind loading? | | | |
| Possible washout of footings? | | | |
| Uplift and overturning moments due to placement of brackets, putlogs or other causes? | | | |
| 20. HAVE PERSONNEL BEEN INSTRUCTED IN THE SAFE USE OF THE EQUIPMENT? | | | |

*Courtesy Safway Steel Products, Milwaukee, Wis. Copyright 1974. (Used with permission.)*

The amount of detail included in the checklist will vary, depending upon the inspector's knowledge of the relevant standards and the nature of the inspection. An experienced inspector with thorough knowledge of the standards will need only sufficient clues to remind him of the items to be inspected. Checklists for infrequent inspections generally will be more detailed than daily or weekly ones.

Checklists should have columns to indicate either compliance or action-date. Space should be provided to cite the specific violation, a way to correct it, and a recommendation that the condition receive more or less frequent attention. Whatever the format of the checklist, space should be provided for the inspector's signature and the inspection date.

Checklists can be prepared by the safety and health committee, by the safety director, or by a subcommittee which includes engineers, supervisors, employees, and maintenance personnel. The safety professional and the department supervisor should monitor development of the checklists and make sure that they cover all applicable standards. In their final form the checklists should conform to the inspection route.

Choosing the inspection route means inspecting an area completely and thoroughly while avoiding:

Time-consuming backtracking and repetitions

Long walks between items

Unnecessary interruptions of the production process

Distracting employees.

Often a closed-loop inspection will give good results. Sometimes it may be valuable to follow the path of the material being processed.

## How often must items be inspected?

The frequency of inspection is determined by four factors.°

1. *What is the loss severity potential of the problem?* Ask yourself, "If the item or critical part should fail, what would happen? What injury, damage, or work interruption would result?" The greater the loss severity potential, the more often the item should be inspected. Because a frayed wire rope on an overhead crane block has the potential to cause a much greater loss than a defective wheel on a wheelbarrow, the rope needs to be inspected more frequently than the wheel.

2. *What is the potential for injury to employees?* If the item or critical part should fail, how many employees would be endangered and how frequently? The greater the probability for injury to employees, the more often the item should be inspected. For example, a stairway used continually by many people needs to be inspected more frequently than one that is seldom used.

3. *How quickly can the item or part become unsafe?* The answer to this question depends on the nature of the part and the conditions to which it is subjected. Equipment and tools that get heavy use can become damaged, defective, or worn more quickly than those used rarely. An item located in a particular spot may be exposed to greater damage than an identical item in a different location. The shorter the time in which it can become unsafe, the more frequently the item should be inspected.

4. *What is the past history of failures? What were the results of these failures?* Maintenance and production records and accident investigation reports can provide valuable information about how frequently items have failed and what were the results in terms of injuries, damage, delays, and shut-downs. The more frequently it failed in the past and the greater the consequences, the more often the item needs to be inspected.

OSHA regulations require inspections at specific intervals; for example, manlifts, not more than 30 days; limit switches, weekly. As a specific example, OSHA regulations dealing with cranes specify daily visual inspection of some aspects, monthly signed reports, semiannual inspection of standby cranes, and periodic inspection of other parts. According to OSHA, the intervals depend on "the nature of the critical components of the crane and the degree of their exposure to wear, deterioration, or malfunction."

The portfolio of checklists has two inspection

---

° Adapted from *Facility Inspection* (see References).

| DEPARTMENT Maintenance | UNIT Workshop | SUPERVISOR RESPONSIBLE J. P. Smith | APPROVED BY Ralph T. Welles | DATE 4/16/72 | PAGE NO. 1 |
|---|---|---|---|---|---|
| 1. PROBLEMS | 2. CRITICAL FACTORS | 3. CONDITIONS TO OBSERVE | 4. FREQUENCY | 5. RESPONSIBILITY | |
| 1. Overhead hoist | Cables, chains, hooks, pulleys | Frayed or deformed cables, worn or broken hooks and chains, damaged pulleys | Daily – before each shift | Operators | |
| 2. Hydraulic pump | High pressure hose | Leaks; broken or loose fittings | Daily | Shift leader | |
| 3. Power generator | High voltage lines | Frayed or broken insulation | Weekly | Foreman | |
| 4. Fire ex- tinguishers | Contents, location, charge | Correct type, fully charged, properly located, corrosion, leaks | Monthly | Area safety inspector | |
| 5. General house- keeping | Passageways, aisles, floors, grounds | Free of obstructions, clearly marked, free of refuse | Daily | Shift leader foreman | |

FIG. 4–7.—Responsibility for each inspection should be assigned in a hazard control inspection inventory. (U.S. Dept. of Labor, Booklet 2215.)

reports for cranes. These forms would meet the OSHA requirement for a monthly signed report. Note that the critical parts are listed and the specific conditions named.

Frequency of inspections should be described in specific terms: for example, before every use, when serviced, daily, monthly, quarterly, yearly.

## Who will conduct the inspection?

Answering the four previous questions—the items to be inspected, the aspects of each item to be inspected, the conditions to be inspected, and the frequency of inspections—will provide a pointer to the persons who are to do the inspecting. No individual or group has exclusive responsibility for inspections. Some things will have to be inspected by more than one person. For example, while an area supervisor may inspect an overhead crane weekly and maintenance personnel inspect it monthly, the operator of the crane will inspect it before each use. When grinding wheels are received, they are inspected by the stock room attendant, but they must be inspected again by the operator before they are used.

As part of the hazard control inspection inventory, responsibility for each inspection should be assigned. Fig. 4–7 shows how the inventory can designate the proper person by title: area supervisor, operator, foreman, maintenance foreman, and so forth.

A suggested guide for planned inspections is as follows:

*Daily*—area supervisor and maintenance personnel; they can also request suggestions from employees in their various work stations.

*Weekly*—department heads

*Monthly*—supervisors, department heads, the safety department, and safety and health committees.

The safety department also may be actively involved in monthly, quarterly, semiannual, and annual inspections.

Five qualifications of a good inspector are:

1. Knowledge of the organization's accident experience

2. Familiarity with accident potentials and with the standards that apply to his area

3. Ability to make intelligent decisions for corrective action

4. Diplomacy in handling personnel and situations.

5. Knowledge of the organization's operations—its workflow, systems, and products.

**Safety professionals.** Clearly the safety professional spearheads the inspection activity. During inspections, whether conducted individually or as part of a group, he can perform an educational function. By using on-the-spot examples and with firsthand contact, supervisors, foremen, and stewards can be taught the fundamentals of hazard identification. Safety and health committeees also can be taught what to look for in making inspections. If there is a fire protection representative or an industrial hygienist in the organization, he will work with the hazard control specialist in inspections.

The number of safety professionals depends on the size of the company and the nature of its operation. Large companies with well organized accident prevention programs usually employ a full-time staff. Sometimes large companies may also have specially designated employees who spend part of their time on inspections.

In organizations where toxic and corrosive substances are present, the industrial hygienist will be part of the inspection team (see also the following section on Measurement and Testing). When an organization uses chemicals, the chief chemist will need to work in close cooperation with the safety professional and fire protection representative in establishing inspection criteria. If the organization has no industrial hygienist, the safety professional must possess special training so that he knows the hazardous properties of the substances, unstable properties of chemicals, and the methods of control. An inspection conducted without this knowledge is only perfunctory.

**Company or plant management.** Safety inspections should be considered part of the duties of company or plant management. By participating in inspections, management evidences its commitment to assuring a safe working environment. But the psychological effects of inspection by senior executives goes beyond merely showing an interest in safety. When employees know that management is coming to inspect their area, things get straightened up in a hurry! Conditions which previously seemed "good enough" quickly are found unsatisfactory and corrective action is taken.

# 4—Acquiring Hazard Information

**First-line supervisor or foreman.** Because supervisors and foremen spend practically all their time in the shop or plant, they are continually monitoring the workplace. At least once a day, supervisors need to check their areas to see that (a) employees are complying with safety regulations, (b) guards and warning signs are in place, (c) tools and machinery are in a safe condition, (d) aisles and passageways are clear and proper clearances maintained, and (e) material in process is properly stacked or stored. Although such a spot check does not take the place of more detailed inspections, it emphasizes the supervisor's commitment to maintaining safety in his area. A supervisor should also conduct regular formal inspections to make certain that all hazards have been detected and that safeguards are in use. Such inspections may be performed weekly as an individual and monthly as part of a safety and health committee.

**Mechanical engineer and maintenance superintendent.** Either as individuals or as members of a committee, the mechanical engineer and the maintenance superintendent also need to conduct regular formal inspections. Necessary work orders for guards or for correcting faulty equipment can be written up on the spot.

**Employees.** As mentioned previously, employee participation in continuous inspection is one goal of an effective hazard control program. Before beginning the work day, the employee should inspect his workplace and the tools, equipment, and machinery that are used. He should immediately report to his supervisor defects that he is not authorized to correct.

**Maintenance personnel.** Maintenance employees can be of great help in locating and correcting hazards. As they work, they can conduct informal inspections and report hazards to the supervisor, who in turn should encourage mechanics to offer suggestions.

**Joint safety and health committees.** Joint safety and health committees (discussed in the previous chapter) conduct inspections as part of their function. They give equal consideration to accident, fire, and health exposures. By visiting areas periodically, members notice changed conditions more readily than someone who is there every day. Another advantage provided by the committee is the various backgrounds, experience, and knowledge represented.

If the committee is large, the territory should be divided among teams of manageable size. Large groups going through the plant are unwieldy and distracting. See the Council's *You Are the Safety and Health Committee.*

**Other inspection teams.** If there is no safety and health committee, a planned formal inspection is still necessary. An inspection team must be assigned, a team that includes the hazard control specialist, production manager, supervisor, employee representative, fire prevention specialist, and industrial hygienist. The important point is that inspections should be under the direction of a responsible executive who will provide the authority necessary to assure effectiveness.

**Outside inspectors** from outside the organization, such as insurance company safety engineers and local, state or provincial, and federal inspectors, may perform inspections.

**Contractors' inspection services.** For some particularly technical systems, notably sprinkler systems, contracting companies furnish inspection services. Companies that do not have qualified safety professionals and a well-established maintenance program can avail themselves of such services.

An example will show how such services operate. A sprinkler contractor arranges with the customer for periodic inspection and test of sprinkler equipment. Frequency of inspection is negotiated between the contractor and the client. In some cases, the inspection can include other items, such as fire extinguishers, hoses, or fire doors. The contractor furnishes a comprehensive written report. The client can request that the contractor send copies of the report to the insurer.

The basic contract does not include maintenance work or materials required for alterations, repairs, or replacement. However, if the report indicates any maintenance needs, the client can have the contractor perform the work.

Although contract service does not relieve management of its primary responsibility for inspection and maintenance, it does provide excellent inspection for small companies, buildings with mixed tenants, and companies with systems too complex for inspection by its own maintenance staff.

## Conducting Inspections

### Preparing to inspect

Inspections should be scheduled at a time that will allow a maximum opportunity to view operations and work practices, with minimum interruption of them. The route to be followed will be planned in advance.

Before making an inspection, the inspector or inspection team should review all accidents that have occurred in the area. At this brief meeting, team members should discuss where they are going and for what they are looking. During the inspection itself, it will be necessary to "huddle" before going into noisy areas in order to avoid arm waving, shouting, and other unsatisfactory methods of communication.

In addition to the regular checklist and accident reports, inspectors should have copies of the previous inspection report for that particular area. Reviewing this report makes it possible to check whether earlier recommendations have been followed and hazards corrected.

Those making inspections should wear the protective equipment required in the areas they enter: safety glasses and shoes, hard hats, acid-proof goggles, protective gloves, respirators, gas masks, and so forth. If inspectors do not have and cannot get special protective equipment, they should not go into the area. They must be careful to "practice what they preach."

Inspectors also should be aware of any special hazards they may encounter. For example, because welding crews and other maintenance crews move from place to place, they may be encountered anywhere in the plant. Inspectors should know what precautions are necessary where these crews are working.

### Relationship of inspector and supervisor

Before inspecting a particular department or area, the inspector should contact the department head, supervisor, foreman, or other person in charge. This person may have information which is important for the inspection, particularly when conditions are temporarily altered because of construction, maintenance, equipment downtime, employee absence, and so forth.

If no rules prohibit it, the person in charge may want to accompany the inspector. Tactfully, the inspector may agree, but will make it clear that no tour guide is needed. The inspector must preserve his independence and make his own observations.

If the supervisor of the area does not accompany the inspector, he should be consulted before the inspector leaves the area. The inspector should discuss each recommendation with the supervisor. Usually an agreement can be reached as to the relative importance of a recommendation. Obviously an inspector should not pick numerous trivial items merely to make the report look good. On the other hand, the inspector does not have the authority to pass up any condition that might result in an accident.

When the supervisor fully understands what is required, he may be able to make corrections quickly and may suggest that the matter need not be reported. Nevertheless the written report should include all items, though it can be noted that the supervisor promises to correct a particular condition. That keeps the record clear and serves as a reminder to check the condition during the next inspection.

An inspector cannot fail to report hazards because a supervisor interprets such reporting as criticism. If a supervisor becomes defensive or resentful, the inspector can only repeat what the supervisor knows: that the purpose of inspection is fact-finding, not fault finding. By retaining his objectivity and refusing to let the issue of safety degenerate into the issue of personality, the inspector keeps matters on the proper professional footing. His attitude should be firm, friendly, and fair.

Sometimes a supervisor may request the inspector's assistance in recommending new equipment, reassignment of space, or transfer of certain jobs from one department to another. When these suggestions deal with safety, the inspector will want to include them in his notes and consider whether to make them part of his report. However the inspector must be careful not to promise either a supervisor or an employee more than he actually can deliver. For example, if a member of the safety and health committee promises that a machine will be replaced by one with an automatic feed and then learns that the funds for equipment replacement in the current budget have all been designated, he unwittingly will have undermined the credibility of the committee.

### Relationship of inspector and employee

Unless company policy or departmental rules prohibit conversation with employees, the inspector may ask questions about operations, being careful, however, not to usurp the responsibility of the supervisor. If, for example, a member of a safety and health committee sees an employee who seems to be working unsafely, it is better to ask the supervisor than the employee about the supposed infraction. The committee member may not fully understand the operation and may be incorrect in his assumption. In another case, the employee may be committing an unsafe act sanctioned by those in authority and could defend himself by arguing that he is only doing what he has been told to do. It is the supervisor's job to require compliance with regulations; it is the inspector's job to do the inspecting and reporting. If, however, the situation appears to present an immediate danger, the employee should be notified.

Chapter 3 differentiated between deviations from accepted practices and workplace-induced human error. The inspection team needs to look for both. The inspector is not concerned with identifying the person who is responsible for the unsafe behavior (fault-finding). His goal is to identify the behavior (fact-finding) and see that it is corrected.

Unsafe behaviors will vary from one area to another. Among common items that might be noted are the following:

1. Using machinery or tools without authority

2. Operating at unsafe speeds or in other violation of safe work practice

3. Removing guards or other safety devices or rendering them ineffective

4. Using defective tools or equipment or using tools or equipment in unsafe ways

5. Using hands or body instead of tools or push sticks

6. Overloading, crowding, or failing to balance materials or handling materials in other unsafe ways, including improper lifting

7. Repairing or adjusting equipment that is in motion, under pressure, or electrically charged

8. Failing to use or maintain (or using improperly) personal protective equipment or safety devices

9. Creating unsafe, unsanitary, or unhealthy conditions by improper personal hygiene, using compressed air for cleaning clothes, poor housekeeping, or smoking in unauthorized areas

10. Standing or working under suspended loads, scaffolds, shafts, or open hatches.

Because the inspector's purpose is to locate unsafe acts, not pinpoint blame, the report should not specify any names. When the report states, "An employee in this area was observed . . . " the supervisor has been advised of the need to enforce safe work practices. The inspector should not be seen as a policeman handing out tickets or, worse, as a snooper from "outside." Information derived from inspections should not be used for punitive measures.

Sometimes it is necessary to observe closely workers at work in order to understand a task. The inspector should explain to the worker the need to observe the task and ask his permission to watch him as he works. When an employee understands that no one is trying to catch him in an error but that, because of his skill, he has been chosen to demonstrate a task, he probably will agree to the observation.

## Recording hazards

Inspectors should locate and describe each hazard found during inspection. A clear description of the hazard should be written down and questions and details recorded for later use. It is important to determine which hazards present the most serious consequences and are most likely to occur. The hazard-ranking scheme described in Chapter 3 will simplify the job of classifying hazards.

Properly classifying hazards places them in the right perspective. A significant benefit is that potential consequences and the probability of such consequences occurring are described without the need for long narrative description. Management should be able to understand and evaluate the problems, assign priorities, and quickly reach decisions.

Unsafe conditions or deviations from accepted practices must be described in detail. Machines and operations must be identified by their correct names. Locations must be accurately named or numbered. Specific hazards must be described. Instead of noting "poor housekeeping," for example, the report should give the details: "Empty pallets left in aisles, slippery spots on the floor from oil leaks, a ladder lying across empty boxes, scrap piled on the floor around machines."

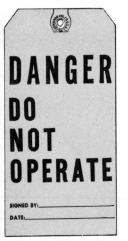

FIG. 4–8.—Front and back views of typical tag used when equipment is taken out of service because it has become unsafe.

Instead of noting "guard missing," the report should read, "Guard missing on shear blade of No. 3 machine, SW corner of Bldg. D."

Some plan should be adopted to note intermediate or permanent corrective measures. For example, if intermediate safety measures have been taken, the item could be circled. When permanent measures are taken, the item can be crossed out or marked with an X. Such a system identifies those items requiring further corrective action.

If the inspection is being performed by a committee, one member can be given the task of keeping notes. Without such notes it is almost impossible to write a satisfactory inspection report.

## Condemning equipment

When a piece of equipment presents an imminent danger, the inspector should immediately notify the supervisor and see to it that the machine or equipment is shut down, tagged, or locked out to prevent its further use. Fig. 4–8 shows both sides of a danger tag that can be used to prevent further use of equipment or materials that have become unsafe through wear, abuse, or defects.

When danger tags are used, those persons authorized to condemn equipment must sign them. Only the inspector who places the tag should be permitted to remove it and only when he is satisfied that the hazardous condition has been corrected.

Lockouts may also be necessary. Before equipment is worked on, the main switch or power source must be locked out. For more on lockouts, see Chapters 8 and 15, *Engineering and Technology* volume of this Manual.

No equipment or materials should be placed out of service without notifying the person in authority in the department affected.

## Writing the inspection report

Every inspection must be followed by a clearly written report. Without a complete and accurate report, the inspection would be little more then an interesting sightseeing tour. Inspection reports are usually of three types:

1. *Emergency*—made without delay when a critical or catastrophic hazard is probable. Using the classification system described in Chapter 3, this category would include any items marked IA or IIA.

2. *Periodic*—covers those unsatisfactory nonemergency conditions observed during the planned periodic inspection. This report should be made within 24 hours of the inspection. Periodic reports may be initial, followup, final, or a combination of all three.

3. *Summary*—lists all items of previous periodic reports for a given time.

The written report should include the name of the department or area inspected (giving the boundaries or location if needed), date and time of inspection, names and titles of those performing the inspection, date of the report, and the names of those to whom the report was made.

One way to make the report is to begin by copying items carried over from the last report because permanent corrective measures had not been taken. Each item is numbered consecutively. The item number can be followed by the hazard classification (IB, IIIC, etc.). Carry-over items can be marked with an asterisk. The narrative should include the date the hazard was first detected. Each hazard should be described and its location given. After the hazard is listed, the recommended corrective action should be specified and a definite abatement date be established. There should follow a space for noting corrective action taken later. Fig. 4–9 is a sample of an

**123**

INSPECTION REPORT

Area Inspected __Building D__

Date and Time of Inspection __11/19/30 – 11:00 a.m.__

Inspector and Title __Ron Baker, Hazard Control Specialist__

Date of Report __11/20/80__

Names of Those to Whom Report Is Sent: __Bob Firenze (Executive Director); Loren Hall (Department Head); file__

No. of Items Carried Over from Previous Report __3__    No. of Items Added to This Report __4__    Total No. of Items on This Report __7__

| Item (asterisk indicates old item) | Hazard Classification | | Hazard Description | Specific Location | Supervisor | Corrective Action Recommended | Corrective Action Taken |
|---|---|---|---|---|---|---|---|
| | Conse- quence | Proba- bility | | | | | |
| *1 | II | B | Guard missing on shear blade #2 machine. Work order issued to engineering for new guard 10/16/80. Wooden barrier guard in temporary use 10/23/79. Guard still missing. | S.W. corner, bay #1 | Jay Rillo | Contact engineering to replace guard | Engineering says they will have guard by 11/24. |
| *2 | IV | C | Window cracked. Work order issued for replacement 10/30/80. | South wall, bay #3 | Joe Whitestone | Have maintenance replace window | maintenance to replace all broken windows starting next week. |
| (3) | II | B | Oil and trash still accumulated under main motor. Was to be cleaned by 10/30/80. | Pump room | Tony Silva | Clean area; have supervisor talk to men | Cleaned out 11/21. Silva told men to keep area clean. |
| 4 | III | B | Mirror at pedestrian walk out of line | North end of machine shop | Tom Schroeder | Post temporary warning sign; call maintenance for adjustment | Sign posted 11/21- Butler has scheduled adjustment for 11/1. |
| 5 | II | A | Three workers at cleaning tank not wearing eye protection | Electric shop | Hank Beine | Have supervisor give more training and education | Discussed with Beine - he held meeting on 11/25. |
| 6 | I | A | Cable on jib crane badly frayed | Bay #3 | Joe Whitestone | IMMEDIATE ACTION REQUIRED | Tapped crane out of service Cable to be replaced 11/21. |
| 7 | II | B | Guard rail damaged on stairway to second floor | Bay #1 | Jay Rillo | Issue work order to carpenter shop to make replacement | Work order issued 11/21. |

FIG. 4-9.—Inspection report form simplifies procedures, and emphasizes carryovers, new items, and responsibilities. Column at right is for noting corrective action taken later.

Courtesy RJF Associates, Inc., Bloomington, Ind.

inspection report made by the organization's hazard control specialist after his weekly inspection. A report should show what is right as well as wrong.

When the report is that of a committee, it is well to have it checked by each member of the inspection team for accuracy, clarity, and thoroughness.

Generally inspection reports are directed to the head of the department or area where the inspection was made. Copies are also directed to executive management and/or the manager to whom the department head reports.

## Followup for corrective action

When the inspection report is written and disseminated, the inspection process starts to return benefits. The information acquired and the recommendations made are without value unless corrective action is taken. Information and recommendations provide the basis for establishing priorities and implementing programs that will reduce accidents, improve conditions, raise morale, and increase the efficiency and effectiveness of the operation.

Recommendations can be listed in the order in which the hazards were discovered or grouped according to the individual responsible for their compliance. Recommendations are then sent to the proper official for approval. Where possible, a definite time limit for compliance should be set for each recommendation, and followed up.

Often the safety professional is authorized to make recommendations directly to the affected foreman, supervisor, or department if such recommendations do not require major capital outlay. One company has simplified the process of making individual safety recommendations by devising special forms (see Fig. 4–10). These forms—which have a carbon attached so that the safety department can keep its records intact—provide a convenient followup file.

Some organizations require that inspection reports be reviewed by the safety and health committee, particularly when recommendations apply to education and training and directly affect employees.

In making recommendations, inspectors should be guided by four rules. (*Facility Inspection*, 1973.)

• Correct the cause whenever possible. Do not merely correct the result, leaving the problem

intact. In other words, be sure you are curing the disease, not just the symptom. If you do not have the authority to correct the real cause, bring it to the attention of the person who does.

• Correct immediately everything possible. If the inspector has been granted the authority and opportunity to take direct corrective action, take it. Delays risk accidents.

• Report conditions beyond your authority and suggest solutions. Relay to management the condition, the potential consequences or hazards found, and solutions for correction. Even when nothing seems to come of a recommendation, it may pay unexpected dividends. A company safety and health committee made a detailed proposal about guarding a particularly hazardous location, only to be told that the engineers had planned to move operations to another location. However, instead of feeling that it had wasted its time, the committee pointed out that organization had serious communication problems, with the right hand not knowing what the left was doing. The committee recommended that effective management techniques be applied to the hazard control program.

• Take intermediate action as needed. When permanent correction takes time, don't simply ignore the hazard. Take any temporary measures you can, such as roping off the area, tagging out equipment or machines, or posting warning signs. These measures may not be ideal, but they are preferable to doing nothing.

Some of the general categories into which recommendations might fall are setting up a better process, relocating a process, redesigning a tool or fixture, changing the operator's work pattern, providing personal protective equipment, and improving personnel training methods. Recommendations may also call for improvements in the system of preventive maintenance and in housekeeping. Cleaning up a lot of dirt may be considered the janitor's job, but *preventing* its accumulation is part of the hazard control program.

Management must realize that employees follow with keen interest the attention it pays to correcting faulty conditions and hazardous procedures. Recommendations approved by management should become part of the organization's program. At regular intervals, supervisors should report progress in complying with the recommen-

---

### SAFETY RECOMMENDATION No. 1053

Date Issued_____19__

Date Ret'd. _____19__

To_____

PLEASE HAVE THE FOLLOWING UNSAFE CONDITION OR
DEVIATION FROM STANDARD PROCEDURE CORRECTED:

_____

_____

_____

_____

Please sign and return to Safety Department within ten days, indicating
below what disposition was made of this recommendation.

SAFETY DEPARTMENT

RECOMMENDATION FOLLOWED ( )   WORK COMPLETED_____
                                                DATE

RECOMMENDATION REJECTED ( )   FOR FOLLOWING REASON:_____

_____

Copy of this recommendation is on
file in the Safety Department. The
Safety Department is instructed to
send a detailed list of all un-
answered recommendations more
than ten days old to the General
Superintendent the first of each     _____
period.                              (SIGNED) DEPARTMENT SUPERINTENDENT

---

FIG. 4–10.—Special form is padded, numbered in pairs, and carboned in order to save office work and permit followup until
recommended work is complete or procedure correction is made.

*Adapted from Tennessee Eastman Corporation form.*

dations to the safety department, the company safety and health committee, or the person designated by management to receive such information. Inspectors should check periodically to see what progress is being made in taking corrective action.

Sometimes management will have to decide among several courses of action. Often these decisions will be based on cost effectiveness. For example, it may be effective and practical, from the standpoint of cost, to substitute a less toxic material that works as well as the highly toxic substance presently in use. On the other hand, replacing a costly but hazardous machine may have to wait until funds can be designated. In this case, the immediate alternative may be to install machine guards.

## Measurement and Testing

Two special sorts of inspection are those made by the industrial hygienist and the medical staff. Testing for exposures to health hazards requires special equipment not always available to the hazard control specialist. Conducting physical examinations of employees exposed to occupational health hazards may require apparatus not available to the organization's medical staff. In such cases assistance frequently can be secured from the industrial hygiene division of the state or provincial department of labor and health. Another source of help can be the industrial hygienists employed by consulting firms and by insurance companies.

The following discussion is a summary of recognition, evaluation, and control of health hazards; details are in *Fundamentals of Industrial Hygiene* (see References). It should help in understanding the role of the safety professional.

### Kinds of measurement and testing

Occupational health surveillance monitors chemical, physical, and biological agents. Four monitoring systems are used: personal, environmental, biological, and medical.

**Personal monitoring.** One example of personal monitoring is measuring the airborne concentrations of contaminants. The measurement device is placed as closely as possible to the site at which the contaminant enters the human body. When the contaminant is noise, the device is placed close to the ear. When a toxic substance is inhaled, the device is placed close to the breathing zone.

**Environmental monitoring.** Environmental monitoring measures contaminant concentrations in the workroom. The measurement device is placed in the general area adjacent to the worker's normal work station or where it can sample the general room air.

OSHA regulations require both personal and environmental monitoring for asbestos exposure.

**Biological monitoring.** Biological monitoring measures changes in composition of body fluid, tissues, or expired air in order to detect the level of absorption of a contaminant. For example, blood or urine may be tested to determine excessive lead absorption. The phenol in urine may be measured to determine excessive benzene absorption.

**Medical monitoring.** When medical personnel examine workers to see their physiological and psychological response to a contaminant, the process is termed medical monitoring. Medical monitoring may include health and work histories, physical examinations, X-rays, blood and urine tests, pulmonary function tests, and vision and hearing tests. The aim of such monitoring is to find evidence of exposure early enough to identify the person especially susceptible and to identify damage before it is irreversible.

Biological and medical monitoring provide information "after the fact." The exposure already has occurred. However, such programs also encompass arrangement to treat an identified health problem and to take corrective action to prevent further damage.

To understand how industrial hygienists measure for health hazards, it is necessary to define some basic terms, to distinguish between acute and chronic effects, and to see how safe exposure levels are established.

### Measuring for toxicity

**Toxicity.** The toxicity of a material is not identical with its potential for being a health hazard. *Toxicity* is the capacity of a material to produce injury or harm. *Hazard* is the possibility that exposure to a material will cause injury and/or illness when a specific quantity is used under certain conditions. The key elements to be considered when evaluating a health hazard are:

1. The amount of material required to be in contact with a body cell in order to produce an injury

2. The total time of contact necessary

3. The probability that the material will be absorbed or come in contact with body cells

4. The rate of generation of airborne contaminants

5. The control measures in use.

Not all toxic materials are hazardous. The majority of toxic chemicals are safe when packaged in their original shipping containers or contained within a closed system. As long as toxic materials are adequately controlled, they can be used safely. For example, many solvents, if not used properly, will cause irritation to eyes, mouth, and throat. Some are also intoxicating and can cause blistering of the skin and other forms of dermatitis. Prolonged exposure may cause more serious illness or genetic changes. But if the solvents are used in a well-ventilated area and the person is provided with protective equipment that prevents the substance from coming in contact with skin, then they can be used without being a hazard.

The toxic action of a substance can be divided into acute and chronic effects:

• *Acute effects.* These involve short-term, high concentrations which cause irritation, illness, or death. They are the result of sudden and severe exposure, during which the substance is rapidly absorbed. Usually acute effects are related to an accident, which disrupts ordinary processes and controls. For example, sudden exposure to a high concentration of zinc oxide fumes in the welding shop can cause acute poisoning.

• *Chronic effects.* These involve continued exposure to a toxic substance over a long time period. When the chemical is absorbed more rapidly than the body can eliminate it, accumulation in the body begins. Since the level of contaminant is relatively low, any effects, even if they are serious and irreversible, may go unnoticed for long periods of time. For example, breathing even low concentrations of carbon monoxide for long periods of time can cause damage to the heart muscles and blood vessels.

**Inhalation as a mode of entry.** In order for a hazardous substance to exert its toxic effects, it must come into contact with a body cell. Chemical compounds—as liquids, gases, mists, dusts, fumes, and vapors—enter the body in three ways:

Ingestion

Skin absorption, and

Inhalation.

Inhalation is a particularly important mode of entry because of the rapidity with which a toxic material can be absorbed in the lungs, pass into the bloodstream, and reach the brain. Had the same material been ingested instead of inhaled, it would have been considerably diluted with the contents of the stomach. Inhalation hazards arise from excessive concentration of mists, vapors, gases, or solids that are in the form of dusts or fumes.

Depending upon the solubility of the material, inhalation of chemical agents may irritate the upper respiratory tract, including the mucous membranes, or it may harm the terminal passages of the lungs and air sacs. Inhaled contaminants fall into three general categories:

1. Particulates which, when deposited in the lungs, may produce rapid local tissue damage, slower tissue reaction, disease, or physical plugging (for example, asbestos fiber)

2. Toxic vapors and gases that produce adverse reaction in the tissue of the lungs (for example, hydrogen fluoride)

3. Aerosols and gases that do not affect the lung tissue locally but may either

   a. Pass from the lungs into the bloodstream, where they are carried to other body organs (for example, cadmium oxide fumes)

   b. Affect adversely the oxygen-carrying capacity of the blood cells themselves (for example, carbon monoxide).

**Threshold Limit Values.** Individual susceptibility to respiratory toxins is difficult to assess. Nevertheless certain safe limits can be established. A Threshold Limit Value (TLV) refers to airborne concentrations of substances and represents an exposure level under which most people can work, day after day, without adverse effect.

Because of wide variations in individual susceptibility, however, an occasional exposure of an individual at or even below the threshold limit may not prevent discomfort, aggravation of a preexisting condition, or occupational illness.

The term TLV refers specifically to limits published by the American Conference of Governmental Industrial Hygienists. These TLV limits are reviewed and updated each year. The National Safety Council's *Fundamentals of Industrial Hygiene* explains this subject in detail. A brief overview follows. There are three categories of Threshold Limit Values:

1. *Time-Weighted Average* (TLV-TWA) is the time-weighted average concentration for a normal eight-hour day or 40-hour week. Nearly all persons can be exposed day after day to airborne concentrations at these limits without adverse effect.

2. *Short-Term Exposure Limit* (TLV-STEL) is the maximal concentration to which persons can be exposed for a period of up to 15 minutes continuously without suffering:

    a. Irritation

    b. Chronic or irreversible tissue change

    c. Narcoses of sufficient degree to reduce reaction time, impair self-rescue, or materially reduce work efficiency. No more than four 15-minute exposure periods per day are permitted with at least 60 minutes between exposure periods.

3. *Ceiling* (TLV-C) is the concentration that should not be exceeded even instantaneously.

**Permissible exposure levels.** The first compilation of health and safety standards from the U.S. Department of Labor's Occupational Safety and Health Administration appeared in 1970. Because it was derived from then-existing standards, it adopted many of the TLVs established in 1968 by the American Conference of Governmental Industrial Hygienists. Thus Threshold Limit Values—a registered trademark of the ACGIH—became, by federal standards, permissible exposure limits (PELs). These PELs represent the legal maximum level of contaminants in the air of the workplace.

The General Industry OSHA Standards as they were in effect on November 7, 1978, are summarized in OSHA Publication 2206. There are about 400 substances for which exposure limits have been established. These are now included in subpart Z, "Toxic and Hazardous Substances," Sections 1910.1000 through 1910.1500.

Most of these exposure limits are tabulated in section 1910.1000. Tables Z–1 and Z–3 in that regulation were originally part of the 1968 TLV list of ACGIH. These limits already had been adopted by the U.S. Department of Labor under provisions of the Walsh-Healey Act before passage of the OSHAct of 1970. Table Z–2 contains limits developed by the American National Standards Institute (ANSI). Sections 6(a) and 4(b) of the OSHAct gave OSHA authority to promulgate these previously established standards without the hearings and waiting periods required in Section 6(b). This authority ended in April 1973, two years after the effective date of the act.

Sections 1910.1001 through 1910.1500 give more detailed standards regarding individual substances. These standards have been developed in conformance with Section 6(b) of the OSHAct. They have been contested by the affected parties in many cases in the U.S. Courts of Appeals. Some of the substances included in this group are asbestos, vinyl chloride, inorganic arsenic, acrylonitrile, cotton dust, and coke oven emissions.

Section 1910.1000 is reproduced in full as Appendix A-2 in the Council's *Fundamentals of Industrial Hygiene*, 2nd ed.. Refer to this book for details on air sampling and industrial toxicology, which are briefly reviewed in this chapter.

**Action level.** A fairly new term has resulted from the Standards Completion Program, a joint effort of NIOSH, OSHA, and the Department of Labor Solicitor's Office. The *action level* is that point at which employers must initiate certain provisions: employee exposure measurement, employee training, and medical surveillance. The action level is defined as one-half of the permissible exposure.

Why is the action level set well below the PEL? Simply stated, setting the action level at one-half the permissible exposure protects employees from overexposure. It provides optimum employee protection with the minimum burden to the employer. Where employee exposure measurements indicate that no employee is exposed to airborne concentrations of a substance in excess of the action level, employers in effect are exempted from initiating certain provisions.

In other words, unless there is a change in production, process, or control measures that could result in an increase in airborne concentrations, employers are not required to monitor employees, provide special training, or provide medical histories. Furthermore, linking the action level to the permissible exposure level avoids confusion and simplifies the measurement.

The action level recognizes that air samples can only estimate the true time-weighted averages. Both employer and employee can be confident that, if the measured exposure level falls *below* the action level, then there is a very high probability that the actual exposure level is below the permissible exposure level. Statistical probability suggests that exposure below the action level will not harm the employee.

## When to measure?

The measurements done by the industrial hygienist can be divided into three phases.

1. Problem definition phase
2. Problem analysis phase
3. Solution phase.

**Problem definition phase.** Frequently measurement is done to see whether there *is* a problem. Because regulations require measurement at certain specified intervals or any time there is a change in production, process, or control measures, measurement often establishes that there is no excessive exposure. Such monitoring of the workplace assures a safe environment.

Monitoring, then, frequently determines that employers are in compliance with OSHAct requirements, state or provincial regulations, commonly accepted standards, Threshold Limit Values, permissible exposure levels, and action levels. Standards published by OSHA usually state:

Each employer who has a place of employment in which [toxic substance name] is released into the workplace air shall determine if there is any possibility that any employee may be exposed to airborne concentrations of [toxic substance name] above the permissible level. The initial determination shall be made each time there is a change in production, process, or control measures that may result in an increase in air-borne concentrations of [toxic substance name.]

When any of the regulated substances are released into the workplace air, the employer must take the first step in the employee exposure monitoring program. He must make an actual exposure determination to see whether any employee may be exposed to concentrations in excess of the action level. This written determination is required even if there is little chance that any employee may be exposed at a level above the permissible exposure level. The exposure determination can be a simple calculation based on such factors as the amount of the substance present, the size of the workplace, the amount and type of ventilation, and the proximity of the employee to the source of the contamination. The written determination is the result of a survey of the workplace. It takes into account:

1. The nature of the substance or agent
2. The intensity of the exposure
3. The duration of the exposure.

Should the measurement determine that an employee might be exposed above the action level, then the employer is required to take the second step in the monitoring program. He is required to determine exposure by taking airborne concentration samples.

But where does sampling begin? Should the sample be taken at the worker's breathing zone? Out in the general air? At the machine or process that is putting out the toxic substance? Air at all three sites should be sampled.

Should the sample be taken for two seconds, two hours, or a whole day? There are two major types of samples:

• *The grab sample*, taken over so short a period of time that the atmospheric concentration is assumed to be constant throughout the sample. This usually will be less than five minutes and usually will cover only part of an industrial cycle. Frequently a series of grab samples will be taken in an attempt to define the total exposure.

• *The long-term sample*, taken over a sufficiently long period of time so that the variations in exposure cycles are averaged.

An adequate number of tests should be taken to define the time-weighted average exposure, in order to relate this to OSHA's permissible exposure levels. But samples also must be taken to characterize the peak emissions during various portions of the process cycle.

When samples indicate that any employee may be exposed at or above the action level, then the employer must take the next higher step in the measurement program. He must make an exposure measurement of the employee who seems to be receiving the greatest exposure. This measurement should represent the maximum eight-hour, time-weighted average exposure of the employee.

When employee measurements indicate exposure at or above the action level, then all employees exposed at or above the action level must be identified and their exposure measured. The population at risk is thus identified. Employees whose exposure measurements exceed the action level need to have medical examinations.

When exposure measurements are at or above action level but not above PEL, the employer needs some statistically reliable means to be certain that exposures exceeding the PEL are not occurring. A sampling every two to three months would be minimal. Medical examinations are necessary to determine if any especially susceptible individuals are exhibiting effects at exposures between the action and permissible levels.

If employees are exposed above the PEL, then a more intensive monitoring program is necessary. Monthly measurements are needed to see that over-exposures do not occur. Medical examinations are required to measure the health effects on those employees exposed in excess of the PEL. Noninhalation exposures—such as skin absorption—also may occur. Therefore, accurate exposure evaluation may require breath, blood, and urine sampling.

The problem definition phase is one of orderly progression. At each step of increasing duties many employers will ascertain that they do not need to proceed to the next higher step.

Only a small number of employers with significant employee exposure problems will need to perform the final steps of the monitoring program.

**Problem analysis phase.** Once the problem has been defined in the first phase of the measurement process, the causes of the problem must be determined. Opportunities for improvement must be identified. The objectives of the solutions must be set. Alternative solutions needs to be determined.

The following nine methods suggest some ways that exposure hazards can be controlled:

1. Substitution of a less harmful material for one that is dangerous to health

2. Change or alteration of a process to minimize worker contact

3. Isolation or enclosure of a process or work operation to reduce the number of persons exposed

4. Wet methods to reduce generation of dust in operations

5. General or dilution ventilation with clean air to provide a safe atmosphere

6. Local exhaust at the point of generation or local dispersion of contaminants

7. Personal protective devices (see Chapter 17 in this volume)

8. Good housekeeping, including cleanliness of the workplace, waste disposal, adequate washing, toilet, and eating facilities, healthful drinking water, and control of insects and rodents

9. Training and education.

**Solution phase.** Once the problem has been analyzed and a number of solutions proposed, the most workable, timely, and practical solution needs to be selected—the solution that provides optimum benefits with minimal risks. The details of the solution should be worked out carefully. In effect, a blueprint needs to be developed, describing what needs to be done, how it is to be done, by whom, and in what sequence the actions are to take place.

Once controls are installed, they must be checked periodically to see that they are functioning properly. Followup monitoring and inspection are necessary to determine that the solution to a given hazardous exposure is controlling it within the specified limits. In other words, the monitoring function should be regarded as circular, not horizontal; if measurement at the solution phase reveals that controls are inadequate, the industrial hygienist must return to the first phase, that of defining the problem.

### Who will do the measuring?

Not every organization requires or can afford the full-time services of an industrial hygienist.

# 4—Acquiring Hazard Information

Independent consultants can be hired to accomplish two major objectives:

1. Identify and evaluate potential health risks and accident hazards to workers in the occupational environment

2. Design effective controls to protect the safety and health of workers.

Because any person can legally offer services as an industrial hygiene consultant, it is important that the consultant who is hired be trained, experienced, and competent. He must have detailed knowledge of proper sampling equipment and analytic procedures.

Good sources of information and assistance regarding consultants are the American Industrial Hygiene Association and the American Society of Safety Engineers, the professional associations related to occupational safety and health; see the descriptive listing in Chapter 24, "Sources of Help." Regional offices of NIOSH usually have lists of consultants in their area. Many insurance companies have loss prevention programs that employ industrial hygienists. The National Safety Council chapters which have offices in major cities, can offer assistance. The Council itself has a consultative service. (Selecting and using a hygiene consultant is covered in detail in the Council's *Fundamentals of Industrial Hygiene,* 2nd ed., Chapter 30, "Sources of Help.")

## Accident Investigation

A fourth function of monitoring in the total hazard control system is accident investigation, the subject of Chapter 7. The following discussion demonstrates how accident investigation fits into the systems approach to hazard control.

### Why accidents are investigated

When viewed as an integral part of the total occupational safety and health program, accident investigation is especially important as a means to determine cause, uncover indirect accident causes, prevent similar accidents from occurring, document facts, provide information on costs, and promote safety.

**Determine cause.** Accident investigation determines cause. At what points did the hazard control system break down? Were rules and regulations violated? Did defective machinery or factors in the work environment contribute to the accident? Poor machinery layout, for example, or the very design of a job process, operation, or task can contribute to an undesirable situation. Chapter 3 outlined the three primary sources of accidents: human, situational, and environmental factors. The accident investigation concentrates on gathering all information about these factors that led up to the accident.

**Uncover indirect accident causes.** Thorough accident investigation is very likely to uncover problems that indirectly contributed to the accident. Such information benefits accident-reduction efforts. For example, a worker slips on spilled oil and is injured. The oil spill is the direct cause of the accident, but a thorough investigation might reveal other factors: poor housekeeping, failure to follow maintenance schedule, inadequate supervision, faulty equipment (such as a lathe leaking oil).

**Prevent similar accidents.** Accident investigation identifies what action can be taken and what improvements made to prevent similar accidents from occurring in the future.

**Document facts.** Accident investigation documents the facts involved in an accident for use in instances of compensation and litigation. The report produced at the conclusion of an investigation becomes the permanent record of facts involved in the accident. Management can breathe more easily when it knows that an accident situation can be reconstructed months or years after the occurrence because the details of the accident have been recorded properly, accurately, and thoroughly.

**Provide information on costs.** Accident investigation provides information on both direct and indirect costs of accidents. Chapter 7 gives details for estimating accident costs.

**Promotes safety.** Accident investigation reaps psychological as well as material benefits. The investigation projects the organization's interest in safety and health. It indicates management's sense of accountability for accident prevention, its commitment to a safe work environment. An investigation in which both labor and management participate promotes cooperation between constituencies too often seen as adversaries.

Despite what many people believe, accident

investigation is a fact-finding, not a fault-finding, process. When attempting to determine the cause of an accident, the novice is tempted to conclude that the person involved in the accident was at fault. But if human error is chosen (and it is not the real cause), the hazard which caused the accident will go unobserved and uncontrolled. Furthermore, the person falsely blamed for causing the accident will respond to the unjustified corrective action with resentment and alienation. Further cooperation will be discouraged, and respect for the organization's safety and health program will be undermined. The intent of accident investigation is to pinpoint causes of error and/or defects so that similar accidents can be prevented.

Conducting an accident investigation is not simple. It can be very difficult to look beyond the incident at hand to uncover causal factors, determine the true loss potential of the occurrence, and develop practical recommendations to prevent recurrence.

A major weakness of many accident investigations is the failure to establish and consider *all* factors—human, situational, and environmental—that contributed to the accident. Reasons for this failure are several:

• Inexperienced or uninformed investigator

• Reluctance of the investigator to accept responsibility

• Narrow interpretation of environmental factors

• Erroneous emphasis on a single cause

• Judging the effect of the accident to be the cause

• Arriving at conclusions too rapidly before all factors can be considered

• Poor interviewing techniques

• Delay in investigating accidents.

The trained investigator must be ready to acknowledge as contributing causes any and all factors that may have, in any way, contributed to the accident. What at first may appear to be a simple, uninvolved accident may, in fact, have numerous contributing factors, which become more complex as analyses are completed.

Immediate, on-the-scene accident investigation provides the most accurate and useful information.

## When to investigate accidents?

The longer the delay in examining the accident scene, interviewing the injured and witnesses, the greater the possibility of obtaining erroneous or incomplete information. The accident scene changes, memories get fuzzy, and people talk to each other. Whether consciously or not, witnesses may alter their initial impressions to agree with someone else's observation or interpretation. Prompt accident investigation also expresses concern for the safety and well-being of employees.

As a general rule, all accidents, no matter now minor, are candidates for thorough investigation. Many accidents that occur in an organization are considered minor because their consequences are not serious. Such accidents—or "incidents," as some people prefer to call them—are taken for granted and often do not receive the attention they demand. Management, safety and health committees, supervisors, and employees must be aware that serious accidents arise from the same hazards as minor "incidents." Usually sheer luck determines whether a hazardous situation results in a minor incident or a serious accident.

## Who should conduct the investigation?

Chapter 7 discusses the question of who is to make the investigation: the supervisor or foreman, the safety professional, a special investigative committee, or a company safety committee. As a supplement to that discussion, the following section will outline the roles played by physicians and management in accident investigation and the responsibility of the safety professional in preventing further accidents from occurring during the investigation itself.

**Physician.** A physician's assistance is particularly important when human factors have been designated as primary or contributing causes of an accident. The physician can assess the nature and degree of injury and assist in determining the source and nature of the forces that inflicted the injury. He can determine what special biomedical studies, if any, are needed. He can establish whether the injured person was physically and mentally fit at the time of the accident and whether the screening, selection, and preplacement process is adequate. He can help judge the adequacy of safety and health protection procedures and equipment. He can help evaluate the effectiveness of the plans, procedures, equipment, training, and response of rescue, first aid, and emergency medical care personnel. The physician also can evaluate the effectiveness of measures aimed at early detection of medical conditions, mental changes, or emotional stress. In fatality cases, a physician can sometimes identify the victim and establish the immediate cause and time of death.

**Management.** Top management and department heads should help investigate accidents that result in lost work days or major property damage. When management actively participates in accident investigation, it can evaluate the hazard control system and determine whether outside assistance is desired or required to upgrade existing structures and procedures. Management also must review accident reports in order to make informed decisions. When accident investigation reveals the need or desirability of specific corrective action, management has the responsibility to determine whether the recommended action has indeed been implemented.

**Safety during the investigation.** In many cases the accident scene is a dangerous place. Electrical equipment may be damaged. Structural members may be weakened by fire or explosion. Radioactive or toxic materials may have been released.

The safety professional must be particularly alert to the hazards encountered by the investigating team. He has the training to provide proper protective equipment and to explain to other investigators the hazards that they may encounter and the emergency procedures they should follow.

See details in Chapter 16, "Planning for Emergencies."

### What to look for

During the accident investigation many questions must be answered. Because of the infinite number of accident-producing situations, contributing factors, and causes, it is impossible to list all questions to apply to all investigations. The following questions are generally applicable, however, and will be considered in most accident investigations (Firenze, 1978).

1. What was the injured person doing at the time of the accident? Performing his assigned task? Maintenance? Assisting another worker?

2. Was the injured employee working on a task

he was authorized to do? Was he qualified to perform the task? Was he familiar with the process, equipment, and machinery?

3. What were other workers doing at the time of the accident?

4. Was the proper equipment being used for the task at hand (screwdriver instead of can opener to open a paint can, file instead of a grinder to remove burr on a bolt after it was cut)?

5. Was the injured person following approved procedures?

6. Is the process, operation, or task new to the area?

7. Was the injured person being supervised? What was the proximity and adequacy of supervision?

8. Did the injured employee receive hazard recognition training prior to the accident?

9. What was the location of the accident? What was the physical condition of the area when the accident occurred?

10. What immediate or temporary action(s) could have prevented the accident or minimized its effect?

11. What long-term or permanent action could have prevented the accident or minimized its effect?

12. Had corrective action been recommended in the past but not adopted?

During the course of the investigation, the above questions should be answered to the satisfaction of the investigators. Other questions that come to mind as the investigation continues should be recorded.

### Conducting interviews

Interviewing accident or injury victims and witnesses can be a very difficult assignment if it is not handled properly. The individual being interviewed often is fearful and reluctant to provide the interviewer with accurate facts about the accident. The accident victim may be hesitant to talk for any number of reasons. A witness may not want to provide information that might place blame on friends, fellow workers, his supervisor, or possibly himself. To obtain the necessary facts during an interview, the interviewer must first eliminate or reduce fear and anxiety by developing rapport with the individual being interviewed. It is essential that the interviewer clear the air, create a feeling of trust, and establish lines of communication before beginning the actual interview.

Once good rapport has been developed, the following five-step method should be followed during the actual interview.

1. Discuss the purpose of the investigation and the interview (fact-finding, not fault-finding).

2. Have the individual relate his version of the complete accident with minimal interruptions. If the individual being interviewed is the one who was injured, ask him to explain where he was, what he was doing, how he was doing it, and what happened. If practical, have the injured person or eyewitness explain the sequence of events that occurred at the time of the accident. When someone is at the scene of the accident, he will be able to relate facts that might otherwise be difficult to explain.

3. Ask questions to clarify facts or fill in any gaps.

4. The interviewer should then relate his understanding of the accident to the injured person or eyewitness. Through this review process, there will be ample opportunity to correct any misunderstanding that may have occurred and clarify, if necessary, any of the details of the accident.

5. Discuss methods of preventing recurrence. Ask the individual for suggestions aimed at eliminating or reducing the impact of the hazards which caused the accident to happen. By asking the individual for his ideas and discussing them with him, the interviewer will show sincerity and place emphasis on the fact-finding purpose of the investigation, as it was explained at the beginning of the interview.

In some cases, contractual agreements may call for an employee representative to be present during any management interview, if the employee so requests.

## Implementing corrective action

Chapters 6 and 7 outline specific ways to record and classify data: how to identify key facts about each injury and the accident that produced it, how to record facts in a form that facilitates analysis and reveals patterns and trends, how to estimate accident costs, how to comply with OSHAct recordkeeping requirements.

An accident in any organization is of significant interest. Employees ask questions that reflect their concern. Is there any potential danger to those in the immediate vicinity? What caused the accident? How many people were injured? How badly?

Those who investigate accidents must be truthful in replying to questions. They should not try to cover up. On the other hand, they must be certain that they are authorized to release information, and they must be sure of their facts.

Because the accident report is the product of the investigation, it should be carefully prepared and adequately justify the conclusions reached. It must be issued soon after the accident. When a report is delayed too long, employees may feel themselves in limbo. If a final report must be postponed pending detailed technical analysis or evaluation, then an interim report should be issued.

Summaries of vital information on major injury, damage, and loss incidents should be distributed to department heads. Such summaries should include information on causes and recommended action for preventing similar incidents. Incident and statistical report files should be maintained for two years or as dictated by company policy.

Supervisors should keep employees informed of significant accidents and preventive measures proposed or executed. Posting accident reports is one way to make information available.

The preceding section on inspection emphasized that hazard control benefits accrue only after the inspection report is written and disseminated. Until corrective action is initiated, recommendations—no matter how earnest, thorough, and relevant—remain "paper promises."

The same truth applies to accident investigation when used as a monitoring technique. Viewed from the perspective of hazard control, accident investigation serves a monitoring function only when it provides the impetus for corrective action.

When management and safety professionals review monthly accident reports, they exercise an essential auditing function. They use accident reports to make decisions to prevent similar accidents from occurring, and they look for answers to certain key questions. Are all signifi-

**135**

cant accidents being reported? Are all parts of the organization equally committed to the hazard control effort? Are there trends or patterns in accidents or injuries? What system breakdowns predominate? What supervisors require additional training? Are employees advised of the results of accident investigation and of preventive measures being instituted?

Accident investigation is a monitoring func-tion that occurs *after* the fact. The hazard control system already has broken down. No amount of investigation can reverse the accident. Nevertheless, accident investigation serves an important monitoring function. Past mistakes are being used to improve future operations. As George Santayana has written, "Those who cannot remember the past are condemned to repeat it."

## References

Boggs, Richard F. "Environmental Monitoring and Control Requirements," *National Safety News*, Vol. 118, No.2 (August 1978).

*Facility Inspection.* Philadelphia, Pa., Insurance Company of North America, 1973.

Factory Mutual Engineering Corporation, *Handbook of Industrial Loss Prevention*, 2nd ed. New York, N.Y., McGraw Hill Book Co., 1967.

Firenze, Robert J. *The Process of Hazard Control*. Dubuque, Iowa, Kendall/Hunt Publishing Co., 1978.

"Industrial Hygiene Instrumentation," *National Safety News*, Vol. 117, No. 3 (March 1978).

Johnson, William G. *MORT Safety Assurance Systems*. New York, N.Y., Marcel Dekker, Inc., 1980. (Also available through National Safety Council.)

National Safety Council, 444 N. Michigan Ave., Chicago, Ill. 60611.
    *OSHA Standards Handbook for Business and Industry.*
    *You Are the Safety and Health Committee.*

Nertney, Robert J. "Practical Applications of System Safety Concepts," *Professional Safety*, Vol. 22, No. 2 (February 1977).

Olishifski, Julian. "Air Sampling Instrumentation," *National Safety News*, Vol. 120, No. 2 (August 1979).

Olishifski, Julian. "Selecting and Using Industrial Hygiene Consultants," *National Safety News*, Vol. 118, No. 3 (September 1978).

Olishifski, Julian, ed. *Fundamentals of Industrial Hygiene*, 2nd ed. Chicago, Ill., National Safety Council, 1979.

Recht, Jack L. "Systems Safety Analysis: A Modern Approach to Safety Problems." Chicago, Ill., National Safety Council, 1966.

Scerbo, Ferdinand A., and Pritchard, James J. "Fault Tree Analysis: A Technique for Product Safety Evaluation," *Professional Safety*, Vol. 22, No. 5 (May 1977).

U.S., Department of Labor, *Principles and Practices of Occupational Safety and Health*, Student Manual, Booklet Three, OSHA Publication 2215.

———. *Safety and Health Inspections for an Effective Safety and Health Program* (February 1977).

# Removing the Hazard from the Job

# Chapter
# 5

# 5—Removing the Hazard from the Job

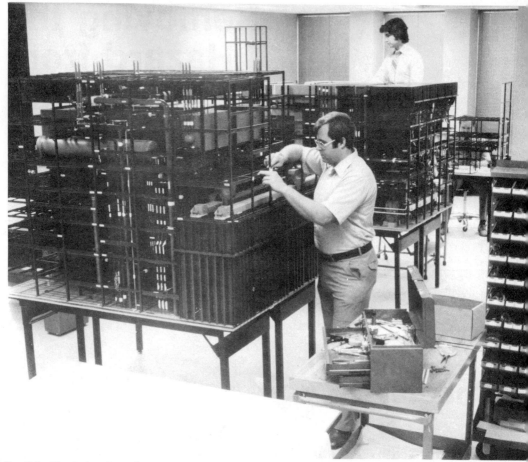

FIG. 5–1.—The drafting board (and sometimes the model shop) is where safety begins as part of the designer's concept. Safety that is designed into equipment, processes, and plants reduces the need for training and supervision of personnel.

*Courtesy Sargent & Lundy, Chicago.*

Once the hazard has been identified and evaluated and management has decided to eliminate it, modify it, or cope with it, then the basic measures for preventing accidental injury and occupational illness, in order of effectiveness and preference, are:

1. Redesign the system to eliminate the hazard from the machine, method, process, or plant structure,

2. Control the hazard by enclosing, safeguarding, or otherwise mitigating it at its source,

3. Train personnel to make them aware of the hazard and to follow safe job procedures to avoid it,

4. Prescribe approved personal protective equipment for personnel to shield them against the hazard.

This chapter will be primarily concerned with the most effective technique—engineering the hazards out of operations before work is performed and, therefore, before accidents or injuries (or illnesses) can occur. If all possibilities have been exhausted and the hazard is still not removed, then every effort should be made to

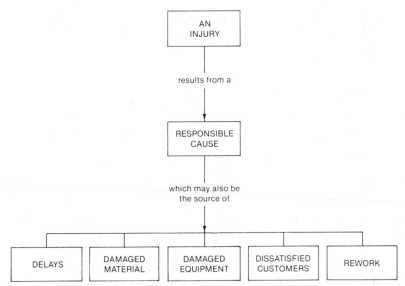

FIG. 5–2.—An injury is significant because it points to its basic cause, which may also be responsible for other operating hindrances (shown at bottom of chart).

*Courtesy Hartford Accident and Indemnity Co.*

enclose, or safeguard the hazard at its source so that exposure to injury or illness is controlled. In some cases, this measure can be just as effective as elimination of the hazard.

If either of the first two measures can be successfully employed, the need for on-the-job training to protect personnel against hazards is greatly reduced, and use of personal protective equipment may not be necessary.

### Reducing Exposure to Injury

Modern industry knows how to engineer the hazards out of jobs. However, on too many jobs, accidents occur because insufficient effort has been put forth to determine the hazards involved. Obviously, until a job has been studied to make these determinations, the hazards cannot be engineered out. (See discussion in Chapter 3.)

Among the jobs or operations that have not been analyzed for hazards are many of a non-repetitive nature, the type of job on which accidents are likely to occur.

### Design for safety

The ultimate goal is to design environments and equipment and to set up job procedures so that employee exposure to injury or illness will be either eliminated or controlled as completely as possible. When a high degree of safety is incorporated into the design of the equipment and the planning of the job procedures, the need for training and supervision to control unsafe acts is reduced.

Company policy should specify that safety must be designed and built into the job before the job is executed. To add safety features after work on a job has begun is usually more costly, less efficient, and less effective.

The most efficient time to engineer hazards out of the plant, product, process, or job is prior to building or remodeling, while a product is being designed, before a change in a process is put into effect, or before a job is started. Every effort, therefore, should be made to find and remove potential hazards at the blueprint or planning stage (Fig. 5–1).

Each level of engineering should be given the responsibility for establishing hazard controls into the job, right through to the production phase. This responsibility should extend to product design, machine design, plant layout and condition of premises, selection and specification of materials, production planning, time study,

**139**

methods, duties of the production supervisor, and the work of employees assigned to the job.

## Production hindrances

In industrial operations, usually the same causes that result in employee injuries are also responsible for damage to materials and equipment and for other hindrances to efficient production, such as:

1. Reduced output

2. Excessive scrap, damaged material, and need for rework

3. Unnecessary material handling

4. Excessive employee time required per unit of production

5. Excessive machine-hours per unit of production

6. Damaged equipment

7. Poor employee morale

8. High labor turnover

These hindrances to production result from accidents—when the term "accident" is used to mean "that occurrence in a sequence of events that usually produces unintended injury or illness, or death, and/or property damage." Thus an accident may cause damage to equipment or material or a production delay, without resulting in an injury. Although an injury may or may not result from a given mishap, interference with the smooth flow of production can be expected.

The significance of an injury (Fig. 5–2), aside from humanitarian considerations, is that it points to a cause that may also be responsible for other operating hindrances. When causes are identified and corrected, the basic source of both the injury or illness and the related production hindrances are eliminated.

## Role of the safety professional

In the removal of hazards from the job, cooperation between the safety professional and engineers in the company is essential. More often than not, the safety professional is not a registered professional engineer; in fact, he or she may have had no academic training in engineering. In such cases, it is especially important that the safety professional seek the advice and help of personnel within the company who are responsible for establishing engineering design criteria and for setting up job procedures.

One important objective of all the company's engineering personnel is to design equipment and processes (including handling and disposal of hazardous substances) and to plan job procedures so that exposure to injury and illness is eliminated or controlled. It is the safety professional's job to see that engineering personnel are acquainted with the particular hazards involved and the methods of eliminating them.

The safety professional must discuss with management and the various supervisors involved the conditions responsible for accidents or potential accidents. He might well remember that, in making his corrective suggestions, he will be more successful if he can demonstrate that an injury is only one of *many* hindrances to efficient production.

The safety professional who has the necessary knowledge and skills for preventing accidents should be able to make recommendations for effective use of the facilities at hand for more efficient as well as safer production.

## Deviation from the standard procedure, and hazardous conditions

In most industrial accidents, *both* hazardous (unsafe) conditions and unsafe acts are contributing factors. In the earlier days of the safety movement, safety professionals were highly concerned with whether it was an unsafe act or an unsafe condition that caused an accident.

The American National Standards Institute Standard Z16.2, *Method of Recording Basic Facts Relating to the Nature of Occupational Work Injuries*, defines an *unsafe act* as being any violation of (or departure from) an accepted, normal, or correct procedure or practice; it could include an unnecessary exposure to a hazard (such as not using protective equipment or a safeguard), or conduct minimizing the degree of safety normally present (such as not taking necessary precautions). A *hazardous condition* is defined as being a physical condition or circumstance that permits or occasions the occurrence of an accident.

It is important to note that every unsafe act does not necessarily result in an accident; a supervisor usually has ample opportunity to correct unsafe acts before an accident occurs. Similarly, it must be kept in mind that most hazardous conditions have been around for some time before an accident occurs; a supervisor again has many opportunities to correct them.

Two historical studies are usually cited to pinpoint the contributing factor(s) to an accident. Both emphasize that most accidents have multiple causes.

- A study of 91,773 cases reported in Pennsylvania in 1953 showed 92 percent of all nonfatal injuries and 94 percent of all fatal injuries were due to hazardous mechanical or physical conditions. In turn, unsafe acts reported in work injury accidents accounted for 93 percent of the notfatal injuries and 97 percent of the fatalities.[*]

- In almost 80,000 work injuries reported in that same state in 1960, unsafe condition(s) was identified as a contributing factor in 98.4 percent of the nonfatal manufacturing cases, and unsafe act(s) was identified as a contributing factor in 98.2 percent of the nonfatal cases.[**]

It must be remembered that a hazardous condition, in addition to being a direct cause of accidents in itself, often can lead people to perform unsafe acts. Many times, an unsafe act is the result of poor machine design, inadequately planned methods, and other engineering deficiencies. Thus, elimination of a hazard caused by an unsafe condition may also reduce the likelihood of injury from an unsafe act.

When an injury occurs, the hazardous condition is often not as glaringly evident as the unsafe act. Unless a careful study is made of the accident, the correctable physical hazard may escape notice.

Many causes for accidents can be found by this technique of finding what elements are involved in accidents, where and when accidents occur, and who is the victim. Engineering for safety should, therefore, have as its objectives both the elimination of hazardous conditions and elimination of unsafe acts.

In the early 1980's, however, an effort was made to discover the *root causes* of accidents—causes that are more difficult to identify. The Council has started a program to obtain improved occupational injury information in order to provide, in turn, even more reliable answers as to *why* the accident occurred in the first place.

As important as engineering is in eliminating the causes of accidents, supervision must continue to deal effectively with both the immediate and the continuing causes of accidents; therefore, as is pointed out in other chapters, the mental and physical condition of both the worker and the supervisor are also important factors in preventing accidents.

## Machine Design

Machinery is one of the top four sources of compensable work injuries, accounting for ten percent of all such injuries. (The other three sources are manual handling of objects—23 percent, falls—20 percent, and struck by falling or moving objects—14 percent.) Further pointing to he need for safe design of machines is the fact that they rank equally with falls and being struck by falling or moving objects as a source of permanent partial injuries (each causing about 19 percent), according to the Council's *Accident Facts*, 1973 edition (the latest edition to report such figures).

The design of machinery and equipment is an evolutionary process. It is always changing and dynamic, because design engineers constantly acquire wider experiences in the course of their everyday work. These experiences give them a broader scope and more initiative at the drawing board. This initiative, however, will be disciplined by the practical consideration of designing the most effective means for controlling hazards in the operation of machines or equipment.

### Basic considerations

Evidently, the design of machinery must be further improved if the number of injuries caused by machines is to be reduced. How hazards can be eliminated from machines in the planning stage is illustrated by much of the evolution in machine design that has thus far occurred (Fig. 5–3). Behind this evolution has been the search for ever-increased efficiency and safety in machines of all types. In repeated instances, innovations in design which improved efficiency also eliminated or lessened a hazard. Conversely, measures taken to prevent accidents also improved production efficiency.

Policy in designing or purchasing should make

---

[*]National Safety Council, Chicago, Ill. *Accident Facts,*1956 Edition, pp. 40-41.

[**]Pennsylvania Department of Labor and Industry, Harrisburg, Pa. *Industrial Injuries in Pennsylvania.* 1960.

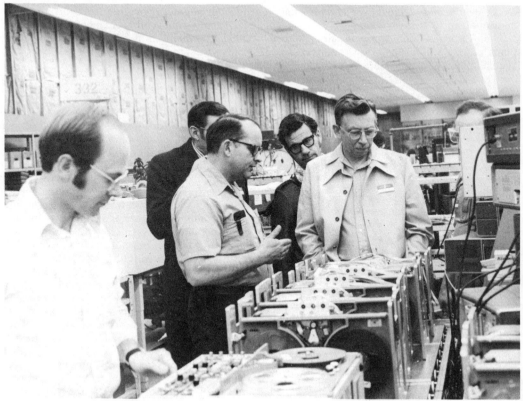

FIG. 5–3.—As a product is being built, toolmakers and designers discuss production and safety features. *Courtesy* Automotive, Tooling, Metalworking and Associated Industries Section Newsletter.

sure that a machine is so designed that it will meet the requirements promulgated under authority of the OSHAct. Adding safeguards to control exposure to injury after the machine has been installed is usually expensive and second best.

• A good example of elimination of hazards by design is the single-point lubricating system installed on many large machines. Use of this system not only eliminates the need to reach remote, and perhaps hazardous, oil points, but also ensures better lubrication.

• The evolution of safe and efficient design of a machine is well exemplified by the engine lathe. This machine was formerly driven by an overhead line shaft with a flat belt, with the spindle speed controlled by changing the belt on the cone pulleys. The feeds were controlled by changing

the gears in the gear box. Since none of these danger points was guarded, the operator or other person standing nearby was exposed to all the hazards.

The modern engine lathe has an individual motor designed to be installed in the frame or structure of the machine. The drive mechanism, fully enclosed in the machine, is operated by V-belts or gears. The speed of the spindle is controlled either by regulating a variable speed motor or by shifting a lever that acts as a clutch (as well as a gear shift). The feed is controlled by a shifting lever also. All the gears, drive belts, and sheaves are fully enclosed. Lubrication is done from a single point rather than at various points on the machine. The new machine is much safer than its predecessor and much more efficient.

## Machine safety checklist

A safety checklist for the use of machine design engineers might well include the following points, to be incorporated in machine design where applicable and possible:

1. Design the machine so that it is impossible for the operator or others to get at the point of operation or any other hazard point while the machine is operating.

2. Design the machine so that corners and edges are rounded.

3. Locate and specify the type of machine controls so that the operator cannot put the machine in motion if he is in the vicinity of the point of operation.

4. Place the controls so that the operator will not have to reach too far or move his body off balance in order to operate the machine.

5. Build power transmission and drive mechanisms as integral parts of the machine.

6. Build overload devices into the machine.

7. Design the machine for single-point lubrication.

8. Design mechanical, instead of manual, holding devices.

9. Design a mechanical device for feeding and ejecting parts so as to eliminate the use of hands for such operations.

10. Minimize motor drift time.

11. Provide fail-safe interlocks so that the machine cannot be started when it is being loaded or unloaded.

12. Build in a lockout system so that unexpected movement of the machine is eliminated when the machine is being worked on. (See Guarding During Maintenance in Chapter 8, "Principles of Guarding," in the *Engineering and Technology* volume.)

13. Provide a grounding system for all electrical equipment.

14. Provide standard access platforms and ladders for inspection and maintenance of equipment.

15. Design component parts of equipment for easy and safe removal and replacement to facilitate maintenance.

16. Reduce sources of excessive noise.

In the past, many investigators of machine accident problems have thought that the practical, perhaps the only, solution was to add a guard here or there. However, installation of an external guard is not always the final, or the best, answer.

When the addition of a guard to a machine is being considered, this question should be asked: "Will this guard afford protection from a hazard but, in so doing, interfere with or defeat the machine's function?" In answer, it can be said that the best solution lies not in a guard that impairs production but rather in a change to a basic design that eliminates the hazard and increases efficiency. There can be little prospect for safe operation of a machine unless the idea of building safety into the machine's function is applied right on the drawing board.

A good illustration of the principle of designing safety into a mechanism is provided by the automatic coupler used on railroad cars. The automatic coupler is a great improvement over the old link and pin coupler, which required an employee to go between the cars to drop the pin and thus be exposed to a crushing hazard when the cars came together. Use of the automatic coupler eliminates exposure to a serious hazard. The device contributes to efficiency, too, by speeding train operation.

## Built-in safety

The machine manufacturer, like any other businessman, wants to have satisfied customers. If his machines cause accidents and thus lead to economic losses, his customers will be unsatisfied. If the purchaser's order for a machine specifies that the machine must meet OSHA regulations and have safety built into it so that the operator will not be exposed to any working hazards, the manufacturer's designers will regard such a specification as a design requirement which they must meet.

In many instances, guards added to a machine after it has been installed in the plant are removed and not replaced. Accidents frequently result from this practice.

If a guard were an aid to production and efficiency rather than a hindrance, it is unlikely that the operator would run the machine without having the guard in place. Machine safety must be improved without either hindering the worker or reducing the efficiency of the machine.

# 5—Removing the Hazard from the Job

## Human factors

When safety is being designed into machines and equipment, special consideration must be given to human factors. Almost every machine requires an operator, and the mechanisms of many machines have become too complex to be understood by the average operator. Therefore, machines and equipment should be designed in terms of human limitations and capabilities, both mental and physical. (Also see Chapter 10, "Human Factors Engineering.")

**Reflex actions.** The employee who reaches into a danger zone, such as a point of operation, to adjust or remove material in process often does so by reflex action. Equipment must be designed so that an operator cannot endanger himself in this way.

**Sensory limitations.** Design engineers must be aware of the limitations of the sensory organs. They must have some idea of the probable ability of the prospective operator to correlate and use the information to be supplied him by the sounds, lights, and other signal devices to be used in the operation of the equipment.

Design engineers must also remember that an operator may react slowly to sensory stimuli simply because he has normal human limitations or is disturbed by special problems, such as trouble at home, poor health, or poor attitude.

The equipment designer must not expect too much of the operator in regard to the sensory responses necessary in operating the machine. For example, each control lever should have a readily identifiable shape and location so that the operator can easily find the one he wants. Occasionally, an operator will inadvertently actuate a wrong control lever because he cannot differentiate between it and the correct one simply by touch. The same point applies to STOP, START, and INCH buttons on electrical controls. (See the discussion in Chapter 10, "Human Factors Engineering.")

**Physical limitations.** In addition to considering sensory limitations, the operator of the equipment may be suffering from temporary ailments, impairment of functions causing inefficiency, or fatigue. The operator's age may also affect his efficiency.

The physical environment in which the operator works must be taken into consideration, too.

Environmental factors may include temperature, humidity, toxic gases, altitude, clothing, and many others. The designer should consider all factors and design the machine or equipment so it will not place unusual demands upon the physical and mental capabilities of the operator.

**Advance analysis.** If there are any defects in the design of a piece of machinery, it is usually only a matter of time before it fails and an accident ensues. Therefore, all possible faults in the design of equipment and all possible hazards in the work area of a machine, as well as the physical and mental capabilities of the operator, should be studied in advance for the purpose of establishing a safe work environment.

An advance analysis can, according to McFarland (see References), be based on the following considerations:

1. Operational job analysis should include a survey of the nature of the task, the work surroundings, the location of controls and instruments, and the duties that the operator must perform.

2. A functional concept of accidents is implied; that is, the errors that may occur while the operator is working on the machine are anticipated. The repetition or recurrence of near or real accidents clearly indicates a need for redesign.

3. From the "human limitations" point of view, it should be assumed that no worker is perfect. In fact, the operator may be far below the ability adjudged by the machine designer. If the worker's duties become too complex, the cumulative burden will probably cause human failures leading to injuries.

4. A wide margin of safety should be provided to eliminate any possible situation that places the operator near his maximum ability with regard to aptitude or effort, especially when adverse factors enter the picture.

## Job Safety Analysis

Job safety analysis (JSA) is a procedure used to review job methods and uncover hazards (a) that may have been overlooked in the layout of the plant or building and in the design of the machinery, equipment, tools, work stations, and processes, or (b) that may have developed after

## JOB SAFETY ANALYSIS WORK SHEET
### JOB: Using a Pressurized Water Fire Extinguisher

| WHAT TO DO (Steps in sequence) | HOW TO DO IT (Instructions) (Reverse hands for left-handed operator.) | KEY POINTS (Items to be emphasized. Safety is always a key point) |
|---|---|---|
| 1. Remove extinguisher from wall bracket. | 1. Left hand on bottom lip, fingers curled around lip, palm up. Right hand on carrying handle palm down, fingers around carrying handle only. | 1. Check air pressure to make certain extinguisher is charged. Stand close to extinguisher, pull straight out. *Have firm grip, to prevent dropping on feet.* Lower, and as you do remove left hand from lip. |
| 2. Carry to fire. | 2. Carry in right hand, upright position. | 2. Extinguisher should hang down alongside leg. (This makes it easy to carry and reduces possibility of strain.) |
| 3. Remove pin. | 3. Set extinguisher down in upright position. Place left hand on top of extinguisher, pull out pin with right hand. | 3. Hold extinguisher steady with left hand. Do not exert pressure on discharge lever as you remove pin. |
| 4. Squeeze discharge lever. | 4. Place right hand over carrying handle with fingers curled around operating lever handle while grasping discharge hose near nozzle with left hand. | 4. Have firm grip on handle to steady extinguisher. |
| 5. Apply water stream to fire. | 5. Direct water stream at base of fire. | 5. Work from side to side or around fire. After extinguishing flames, play water on smouldering or glowing surfaces. |
| 6. Return Extinguisher. Report Use. | | |

FIG. 5–4.—Here is the first step in preparing a job safety analysis. The work sheet is then broken down as shown in Figs. 5–5 and -6.

production started, or (c) that resulted from changes in work procedures or personnel. It is one of the first steps in hazard and accident analysis and in safety training (see Chapter 9, "Safety Training").

Once the hazards are known, the proper solutions can be developed. Some solutions may be physical changes that eliminate or control the hazard, such as placing a safeguard over exposed moving machine parts. Others may be job procedures that eliminate or minimize the hazard, for example, safe piling of materials. These will require training and supervision.

A job safety analysis can be written up in the manner shown in Fig. 5–4. In the left-hand column, the basic steps of the job are listed in the

| JOB SAFETY ANALYSIS TRAINING GUIDE | JOB: | | DATE: |
|---|---|---|---|
| | TITLE OF MAN WHO DOES JOB: | FOREMAN/SUPR: | ANALYSIS BY: |
| DEPARTMENT: | SECTION: | | REVIEWED BY: |
| REQUIRED AND/OR RECOMMENDED PERSONAL PROTECTIVE EQUIPMENT: | | | APPROVED BY: |

| SEQUENCE OF BASIC JOB STEPS | POTENTIAL ACCIDENTS OR HAZARDS | RECOMMENDED SAFE JOB PROCEDURE |
|---|---|---|
| Break the job down into its basic steps, e.g., what is done first, what is done next, and so on. You can do this by 1) observing the job, 2) discussing it with the operator, 3) drawing on your knowledge of the job, or 4) a combination of the three. Record the job steps in their normal order of occurrence. Describe what is done, not the details of how it is done. Usually three or four words are sufficient to describe each basic job step. | For each job step, ask yourself what accidents could happen to the person doing the job step. You can get the answers by (1) observing the job, (2) discussing it with the operator, (3) recalling past accidents, or (4) a combination of the three. Ask yourself: can he be struck by or contacted by anything; can he strike against or come in contact with anything; can he be caught in, on, or between anything; can he fall; can he overexert; is he exposed to anything injurious such as gas, radiation, welding rays, etc.? for example, acid burns, fumes. | For each potential accident or hazard, ask yourself how should the worker do the job step to avoid the potential accident, or what should he do or not do to avoid the accident. You can get your answers by (1) observing the job for leads, (2) discussing precautions with experienced job operators, (3) drawing on your experience, or (4) a combination of the three. Be sure to describe specifically the precautions a man must take. Don't leave out important details. Number each separate recommended precaution with the same number you gave the potential accident (see center column) that the precaution seeks to avoid. Use simple do or don't statements to explain recommended precautions as if you were talking to the person.<br><br>For example: "Lift with your legs, not your back." Avoid such generalities as "Be careful," "Be alert," "Take caution," etc. |

Fig. 5–5.—Job safety analysis training guide. Use these guidelines when preparing a JSA.

order in which they occur. The middle column describes all hazards, both those produced by the environment and those connected to the job procedure. The right-hand column gives the safe procedures that should be followed to guard against the hazards and to prevent potential accidents.

For convenience, both the job safety analysis procedure and the written description are commonly referred to as JSA. Health hazards are also considered when making a JSA.

The four basic steps in making a job safety analysis are:

1. Select the job to be analyzed.

2. Break the job down into successive steps or activities and observe how these actions are performed.

3. Identify the hazards and potential accidents. (This is the critical step because only an identified problem can be eliminated.)

4. Develop safe job procedures to eliminate the hazards and prevent the potential accidents.

Each step will be discussed in detail.

## Select the job

A job is a sequence of separate steps or activities that together accomplish a work goal. Some jobs can be broadly defined in general terms of what is accomplished. Making paper, building a plant, mining iron ore are examples. Such broadly defined jobs are not suitable for JSA. Similarly, a job can be narrowly defined in terms of a single action. Pulling a switch, tightening a screw, pushing a button are examples. Such narrowly defined jobs also are not suitable for JSA.

Jobs suitable for JSA are those job assignments that a line supervisor may make. Operating a machine, tapping a furnace, piling lumber are good subjects for job safety analyses. They are neither too broad nor too narrow.

Jobs should not be selected at random—those with the worst accident experience should be analyzed first if JSA is to yield the quickest possible results. In fact, some companies make this the focal point of their accident prevention program.

In selecting jobs to be analyzed and in establishing the order of analysis, top supervision of a department should be guided by the following factors:

1. FREQUENCY OF ACCIDENTS. A job that has repeatedly produced accidents is a candidate for a JSA. The greater the number of accidents associated with the job, the greater its priority claim for a JSA.

2. PRODUCTION OF DISABLING INJURIES. Every job that has produced disabling injuries should be given a JSA. Subsequent injuries prove that preventive action taken prior to their occurrence was not successful.

3. SEVERITY POTENTIAL. Some jobs may not have a history of accidents but may have the potential for severe injury.

4. NEW JOBS created by changes in equipment or in processes obviously have no history of accidents, but their accident potential may not be fully appreciated. A JSA of every new job should be made as soon as the job has been created. Analysis should not be delayed until accidents or near misses occur.

## Break the job down

Before the search for hazards begins, a job should be broken down into a sequence of steps, each describing what is being done. Avoid the two common errors: (a) making the breakdown so detailed that an unnecessarily large number of steps results, or (b) making the job breakdown so general that basic steps are not recorded.

The technique of making a job safety analysis involves these steps:

1. Selecting the right person to observe

2. Briefing him on the purpose

3. Observing him perform the job, and trying to break it into basic steps

4. Recording each step in the breakdown

5. Checking the breakdown with the person observed

Select an experienced, capable, and cooperative person who is willing to share ideas. If the employee has never helped on a job safety analysis, explain the purpose—to make a job safe by identifying hazards and eliminating or controlling them—and show him a completed JSA. Reassure the employee that he was selected because of his experience and capability.

To determine the basic job steps, ask "What step starts the job?" Then, "What is the next basic

| JOB SAFETY ANALYSIS TRAINING GUIDE | JOB: DIE CHANGING | | DATE: MAY 4, 19 -- |
|---|---|---|---|
| | TITLE OF PERSON WHO DOES JOB: DIE SETTER | SUPERVISOR: J. JONES | ANALYSIS BY: DIE SETTER, OPERATOR, SUPERVISOR |
| DEPARTMENT: LADDER FABRICATION | | SECTION: POWER PRESSES | REVIEWED BY: J. JONES, SUPERVISOR |
| REQUIRED AND/OR RECOMMENDED PERSONAL PROTECTIVE EQUIPMENT: FOOT AND EYE PROTECTION | | | APPROVED BY: S. SMITH, Plt. Supt. |

| SEQUENCE OF BASIC JOB STEPS | POTENTIAL ACCIDENTS OR HAZARDS | RECOMMENDED SAFE JOB PROCEDURE |
|---|---|---|
| 1. Check the die number. | 1. Damage to die and to press from use of wrong die. | 1. Supervisor should recheck the die number before change. |
| 2. Move the lift to the die bin. | 2. a) Injure die setter: struck by or caught between lift. | 2. a) Be familiar with operation and controls of the lift, stay clear of moving lift. |
| | b) Injure another employee. | b) Be familiar with operation and controls of the lift, clear out other employees. |
| | c) Damage to property: struck by lift. | c) Be familiar with operation and controls of the lift, make certain path is clear of obstacles. |
| 3. Remove the die from bin. | 3. a) Strain from transferring the die to the lift. | 3. a) Position lift abutting bin, keep lift slightly lower than bin, and make certain die can be removed by one person. |
| | b) Injury from falling die. | b) Same as a), and lock lift to prohibit moving. |
| 4. Move lift from bin to press. | 4. Same as 2a,b,c. | 4. Same as 2a,b,c. |
| 5. Move die from table to press. | 5. Injure die setter. | 5. Position lift abutting press, keep lift slightly higher than press, and lock lift to prohibit moving. |
| 6. Remove die from press to table. | 6. Injure die setter. | 6. Position lift abutting press, keep lift slightly lower than press, and lock lift to prohibit moving. |
| 7. Move lift from press to bin. | 7. Same as 2a,b,c. | 7. Same as 2a,b,c. |

step?" and so on.

In recording the job steps, each should be described completely and the employee should be asked to verify the written job description; possible deviations from the regular procedure should be recorded because it may be this irregular activity that leads to an accident.

To record the breakdown, number the job steps consecutively as illustrated in the first column of the JSA training guide, illustrated in Fig. 5–5. Each step tells what is done, not how.

The wording for each step should begin with an "action" word, like "remove," "open," or "weld." The action is completed by naming the item to which the action (expressed by the verb) applied, for example, "remove extinguisher," "carry to fire."

In checking the breakdown with the person observed, obtain his agreement of what is done and the order of the steps. Thank the employee for his cooperation.

## Identify hazards and potential accidents

Before filling in the next two columns of the JSA—"Potential Accidents or Hazards" and "Recommended Safe Job Procedure"—begin the search for hazards. The purpose is to identify all hazards—both those produced by the environment and those connected with the job procedure. Each step, and thus the entire job, must be made safer and more efficient. To do this, ask yourself these questions about each step:

1. Is there a danger of striking against, being struck by, or otherwise making injurious contact with an object?

2. Can the employee be caught in, by, or between objects?

3. Is there a potential for a slip or trip? Can he fall on the same level or to another?

4. Can he strain himself by pushing, pulling, lifting, bending, or twisting?

5. Is the environment hazardous to safety and/or health (toxic gas, vapor, mist, fume, or dust, heat or radiation)? (See discussion in the National Safety Council book *Fundamentals of Industrial Hygiene.*)

Close observation and job knowledge are required. The job observation should be repeated as often as necessary until all hazards and potential accidents have been identified.

Include hazards that might result. Record the type of accident and the agent involved. To note that the employee might injure a foot by dropping a fire extinguisher, for example, write down "struck by extinguisher."

Again check with the observed employee after the hazards and potential accidents have been recorded. The experienced employee will probably suggest additional ideas. You should also check with others experienced with the job. Through observation and discussion, you will develop a reliable list of hazards and potential accidents.

## Develop solutions

The final step in a JSA is to develop a recommended safe job procedure to prevent occurrence of potential accidents. The principal solutions are:

1. Find a new way to do the job.

2. Change the physical conditions that create the hazards.

3. To eliminate hazards still present, change the work procedure.

4. Try to reduce the necessity of doing a job, or at least the frequency that it must be performed. This is particularly helpful in maintenance and material handling.

• To find an entirely new way to do a job, determine the work goal of the job, and then analyze the various ways of reaching this goal to see which way is safest. Consider work-saving tools and equipment.

• If a new way cannot be found, then ask this question about each hazard and potential accident listed: "What change in physical condition (such as change in tools, materials, equipment, layout, or location) will eliminate the hazard or prevent the accident?"

When a change is found, study it carefully to find what other benefits (such as greater production or time saving) will accrue. These benefits should be pointed out when proposing the change to higher management. They make good selling points.

• The third solution in solving the job-hazard problem is to investigate changes in the job procedure. Ask of each hazard and potential accident listed: "What should the employee do—or not do—to eliminate this particular hazard or prevent this potential accident?" Where appropriate, ask an additional question, "How should it be done?" Because of his experience, the supervisor can answer these questions, in most cases.

Answers must be specific and concrete if new procedures are to be any good. General precautions—"be alert," "use caution," or "be careful"—are useless. Answers should precisely state what to do and how to do it. This recommendation—"Make certain the wrench does not slip or cause loss of balance"—is only "half good." It does not tell how to prevent the wrench from slipping.

Here, in contrast, is an example of a good recommended safe procedure that tells both "what" and "how": "Set wrench properly and securely. Test its grip by exerting a slight pressure on it. Brace yourself against something immovable, or take a solid stance with feet wide apart, before exerting full pressure. This prevents loss of balance if the wrench slips."

• Often a repair or service job has to be repeated frequently because a condition needs correction again and again. To reduce the necessity of such a repetitive job, ask "What can be done to eliminate the cause of the condition that makes excessive repairs or service necessary?" If the cause cannot be eliminated, then ask "Can anything be done to minimize the effects of the condition?"

Machine parts, for example, may wear out quickly and require frequent replacement. Study of the problem may reveal excessive vibration is the culprit. After reducing or eliminating the vibration, the machine parts last longer and require less maintenance.

Reducing frequency of a job contributes to safety only in that it limits the exposure. Every effort still should be made to eliminate hazards and to prevent potential accidents through changing physical conditions or revising job procedures or both.

• A job that has been redesigned may require going beyond the immediate boundaries of the specific job—affecting other jobs and even the entire work process. Therefore, the redesign should be discussed not only with the worker involved, but also co-workers, the supervisor, the plant engineer, and others who are concerned. In all cases, however, check or test the proposed changes by reobserving the job and discussing the changes with those who do the job. Their ideas about the hazards and proposed solutions may be of considerable value. They can judge the practicality of proposed changes and perhaps suggest improvements. Actually these discussions are more than just a way to check a JSA. They are safety contacts that promote awareness of job hazards and safe procedures.

A final version of a JSA is shown in Fig. 5–6.

## Use JSA effectively

The major benefits of a job safety analysis come after its completion. However, benefits are also to be gained from the development work itself.

While making job safety analyses, supervisors learn more about the jobs they supervise. When employees are encouraged to participate in job safety analyses, their safety attitudes are improved and their safety knowledge is increased. As a JSA is worked out, safer and better job procedures and safer working conditions are developed.

But these important benefits are only a portion of the total benefits to be derived from the JSA program. The principal benefits were listed at the beginning of this discussion.

When a JSA is distributed, the supervisor's first responsibility is to explain its contents to employees and, if necessary, to give them further individual training. The entire JSA must be reviewed with the employees concerned so that they will know how the job is to be done—without accidents.

The JSA can furnish material for planned safety contacts. All steps of the JSA should be used for this purpose. The steps that present major hazards should be emphasized and reviewed again and again in subsequent safety contacts.

New employees on the job must be trained in the basic job steps. They must be taught to recognize the hazards associated with each job step and must learn the necessary precautions. There is no better guide for this training than a well-prepared JSA.

Occasionally, the supervisor should observe his employees as they perform jobs for which job analyses have been developed. The purpose of these observations is to determine whether or not the employees are doing the jobs in accordance with the safe job procedures. Before making such observations, the supervisor should prepare himself by reviewing the JSA in question so that he will have firmly in mind the key points that should be part of his observations.

Many jobs, such as certain repair or service jobs, are done infrequently or on an irregular basis. The employees who do them will benefit from pre-job instruction that reminds them of the important hazards and the necessary precautions. Using the JSA for the particular job, the supervisor should give this instruction at the time he makes the job assignment.

Whenever an accident occurs on a job covered by a job safety analysis, the JSA should be reviewed to determine whether or not it needs revision. If the JSA is revised, all employees concerned with the job should be informed of the changes and instructed in any new procedures.

When an accident results from failure to follow JSA procedures, the facts should be discussed with all those who do the job. It should be made clear that the accident would not have occurred had the JSA procedures been followed.

All supervisors are concerned with improving job methods to increase safety and health, reduce costs, and step up production. The job safety analysis is an excellent starting point for questioning the established way of doing a job. And study of the JSA may well suggest definite ideas for improvement of job methods.

## Purchasing

The safety department should have excellent liaison not only with the engineering department but also with the purchasing department.

It should be the duty of the safety department to devise and put in writing the safety standards that will guide the purchasing department. These standards should be set up so that the hazards involved in a particular kind of equipment or material being purchased are eliminated (as by substitution of a safe material for a dangerous one) or safeguarded for the protection of the worker, the machine, and the product.

The purchasing agent is not concerned closely with educational and enforcement activities, but he is vitally concerned with many phases of the engineering activities. It is the agent's duty to select and purchase the various items of machinery, tools, equipment, and materials used in the organization; and it is his responsibility—at least in part, and often to a considerable degree—to see that in design, manufacture, and particulars of shipment of all these items, safety has received adequate attention.

In one example, a lead hazard occurred in the unloading of litharge (PbO), which was shipped in 10-gallon paint pails with covers. These pails arrived, either in trucks or in boxcars, with a film of litharge on the outside. When they were moved, a lead concentration in the air 30 to 40 times the permissible limit was produced.

Several possible solutions were considered and tried, but the fundamental answer was to eliminate the hazard by having the purchasing department specify a rubber gasket under the pail lid as a part of the purchasing requirements. Thus the leakage, which created a serious health hazard, was easily controlled.

### Specifications

The engineering department, with the help of the safety department, should specify to the purchasing department all the necessary safeguarding to be built into a machine before it is purchased.

Persons responsible for purchasing in an industrial plant are necessarily cost conscious. Consequently, the safety professional must have as complete a grasp as possible of the accident losses to the company in terms of specific machines, materials, and processes. For instance, if he is to recommend the expenditure of several thousand dollars for a superior grade of tool to be used throughout the plant, the evidence must justify the investment.

Because of highly competitive marketing, manufacturers of machine tools and processing equipment often list safety devices designed for the protection of operators as separate auxiliary equipment. It is important that the safety professional be familiar with such auxiliary equipment and satisfy the purchasing agent of the need for its inclusion in the original order.

In some large organizations, the safety professional is charged with checking all plans and specifications for machinery and other equipment. In many organizations, particularly where certain items, such as goggles or safety shoes, are to be reordered from time to time, standard lists have been prepared through the cooperation of various operating officials, and purchases are selected only from among the types and from the companies shown on these approved lists. In still other establishments, the responsibility for design, quality, safety, and other features rests entirely on the employees who are to use the

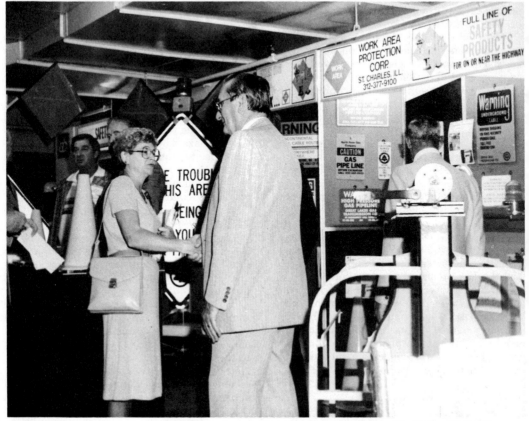

FIG. 5-7.—Twice each year, thousands of persons glean product and service information at the National Safety Congress and Exhibition in the fall and the Regional Safety Congress and Exposition in the spring.

articles. In such cases, the purchasing agent is responsible only for price, date of delivery, and similar details.

In many companies where purchases are made in enormous quantities and at a great investment of money, important duties are placed in three coordinate departments: (a) engineering department, where plans and specifications are prepared for all machinery and equipment to be purchased; (b) safety department, where these plans and specifications are carefully checked for safety and final inspections of articles purchased are carried out; and (c) purchasing department, which still has latitude in making selections as well as in determining standards of quality, efficiency, and price.

Still another variable must be mentioned. Many companies have both a full-time purchas-

ing agent and a full-time safety professional. However, in many other companies, especially smaller ones, these important duties are assumed by executives who devote part of their time to other activities. Nevertheless, the measures that should be taken to prevent accidents in the small plant are substantially the same as those in the large plant. The part that the purchasing agent can take in the safety program is similar; his interest will be the same and his activities will vary only in degree. His opportunity will lie in accepting as fully as possible all the suggestions that are presented here and in cooperating as closely as possible with others for the safety of all the workers in the establishment.

**Specification of shipping methods.** When materials are ordered, it may be desirable to specify that they be shipped in a particular manner. If safe and efficient shipping methods are worked out and then specified in the orders, the suppliers will be better able to deliver materials on time, in good condition, and in a shape or form that can be easily and safely handled by employees. Labeling of hazardous materials should be specified. Use DOT-authorized shipping labels.

## Codes and standards

In purchasing, as in no other aspect of his job, the safety professional will find a need for thorough knowledge of the accident history of his plant, the costs involved in accidents, and the probable benefits of the changes he advocates.

To fulfill his function in cooperation with the purchasing department, it is important that the safety professional be familiar with codes and standards. When a specific item of equipment is recommended, the safety professional should be able to state that it is a type approved by authoritative bodies and that it meets OSHA requirements.

It is usually necessary for the safety professional to consult with everyone concerned before setting up company standards for the guidance of the purchasing department.

There are many guides and standards that can be used as models. Accordingly, the safety professional (and all others concerned with setting company standards) should be familiar with the following:

1. Codes and standards approved by the American National Standards Institute and other standards and specifications groups—see Chapter 24, "Sources of Help."

2. Codes and standards adopted or set by federal, state, and local governmental agencies, such as the Occupational Safety and Health Administration, the Bureau of Mines, and the National Bureau of Standards.

3. Codes, standards, and lists of approved or tested devices published by such recognized agencies as the National Institute of Occupational Safety and Health, the Mining Safety and Health Administration, Underwriters Laboratories Inc., and fire protection organizations. For fire protection, the standards and codes of the National Fire Protection Association should be followed. (See Chapter 24.)

4. Safe practice recommendations of such agencies as the National Safety Council, insurance carriers or their associations, and trade and industrial organizations.

## Purchasing–safety liaison

With a background of knowledge gathered from such materials as those listed above, the safety professional should be well prepared to advise the purchasing department when required to do so.

**What purchasing can expect.** The purchasing agent can reasonably expect that the safety professional will:

1. Give specific information about machine and process hazards that can be eliminated by change in design or by guarding by the manufacturer.

2. Supply similar information about other equipment, tools, and materials, with the facts about injuries suffered and their causes.

3. Give specific information about health and fire hazards in the workplaces.

4. Provide information on federal and state safety requirements.

5. Supply on request additional special information on accident experience with machines, equipment, or materials when such articles are about to be reordered.

6. Request assistance in the investigation of accidents that may have been caused by faulty equipment or material.

**What the safety department can expect.** Where there is effective liaison between the safety and purchasing departments, the safety professional can expect that the purchasing agent will:

1. Become familiar with the departmental and plant process hazards, especially in relation to machinery, other equipment, and materials.

2. Ask the safety department for information on hazards and accident costs, for federal and state safety requirements, and for lists of approved devices and appliances that may be helpful to him in considering purchases.

3. Become acquainted with the specific location and departmental use of machinery or equip-

**153**

ment that is about to be ordered.

4. Participate in accident investigations where injuries may have been caused through the failure of machinery, equipment, or materials.

### Safety considerations

In the purchase of many articles, there is no need to consider safety. Some items, however, have a more important bearing upon safety than was at first suspected.

Utmost caution will be observed, of course, in the purchase of personal protective equipment, such as eye protection, respirators, masks, and the like; of equipment for the movement of suspended loads, such as ropes, chains, and cables; of equipment for the movement and storage of materials; of miscellaneous substances and fluids for cleaning and other purposes that might constitute or aggravate a fire or health hazard. Adequate labeling, identifying contents and calling attention to hazards, should be specified.

Investigation, however, may show that unsuspected hazards also lie in the purchase of very ordinary items, such as common hand tools, reflectors, tool racks, cleaning rags, paint for shop walls and machinery, and even filing cabinets. Among the factors to be considered by the purchasing agent are, for example, maximum load strength; long life without deterioration; sharp, rough, or pointed characteristics of articles; need for frequent adjustment; ease of maintenance; production of excessive fatigue; and hazard to the worker's health.

Here are a few examples of hazards created by purchased items that were thought to be safe. Goggles supplied to one group of workers were found to have imperfections in the lenses that caused eyestrain and headache, which led to fatigue and accidents. The toes of a laborer were crushed because the safety shoe he was wearing had an inferior metal cap and collapsed under a weight that should have been supported easily by a well-made shoe. Men were supplied with wooden carrying boxes in another plant, when a proper type of metal box could have eliminated the hazard of splinters and perhaps an infected hand.

It is in the purchase of larger items, however, and especially in the buying of machines, that the more spectacular examples of purchasing for safety are found. Today, machines of many types are manufactured and may be purchased with adequate safeguards in place as integral parts of the machines. The enclosed motor drive is an outstanding example of such engineering for safety in machine construction.

When an order for equipment is about to be placed, the purchasing agent, if possible, will not consider any machine which has been only partly guarded by the manufacturer and which, therefore, will need to be fitted with makeshift safeguards after it has been installed. The agent should be in frequent consultation with the safety department before making all purchases where safety is a factor. He will also be particularly careful to see that every purchased machine complies fully with the safety regulations of the state in which it is to be operated.

### Price considerations

When considering plant purchases from the standpoint of safety, the item of cost cannot be minimized. There is a constant struggle in the mind of the purchasing agent to reconcile quality, work efficiency, and safety with the price of an item.

Sometimes it may seem that the cost of an adequately safeguarded machine is out of all proportion to the cost of an unguarded machine plus the estimated cost of adding home-made safeguards. But the experience of many industrial plants has proved again and again that the best time to safeguard a machine or process is in the design stage. Safeguards planned and built as integral parts of a machine are the most efficient and durable.

The purchasing agent, through accident information supplied by the safety department, will be familiar with the costs of specific accidents in the plant, especially those in which an "unsafe condition" caused by a purchased item has been found to contribute to an accident.

The purchasing agent should be able to defend the decision to buy a slightly higher priced component, if that is necessary. Cooperation between the safety, engineering, manufacturing, and purchasing departments is absolutely necessary if accidents are to be eliminated.

These are arguments that must appeal to all executives who are responsible for the success of the industrial organization. The executive who is already sold on safety will be favorable to expenditures reasonably justified in the interest of accident prevention. If an executive does not have this attitude, means of increasing his interest and of broadening his understanding of the accident situation must be sought. In this undertaking, the purchasing agent can undoubtedly count upon the active cooperation of the safety professional.

In some instances, the purchase of machinery or equipment involves engineering details of great importance. For such purchases, the industrial establishment will undoubtedly have a system whereby definite specifications, perhaps including drawings, will first be prepared by engineers. These plans and specifications will then be carefully checked by the safety professional before bids and estimates of cost are solicited.

The purchasing agent will have the plans and specifications at hand when asking for prices. However, he will want to keep in close touch with the safety professional throughout the negotiations in order to use the latter's knowledge and experience in accident prevention.

After the purchase order has been made out and before it is signed, one other most important detail should not be overlooked. This is a statement, in language that cannot possibly be misinterpreted, that the articles ordered must comply fully with the applicable federal and state safety laws and regulations of the locality in which they are to be used.

This statement must be made a part of the purchase order.

## References

Bethlehem Steel Company, Bethlelem, Pa. "Job Safety Analysis." *Bethlehem Steel's Supervisory Safety Manual.* Chapter 5.

National Safety Council, 444 North Michigan Ave., Chicago, Ill. 60611
*Accident Facts* (published annually).
*OSHA Standards Handbook for Business and Industry.*

Pennsylvania Department of Labor and Industry, Harrisburg, Pa. *Industrial Injuries in Pennsylvania.* 1960.

U.S. Department of Transportation, Office of Hazardous Materials, Washington, D.C. 20590. "Newly Authorized Hazardous Materials Warning Labels." (Latest edition.) (Based on Title 49, *Code of Federal Regulations,*sections 173.402,—403, and—404; import or export shipments are covered in Title 14, C.F.R., section 103.13.)

# Accident Records
# and
# Incidence Rates

# Chapter
# 6

# 6—Accident Records and Incidence Rates

In this chapter, the terms *accident, incident,* and *injury* are restricted to those that include occupational injuries and illnesses. In other chapters, accident and incident are used in their broad meanings— "unplanned events that interrupt the completion of an activity, and that may (or may not) include property damage or injury."

With the Williams-Steiger Occupational Safety and Health Act of 1970, a majority of employers are required by law to maintain certain records of work-related employee injuries and illnesses. In addition to these records, many employers are also required to make reports to state compensation authorities. Insuring agencies may also require reports. For contest and award programs, further reports also based on OSHA recordkeeping requirements, may be filed. Occupational injury and illness reports and records are now required of nearly every establishment by management or government.

Safety personnel are faced with two tasks—maintaining those records required by law and by their management, and maintaining records that are useful to an effective safety program. In general, unfortunately, the two are not always synonymous. A good recordkeeping system necessitates more data than that contained in almost all required forms.

This chapter deals with both aspects of recordkeeping. Specific legal requirements are beyond the scope of this volume because they differ from industry to industry and state to state and are subject to change with time. The appropriate federal and state authorities need to be contacted in order to obtain the most current requirements. An outline of the general recordkeeping requirements under the OSHAct, as it exists at this time, is presented in this chapter. The basic definitions and the method of keeping records under the American National Standards Institute Z16.1 Standard are also presented, in the last section of this chapter, for those employers not using the OSHA recordkeeping system.

Although this chapter covers injuries and illnesses occurring to employees while on the job, standards exist both for off-the-job injuries to employees (ANSI Z16.3) and for injuries occurring to nonemployees in establishments (ANSI Z108). Both standards are briefly summarized in the off-the-job and patron injuries section. The standards themselves should be consulted by the safety personnel concerned with those aspects of the overall safety program.

The first section deals with recordkeeping systems in general and contains sample forms and recommendations for establishing a good recordkeeping system.

## Accident Records

Records of accidents and injuries are essential to efficient and successful safety programs, just as records of production, costs, sales, and profits and losses are essential to efficient and successful operation of a business. Records supply the information necessary to transform haphazard, costly, ineffective safety work into a planned safety program that controls both conditions and acts that contribute to accidents. Good recordkeeping is the foundation of a scientific approach to occupational safety.

### Uses of records

A good recordkeeping system can help the safety professional in the following ways:

1. Provide safety personnel with the means for an objective evaluation of the magnitude of their accident problems and with a measurement of the overall progress and effectiveness of their safety program.

2. Identify high-rate units, plants, or departments and problem areas so that extra effort can be made in those areas.

3. Provide data for an analysis of accidents and illnesses that can point to specific circumstances of occurrence which can then be attacked by specific countermeasures.

4. Create interest in safety among supervisors by furnishing them with information about the accident experience of their own departments.

5. Provide supervisors ad safety committees with hard facts about their safety problems so that their efforts can be concentrated.

6. Measure the effectiveness of individual countermeasures and determine if specific programs are doing the job that they were designed to do.

### Recordkeeping systems

The system presented in this section is a model that can be used to provide the basic items necessary for good recordkeeping. It is designed to dovetail with the present recordkeeping requirements of the OSHAct and attempts to avoid a duplication of effort on the part of the personnel responsible for keeping records and filing reports. Provision is also made for easily entering the data necessary for those organizations using the Z16.1 Standard and computing those frequency and severity rates without the necessity of a separate set of records. Some of the forms presented in this section are also constructed with modern data processing methods in mind. In general, a self-coding, check-off form can save time for both the person who fills out the report and the person who is responsible for tabulating and processing the data on the forms.

A well-designed form takes into account the person who will fill it out and the way in which the forms will be processed. It more likely will be filled out accurately and will present fewer problems for those who process and analyze the data. Care in the choice and design of forms will pay dividends in better, more reliable data.

The recordkeeping system in this section is not presented as the only way to keep records but rather as an example. The accident problems of individual establishments are unique and no one form or set of forms can possibly provide every establishment with all the data for solving all of its individual problems. A system that does a good job of collecting the basic facts, however, makes it easier to zero-in later on the specific data about a specific problem.

The following sections deal with occupational injuries and illnesses. Property-damage accidents are covered in Chapter 7. Nonemployee accidents are covered in Chapter 21. Specific recordkeeping requirements were explained in Chapter 2, "Federal Legislation."

## Accident reports and injury records

To be effective, preventive measures must be based on complete and unbiased knowledge of the causes of accidents. The primary purpose of an accident report is to obtain such information and not to fix blame. Since the completeness and accuracy of the entire accident record system depend upon information in the individual accident reports, be sure that the forms and their purpose are understood by those who must fill them out. Necessary training or instruction should be made available to these personnel.

**The first aid report.** The collection of injury data generally begins in the first aid department. The first aid attendant or nurse fills out a first aid report for each new case. Copies are sent to the safety department or safety committee, the worker's supervisor, and other departments as management may wish. See Fig. 6–1.

The first aid attendant or the nurse should know enough about accident analysis and investigation to be able to record the principal facts about each case. The physician engaged or authorized by the employer to treat injured employees also should be informed of the basic rules for classifying cases since, at times, his opinion of the seriousness of an injury may be necessary to record the case accurately.

**Supervisor's accident report.** It is recommended that the supervisor make a detailed report about each accident, even when only a minor injury or no injury is the result. For purposes of OSHA or ANSI Z16.1 summaries, only those reports that meet the minimum severity level can be separated and tallied. Minor injuries occur in greater numbers than serious injuries and records of these injuries can be helpful in pinpointing problem areas. By working to alleviate these problems, serious injuries can sometimes be prevented. Furthermore, complications may arise out of the less serious injuries and their end result may be quite serious.

The supervisor's accident report form should be completed as soon as possible after an accident occurs. Copies of these reports should be sent to the safety department and to other designated persons. Information concerning activities and conditions that preceded an occurrence is important in the prevention of future accidents. This information is particularly difficult to get unless it is obtained promptly after the accident occurs.

Generally, analyses of accidents are made only periodically, and often long after the accidents have occurred. Because it is often impossible to recall with accuracy the details of an accident, if details are not recorded accurately and completely at once, they may be lost forever.

Although all information may not be available at the time that the accident report is being filled out, items such as total time lost and amount of dollars of damage can be added later. This should not, however, prevent the other items from being answered as soon as possible after the accident occurs.

Three different supervisor's report forms are

Case No. 164          Date 2-12-

### First Aid Report

Name S. D. Smith _____ Department Shipping

Male ☒  Female ☐  Occupation Packer ___ Foreman Miller

Date of
Occurrence 2-12 Time 10 a.m. p.m.   Date of
First Treatment 2-12 Time 10 a.m. p.m.

Nature of
Occurrence Splinter in index finger of left hand

Sent: Back to Work ☒    Doctor ☐    Home ☐    Hospital ☐

Estimated Disability 0 days

Employee's Description of Occurrence Handling wooden crates
without gloves, ran splinter into finger

Signed *M. Miller*
First Aid

**Issued by National Safety Council, Inc.**
Form IS-6          Printed in U.S.A.          STOCK No. 129.26

Fig. 6-1.—A "First Aid Report" (4 × 6 in. or 10 × 15 cm) is prepared by the first aid attendant at the time an injured or ill person comes for treatment. A report should be prepared for each case, whether minor or serious. The report serves as a record and permits quick tabulation of such data as department, occupation, and the key facts of the occurrence.

presented. They fulfill all of the information requirements of the present OSHA 101 form. Provision is also made to easily enter ANSI Z16.1 information, which allows both types of record-keeping to be accomplished in one form, without any duplication of effort. The forms also include questions in addition to those contained in the present OSHA 101 form (Fig. 6-8, p. 178). These questions ask for additional basic data that should be known about each accident.

The first supervisor's report form (Fig. 6-2) is an open end, narrative type of form. The next forms (Figs. 6-3 and -4) are self-coding to allow key-punching of data items directly from the form without the extra step of recoding this information for data processing equipment. By using self-coding forms, data processing equipment can be easily used to process the information and produce a variety of summary reports (such as summaries by department, by type of accident, etc.).

Detailed cross tabulations can thus be produced with little effort.

For defintions of the terms regarding severity of injury, what cases are recordable, and the like, please consult the OSHA and Z16.1 sections of this chapter. For further clarification of OSHA definitions, see the guidelines section of this chapter. You may also want to consult federal or state authorities (if your state has an approved plan in effect).

**Injury and illness record of employee.** After cases are closed, the first aid report and the supervisor's report are filed by agency of injury (type of machine, tool, material, etc.), type of accident, or other factor that will facilitate use of the reports for accident prevention. Another form, therefore, must be used to record the injury experience of individual employees. (See Fig. 6-5.)

This form helps supervisors remember the experience of individual employees. Particularly in large establishments or plants where supervisors may have many people working for them, they probably cannot recall from memory the total number of injuries—especially if the injuries are minor—that are suffered by individual employees.

The employee injury card, therefore, fills a real need. It has space for recording such factors about the injury as date, classification, days charged, costs, and OSHA lost workdays.

Because of the importance of the personal factor in accidents, much may be learned about accident causes from studying employee injury records. If certain employees or job classifications have frequent injuries, a study of employee working habits, physical and mental abilities, training, job assignments, working environment, and the instructions and supervision given them may reveal more than a study of accident locations, agencies, or other factors.

**Filing reports.** After injury reports have been used to compile monthly summaries, the incomplete reports may be kept in a temporary file for convenient reference as later information about the injuries becomes available.

After the injury reports are complete, they should be filed in a way that will permit ready use of them for making special studies of accident conditions. To facilitate this work, the reports may be filed by agency of the injury, by occupation of the injured person, by department, or by some similar item.

The employee injury card should be cross referenced to the file location of the detailed accident report.

### Periodic reports

The forms discussed in the preceding paragraphs are prepared when the accidents occur; they are used to record the accidents and preserve information about contributing circumstances. Periodically, this information should be summarized and related to department or plant exposure so that the safety work can be evaluated and the principal accident causes brought into proper focus.

**Monthly summary of injuries and illnesses.** A summary of injuries and illnesses should be prepared monthly to reveal the current status of accident experience. This monthly summary of injury and illness cases (Fig. 6–6) allows for tabulating monthly and cumulative totals and the computation of OSHA incidence rates as well as ANSI Z16.1 frequency and severity rates (for those organizations still using that standard). Space is also provided for yearly totals and rates. This form would be filled out on the basis of the individual report forms that were processed during the month or from form OSHA No. 200, Log and Summary of Occupational Injuries and Illnesses. (See Fig. 6–7, pp. 176-177.)

The monthly summary should be prepared as soon after the end of each month as the information becomes available, but not later than the 20th of the following month. Because this report is prepared primarily to reveal the current status of accident experience, it is essential that this information be determined as soon as possible.

If an accident report is still incomplete on the 20th of the following month because the employee has not returned to work, or if the classification of an injury is still in doubt at that time, an estimate of the outcome should be made by the company physician and the report included with the completed cases in the monthly summary.

When definite information becomes available for estimated cases, any change in classification or OSHA lost workdays should be entered in the appropriate columns in the month of closing of the case, and the adjustment included in the cumulative figures for the year through that month. This procedure provides reliable monthly data and an easy method of adjusting cumulative data.

**Annual report.** Every establishment that is subject to the OSHAct is obliged to post its annual report on February 1st. The cumulative totals on form OSHA No. 200, Log and Summary of Occupational Injuries and Illnesses, serve as the annual report. Those establishments designated as part of the annual Bureau of Labor Statistics sample must also send a copy of this report to Washington.

For management purposes, however, the annual report fulfills a more direct function. Whereas monthly summaries of injuries and illnesses are prepared primarily to show the trend of safety performance during the year, annual reports are prepared so that comparisons for the longer period may be made with the experience of

*(Text continues on page 173.)*

# 6—Accident Records and Incidence Rates

1. <u>ACCIDENT CATEGORY</u> ☐ Injury; ☐ Illness; ☐ Property Damage; ☐ Fire; ☐ Other

    Company name and address _____

    Plant location (if different from above) _____

2. Name and address of injured (or ill) person _____

    _____ SSN _____ 3. Age _____

4. Sex _____ 5. Years of service _____ 6. Time on present job _____

7. Title/occupation (at time of occurrence)_____

8. Department _____ 9. Date of incident _____

10. Time of incident _____ a.m. - p.m.

11. <u>SEVERITY OF INJURY OR ILLNESS</u> ☐ First-aid; ☐ Medical treatment; ☐ Lost workday case;

    ☐ Restricted work case; ☐ Time away from work case; ☐ Fatality

12. Estimated number of days on restricted work _____

13. Estimated number of days away from work _____

14. <u>INJURY DESCRIPTION</u> Describe nature of injury or illness _____

15. Part of body affected _____

16. Degree of disability (describe) _____

                   (Temporary total; permanent partial; permanent total)

17. <u>ACCIDENT DESCRIPTION</u> Place incident occurred _____

18. What part of job was being performed at time of incident? _____

19. What happened? Describe in sequence: _____

20. Physical surroundings at time of incident: (weather, equipment, machinery, aisles, features, etc.) _____

21. How was work being done? _____

22. What happened to cause incident? _____

23. Other factors necessary to fully describe incident _____

24. <u>PERSONAL PROTECTIVE EQUIPMENT</u> required (Protective glasses, safety shoes, safety hat, hearing protection, respirator, etc.) _____

25. Was injured using required safety equipment? _____

26. Date employee was last trained in proper use of required safety equipment _____

27. <u>WAS THERE A VIOLATION</u> of a published safety/health rule, regulation, procedure or specific instructions? (Explain) _____

28. <u>WAS EMPLOYEE PROPERLY INSTRUCTED</u> on how to do the job safely and properly exposed in training to those items listed in previous question? (Explain) _____

FIG. 6–2.—Supervisor's Accident Report ($8^1/_2 \times 11$ in. or $22 \times 28$ cm) provides a record of contributing circumstances to provide a basis for specific remedial action. Supervisors should be trained to fill it in properly. The bottom portion of the second page (*at right*) is filled in by higher management. Details of the unsafe acts and conditions are important in preventing future accidents; often even more important is information that shows *why* the unsafe condition existed and *why* the injured person acted unsafely.

29. WERE INSTRUCTIONS ADEQUATELY related to the specific hazards involved? (Explain)
_____
_____

30. WERE MECHANICAL/PHYSICAL/ENVIRONMENTAL conditions safe at the time of the incident?
(Explain) _____
_____

31. DETAILED NARRATIVE DESCRIPTION: (How did accident occur; why; objects, tool, equipment, tools used, etc.) _____
_____
_____
_____

32. WHAT CORRECTIVE ACTION should be taken to avoid a reoccurence of this type of injury
(state who - what - engineering changes; written procedure development or improvement,
enforcement of safety rules, regulations, instructions or procedures or specific training) _____
_____
_____

33. ACTIONS TAKEN ALREADY to correct and/or eliminate the hazard, injury causing agent(s)
_____
_____
_____

34. WITNESS TO ACCIDENT _____
    Date report prepared _____
       Signature of investigating Foreman/Supervisor _____
       Signature of reviewing Supervisor _____


SUPERINTENDENT'S APPRAISAL AND RECOMMENDATION

MANAGEMENT COMMENTS AND ADDITIONAL CORRECTIVE/PREVENTIVE ACTION REQUIRED

_____
_____
_____
_____
_____

                              Signature of Superintendent/Plant Manager

Date: _____

                                              Stock No. 129.21

# 6—Accident Records and Incidence Rates

SERVICE NO. (NSC)
► 1-9 _____

CASE OR FILE NO.
► 10-15 _____

**SUPPLEMENTARY RECORD OF**
**OCCUPATIONAL INJURIES AND ILLNESSES**

OSHA No. 101   NSC revision
(Meets OSHA requirements
when Instruction 1. has
been followed.)

## THIS REPORT IS

► 16, 1 ☐ First report   2 ☐ Revised report

## EMPLOYER

1. NAME _____

2. MAIL ADDRESS _____

3. LOCATION, if different
   from mail address _____

## INJURED OR ILL EMPLOYEE

4. NAME _____

   SOCIAL SECURITY NO. _____

   ► EMPLOYEE NO.  17-26 _____

5. HOME ADDRESS _____

► 6. AGE  27-28 _____

► 7. SEX  29, 1 ☐ Male   2 ☐ Female

► 8. OCCUPATION (specify) _____

   30-31, 01 ☐ Manager, official, proprietor
   02 ☐ Professional, technical
   03 ☐ Foreman, supervisor
   04 ☐ Sales worker
   05 ☐ Clerical worker
   06 ☐ Craftsman—construction
   07 ☐ Craftsman—other
   08 ☐ Machinist
   09 ☐ Mechanic
   10 ☐ Operative (production worker)
   11 ☐ Motor vehicle driver
   12 ☐ Laborer
   13 ☐ Service worker
   14 ☐ Agricultural worker
   15 ☐ Other
   16 ☐ Unknown

9. DEPARTMENT _____
   (Enter the name of department or division in which
   the injured person is regularly employed.)

## CLASSIFICATION OF CASE

A. INJURY OR ILLNESS (see code on Log, OSHA No. 100)

   ► 32, 1 ☐ Injury (10)
   2 ☐ Occupational skin disease or disorder (21)
   3 ☐ Dust disease of the lungs (pneumoconioses) (22)
   4 ☐ Respiratory conditions due to toxic agents (23)
   5 ☐ Poisoning (systemic effects of toxic materials) (24)
   6 ☐ Disorder due to physical agents
       (other than toxic materials) (25)
   7 ☐ Disorder due to repeated trauma (26)
   8 ☐ All other occupational illnesses (29)

B. EXTENT OF INJURY OR ILLNESS

   ► 33, 1 ☐ Fatality
   2 ☐ Lost workday case
   3 ☐ Nonfatal case without lost workdays

► C. Number of workdays lost  34-36 _____

D. Permanently transferred or terminated

   ► 37, 1 ☐ Yes   2 ☐ No

**164**

## INSTRUCTIONS

1. Type or print the narrative where requested.
2. Check the one box which most clearly describes
   each narrative statement.
3. See also original OSHA No. 101 for more details.
4. Complete form in duplicate. Retain original.
   Mail duplicate to:  National Safety Council,
   Chicago IL 60611.

## THE ACCIDENT OR EXPOSURE TO OCCUPATIONAL ILLNESS

10. PLACE OF ACCIDENT
    OR EXPOSURE _____
    (mail address)

11. WHERE DID ACCIDENT OR EXPOSURE OCCUR?
    a. On employer premises
    ► 38, 1 ☐ Yes   2 ☐ No   3 ☐ Unknown

    b. Place (specify) _____

    ► 39-40, 01 ☐ Office
    02 ☐ Plant, mill
    03 ☐ Shipping, receiving, warehouse
    04 ☐ Maintenance shop
    05 ☐ General or public area of employer premises
        (corridor, washroom, lunchroom, parking lot, etc.)
    06 ☐ Retail establishment
        (store, restaurant, gasoline station, etc.)
    07 ☐ Farm
    08 ☐ Motor vehicle accident
    09 ☐ Other
    10 ☐ Unknown

12. WHAT WAS THE EMPLOYEE DOING WHEN INJURED? (Be specific)

    _____
    _____
    _____

    a. Task performed at time of accident
    ► 41-42, 01 ☐ Operating machine
    02 ☐ Operating hand tool (power or nonpower)
    03 ☐ Materials handling
    04 ☐ Maintenance & repair—machinery
    05 ☐ Maintenance & repair—building & equipment
    06 ☐ Motor vehicle driver, operator or passenger
    07 ☐ Office and sales tasks, except above
    08 ☐ Service tasks, except above
    09 ☐ Other
    10 ☐ Not performing task
    11 ☐ Unknown

    b. Activity at time of accident
    ► 43-44, 01 ☐ Climbing
    02 ☐ Driving
    03 ☐ Jumping
    04 ☐ Kneeling
    05 ☐ Lying down
    06 ☐ Lifting
    07 ☐ Reaching, stretching
    08 ☐ Riding
    09 ☐ Running
    10 ☐ Sitting
    11 ☐ Standing
    12 ☐ Walking
    13 ☐ Other
    14 ☐ Unknown

FIG. 6-3.

**13. HOW DID THE ACCIDENT OCCUR?** (Describe fully the events)

_____
_____
_____
_____
_____

**a. AGENCY.** (Object or substance involved)

**ACCIDENT AGENCY** (1st column). The first object or substance involved in accident sequence.

**INJURY AGENCY** (2nd column). The agency inflicting the injury. See also section 15.

(Example: Worker fell from ladder and struck head on machine. Check "Ladder" under accident and check "Machine" under injury.)

| ACCIDENT | INJURY | (Check one box in each column) |
|---|---|---|
| 45-46, 01 ☐ | 47-48, 01 ☐ | Machine |
| 02 ☐ | 02 ☐ | Conveyor, elevator, hoist |
| 03 ☐ | 03 ☐ | Vehicle |
| 04 ☐ | 04 ☐ | Electrical apparatus |
| 05 ☐ | 05 ☐ | Hand tool |
| 06 ☐ | 06 ☐ | Chemical |
| 07 ☐ | 07 ☐ | Working surface, bench, table, etc. |
| 08 ☐ | 08 ☐ | Floor, walking surface |
| 09 ☐ | 09 ☐ | Bricks, rocks, stones |
| 10 ☐ | 10 ☐ | Box, barrel, container (empty or full) |
| 11 ☐ | 11 ☐ | Door, window, etc. |
| 12 ☐ | 12 ☐ | Ladder |
| 13 ☐ | 13 ☐ | Lumber, woodworking materials |
| 14 ☐ | 14 ☐ | Metal |
| 15 ☐ | 15 ☐ | Stairway, steps |
| 16 ☐ | 16 ☐ | Other |
| 17 ☐ | 17 ☐ | Unknown |
| 18 ☐ | 18 ☐ | None |

**b. ACCIDENT TYPE.** (First event in the accident sequence)

49-50, 01 ☐ Fall from elevation
02 ☐ Fall on same level
03 ☐ Struck against
04 ☐ Struck by
05 ☐ Caught in, under or between
06 ☐ Rubbed or abraded
07 ☐ Bodily reaction
08 ☐ Overexertion
09 ☐ Contact with electrical current
10 ☐ Contact with temperature extremes
11 ☐ Contact with radiations, caustics, toxic and noxious substances
12 ☐ Public transportation accident
13 ☐ Motor vehicle accident
14 ☐ Other
15 ☐ Unknown

## ANSI Z16.1 INFORMATION

**A. DEGREE OF DISABILITY UNDER Z16.1**

60, 1 ☐ Not a recordable case under Z16.1
2 ☐ Temporary total disability
3 ☐ Permanent partial disability
4 ☐ Permanent total disability
5 ☐ Fatality

**B. DAYS CHARGED UNDER Z16.1** 61-64 _____

## OCCUPATIONAL INJURY OR ILLNESS

**14. DESCRIBE THE INJURY OR ILLNESS** in detail and indicate the part of the body affected.

_____
_____
_____
_____

**a. NATURE OF INJURY OR ILLNESS.** (Check most serious one)

51-52, 01 ☐ Amputation
02 ☐ Burn and scald (heat)
03 ☐ Burn (chemical)
04 ☐ Concussion
05 ☐ Crushing injury
06 ☐ Cut, laceration, puncture, abrasion
07 ☐ Fracture
08 ☐ Hernia
09 ☐ Bruise, contusion
10 ☐ Occupational illness
11 ☐ Sprain, strain
12 ☐ Other

**b. PART OF BODY.** (Check most serious one)

53-54, 01 ☐ Eyes
02 ☐ Head, face, neck
03 ☐ Back
04 ☐ Trunk (except back, internal)
05 ☐ Arm
06 ☐ Hand and wrist
07 ☐ Fingers
08 ☐ Leg
09 ☐ Feet and ankles
10 ☐ Toes
11 ☐ Internal and other

**15. NAME THE OBJECT OR SUBSTANCE WHICH DIRECTLY INJURED THE EMPLOYEE.** Also check one box in injury column under 13a.

_____
_____
_____

**16. DATE OF INJURY OR INITIAL DIAGNOSIS OF OCCUPATIONAL ILLNESS.**

**a. MONTH**

| | | | |
|---|---|---|---|
| 55-56, 01 ☐ Jan. | | 07 ☐ July |
| 02 ☐ Feb. | | 08 ☐ Aug. |
| 03 ☐ March | | 09 ☐ Sept. |
| 04 ☐ April | | 10 ☐ Oct. |
| 05 ☐ May | | 11 ☐ Nov. |
| 06 ☐ June | | 12 ☐ Dec. |

**b. DATE OF MONTH** 57-58 _____

**17. DID EMPLOYEE DIE?**

59, 1 ☐ Yes    Date of Death _____
2 ☐ No

## OTHER

**18. NAME AND ADDRESS OF PHYSICIAN** _____
_____

**19. IF HOSPITALIZED, NAME AND ADDRESS OF HOSPITAL** _____
_____

DATE OF REPORT _____

PREPARED BY _____

OFFICIAL POSITION _____

NSC will use for statistics only and hold report confidential.

Fig. 6–4.—This 6-page "Form 2020, Supervisor's Injury/Illness Investigation Report" is well designed to solicit additional information for causal and cost analyses. The pages fold to open as illustrated here, so that instructions can easily be followed.

*Reprinted with permission of Air Products and Chemicals, Inc.*

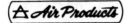

---

**FORM 2020**
**SUPERVISOR'S INJURY / ILLNESS**
**INVESTIGATION REPORT**

---

## GENERAL INSTRUCTIONS

### WHEN MUST FORM 2020 BE USED?

All accidents and near-miss accidents should be investigated. Form 2020 must be completed and forwarded to Corporate Safety in Trexlertown within **48 hours** in the following circumstances:

1. When near-miss accidents, with the potential for serious injury occur.

2. All accidents involving personnel injury or illness serious enough to require a State Workmen's Compensation Insurance Report (an Employer's First Report of Injury). This includes injuries sustained in automobile accidents while the employee is on company business.

3. All suspected OSHA recordable injuries / illnesses.

4. All known injuries or illnesses to non-employees that involve our products, facilities, or employees.

ONE FORM MUST BE COMPLETED FOR EACH PERSON INJURED / ILL AS DESCRIBED IN 2, 3 & 4 ABOVE.

### WHO MUST FILL OUT FORM 2020?

Section I on Form 2020 is all coded indexing information for the computer system. This section will be completed by Corporate Safety.

Sections II through V will be filled out by the injured / ill person's supervisor.

Sections VI will be filled out by the Supervisor's Manager, after Sections II through V have been completed.
When the injured / ill person is not an employee, Sections II through V will be filled out by the person investigating the accident and Section VI by the Supervisor's Manager.
Each line on the form is keyed to the appropriate instruction by the circled numbers e.g.⑤

PLEASE NOTE: The format of some of the entries, such as the date, etc. is very critical. PLEASE FOLLOW THE DETAILED INSTRUCTIONS IN THIS PAMPHLET CAREFULLY WRITING ONLY IN THE UNSHADED AREAS.
FILL IN ALL APPLICABLE BOXES — ONE ENTRY — ONE BOX.

### WHAT TO DO WHEN THE FORM IS COMPLETED?

When Sections II through V are completed, the form should be sent to the Supervisor's Manager who will complete Section VI.
When Section VI is completed, the form should be detached from the instructions, copied and the following distribution made:

1. The original 2020 and a copy of the State Workmen's Compensation Insurance Report (Employer's First Report of Injury) should be sent to Corporate Safety, Trexlertown. (A copy of the State Workmen's Compensation Insurance Report should also be sent to Corporate Risk Management, Trexlertown).

2. One copy should be retained in the facility's file.

3. One copy should be sent to Group / Division Safety.

4. Other copies as required by Group / Division or Local requirements.

### WHAT IS FORM 2020 USED FOR?

Form 2020 will be used as the data entry form for the computerized Safety Information System (SINS). SINS will compile accident information and allow us to determine, among other things, what kind of accidents and injuries are occurring, their causes, and how much they cost. With this information, which is available to all supervisors and managers in the company, we can develop specific programs to help you solve your particular safety problems.

### NOTICE!

**THIS FORM MUST BE SUBMITTED IN**
**ORDER FOR INSURANCE CLAIMS TO BE PAID.**

FORM 2020 (REV 1 / 81)

# 6—Accident Records and Incidence Rates

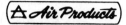

To start—
Match this
Arrow with
Arrow on
Page 3

**FORM 2020**
**SUPERVISOR'S INJURY / ILLNESS INVESTIGATION REPORT**

## INSTRUCTIONS

### SECTION I — TO BE COMPLETED BY CORPORATE SAFETY, TREXLERTOWN

### SECTION II — ACCIDENT INFORMATION

(1) Give **Date, Time** and **Day of Week** accident occured:
Date: Use 2 digits for day, first 3 letters of month, last 2 digits of year:  July 2, 1980 = 02 Jul 80
Time: Use military time:  11:38 P.M. = 23 38; 11:38 A.M. = 11 38.
Day of week: Use first 3 letters of day of week:  Thursday = THU.

(2) **Complete for Company employees only:**
Give **Name** of injured / ill employee; **Employee Number; Sex; Age**
Was employee on **Overtime?** (Y = Yes; N = No)
How **long** has employee held **this job title?**
  [1] less than 1 month
  [2] 1 month through 5 months
  [3] 6 months through 5 years
  [4] more than 5 years

(3) **Complete for Non-Company employees only:**
Give **Name** of injured / ill person; **Sex** (M = Male; F = Female); **Age; Address.**

(4) Give the name of the **Reporting Facility and the location of the accident.**

(5) Give number of **People injured / ill** due to this accident. Break down number of injured / ill people into **Company employees** and **Non-Company employees.** Indicate if property was damaged (applies only to **Damage more than $10,000** replacement and / or repair cost).

### SECTION III — ACCIDENT SEQUENCE

(6) Describe **How accident resulted in injury / illness** (e.g.; hit head on floor). Describe the physical condition or contact that actually produced the injury.

(7) Describe the **Actual Events that occurred during the accident.** (e.g.; forklift hit ladder and employee fell; valve broke and employee was struck by flying object). Include any equipment or substances involved, any actions, movements or conditions which may have led to the accident or increased its severity.

(8) Choose an **Accident Type Code** from one of the major categories below (e.g.; dust in eye, code 201).
If **"other" describe.** If no code is appropriate, provide a written description of the accident type.

| ACCIDENT TYPE CODES | | | |
|---|---|---|---|
| **FALLS, SLIPS, TRIPS** (off, on, over) | **STRUCK, CAUGHT** (by, against, between) **OBJECT** | **CONTACT WITH MATERIAL. CONDITION** (Touching, breathing, swallowing, absorbing). | **OVEREXERTION, STRAIN** (load, no load) |
| 101 Off chair, furniture | 201 By airborne dust, particles | | 401 Load-carrying, holding twisting, reaching |
| 102 Off dock, opening excavation | 202 By another person, object being held | 301 Chemicals - corrosive, irritating substances in, around or from process equipment | 402 Load-lifting |
| 103 Off ladder, scaffold | 203 By chips/particles from use of powered hand tools, machinery or equipment. | 302 Chemicals - corrosive, irritating substances while handling or transferring bulk quantity | 403 Load-pulling, pushing turning |
| 104 Off machinery, equipment | 204 By chips / particles from use of non-powered hand tools. | 303 Chemicals - corrosive, irritating substances - in small laboratory quantity | 449 Load - other |
| 105 Off vehicle | | | 450 No load - bending |
| 109 Off other high place | 210 By object - blown off pressurized system | 304 Commercial cleaning materials | 451 No load - reaching, twisting |
| 141 On stairs, steps-indoors | | 329 Chemicals - other | 499 No load - other |
| 142 On paved surfaces-indoors | 211 By object - broken off, vibrated loose, mobilized | 330 Electricity, power hand tools | |
| 149 On other flat surfaces-indoors | 212 By object - collapse, cave-in | 339 Electricity, other | |
| 151 On stairs, steps-outdoors | 213 By object - dropped, released by self during handling | 340 Exposure to natural elements | |
| 152 On paved surfaces-outdoors | | 351 Fire flame, intense heat | |
| 153 On loose ground covers-outdoors | 214 By object - from explosion, overpressure | 352 Hot, cold surface | |
| 159 On other flat surfaces-outdoors | 215 By object- dropped, released or thrown by another person | 353 Non pressurized hot liquid, hot material | |
| | 219 By - other | 354 Pressurized hot liquid, gas | |
| | 240 By / against handtool, non-powered | 355 Pressurized cold liquid, gas | **MISCELLANEOUS** |
| | 241 By / against handtool, powered | 360 Noise | 501 Animal, insects, plants |
| | | 370 Radiation | 521 Public transportation |
| | 242 By / against moving equipment / machinery | 380 Smoke, gas | 541 Sports activity |
| | 250 Against stationary, sharp object | 390 Welding flash | 561 Vehicle passenger, driver |
| | 259 Against other | 399 Other material or condition | 599 Other |
| | 280 Caught in moving machinery, equipment | | |
| | 281 Caught, pinched between objects | | |
| | 299 Other - struck by or against | | |

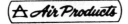

**FORM 2020**
**SUPERVISOR'S INJURY / ILLNESS INVESTIGATION REPORT**

## SECTION I — TO BE COMPLETED BY CORPORATE SAFETY, TREXLERTOWN

IND

ICIS NO.  SINS NO.

15A  A  B  C  D  E  F  G  H  I

10A  ORGANIZATION NO.  CASE / IDENTIFIER

## SECTION II — ACCIDENT INFORMATION

(1) DATE OF ACCIDENT (DDMMMYY)  TIME OF ACCIDENT  DAY OF WEEK OF ACCIDENT

(2) COMPLETE FOR COMPANY EMPLOYEE ONLY

FIRST NAME  INITIAL  LAST NAME

20A  EMPLOYEE NO.  SEX  AGE  O/T (Y or N)  TIME IN JOB ★

(3) COMPLETE FOR NON-COMPANY EMPLOYEE ONLY

FIRST NAME  M.I.  LAST NAME  SEX  AGE

ADDRESS

(4) FACILITY / ACCIDENT LOCATION

(5) TOTAL PEOPLE INJURED / ILL  CO. EMPLOYEES INJURED / ILL  NON-CO. EMPLOYEES INJURED / ILL  (✓) IF PROPERTY DAMAGE EXCEEDS $10,000.

## SECTION III — ACCIDENT SEQUENCE

(6) HOW ACCIDENT RESULTED IN INJURY / ILLNESS (e.g. hit head on floor)

(7) ACTUAL EVENTS THAT OCCURRED DURING THE ACCIDENT (e.g. forklift hit ladder - employee fell)

(8) ACCIDENT TYPE CODE ★  IF "OTHER", DESCRIBE

★ SEE INSTRUCTIONS FOR CODES  FILE _____

**169**

# 6—Accident Records and Incidence Rates

## SECTION IV — ACTIVITY INFORMATION

9  What was the injured / ill person doing? (e.g. bolting a flange).

10  How often has the person done this activity? { ( 1 DAILY          2 WEEKLY          3 MONTHLY
                                                     4 LESS THAN ONCE PER MONTH    5 NEVER BEFORE )

Was this activity a normal part of the job? (Y = Yes; N = No).
Was person adequately trained for this activity in your opinion? (Y = Yes; N = No)

11  Do standard methods or procedures exist for the task the person was doing? (Y = Yes; N = No) If Yes,
Were they followed? (Y = Yes; N = No) If procedures were not followed,

Did something discourage following procedures? (Y or N)

12  If procedures were not followed, what was done differently than called for by the procedure?

## SECTION V — INJURY / ILLNESS INFORMATION

13  Was person using equipment to protect against this injury / illness? (Y = Yes; N = No)
Was person supposed to be using protective equipment? (Y = Yes; N = No)
Describe the Type of protective equipment required and actually used.

14  Select the most serious and second most serious Nature of Injury / Illness code from below.

### NATURE OF INJURY / ILLNESS CODES

| INJURY | | OCCUPATIONAL ILLNESS |
|---|---|---|
| 101 Amputation | 110 Foreign Body, Sliver, Chip, Dust | 201 Skin Disease, Disorder |
| 102 Bite, Sting | 111 Fracture, Crush, Dislocate | 202 Lung Problem, Dust-Related |
| 103 Bruise, Contusion | 112 Internal Injury, Hernia, Heart | 203 Lung Problem, Toxic-Agent Related |
| 104 Burn, Hot, Cold, Chemical, Scald | 113 Loss of Senses, Faculties | 204 Poisoning |
| 105 Concussion, Unconscious | 114 Scrape, Scratch, Abrasion | 205 Disorders Due To Physical Agents |
| 106 Cut, Laceration, Puncture | 115 Sprain, Strain, Torn | (Other Than Toxic Agents) |
| 107 Exhaustion, Heat Stroke | 116 Suffocation, Drowning | 206 Disorders Associated With Repeated Trauma |
| 108 Electric Shock | 199 All Other | 299 All Other |

15  Select the Part of Body Code from below corresponding to the most serious and second most serious injury / illness.
For 14 and 15, Describe each injury / illness and how each part of the body was affected.

### PART OF BODY CODES

| HEAD / NECK | ARM / SHOULDER | TORSO | LEG | FACULTY / SYSTEM |
|---|---|---|---|---|
| 301 Scalp | 401 Shoulder | 501 Chest / Ribs | 601 Thigh | 701 Hearing |
| 302 Skull | 402 Upper Arm | 502 Back-Muscles | 602 Knee | 702 Vision |
| 303 Ears | 403 Elbow | 508 Back-Skeletal / Nervous | 603 Shin, Calf | 703 Smell |
| 304 Eyes | 404 Forearm | 503 Heart | 604 Ankle | 704 Taste |
| 305 Face | 405 Wrist | 504 Abdomen | 605 Foot | 705 Touch |
| 306 Nose | 406 Hand | 505 Groin | 606 Toe | 706 Respiratory |
| 307 Mouth / Teeth | 407 Finger | 506 Hip | 610 Whole Leg | 707 Circulatory |
| 308 Neck | 410 Whole Arm | 507 Buttocks | | 708 Digestive |
| 310 Whole Head | | 510 Whole Torso | | 710 Nervous |

16  Describe Treatment provided (e.g. X-rayed and released; 6 stitches; hospitalized).

17  Print and sign name of Supervisor preparing this report; give Telephone Number at work (include area code); Date Report was prepared.

## STOP — FORWARD TO YOUR MANAGER FOR COMPLETION

## SECTION VI — CLASSIFICATION, PREVENTION RECOMMENDATIONS — To be completed by supervisors' manager

18  Select the appropriate Injury / Illness Classification Code
0 First aid case, treated at plant—Form 2020 not required by Corporate Safety.
1 Near miss-no injury but serious potential for fatality or disability.
2 Injury requiring first aid, with outside professional attention - Workmen's Compensation Claim.
3 Medical treatment without restricted or lost workdays but OSHA recordable
4 Restricted and / or lost work day case.
5 Partial or total permanent disability
6 Fatality

Estimate number of Days Away From Work; number of Days of Restricted Duty; number of Hospital Days. If "none", leave blank.

19  Indicate if permanent non-disciplinary T Transfer or D Dismissal (Termination) is required.
If neither, leave blank, Give Group, Division, Department of injured / ill person.

20  Was accident, injury, illness preventable? Explain.

21  Circle all realistic areas for corrective Action (By Management) to prevent recurrence. Circle all realistic areas for corrective Action (By Worker)
to prevent recurrence.

22  Give Recommendations to prevent similar problems in the future.

23  Assign specific Tasks, Responsibilities, and Completion Dates for implementation of recommendations.

24  Obtain Management Approvals in accordance with local requirements.

## SECTION IV — ACTIVITY INFORMATION

⑨ WHAT WAS PERSON DOING? (e.g. bolting a flange)

**30A**

⑩ [A] How often has person done this activity? ✱    [B] Was activity a normal part of job? (Y or N)    [C] Was person adequately trained? (Y or N)

⑪ [D] Do standard methods / procedures exist? (Y or N)   **If Yes,** ➡   [E] Were they followed? (Y or N)   **If No,** ➡   [F] Did something discourage following procedures. (Y or N)

⑫ IF PROCEDURES WERE NOT FOLLOWED, WHAT WAS DONE DIFFERENTLY?

## SECTION V — INJURY / ILLNESS INFORMATION

⑬ [G] Was person using it? (Y or N)   **EQUIPMENT TO PROTECT AGAINST THIS INJURY**   Was Person supposed to be using it? (Y or N) [H]   TYPE REQUIRED   TYPE USED

⑭ [I] **NATURE OF INJURY ✱ ILLNESS CODE** MOST SERIOUS   SECOND MOST SERIOUS [J]   DESCRIPTION

⑮ [K]   **PART OF BODY CODE ✱** [L]

⑯ TREATMENT PROVIDED

⑰ SUPERVISOR: PRINT NAME AND SIGN    WORK TELEPHONE NO. ( )  —   DATE OF REPORT

**STOP — FORWARD TO YOUR MANAGER FOR COMPLETION**

## SECTION VI — CLASSIFICATION, PREVENTION, RECOMMENDATIONS — To be completed by Supervisor's Manager

⑱ [M] INJURY / ILLNESS CLASSIFICATION CODE ✱   [N] DAYS AWAY FROM WORK   [O] DAYS OF RESTRICTED DUTY   [P] HOSPITAL DAYS

⑲ [Q] (T) TRANSFER OR (D) DISMISSAL   GROUP, DIVISION, DEPARTMENT OF INJURED / ILL

⑳ WAS ACCIDENT, INJURY, ILLNESS PREVENTABLE? EXPLAIN

### CIRCLE ALL REALISTIC ACTIONS MANAGEMENT AND WORKERS CAN TAKE TO PREVENT RECURRENCE

㉑

**MANAGEMENT (CIRCLE)**
A. Emergency Procedures Training Equipment
B. Facilities, Lighting, Ventilation
C. Guarding, Safety Devices
D. Housekeeping
E. Maintenance
F. Methods Safety Work Practice
G. Personal Protective Equipment
H. Process Engineering, Hazard Analysis
I. Staffing-Quality, Quantity
J. Supervision
K. Training
L. Working Conditions - Hours, Etc.

**WORKER ACTIONS (CIRCLE)**
A. Follow Instructions, Work Permits
B. Follow Safe Work Practices
C. Follow Training Program Directives
D. Operate Tools / Equipment Properly, Safely
E. Secure, Shut-off, Disconnect Systems
F. Stop Horseplay With Others
G. Stop Recklessness, Inattentiveness
H. Stop Unauthorized Work
I. Use Common Sense, Good Judgement
J. Use Guards, Safety Equipment Properly
K. Wear Personal Protective Equipment
L. Wear Proper Clothing

㉒ DETAILED RECOMMENDATIONS TO PREVENT RECURRENCE

㉓ TASK    PERSON REPONSIBLE    COMPLETION DATE

㉔ LOCAL APPROVALS    FACILITY MANAGER

✱ SEE INSTRUCTIONS FOR CODES

**171**

# 6—Accident Records and Incidence Rates

**A. CONTROL THE ACCIDENT SITUATION · PEOPLE ARE THE FIRST PRIORITY**
- ☐ Send For Help · Notify Management.
- ☐ "Safe" The Area and Administer First-aid.

**To Stop Ongoing Hazards To Rescue Personnel you _may_ have to...**
- ☐ Shut off electrical power
- ☐ Bleed or isolate pressurized systems
- ☐ Block mechanical equipment · prevent movement
- ☐ Check air quality
- ☐ Issue personal protective equipment
- ☐ Provide emergency lighting, power, air, etc.

**Secure the Scene and Protect Evidence**
- ☐ Rope off area or Station a guard
- ☐ Issue tagouts, lockouts, permits

**B. COLLECT EVIDENCE**

**Identify Transient Evidence · Make notes, take pictures or provide sketches of the following...**
- ☐ Positions of tools, equipment, layout, etc.
- ☐ Note air quality, things that evaporate or melt, etc.
- ☐ Tire tracks, foot prints, loose material on floor, etc.
- ☐ Collect operating logs, charts, records
- ☐ Identification numbers of the equipment and maintenance records

Note: Put dimensions on all sketches, sign and date all photos

**Note General Conditions · Yes or No (Y or N) · Did the following factors contribute to the accident?**

| | |
|---|---|
| Housekeeping | Equipment Condition or Malfunction History |
| Work Environment or Layout | Training, Experience or Supervision |
| Floor or Surface Condition | Periodic Rule or Procedure Violations |
| Lighting or Visibility | Employee Morale or Attitude |
| Noise or Distractions | Health or Safety Record |
| Air Quality, Temperature or Weather | Alcohol or Drug Abuse |

**C. GET THINGS BACK TO NORMAL**

**D. INTERVIEW WITNESSES**

**DO...**
- Interview as soon as possible
- Interview at the accident scene
- Take notes or use a tape recorder
- Put the witness at ease
- Ask open ended questions
- Repeat the story back to the witness
- End the interview on a positive note

**DON'T...**
- Pressure the witness
- Blame the witness for the accident
- Interrupt an answer
- Ask questions that can be answered "yes or no"
- Ask "why" questions and "opinion" questions first

**ALWAYS...**
- Stress that you only want the facts
- Stress that you want to prevent the next accident
- Take the extra time to get understanding

**E. ANALYSIS**
- Write down the accident story
- List the facts (parts of the story) which are in dispute
- Compare the facts and dispute with the physical evidence to establish the best answer
- Finalize the story and identify accident causes with your Manager

**F. REPORT**
- Form 2020 for each person injured
- Form 2021 for accidental property loss in excess of $10,000 · 1 per occurrence
- Form 3175 for vehicle accidents · 1 per occurrence

## INJURY AND ILLNESS RECORD OF EMPLOYEE

S. S. Jones                                              845

_(Name)_                                          _(Employee Number)_

Occupation ___Packer___  Department ___Shipping___  Date Employed ___1-23-69___

| Case Number | Injury or Illness | Date of Occurrence | Z16 Type (Fatal, Permanent, Temporary, Non-disabling) | Z16 Days Charged | Comp. and Other Costs | OSHA Type (Fatal, Lost Workday, Non-Lost Workday) | OSHA Lost Workdays |
|---|---|---|---|---|---|---|---|
| 164 | Inj. | 2-12-70 | Non-disab. | 0 | 0 | | |
| 349 | Inj. | 3-16-73 | Temporary | 3 | 0 | Lost workday | 1 |
| 766 | Ill. | 8- 3-79 | Temporary | 8 | 0 | Lost workday | 6 |
| | | | | | | | |
| | | | | | | | |
| | | | | | | | |
| | | | | | | | |
| | | | | | | | |

_(Reverse side may be used for remarks)_

Issued by NATIONAL SAFETY COUNCIL, 444 N. Michigan Ave., Chicago, Ill. 60611

IS3 Rev. 10M17499'          Printed in U.S.A.          Stock No. 129.23

Fig. 6-5.—Injury and Illness Record of Employee is a 4 × 6 in. (10 × 15 cm) card for recording injuries.

previous years, and with the experience of similar organizations and of the industry as a whole.

Especially in smaller companies, monthly injury rates often show wide variations that make it difficult to evaluate the safety performance correctly. If a small company has only two or three injuries in a year, in the months in which these injuries occur, the rates will jump to extreme highs; but in the other months, the rates will be zero. These variations will be smoothed out in annual totals, however, and the rate for the longer period will have increased significance.

Annual reports should be prepared as soon after the close of the year as information becomes available, but again not later than the twentieth of the month following. If any injury report is still incomplete twenty days after the close of the year because the employee has not returned to work, or if the classification of any injury is in doubt at that time, an estimate of the outcome should be made by the company physician and the report included with the completed cases.

When annual records are closed, the estimated charges or OSHA lost workdays on cases still pending become final for that year, and any injuries or time charges reported later are considered only in rates for two or three years of which that year is a part. They need not be added to the record of that year, and they should _not_ be added to the record of the succeeding year.

If time charges or OSHA lost workdays that occurred in one year were included in the record for the next year, the latter year's experience would be biased and the record would fail to give a true picture of the severity of injuries or OSHA lost workdays which actually happened during that time.

On the other hand, absolute accuracy in rates does not justify delaying the annual report more than twenty days after the end of the year in order to get exact time charges or OSHA lost workdays, or to make sure that there are no delayed cases. It is better to omit such delayed cases from the rates

_(Text continues on page 179.)_

**MONTHLY SUMMARY OF**

Company _ABC Mfg. Co._     Plant _____

| Period | Average Number of Employees | Number of Man-Hours Worked | Fatal, Permanent Total | Permanent Partial | Temporary Total | Total Z16 Cases | Frequency Rate* | Fatal, Permanent Total | Permanent Partial | Temporary Total |
|---|---|---|---|---|---|---|---|---|---|---|
| | | | Disabling Injuries and Illnesses | | | | | Time Charges (Z16.1 CASES) | | |
| Jan. | 2,060 | 345,000 | 0 | 1 | 1 | 2 | 5.80 | 0 | 150 | 18 |
| Feb. | 2,010 | 298,000 | 0 | 0 | 3 | 3 | 10.07 | 0 | 0 | 22 |
| Cum. | | 643,000 | 0 | 1 | 4 | 5 | 7.78 | 0 | 150 | 40 |
| Mar. | 2,080 | 353,000 | 0 | 0 | 1 | 1 | 2.83 | 0 | 0 | 42 |
| Cum. | | 996,000 | 0 | 1 | 5 | 6 | 6.02 | 0 | 150 | 78/82 |
| Apr. | 2,000 | 332,000 | 0 | 0 | 4 | 4 | 12.05 | 0 | 0 | 47 |
| Cum. | | 1,328,000 | 0 | 1 | 9 | 10 | 7.53 | 0 | 150 | 125 |
| May | 2,150 | 375,000 | 0 | 0 | 5 | 5 | 13.33 | 0 | 0 | 63 |
| Cum. | | 1,703,000 | 0 | 1 | 14 | 15 | 8.81 | 0 | 150 | 203/188 |
| June | 1,900 | 303,000 | 0 | 1 | 0 | 1 | 3.30 | 0 | 1,000 | 0 |
| Cum. | | 2,006,000 | 0 | 2 | 14 | 16 | 7.98 | 0 | 1,150 | 203 |
| July | 1,825 | 295,000 | 0 | 1 | 3 | 4 | 13.56 | 0 | 250 | 23 |
| Cum. | | 2,301,000 | 0 | 3 | 17 | 20 | 8.69 | 0 | 1,400 | 226 |
| Aug. | 1,800 | 285,000 | 0 | 0 | 4 | 4 | 14.04 | 0 | 0 | 31 |
| Cum. | | 2,586,000 | 0 | 3 | 21 | 24 | 9.28 | 0 | 1,400 | 257 |
| Sept. | 1,875 | 301,000 | 0 | 0 | 0 | 0 | 0.00 | 0 | 0 | 0 |
| Cum. | | 2,887,000 | 0 | 4/3 | 20/21 | 24 | 8.31 | 0 | 2,300/1,400 | 215/254 |
| Oct. | 1,795 | 302,000 | 0 | 0 | 1 | 1 | 3.31 | 0 | 0 | 14 |
| Cum. | | 3,189,000 | 0 | 4 | 21 | 25 | 7.84 | 0 | 2,300 | 229 |
| Nov. | 1,665 | 280,000 | 0 | 0 | 2 | 2 | 7.14 | 0 | 0 | 17 |
| Cum. | | 3,469,000 | 0 | 4 | 23 | 27 | 7.78 | 0 | 2,300 | 246 |
| Dec. | 1,620 | 275,000 | 1 | 0 | 0 | 1 | 3.64 | 6,000 | 0 | 0 |
| YEAR | | 3,744,000 | 1 | 4 | 23 | 28 | 7.48 | 6,000 | 2,300 | 246 |

*Z16 Rates: Frequency rate is the total number of Z16 cases per 1,000,000 man-hours worked. Severity rate is the total Z16
†OSHA Rate: Incidence rate is the total number of OSHA cases per 200,000 man-hours worked.
Issued by NATIONAL SAFETY COUNCIL, 425 N. Michigan Ave., Chicago, Illinois 60611

Printed in U.S.A.

Fig. 6–6.—Results of the safety program may be gaged from data on this "Monthly Summary of Injuries and Illnesses" form (8½ × 14 in.). Rates computed for the month, year to date (cumulative), and year permit comparisons between time

# INJURIES AND ILLNESSES, 19____

_Dayton, Ohio_ _____ Department ___ _All_ _____

| Total Z16 Charges | Severity Rate* | COSTS (Compensation, Other) | OSHA CASES | | | | | | FIRST AID CASES ONLY |
| --- | --- | --- | --- | --- | --- | --- | --- | --- | --- |
| | | | Fatals | Lost Workday Cases | Non Lost Workday Cases | Total OSHA Cases | Incidence Rate† | Total Lost Workdays | |
| 168 | 487 | #284.50 | 0 | 3 | 18 | 21 | 12.2 | 42 | 20 |
| 22 | 74 | 42.65 | 0 | 4 | 27 | 31 | 20.8 | 34 | 36 |
| 190 | 295 | 327.15 | 0 | 7 | 45 | 52 | 16.2 | 76 | 56 |
| 42 | 119 | 77.82 | 0 | 1 | 9 | 10 | 5.7 | 12 | 10 |
| 228/232 | 229 | 404.97 | 0 | 8 | 54 | 62 | 12.4 | 88 | 66 |
| 47 | 142 | 92.64 | 0 | 5 | 35 | 40 | 24.1 | 64 | 42 |
| 275 | 207 | 497.61 | 0 | 13 | 89 | 102 | 15.4 | 152 | 108 |
| 63 | 168 | 123.24 | 0 | 7 | 45 | 52 | 27.7 | 88 | 55 |
| 353/338 | 207 | 620.85 | 0 | 20 | 134 | 154 | 18.1 | 240 | 163 |
| 1,000 | 3,300 | 985.56 | 0 | 1 | 13 | 14 | 9.2 | 25 | 15 |
| 1,353 | 674 | 1,606.41 | 0 | 21 | 147 | 168 | 16.7 | 265 | 178 |
| 273 | 925 | 368.18 | 0 | 5 | 40 | 45 | 30.5 | 91 | 51 |
| 1,626 | 707 | 1,974.59 | 0 | 26 | 187 | 213 | 18.5 | 356 | 229 |
| 31 | 109 | 63.24 | 0 | 5 | 43 | 48 | 33.7 | 123 | 53 |
| 1,657 | 641 | 2,037.83 | 0 | 31 | 230 | 261 | 20.2 | 479 | 282 |
| 0 | 0 | 843.66 | 0 | 0 | 9 | 9 | 6.0 | 0 | 12 |
| 2,515/1,657 | 871 | 2,881.49 | 0 | 31 | 239 | 270 | 18.7 | 479 | 294 |
| 14 | 46 | 45.60 | 0 | 1 | 5 | 6 | 4.0 | 10 | 6 |
| 2,529 | 793 | 2,927.09 | 0 | 32 | 244 | 276 | 17.3 | 489 | 300 |
| 17 | 61 | 36.76 | 0 | 2 | 23 | 25 | 17.9 | 13 | 26 |
| 2,546 | 734 | 2,963.85 | 0 | 34 | 267 | 301 | 17.4 | 502 | 326 |
| 6,000 | 21,818 | 6,785.25 | 1 | 1 | 7 | 9 | 6.5 | 2 | 8 |
| 8,546 | 2,283 | 9,749.10 | 1 | 35 | 274 | 310 | 16.6 | 504 | 334 |

charges per 1,000,000 man-hours worked.

Stock No. 129.25

periods, and departments, plants, and companies during the same period. Changes in the classification of injuries and other adjustments can be made easily. Details on this form are on page 161.

# 6—Accident Records and Incidence Rates

Bureau of Labor Statistics
Log and Summary of Occupational
Injuries and Illnesses

| NOTE: | This form is required by Public Law 91-596 and must be kept in the establishment for 5 years. Failure to maintain and post can result in the issuance of citations and assessment of penalties. (See posting requirements on the other side of form.) | RECORDABLE CASES: You are required to record information about every occupational death; every nonfatal occupational illness; and those nonfatal occupational injuries which involve one or more of the following: loss of consciousness, restriction of work or motion, transfer to another job, or medical treatment (other than first aid). (See definitions on the other side of form.) | Company |
| --- | --- | --- | --- |
| | | | Establishm |
| | | | Establishm |

| Case or File Number | Date of Injury or Onset of Illness | Employee's Name | Occupation | Department | Description of Injury or Illness | Extent of |
| --- | --- | --- | --- | --- | --- | --- |
| | | | | | | Fatalities |
| Enter a nondupli-cating number which will facilitate com-parisons with supple-mentary records. | Enter Mo./day. | Enter first name or initial, middle initial, last name. | Enter regular job title, not activity employee was per-forming when injured or at onset of il'ness. In the absence of a formal title, enter a brief description of the employee's duties. | Enter department in which the employee is regularly employed or a description of normal workplace to which employee is assigned, even though temporarily working in another depart-ment at the time of injury or illness. | Enter a brief description of the injury or illness and indicate the part or parts of body affected. | Injury Related |
| | | | | | | Enter DAT of death. |
| | | | | | Typical entries for this column might be: Amputation of 1st joint right forefinger; Strain of lower back; Contact dermatitis on both hands; Electrocution—body. | Mo./day/y |
| (A) | (B) | (C) | (D) | (E) | (F) | (1) |
| | | | | | PREVIOUS PAGE TOTALS ⟶ | |
| | | | | | | |
| | | | | | | |
| | | | | | | |
| | | | | | | |
| | | | | | | |
| | | | | | | |
| | | | | | | |
| | | | | | | |
| | | | | | | |
| | | | | | | |
| | | | | | TOTALS (Instructions on other side of form.) ⟶ | |

OSHA No. 200

FOLD

Certifi

OSHA

FIG. 6-7.—Log of Occupational Injuries and Illnesses, Form OSHA No. 200, is used to record injuries or illnesses that result in fatalities, lost workdays, require medical treatment, involve loss of consciousness, or restrict work or motion. Complete

S. Department of Labor

For Calendar Year 19 _____          Page ___ of ___

Form Approved
O.M.B. No. 44R 1453

me

dress

| tcome of INJURY | | | | | Type, Extent of, and Outcome of ILLNESS | | | | | | | | | | | | | |
|---|---|---|---|---|---|---|---|---|---|---|---|---|---|---|---|---|---|---|
| fatal Injuries | | | | | Type of Illness | | | | | | | Fatalities | Nonfatal Illnesses | | | | |
| ries With Lost Workdays | | | | Injuries Without Lost Workdays | CHECK Only One Column for Each Illness *(See other side of form for terminations or permanent transfers.)* | | | | | | | !llness Related | Illnesses With Lost Workdays | | | | Illnesses Without Lost Workdays |
| er a CK jury lves away k, or s of icted rity, oth. | Enter a CHECK if injury involves days away from work. | Enter number of DAYS *away from work.* | Enter number of DAYS of *restricted work activity.* | Enter a CHECK if no entry was made in columns 1 or 2 but the injury is recordable as defined above. | Occupational skin diseases or disorders | Dust diseases of the lungs | Respiratory conditions due to toxic agents | Poisoning (systemic effects of toxic materials) | Disorders due to physical agents | Disorders associated with repeated trauma | All other occupational illnesses | Enter DATE of death. Mo./day/yr. | Enter a CHECK if illness involves days away from work, or days of restricted work activity, or both. | Enter a CHECK if illness involves days away from work. | Enter number of DAYS *away from work.* | Enter number of DAYS of *restricted work activity.* | Enter a CHECK if no entry was made in columns 8 or 9. |
| | (3) | (4) | (5) | (6) | | | | (7) | | | | (8) | (9) | (10) | (11) | (12) | (13) |
| | | | | | (a) | (b) | (c) | (d) | (e) | (f) | (g) | | | | | | |

INJURIES

ILLNESSES

Annual Summary Totals By _____ Title _____ Date _____

**POST ONLY THIS PORTION OF THE LAST PAGE NO LATER THAN FEBRUARY 1.**

instructions for using the Log are on its reverse side (not shown here). The form measures $10\frac{1}{2} \times 20$ in. ($26 \times 49$ cm). Because forms are subject to change, be sure to check your OSHA Area Office for the latest forms.

OSHA No. 101
Case or File No. _____

Form approved
OMB No. 44R 1453

## Supplementary Record of Occupational Injuries and Illnesses

**EMPLOYER**

1. Name _____

2. Mail address _____
                (No. and street)         (City or town)        (State)

3. Location, if different from mail address _____

**INJURED OR ILL EMPLOYEE**

4. Name _____ Social Security No. _____
       (First name)      (Middle name)    (Last name)

5. Home address _____
           (No. and street)        (City or town)   (State)

6. Age _____    **7. Sex: Male**_____ Female_____ (Check one)

8. Occupation _____
           (Enter regular job title, *not* the specific activity he was performing at time of injury.)

9. Department _____
           (Enter name of department or division in which the injured person is regularly employed, even
           though he may have been temporarily working in another department at the time of injury.)

**THE ACCIDENT OR EXPOSURE TO OCCUPATIONAL ILLNESS**

10. Place of accident or exposure _____
            (No. and street)      (City or town)     (State)
    If accident or exposure occurred on employer's premises, give address of plant or establishment in which
    it occurred. Do not indicate department or division within the plant or establishment. If accident oc-
    curred outside employer's premises at an identifiable address, give that address. If it occurred on a pub-
    lic highway or at any other place which cannot be identified by number and street, please provide place
    references locating the place of injury as accurately as possible.

11. Was place of accident or exposure on employer's premises? _____ (Yes or No)

12. What was the employee doing when injured? _____
            (Be specific. If he was using tools or equipment or handling material,
    _____
            name them and tell what he was doing with them.)
    _____

13. How did the accident occur? _____
            (Describe fully the events which resulted in the injury or occupational illness. Tell what
    _____
    happened and how it happened. Name any objects or substances involved and tell how they were involved. Give
    _____
    full details on all factors which led or contributed to the accident. Use separate sheet for additional space.)

**OCCUPATIONAL INJURY OR OCCUPATIONAL ILLNESS**

14. Describe the injury or illness in detail and indicate the part of body affected. _____
    _____
            at second joint; fracture of ribs; lead poisoning; dermatitis of left hand, etc.)

15. Name the object or substance which directly injured the employee. (For example, the machine or thing
    he struck against or which struck him; the vapor or poison he inhaled or swallowed; the chemical or ra-
    diation which irritated his skin; or in cases of strains, hernias, etc., the thing he was lifting, pulling, etc.)
    _____
    _____

16. Date of injury or initial diagnosis of occupational illness _____
            (Date)

17. Did employee die? _____ (Yes or No)

**OTHER**

18. Name and address of physician _____

19. If hospitalized, name and address of hospital _____
    _____

Date of report _____ Prepared by _____
Official position _____

FIG. 6–8.—Supplementary Record of Occupational Injuries and Illnesses, Form OSHA No. 101, gives details of each
recordable occupational injury or illness. Records must be available for examination by representatives of the U.S.
Department of Labor and the Department of Health and Human Services and states accorded jurisdiction under the
OSHAct. Records must be kept at least five years following the calendar year to which they relate.

**178**

entirely, unless a two- or three-year rate is calculated, or unless the company wishes to make revisions for its own information.

## Use of reports

**Reports to management.** Management is increasingly interested in the accident experience of its companies. Therefore, monthly and other periodic summary reports, which show the results of the safety program, should be furnished to the responsible executive. Such reports need contain no details nor technical language and may be supplemented by simple charts or graphs to show the recent accident experience in relation to that of the preceding period and that of companies engaged in similar work.

In a large company, departmental data help the executive visualize accident experience in various plant operations and provide a yardstick for better evaluation of progress made in the elimination of accidents. If cost figures are obtained, comparisons of such figures for different periods are of particular interest.

**Bulletins to supervisors.** A supervisor is primarily interested in his own department and workers. One of the most effective ways to create and maintain the interest of supervisors in accident prevention is to keep them informed about the accident records of their departments. Department injury rates based on sufficient amounts of exposure reflect the effectiveness of the supervisors' safety activities.

Because interest increases with knowledge, bulletins containing analyses of the principal causes of accidents in each department not only will maintain the supervisors' interest at a high level, but will provide the supervisors with the type of information that will help them to effect further reductions in injuries.

The agenda for employee safety meetings should particularly include information about the outstanding injury and illness problems, frequent unsafe practices, hazardous types of equipment, and similar data disclosed by analysis of the accidents that have occurred in the department and plant.

**Bulletin board publicity.** Posting a variety of materials on bulletin boards is one of the best ways to maintain the interest of employees in safety. Accident records furnish many items, such as the following:

NO-INJURY RECORDS
UNUSUAL ACCIDENTS
FREQUENT CAUSES OF ACCIDENTS
CHARTS SHOWING REDUCTIONS IN ACCIDENTS
SIMPLE TABLES COMPARING DEPARTMENTAL RECORDS
STANDINGS IN CONTESTS

**Reports to National Safety Council.** Each year the National Safety Council requests an annual summary report of occupational injury and illness experience from each member. These reports are tabulated to determine accident rates by industry.

An annual "Work Injury and Illness Rates" pamphlet containing these incidence rates by industry is published and distributed to members, so that each company may compare its experience with the average experience of other companies in the same industry. These reports (along with data from the Bureau of Labor Statistics, state and national vital statistics authorities, state compensation authorities, and other federal, state, and private agencies) are also tabulated and shown in *Accident Facts*, the Council's annual statistical publication.

These annual summary reports are also used by the National Safety Council to evaluate members' experience for the presentation of awards under the Council's "Award Plan for Recognizing Good Occupational Safety Records."

National Safety Council members may also, according to a vote by their section membership, establish and compete in safety contests that are administered by the Council. Monthly bulletins are sent to contestants so that they can compare their experience with other competitors. Awards are made to the leaders of the individual contests at the end of each contest year.

## The concept of bilevel reporting

As mentioned earlier in this chapter, each establishment has accident problems that are different from those of establishments in other industries and, in many cases, different from those of other establishments in the same industry. No individual form or set of forms can possibly include all of the information necessary to fully investigate the causes of all accidents. With this in mind and because very long forms are rarely completed accurately and are, very often, received with much resistance by those persons

**179**

who must fill them out, the concept of bilevel reporting has arisen.

The basic idea of bilevel reporting is that in addition to the general information contained in the standard report form (such as the Supervisor's Report Form), further facts are necessary concerning specific types of accidents. To obtain this additional data, a supplementary form, containing a few specific questions about the accident type under investigation, is prepared and made available. This supplementary form is then filled out, and attached to the regular report—only for those accidents about which the investigator is trying to obtain in-depth data.

When a sufficient number of the bilevel forms have been collected, the supplementary form is discontinued and the results can be analyzed. In this way, a minimum of time needs to be spent by the persons who fill out the forms in order to obtain useful information. Several bilevel forms, each a different color for easy handling, can be used at any one time. They can be discontinued when their job is done and replaced by other supplementary forms, while the basic report form remains unchanged and in use.

## OSHA Recordkeeping and ANSI Z16

The OSHA Recordkeeping system is mandatory for all establishments subject to the OSHAct. However, not all workplaces come under this Act and there are many establishments who continue to use the ANSI Z16.1 standard for their management reports. Some do so to maintain continuity with past records of accident experience and others find parts of the standard valuable since it provides information not specified in the OSHA system. Many organizations want a separate record of permanent impairments, for example. In addition, many safety people feel that the Z16.1 severity rate provides a better measurement of severity than the lost work day incidence rate.

The National Safety Council changed from the ANSI Z16.1 standard to the OSHA Recordkeeping system beginning with January 1, 1977 for all its data gathering and for contests and awards. However, for the benefit of those organizations still using all or part of the Z16.1, the basic elements of the standard have been included in this chapter.

It should also be noted that in July 1977, a new standard Z16.4 was approved by the American National Standards Institute. This standard conforms to the OSHA Recordkeeping system but in the appendix, it provides the details needed to compute the Z16.1 severity rate.

## Guidelines to Occupational Safety and Health Act (OSHAct) Recordkeeping

The following material provides (a) the basic definitions and recordkeeping requirements of the OSHAct, as they existed at the time this volume was prepared, and (b) guidelines to implementing these recordkeeping procedures. The requirements and definitions are subject to change; the individual states, which may implement the Act in their own jurisdiction, may make modifications. To determine the most current definitions and requirements, safety personnel should contact the appropriate state or federal authorities.

Regulations issued under the Occupational Safety and Health Act of 1970 require all establishments subject to the Act to maintain records of recordable occupational injuries and illnesses occurring on or after July 1, 1971. Such records must consist of: (a) a log of occupational injuries and illnesses; (b) a supplementary record of each occupational injury and illness; and (c) an annual summary of occupational injuries and illnesses. The log and summary comprise form OSHA No. 200 (Fig. 6–7); and the supplementary record is form OSHA No. 101 (Fig. 6–8).

The recordkeeping requirements as written in the *Code of Federal Regulations*, as well as the burden placed on the employer to record those cases where there is doubt, make it impossible to get perfectly uniform recordkeeping. There will always be cases that fall into a gray area and are subject to varying interpretations. The following guidelines, however, can reduce the number of such cases and increase the consistency and uniformity of reporting using the OSHA recordkeeping system. This in turn will increase the usefulness of these records in accident and illness prevention.

It must be stressed that these guidelines are not a replacement for the present *OSHA Recordkeeping Requirements* nor are they meant to change them. Rather, these guidelines are a clarification of and an adjunct to the requirements. As such, the guidelines should be used in conjunction with such federal publications as *Recordkeeping*

*Requirements Under the Occupational Safety and Health Act of 1970* (Revised 1978),° U.S. Department of Labor, Occupational Safety and Health Administration, and *What Every Employer Needs to Know about OSHA Record-keeping,* U.S. Department of Labor, Bureau of Labor Statistics, Report 412-3 (Revised), 1978.°°

Records are to be kept on the establishment level. An establishment is defined as a single physical location where business is conducted or where services or industrial operations are performed (for example: a factory, mill, store, hotel, restaurant, movie theater, farm, ranch, bank, sales office, warehouse, or central administrative office). Where distinctly separate activities are performed at a single physical location, such as construction activities operated from the same physical location as a lumber yard, each activity shall be treated as a separate establishment.

For firms engaged in activities that may be physically dispersed, such as agriculture; construction; transportation; communications; and electric, gas, and sanitary services; records may be maintained at a place to which employees report each day.

Records for personnel who do not primarily report or work at a single establishment, such as traveling salesmen, technicians, engineers, etc., shall be maintained at the location from which they are paid or the base from which personnel operate to carry out their activities.

## How the guidelines are organized

Three decisions must be made in recording a case. First, it must be determined if the case is work-related. Second, it must be decided whether the case meets the criteria for recordability. If a case is recordable, a third decision must be made to determine the proper injury or illness classification. These guidelines consist of three sections that correspond to these three decisions:

Section I—Work-related cases;

Section II—Recordability;

Section III—Classification by extent of injury or illness.

The first section deals with the concept of work-related injuries and illnesses and the determination of what cases occur in the work environment. The second section discusses which work-related injuries and illnesses are to be recorded and presents information useful in distinguishing between *first aid* and *medical treatment.* The third section covers classification by extent of injury or illness:

- Deaths;

- Lost workday cases involving days away from work;

- Lost workday cases with days of restricted work activity;

- Non-fatal cases without lost workdays.

Definitions of these classifications and points to be considered in making the distinctions between them are included.

In using these guidelines, remember that the final decision of whether to record a case and how to classify a recordable case rests with the employer. When the employer is in doubt about recordability or the extent of injury or illness, the case should be recorded and classified to the higher extent of injury or illness.

## Section I—Work-related cases

Cases that are work-related and meet the criteria discussed in Section II should be recorded. No detailed definition of work-related is contained in any of the OSHA publications or in the law itself.

The broad concept is that any injury or illness "occurring in the work environment" is *work-related.* The Form OSHA No. 200, Log and Summary of Occupational Injuries and Illnesses, provides the following definition:

WORK ENVIRONMENT is comprised of the physical location, equipment, materials processed or used, and the kinds of operations performed by an employee in the performance of his work, whether on or off the employer's premises.

There are *no stated exclusions* of place or circumstance. Therefore, injuries or illnesses occurring in such places as the employee parking lot, lunch room or rest room, or during rest or lunch period on the employer's premises, can be *work-related.* The final determination of whether any case is *work-related* must be made by the

―――
°U.S. Department of Labor, Occupational Safety and Health Administration, Washington, D.C. 20210.

°°U.S. Department of Labor, Bureau of Labor Statistics, Washington, D.C. 20212.

employer. Responsibility or fault *does not* enter into the decision of whether a case is *work-related*. In doubtful situations, a case should be recorded.

## Section II—Recordability

Recordable Cases. Work-related cases are recordable that involve any of the following:

*Deaths*—All occupational deaths regardless of the time between injury and death or length of illness.

*Injuries*—All occupational injuries resulting in any of the following:

• Lost Workdays (either Days away from work or Days of restricted work activity);

• Medical treatment other than first aid;

• Loss of consciousness;

• Restriction of work or motion;

• Transfer. Temporary or permanent transfer to another job;

• Termination of the injured or ill employees.

*Illnesses*—All occupational illnesses including, but not limited to, the following categories and examples:

• Occupational skin diseases or disorders—Examples: contact dermatitis, eczema, or rash caused by primary irritants and sensitizers or poisonous plants; oil acne; chrome ulcers; chemical burns or inflammations; etc. (Direct contact causing tissue damage only, resulting from a thermal or chemical burn, is classified as an injury, not an illness case.)

• Dust diseases of the lungs (Pneumoconioses)—Examples: silicosis, asbestosis, coal worker's pneumoconiosis, byssinosis, and other pneumoconioses.

• Respiratory conditions due to toxic agents—Examples: pneumonitis, pharyngitis, rhinitis or acute congestion due to chemicals, dusts, gases, or fumes; and farmer's lung.

• Poisoning (systemic effects of toxic materials)—Examples: poisoning by lead, mercury, cadmium, arsenic, or other metals; poisoning by carbon monoxide, hydrogen sulfide or other gases; poisoning by benzol, carbon tetrachloride, or other organic solvents; poisoning by insecticide sprays such as parathion, lead arsenate; and poisoning by other chemicals such as formaldehyde, plastics and resins.

• Disorders due to physical agents (other than toxic materials)—Examples: heatstroke, sunstroke, heat exhaustion and other effects of environmental heat; freezing, frostbite and effects of exposure to low temperatures; caisson disease; effects of ionizing radiation (isotopes, X-rays, radium); and effects of nonionizing radiation (welding flash, ultraviolet rays, microwaves, sunburn).

• Disorders associated with repeated trauma—Examples: Noise-induced hearing loss; synovitis, tenosynovitis, and bursitis; Raynaud's phenomena; and other conditions due to repeated motion, vibration, or pressure.

• All other occupational illnesses—Examples: anthrax, brucellosis, infectious hepatitis, malignant and benign tumors, food poisoning, histoplasmosis, and coccidioidomycosis.

Conditions resulting from animal bites, such as insect or snake bites, or from one-time exposure to chemicals are considered to be injuries.

A discussion of what constitutes Days away from work, Days of restricted work activity, Temporary transfers, Permanent transfers, and Terminations is contained in Section III—Classification by extent of injury or illness.

Loss of consciousness of the employee for any period of time is self-explanatory. Restriction of motion is not defined specifically in the OSHA publications or in the law. Each case must be judged individually to determine if there is more than a trivial amount of restricted motion, such as would occur when a small adhesive bandage was placed on the second joint of the finger. It should be noted here that damage to prostheses (such as false teeth) is not in and of itself grounds for recordability unless accompanied by other damage to the body that meets the recordability criteria.

The distinction between *medical treatment* and *first aid* is probably the most difficult of the recordability criteria to interpret. Medical treatment and first aid are defined in the same paragraph of the Form OSHA No. 200, Log and Summary of Occupational Injuries and Illnesses, as follows:

MEDICAL TREATMENT *includes treatment (other than first aid) administered by a physician or by registered professional personnel under the standing orders of a physician. Medical treatment does* NOT *include first aid treatment (one-time treatment and subsequent observation of minor scratches, cuts, burns, splinters, and so forth, that do not ordinarily require medical care), even though provided by a physician or registered professional personnel.*

The important point to be stressed is that the decision as to whether a case involves medical treatment should be made on the basis of whether the case *normally* would require medical treatment. The decision cannot be made on the basis of who treats the case. First aid can be administered by a physician and medical treatment by someone other than a physician.

It is not possible to list all types of medical procedures and treatments and *on that basis alone* determine if first aid or medical treatment was involved. For example, whirlpool treatments, heat treatments, application of hot or cold compresses, or elastic bandages are not in and of themselves either first aid or medical treatment.

What follows is a discussion of diagnostic procedures and preventive procedures and treatments, both of which are not in and of themselves medical treatment. Next is a discussion of treatments that are almost always medical treatment, and, finally, comments on medical treatment and first aid for certain types of injuries.

### Diagnostic procedures.

*Hospitalization* for observation, where no medical treatment is rendered other than first aid, is *not* considered medical treatment. However, if the employee misses any part of his next scheduled shift, the case would become recordable because of lost workdays.

*Visits to a physician* or nurse for observation *only* or for a routine change of dressing are *not* medical treatment.

*X-ray examination* for fractures is considered diagnostic procedure and as such is *not* medical treatment or first aid. Where the X-ray is negative, the case is not recordable, unless the injury required other medical treatment or met one of the other criteria for recordability.

*Physical examination* yielding few or no findings, and not substantiating subjective complaints in questionable cases, is *not* medical treatment.

*Reactions* to or side effects of diagnostic procedures, which are necessitated by a work-related injury or illness and which meet the criteria for recordability, *should* be recorded.

### Preventive procedures and treatments.

*Tetanus shots*—Either initial tetanus shots or boosters are considered preventive in nature and are *not* in and of themselves considered medical treatment. However, treatment of a reaction to a tetanus shot administered because of an injury *would* be considered medical treatment, and would make the case recordable.

*Prescription medication*—Any use of prescription medication normally constitutes medical treatment. However, it should be considered first aid when a single dose or application of a prescription medication is given on the first visit merely for relief of pain or as preventive treatment for a minor injury. This situation can occur at facilities having dispensaries stocked with prescription medications frequently used for preventive treatment and relief of pain and attended by a physician or nurse operating under the standing orders of a physician. The administration of nonprescription medication in similar circumstances would be considered first aid.

*Ointments and salves*—The application of ointments and salves to prevent the drying or cracking of skin at the site of a minor injury can be considered first aid.

*Antiseptics and dressings*—The application of antiseptics to minor injuries, which do not themselves require medical treatment, can be considered first aid. Changing the bandage or dressing on an injury, which did not require medical treatment, because the bandage or dressing has become dirty, is considered to be first aid.

*Preventive medication*—Reaction to preventive medication (not administered because of an occupational injury or illness) administered in plant (such as flu shots) would not constitute a recordable case.

*Off-the-job cases*—In-plant treatment of off-the-job injuries and illnesses is not recordable.

### Treatments that are almost always medical treatment.

*Sutures*—The suturing of any wound.

*Fractures*—Treatment of fractures.

**183**

*Casts*—Application of a cast or other professional means of immobilizing an injured part of the body.

*Infections*—Treatment of infection arising out of an injury.

*Bruises*—Treatment of a bruise by drainage of blood.

*Debridement*—Surgical debridement, that is, the removal of dead or damaged skin.

*Abrasions*—Treatment of abrasions that occur to greater than full skin depth.

*Prescriptions*—Administration of prescription medicines are usually *medical treatment.* (See also the preceding section, Preventive procedures and treatments.)

*Burns*—The treatment of second and third degree burns is almost always medical treatment.

**Medical treatment and first aid for certain types of injuries.**

*Cuts and lacerations.*

First Aid treatment is limited to cleaning wound, soaking, applying antiseptic and nonprescription medication and bandaging on first visit. Followup visits limited to observation including changing dressing and bandage. Additional cleaning and application of antiseptic permissible as first aid where it is required by work duties that are likely to soil the bandage. The application of butterfly closures for *cosmetic purposes only* can be considered first aid.

Medical treatment includes the application of butterfly closures for noncosmetic purposes, sutures (stitches), surgical debridement (cutting away dead skin), treatment of infection, or other professional treatment.

*Abrasions.*

First Aid treatment for abrasions is the same as for cuts and lacerations except ointments can be added on follow up visits to prevent drying and cracking of skin.

Medical treatment includes careful examination for removal of imbedded foreign material, multiple soakings, whirlpool treatment, treatment of infection, or other professional treatment. Any case involving more than a minor, spot-type injury, such as treatment of abrasions occurring to greater than full skin depth, is

considered medical treatment.

*Bruises.*

First Aid treatment is limited to a single soaking or application of cold compresses. Followup visits limited only to observation.

Medical treatment includes multiple soakings, draining of collected blood, or other extended care beyond observation.

*Splinters and puncture wounds.*

First Aid treatment is limited to cleaning the wound, removal of foreign object(s) by tweezers or other simple techniques, application of antiseptics and nonprescription medications, and bandaging on first visit. Followup visits are limited to observation including changing bandage. Additional cleaning and application of antiseptic permissible as first aid where it is required by work duties that are likely to soil the bandage.

Medical treatment consists of removal of foreign object(s) by physician due to depth of imbedment, size or shape of object(s) or location of wound. Treatment for infection, treatment of a reaction to tetanus booster, or other professional treatment is considered medical treatment.

*Burns, thermal and chemical* (resulting in destruction of tissue by direct contact).

First Aid treatment is limited to cleaning or flushing the surface, soaking, applying cold compresses, antiseptics and/or nonprescription medications and bandaging on a first visit. Follow up visits are restricted to observation, changing bandages or additional cleaning. Most first-degree burns are amenable to first aid treatment.

Medical treatment includes a series of treatments including soaks, whirlpool, and surgical debridement (cutting away dead skin). Most second and third degree burns require medical treatment.

*Sprains and strains.*

First Aid treatment is limited to soaking, application of cold compresses, and use of elastic bandage on first visit. Followup visits for observation, possibly including reapplying bandage, are first aid.

Medical treatment includes a series of hot and cold soaks, use of whirlpools, diathermy treatment, or other professional treatment.

*Eye injuries.*

FIRST AID treatment is limited to irrigation, removal of foreign material not imbedded in eye, and application of nonprescription medications. A precautionary visit (special examination) to a physician is considered as first aid if treatment is limited to above items. Followup visits for observation only are also considered as first aid.

MEDICAL TREATMENT cases involve removal of imbedded foreign objects, use of prescription medications, or other professional treatment.

*Inhalation of toxic or corrosive gases.*

FIRST AID treatment is limited to removal of the employee to fresh air or the one-time administration of oxygen for several minutes.

MEDICAL TREATMENT consists of any professional treatment beyond that mentioned under first aid, and all cases involving loss of consciousness.

## Section III—Classification by extent of injury or illness

There are four classes, based on extent of injury, used in the OSHA recordkeeping system as defined next. An injury or illness should be classified according to its most severe consequence. For example, a case might first become recordable as a Nonfatal case without lost workdays. Subsequently, the injured or ill employees may lose workdays because of the injury or illness. The case then becomes a Lost workday case and should be counted under that classification. Because a particular injury or illness should be counted in *only one* of the four classifications, this case would be removed from the total of Nonfatal cases without lost workdays when the employer becomes aware of the lost workdays.

There is an additional category for those cases where injury or illness resulted in termination or permanent transfer. Any case involving termination or permanent transfer must *also* be classified by extent of injury or illness.

Any case that results in death is counted in that classification *only*. Any lost workdays, transfers, or terminations, which have been recorded prior to the occurrence of death, should be lined out on the form OSHA 200 and not included in the totals for those classifications when summaries are made or reported to the National Safety Council.

**Deaths.** Any work-related injury or illness that results in the death of the employee, regardless of the length of time between injury and death, or the length of illness is recordable.

**Lost workday cases involving days away from work.** Cases that result in one or more Days away from work are recordable. Days away from work are those workdays (consecutive or not) on which the employee would have worked but could not because of occupational injury or illness. The number of lost workdays should *not* include the day of injury or onset of illness or any days on which the employee would not have worked even though able to work.

*Weekends.* For example, if an employee, who is scheduled to work Monday through Friday, is injured on Friday and returns to work on Monday, the case does not involve any Days away from work even if the employee was unable to work on Friday, Saturday, or Sunday. If this same employee had been scheduled to work on Saturday, even if that Saturday constituted overtime, the Saturday would be counted in the Days away from work, and the case would be classified as a Lost workday case with Days away from work.

*Irregular shifts.* For employees not having a regularly scheduled shift, *i.e.*, certain truck drivers, construction workers, farm labor, casual labor, part-time employees, and the like, it may be necessary to estimate the number of lost workdays. Estimates of the number of days that the employee would have worked should take into account the prior work history of the employee and days worked by fellow employees, not ill or injured, working in the same department or occupation as the ill or injured employee.

*Doubtful cases.* In some cases an injured or ill employee will miss one or more scheduled days or shifts beside the day of injury or onset of illness, but it will be uncertain whether the employee was truly unable to work on the days missed. Such cases may arise when a physician judges that the employee is able to work but the employee decides that he is not. In such cases, the employer should not rely solely on the physician's opinion. He should make the final judgment himself, based on all the evidence at his disposal. Again, the rule should be "when in doubt, record the case."

*Full shifts only.* Days away from work should include only those full days or shifts that are missed by the employee. The loss of a part of a day or shift would be counted under Days of restricted work activity as defined next.

*Restricted days.* A Lost workday case involving days away from work may also result in Days of restricted activity. Such a case will be recorded as only one case, but will have days recorded under both categories of recordable days.

**Lost workday cases with days of restricted work activity only** are cases that result in one or more days of Restricted Work Activity but do not result in any Days away from work. Although the OSHA Log and Summary of Occupational Injuries and Illnesses contains a separate classification for Days of restricted work activity, the Summary does not provide a separate column for entering the number of such cases. This number can be arrived at by subtracting the number of Cases involving days away from work (columns 3 and 10 on the OSHA 200 form) from the number of Total lost workday cases (Columns 2 and 9 on the OSHA 200 form). Days of restricted work activity include those days (consecutive or not, but *excluding* the day of injury or onset of illness) on which one of the following occurred:

• Temporary assignment. The employee was assigned to another job on a temporary basis. Even if the employee normally shifts from job to job within an occupational classification, if any switch or transfer is occasioned by a work-related injury or illness, the case involves Days of restricted work activity. Such days are meant to cover all days on which the employee was unable to contribute a full day's work on all parts of his permanent job. In cases where an employee is not working at his regular job and is injured or becomes ill and is transferred back to his original job, which he can perform without limitation, there are no Days of restricted work activity.

• Loss of part of shift. The employee worked at a permanent job less than his full shift or normal day. Loss of a *full* day or shift would constitute a Lost Workday Away From Work.

• Restricted work activity. The employee worked at a permanently assigned job but could not perform all duties normally connected with it. All days (excluding the day of injury or onset of illness), for which the employee was scheduled to work, and could not perform *all or any part* of his normal assignment during *all or any part* of the workday or shift, should be considered Days of restricted work activity.

*Estimating days lost.* As in determining whether or not a case involves Days away from work, there may be cases where the employer must estimate the number of days for those employees working irregular or unusual shifts. Again, the final determination as to whether a case involves Days of restricted work activity must be made by the employer, considering all evidence, and recording the case if there is any doubt.

*Precautionary transfers.* If an employee is transferred to another job as a *precautionary* measure while his case is being diagnosed, the case should be included under Lost workday cases with Days of restricted work activity only if the transfer proves necessary (that is, the diagnosis indicates that such a transfer was indeed necessary).

*When to stop counting.* The number of Days of Restricted Work Activity can end for a particular case in the following ways:

• The employee is able to return to his regularly scheduled job and is able to perform all of its duties for a full day or shift.

• The employee is *permanently* transferred to another permanent job (which would be recorded under Permanent transfers and terminations). If this happens, even though the employee could not perform his original job any longer, the Days of restricted work activity will stop.

• The employee is terminated or leaves the job. (Terminations would also be recorded under Permanent transfers and terminations.)

• If the employee continues on his regular job for a long period of time, even though he cannot perform all parts of it, the job can be considered to be redefined after a reasonable period of time and the Days of restricted work activity will stop. It is not practical to continue to count Lost workdays for the rest of the work life of such employees.

**Nonfatal cases without lost workdays.** This classification would include those cases that are recordable (as defined in Section II) but do not result in Death or Lost workdays (either Days away from work or Days of restricted work activity) as discussed earlier. These are primarily cases involving medical treatment only.

*Restriction of motion.* One of the criteria for recordability, as opposed to classification, is any restriction of motion. As some restrictions of motion may not affect the employee's ability to perform all the duties normally connected with his job, it is possible to record a case because of restriction of motion as a Nonfatal case without lost workdays.

**Date of recordability.** *Injury.* An injury should be charged to the date on which it occurred, not the date when it is reported or brought to the attention of the employer. If the extent of injury changes, such as a case originally recorded as a Nonfatal case without lost workdays which subsequently results in Lost workdays, the date of recordability does not change.

*Illness.* For occupational illnesses, the case is charged to the date on which the illness is diagnosed or brought to the attention of the employer. As with injuries, as outlined above, any changes in the outcome of the case would not change the date against which the illness is charged.

## OSHA incidence rates

Safety performance is *relative.* Only when a company compares its injury experience with that of similar companies, or with that of the entire industry of which it is a part, or with its own previous experience can it obtain a meaningful evaluation of its safety accomplishments.

To make such comparisons, a method of measurement is needed that will adjust for the effects of certain variables which contribute to differences in injury experience. For two reasons, injury totals alone cannot be used.

First, a company with many employees may be expected to have more injuries than a company with few employees. Second, if the records of one company include all the injuries treated in the first aid room, whereas the records of a similar company include only injuries serious enough to cause lost time, obviously the first total will be larger than the second.

A standard procedure for keeping records, which provides for these variables, is included in the OSHA recordkeeping requirements. First, this procedure uses incidence rates which relate injury and illness cases, and days lost as a result of them, to the number of employee-hours worked; thus these rates automatically adjust for differences in the hours of exposure to injury. Second, this procedure specifies the kinds of injuries and illnesses that should be included in the rates.

These standardized rates, which are easy to compute and to understand, have been accepted generally as uniform procedure in industry and permit the necessary and desired comparisons.

A chronological arrangement of these rates for a company will show whether its level of safety performance is improving or getting worse. Within a company, the same sort of arrangement by departments will not only show the trend of safety performance for each department, but may reveal to management information which will make safety work more efficient.

If it is found, for example, that the trend of incidence rates in a company is up, a review of the rate trends by department may reveal that this adverse change is accounted for by the rates of just a few departments. With the source of the highest company rates thus isolated, safety efforts may be concentrated at the points of worst experience.

A comparison of current incidence rates with those of similar companies and with those of the industry as a whole will provide the safety professional with a more reliable evaluation of the safety performance of his company than he could obtain merely by reviewing numbers of cases.

**Formulas for rates.** Incidence rates are based on the exposure of 100 full-time workers using 200,000 employee-hours as the equivalent (100 employees working 40 hours per week for 50 weeks per year). An incidence rate can be computed for each category of cases or days lost depending on what number is put in the numerator of the formula. The denominator of the formula should be the total number of hours worked by all employees during the same time period as that covered by the number of cases in the numerator.

Incidence Rate =

$$\frac{\text{No. of injuries \& illnesses} \times 200{,}000}{\text{Total hours worked by all employees during period covered}}$$

or

$$\frac{\text{No. of lost workdays} \times 200{,}000}{\text{Total hours worked by all employees during period covered}}$$

There are two other formulas that can be used

**187**

to measure the average severity of the recorded cases:

$$\begin{array}{l}\text{Average lost workdays} \\ \text{per total lost} \\ \text{workday cases}\end{array} = \dfrac{\text{Total lost workdays}}{\text{Total lost workday cases}}$$

$$\begin{array}{l}\text{Average days away} \\ \text{from work}\end{array} = \dfrac{\text{Total days away from work}}{\begin{array}{c}\text{Total cases involving days} \\ \text{away from work}\end{array}}$$

If these numbers are small, then it is known that the cases are relatively minor. If, however, they are large, then the cases are of greater average severity and should receive serious attention.

For example, to calculate the incidence rate for total recordable cases at the end of the year, one would simply multiply the number of recordable cases by 200,000 and divide that by the number of hours worked by all employees for the whole year.

The incidence rates may also be interpreted as the percentage of employees that will suffer the degree of injury for which the rate was calculated. That is, if the incidence rate of lost workday cases is 5.1 per 100 full-time workers, then about 5 percent of the establishment's employees incurred a lost workday injury.

## Significance of Changes in Injury and Illness Experience

The incidence rate for lost workday cases is the best measure for comparing the occupational injury and illness experience between companies of various sizes, although it is often not sufficient for determining the significance of month-to-month changes in the actual number of cases within a single company. For comparing month-to-month changes within a company, it is usually necessary to use all cases, not only the lost workday cases. This provides a more objective measure for determining the significance of month-to-month fluctuations in the number of cases, especially when there is an apparently large increase or decrease from the monthly average.

Since the average number of cases per month is calculated from numbers of cases that are larger and smaller than the average itself, variation from the average is to be expected. The variation can be either random or caused; caused variation is significant and random variation is nonsignificant. Therefore, the significance of variations can easily be determined by distinguishing between those which are random and those which are caused.

Manufacturing organizations are already faced with the task of determining the significance of variations in such things as dimensions, weight, or performance of their products. To ease this task, they frequently employ a tool known as a "quality control chart." The quality control chart identifies and distinguishes between a *random* variation, which is said to be "in control," and *caused* variation, which is said to be "out of control." Being able to distinguish between the two types of variation permits management to concentrate its efforts on those variations that are "out of control."

A similar control chart can be developed to evaluate the significance of changes in injury and illness experience. The first step in developing the chart is to calculate the average number of cases per month. Because this monthly average will fluctuate from year to years, several years' experience should be used to develop a stable average. Preferably, the average should be calculated using 60 months' experience. After the average number of cases per month has been determined, the upper and lower control limits (UCL and LCL, respectively) are calculated using the following equation:

$$\text{UCL and LCL} = n \pm 2\sqrt{n}$$

where $n$ is the average number of cases per month.

Fig. 6–9 shows a control chart developed for one company. Using 60 months' experience, it was determined that the company had an average of 25 cases per month. Substitution of 25 for $n$ in the equation yielded the upper and lower control limits shown below:

$$25 \pm 2\sqrt{25} = 25 \pm 10 = \begin{cases} 25 + 10 = 35 \text{ for the Upper limit} \\ 25 - 10 = 15 \text{ for the Lower limit} \end{cases}$$

The control chart was then constructed and the company recorded the actual number of cases each month. Note that the actual monthly number of cases, with the exception of February, fall within the upper and lower control limits. These variations are random and do not represent significant changes from the monthly average of 25 cases. The variation for February, probably, is a caused variation indicating that the experience for February is "out of control" and that corrective measures should be taken. Suppose, for example, an investigation revealed that an unguarded

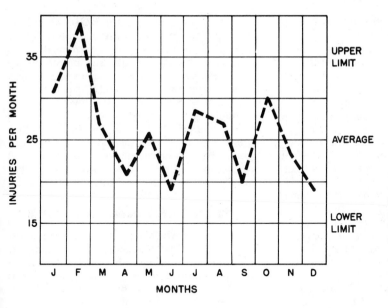

FIG. 6–9.—Upper and lower control limits of this control chart were based on 60 months' experience, and show points at which the number of injuries can statistically be shown to have a "contributing cause" rather than be "by chance." Thus action can be taken where it will be most effective.

machine was the cause of the increase in cases for the month of February. It can be assumed that the installation of a mechanical guard corrected this cause and brought the injury and illness experience for March back "in control."

The control chart can be a useful tool when it is used properly. As with any tool, it will depend on the skill of the user to yield good results. Follow these rules when constructing a control chart:

1. Always use several years' experience when calculating the average number of cases per month to assure that a stable average will be developed. Sixty months' experience is preferable, except as noted in (3), (4), and (5) following.

2. Count *all* cases when constructing a control chart. The use of lost workday cases alone may not provide enough data. A control chart cannot be constructed if the average number of cases per month is less than four because the lower limit will be negative. Since a plant cannot experience a negative number of cases per month, a chart based on an average of less than four would not yield meaningful results.

3. Calculate a new average each year—adding the latest year's cases and subtracting the oldest year's cases—to reflect any change in the monthly average number of cases.

4. Construct more than one chart if there are seasonal changes in employment. For example, if an operation employs one hundred people for the first 6 months of each year and four hundred people for the last 6 months, a separate chart must be constructed for each 6–month period.

5. Construct a new control chart if external factors, such as a change in the level of employment, a change in the work environment, or a change in work hazards, bring about a permanent change in injury and illness experience. When calculating a new average in such a situation, *do not* use experience prior to the change.

### Off-the-Job and Patron Injuries

#### Accidental injury experience of employees

In recent years, off-the-job disabling injuries of employees have exceeded on-the-job disabling injuries by 30 to 40 percent. Since the unscheduled absence of employees for any reason can cause production slowdowns and delays, costly retraining and replacement, or costly overtime by remaining employees, many safety specialists are concerned with the off-the-job injuries that occur to their employees. Moreover, activity

**189**

to reduce off-the-job accidents should help promote interest in on-the-job safety.

The ANSI Z16.3 Standard provides a means for recording and measuring these off-the-job injuries—those injuries suffered by an employee that do *not* arise out of and in the course of employment. Definitions and rates used under the ANSI Z16.3 Standard are very similar to those used under ANSI Z16.1. Because the data on off-the-job injuries is not as easy to obtain, however, certain simplifications are introduced in ANSI Z16.3. Exposure (for use in rates per million employee-hours) is standardized at 312 employee-hours per employee per month (equal to four and one-third weeks less forty hours per week at work and 56 hours per week for sleeping). For the calculation of severity rates, each permanent partial disability is recorded at 390 days of disability (based upon Bureau of Labor Statistics averages for all permanent partial disabilities). Provision is also made in ANSI Z16.3 for recording home, public, and transportation injuries separately to allow for concentrated effort in problem areas.

## Patron and nonemployee injury statistics

Many safety professionals concerned with employee injuries and workers' compensation have a similar or even greater concern about injuries to customers, patients, hotel guests, diners, tenants or others not employed by the reporting facility. For this reason the Trades and Services Section of the National Safety Council initiated and sponsored the American National Standard Z108.1. See Chapter 21, "Nonemployee Accident Prevention," for a discussion of applicable control activities.

A reportable patron injury is defined as one which occurs to a patron in the service environment (such as a store, parking lot, hotel, office, or restaurant) or from a "service"-connected accident or illness resulting from the use of a service or product, and which requires professional medical or dental treatment or examination. Property damage or injuries not serious enough to warrant professional attention (or which upon examination reveal no actual injury) need not be recorded. Accidents involving street and highway vehicles and passenger carrying operations subject to federal reporting systems would also be excluded.

Since the exposure base would vary widely between services such as theaters, with fairly consistent exposure time, and bus terminals, with inconsistent exposure, the ANSI Z108.1 Standard provides that the trade association or other national representative group determine its exposure base. In other words, the patron injury frequency rate may use as an exposure base 10,000 sales transactions, 100,000 patron-days, $1 million gross sales, or other common denominator.

The measure of severity (patron loss injury rate) is also chosen by the industry or business group. It might be the dollar value of incurred losses (claims) per $1 million sales or some other basis, generally over a twelve-month time span.

## ANSI Z16.1 Recordkeeping and Rates

Work on the ANSI Z16.1 standard goes back to Bulletin No. 276, "Standardization of Industrial Accident Statistics," published by the U.S. Bureau of Labor Statistics in 1920. Although developed by a body representing governmental statistical agencies, the rate provisions of this Bulletin were widely followed in whole or part by private agencies. At a national conference on Industrial Accident Prevention, called by the U.S. Secretary of Labor in Washington in 1926, a resolution was adopted in favor of a revision of Bulletin 276 by a committee set up under the procedures of the American Standards Association (presently the American National Standards Institute). As a result of the work of this committee, the first edition of this standard was completed and approved in 1937 as Z16.1-1937. Since then this standard has been reviewed and revised.

**Dates for compiling rates.** Injury rates should be determined as soon after each period (month or year, for example) as the information becomes available. A reasonable time may be allowed for completion of reports. However, absolute accuracy in rates does not justify long delays.

The ANSI Z16.1 Standard suggests the following schedule for compiling injury rates:

1. Annual frequency rates should be based on all disabling injuries occurring within the year and reported within twenty days after the close of the year. Monthly frequency rates should be based on all disabling injuries occurring within the month and reported within twenty days after the close of the month.

2. Days charged for reported cases in which disability continues beyond the closing dates

in (1) should be estimated on the basis of medical opinion of probable ultimate disability.

3. Cases first reported after closing dates stated in (1) need not be included in the rates for that period, or for any similar subsequent period. However, they should be included, and should replace estimates, in rates for longer periods of which that period is a part.

A disabling injury, and all days lost or charged because of it, should be charged to the date on which the injury occurred, except that for injuries, such as bursitis, tenosynovitis, pneumoconiosis ("black lung"), or silicosis, which do not arise out of specific accidents, the date of the injury should be the date when the injury is first reported. (Remember, OSHA calls these "occupational illnesses.")

## Standard formulas for rates

The injury frequency rate and the injury severity rate are based on standard formulas as set forth in ANSI Z16.1.

**Frequency rate.** The disabling injury frequency rate relates the injuries to the hours worked during the period and expresses them in terms of a million-hour unit by use of the following formula:

$$\frac{\text{Number of disabling injuries} \times 1,000,000}{\text{Employee-hours of exposure}}$$

**Severity rate.** The disabling injury severity rate relates the days charged to the hours worked during the period and expresses them in terms of a million-hour unit by use of the following formula:

$$\frac{\text{Total days charged} \times 1,000,000}{\text{Employee-hours of exposure}}$$

**Average days charged.** The frequency and severity rates show, respectively, the rate at which disabling injuries occur and the rate at which time is charged. A third measure included in the standard procedure shows the average severity of the disabling injuries. It is called the average days charged per disabling injury and may be calculated by either of the following formulas:

I. $$\frac{\text{Total days charged}}{\text{Total disabling injuries}}$$

or

II. $$\frac{\text{Severity rate}}{\text{Frequency rate}}$$

## Calculation of employee-hours

Employee-hours used in calculating injury rates is the total number of hours worked by all employees, including those of operating, production, maintenance, transportation, clerical, administrative, sales, and other departments.

Employee-hours should be calculated from the payroll or time clock records. If this method cannot be used, they may be estimated by multiplying the total employee-days worked for the period covered by the number of hours worked each day.

The experience of a central administrative office or central sales office of a multi-establishment should not be included in the experience of any one establishment, nor should it be prorated among the establishments, but it should be included in the overall experience of the concern.

In calculating hours for employees who live on company property, only those hours are counted during which the employee is on duty.

For traveling personnel, such as salesmen, executives, and others whose working hours are not defined, an average of 8 hours per day should be used in computing the hours worked.

For standby employees who are restricted to the confines of the employer's premises, including seamen aboard vessels, all stand-by hours should be counted, as well as all work injuries occurring during such hours.

## Disabling injuries

The standard specifies that a work injury is any injury, including occupational disease and other work-connected disability, which arises out of and in the course of employment. The following descriptions paraphrase the standard. For full details, refer to the standard.

**Occupational disease** is a disease caused by exposure to environmental factors associated with employment. Work-connected disability includes such ailments as silicosis, pneumoconiosis, tenosynovitis, bursitis, and loss of hearing. Even though there is no traumatic injury in such

**191**

disabilities, if they are work connected, they are considered work injuries.

**Definitions.** To ensure uniformity in the computation of injury rates and thereby provide for comparison among rates, the standard specifies that only *disabling injuries* shall be counted in the computation of standard injury rates. In general terms, a disabling injury is one which results in death or permanent impairment or which renders the injured person unable to work for a full day on any day after the day of injury. Disabling injuries are of four classes, as follows:

1. *Death* is any fatality resulting from a work injury, regardless of the time intervening between injury and death.

2. *Permanent total disability* is an injury other than death which permanently and totally incapacitates an employee from following any gainful occupation, or which results in the loss (or the complete loss of use) of any of the following in one accident: (*a*) both eyes; (*b*) one eye and one hand, or arm, or foot, or leg; (*c*) any two of the following not on the same limb, hand, arm, foot, leg.

3. *Permanent partial disability* is any injury other than death or permanent total disability which results in the complete loss or loss of use of any member or part of a member of the body, or any permanent impairment of functions of the body or part thereof, regardless of any preexisting disability of the injured member or impaired body function.

4. *Temporary total disability* is any injury which does not result in death or permanent impairment, but which results in one or more days of disability.

**Temporary total disability—key points.** Of the four classes of disabling injuries used in calculating standard injury rates, temporary total disability is the most difficult to interpret uniformly. Key points in the definition are:

- *Day of disability.* A day of disability is any day on which an employee is unable, because of injury, to perform effectively throughout a full shift the essential functions of a regularly established job which is open and available to him. Days include Sundays, days off, plant shutdowns, and other nonwork days subsequent to the day of injury. (Note: Disability days for an injury are not counted when scheduled charge(s) apply.)

Here is how the standard describes it.

**1.5.1.1.** The day of injury and the day on which the employee was able to return to full-time employment shall not be counted as days of disability; but all intervening calendar days, or calendar days subsequent to the day of injury (including weekends, holidays, other days off, and other days on which the plant may be shut down), shall be counted as days of disability provided they meet the criteria of the preceding paragraph.

**1.5.1.2.** Time lost on a workday, or on a nonworkday, subsequent to the day of injury, ascribed solely to the unavailability of medical attention or of necessary diagnostic aids, shall be considered disability time, unless in the opinion of the physician authorized by the employer to treat the case the person was able to work on all days subsequent to the day of injury.

**1.5.1.3.** If the physician authorized by the employer to treat the case is of the opinion that the injured employee is actually capable of working a full normal shift at a regularly established job, but has prescribed certain therapeutic treatments, the employee may be excused from work for those treatments without counting the excused time as disability time, provided: (*a*) the time required to obtain the treatments does not, on any workday, prevent him from performing effectively the essential functions of his job assignment on that day, and (*b*) the treatments are professionally administered and constitute more than simple rest.

**1.5.1.4.** If the physician authorized by the employer to treat the case is of the opinion that the injured employee was actually capable of working a full normal shift at a regularly established job, but because of transportation problems, associated with his injury, the employee is forced to arrive at his place of work late, or to leave the workplace before the established quitting time, such lost time may be excused and not counted as disability time, provided: (*a*) that the excused time does not materially reduce his working time, and (*b*) that it is clearly evident that this failure to work the full shift hours is the result of a bona fide transportation problem and not a deviation from the "regularly established job."

**1.5.1.5.** If the injured employee receives medical treatment for his injury, the determination of his ability to work shall rest with the physician authorized by the employer to treat the case. If the employee rejects medical attention offered by the employer, the determination may be made by the employer based upon the best information available to him. If the employer fails to provide medical attention, the employee's decision shall be controlling.

○ ○ ○

• *Specific disabilities.* Following are examples of specific disabilities and the standard procedures for handling them. In all these cases, the regular shift is assumed to be 8:00 A.M. to 5:00 P.M.

1. Injury occurred at 4:30 P.M. on Monday. The employee worked on Tuesday and Wednesday, but delayed infection prevented him from working from Thursday through the following Monday. He returned to work on Tuesday at 11:00 A.M. after seeing his doctor. This is a disabling injury with five chargeable days of disability (Thursday through Monday).

2. Injury occurred at 1:00 P.M. on Friday. Saturday was not a workday, but the doctor certified that the employee could not have worked on that day if it had been, although he could have worked on Sunday and thereafter. The employee returned to work on Monday. This is a disabling injury with one day of disability (Saturday), even though the employee lost no actual work time except Friday afternoon.

3. Injury occurred at 4:00 P.M. on Tuesday. The employee was hospitalized for treatment of his injury until noon on Wednesday when the doctor released him with permission to resume work on Thursday morning. This is a disabling injury with one day of disability.

4. Injury occurred at 11:00 A.M. on Tuesday. The employee was treated by the doctor and sent home with instructions not to work Wednesday, but to report to the doctor's office Wednesday afternoon. At 5:30 P.M. Wednesday the employee was seen by the doctor, who discharged him as fit to work immediately. This is a disabling injury with one day of disability.

5. The doctor determined that an injury would not allow an employee to return to his own job for at least a week. On checking with the personnel department, the doctor learned that

another job was open which the employee could handle, and the employee was cleared for this work. This is not a disabling injury because the employee could perform another regularly established job which was open and available to him.

• *Additional key points* with regard to all the classifications of disabling injuries are:

1. An injury need not be traumatic—there does not have to be a visible wound. More precisely, the standard covers work-connected *disabilities,* which may include such conditions as bursitis, tenosynovitis, loss of hearing, and similar ailments.

2. An injury need not arise out of an accident, although it must be work connected. Examples of such injuries would be dermatitis, silicosis, and bursitis. A strain resulting from overlifting would be a work injury even though there was no accident.

3. The classification of an injury is entirely independent of workers' compensation laws, and rulings of workers' compensation agencies. This provision is necessary to promote uniformity in injury classification. Otherwise, similar injuries, might be classified differently in different states.

As may readily be seen, minor injuries are excluded in the calculation of the standard injury rates. The reason is that it is impossible to obtain standardization of minor cases. The standard does provide classification for minor injuries, though, as *medical treatment injuries,* and identifies them as injuries that do not result in death, permanent impairment, or temporary total disability, but which require medical treatment, including first aid.

Although these nondisabling injuries are not included in the standard injury rates, they should be given consideration and attention by the safety professional. He may well keep totals of them, and note their frequency, the departments in which they occur, the types of injuries, and the relationship between them and disabling injuries.

## Classification of special cases

**Work injuries.** In addition to the usual injuries and occupational diseases, the following are specifically identified as work injuries for statistical purposes:

# 6—Accident Records and Incidence Rates

1. Inguinal hernia, if it is precipitated by an impact, sudden effort, or severe strain and meets *all* of the following conditions:

   a). There is a clear record of an accident or an incident, such as a slip, trip, fall, sudden effort, or overexertion;

   b). There is actual pain in the hernial region at the time of the accident or incident;

   c). The immediate pain was so severe that the injured employee was forced to stop work long enough to draw the attention of his supervisor or fellow employee to his condition, or the attention of a physician was secured within twelve hours.

2. Back injury, if:

   a). There is a clear record of an accident or an incident, such as a slip, trip, or fall, sudden effort or blow on the back; or

   b). The employee was engaged in a work activity which, in the opinion of the physician authorized by the employer to treat the case, produced a physical condition resulting from overexertion.

A back condition which is revealed in the course of employment, but which does not satisfy *either* of these conditions, should not be considered a work injury.

3. Aggravation of a pre-existing physical deficiency, if the aggravation arises out of and in the course of employment.

4. Aggravation of a minor work injury, whether due to improper diagnosis or treatment or to infection either on the job or off the job.

5. Animal and insect bites incurred in the performance of duties of employment.

6. Skin irritations and infections, such as poison ivy or dermatitis, when the employee is exposed to irritants in connection with his work.

7. Exposure to temperature extremes in the course of employment.

8. Muscular disability, such as bursitis or tenosynovitis, if it arises out of duties of employment.

**Nondisabling injuries.** The following cases

## TABLE 6–A.* SCHEDULED CHARGES
### (See Fig. 6–10 for bone location)

### A. FOR LOSS OF MEMBER – TRAUMATIC OR SURGICAL

(For loss of use of member, see footnote°°)

*Fingers, Thumb, and Hand*

Amputation Involving All or Part of Bone°°

|  | Thumb | Fingers | | | |
|---|---|---|---|---|---|
|  |  | Index | Middle | Ring | Little |
| Distal phalange ..... | 300 | 100 | 75 | 60 | 50 |
| Middle phalange ... .. | | 200 | 150 | 120 | 100 |
| Proximal phalange.. | 600 | 400 | 300 | 240 | 200 |
| Metacarpal ........... | 900 | 600 | 500 | 450 | 400 |

Hand at wrist.............................................3000

*Toe, Foot, and Ankle*

| Amputation Involving All or Part of Bone°° | Great Toe | Each of Other Toes |
|---|---|---|
| Distal phalange........................150 | | 35 |
| Middle phalange .................... . . | | 75 |
| Proximal phalange.................300 | | 150 |
| Metatarsal..............................600 | | 350 |

Foot at ankle ...............................................2400

*Arm*

Any point above°°° elbow, including
   shoulder joint ...........................................4500
Any point above wrist and at or
   below elbow...............................................3600

*Leg*

Any point above°°° knee...............................4500
Any point above ankle and at or
   below knee ...............................................3000

### B. IMPAIRMENT OF FUNCTION
One eye (loss of sight), whether or not
   there is sight in the other eye....................1800
Both eyes (loss of sight), in one accident .......6000
One ear (complete industrial loss of
   hearing), whether or not there is
   hearing in the other ear ............................ 600
Both ears (complete industrial loss of
   hearing), in one accident...........................3000
Unrepaired hernia (for repaired
   hernia, use actual days lost)....................... 50

### C. FATAL OR PERMANENT TOTAL DISABILITY
   ............6000

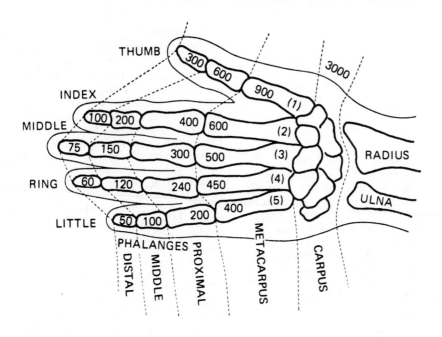

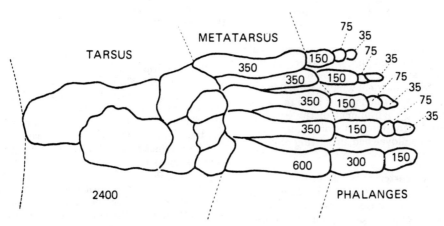

FIG. 6–10.—Chart of scheduled charges for hand (*above*) and foot (*below*). Numbers on the bones are the charges (in days) for loss involving part or all of the bone. (See also Table 6–A at left.)

*Courtesy American National Standards Institute.*

## Footnotes to Table 6–A

°Source: ANSI Z16.1, *Method of Recording and Measuring Work Injury Experience.*

°°For loss of use, without amputation, use a percentage of the scheduled charge corresponding to the loss of use as determined by the physician authorized to treat the case. If the bone is not involved, use actual days lost and classify as temporary total disability.

°°°The term "above" when applied to the arm means toward the shoulder, and when applied to the leg means toward the hip.

resulting in lost time are not classified as disabling:

1. Hospitalization for observation, for a period not to exceed 48 hours from the time of injury, or of suspected injury known to have a delayed effect, from such accidents as:

   a) A blow on the head

   b) A blow to the abdomen

   c) The inhalation of harmful gases

   provided that in every such case, the physician determines that the injury was in reality slight and that the injured person could have returned to work without permanent impairment or temporary total disability. In cases of exposure to ionizing radiation, the period of observation may be extended to ten days. NOTE: if *any* treatment or medication is given for a confining injury (or the suspected confining injury) after the first 24 hours of observation, the injury shall be classified as a work injury.

2. Illness from antitoxin, provided that the illness results *solely* from the antitoxin, vaccines, or drugs used in the treatment of a nondisabling injury.

3. Disability arising solely out of a physical deficiency, provided that a worker without such physical deficiency would not have experienced the incident which resulted in the injury. (An injury which results from the work activity or the environment of the employment shall be considered a work injury, even though the employee had an existing physical deficiency.)

4. Injury from an external event of such proportions and character as to be beyond the control of the employer, such as a tornado, "twister," hurricane, earthquake, flood, conflagration, or explosion originating outside of employment, or from an immediate secondary event, such as a fire, boiler explosion, or falling electric wire. (An injury would be reportable, though, if the victim were a policeman, firefighter, member of a disaster or emergency squad, utility line worker, or other employee who is assigned duties in connection with such events. An injury also would be reportable if it arose out of activities necessitated by an external event, such as fighting a fire, cleaning up debris, or repairing equipment.)

### Days charged

Losses from work injuries are evaluated in terms of days of disability, or inability to produce, either actual or potential. These losses are referred to simply as "days charged." For the first three classes of injuries—death, permanent total disability, and permanent partial disability—the number of days charged is a predetermined total. For permanent partial disability, the predetermined total usually exceeds the actual time lost to reflect potential future losses of productive capacity. The predetermined totals are referred to as "scheduled charges."

This procedure is based on the philosophy of economic loss which reasons, for example, that a worker who has a hand amputated will produce less during his remaining working years than a worker who completely recovers from a hand injury, even though both injuries resulted in the same number of actual days lost at the time of the injury. If both injuries resulted in, say, 60 days lost at the time of the injury, the injury from which the victim completely recovers would be charged only the 60 days, whereas the amputation would be charged 3000 days, the scheduled charge for this kind of injury.

**Death and permanent total disabilities.** For death and permanent total disabilities, a scheduled charge of 6000 days is made in each case. There are no variations in this amount. If the injury is fatal, or if it results in any of the losses specified as constituting permanent total disability, the charge is the same—6000 days.

The original basis for measuring the permanent disability of an injured worker was that, on the average, death or permanent total disability of a worker resulted in his losing 20 years of productive labor at 300 days per year, or 6000 days. Today, the death or permanent total disability of a worker would, on the average, result in his losing about 24 years of productive labor at 250 days per year, giving approximately the same total loss. Time charges for permanent partial disabilities are partly related to this possible total.

**Permanent partial disabilities.** For permanent partial disabilities, the scheduled charges vary depending on the specific loss. For example, amputation of the index finger at the first joint has a scheduled charge of 100 days; at the second joint, 200 days; and at the third joint, 400 days.

Scheduled charges for permanent partial injuries are shown in Table 6–A. Fig. 6–10 illustrates pictorially the charges for various hand and foot losses.

For permanent partial injuries that result in loss of use of an injured member, a percentage of the scheduled charge is used which corresponds to the percentage loss of use, as determined by the physician authorized to treat the injury.

For fatal, permanent total, and permanent partial disabilities, only the scheduled charges are used—the actual days of disability are disregarded. In some permanent partial injuries, there may be no losses at all, or there may be losses which exceed the scheduled charge. In either of these cases, though, disregard the number of days lost and *use only the scheduled charge.*

**Temporary total disabilities.** For temporary total disabilities, the fourth class of injuries, the number of days charged is the total number of full calendar days on which the injured person was unable to work as a result of the injury. The total does not include the day the injury occurred nor the day the injured person returned to work, but it does include all intervening calendar days (including Sundays, days off, or plant shutdowns). It also includes any other full days of inability to work because of the specific injury, subsequent to the injured person's return to work.

**Days charged in special cases** are indicated in the following paragraphs.

If a hernia is unrepaired (whether or not it can be repaired), it is classified as a permanent partial disability and carries a scheduled charge of 50 days. If a hernia is repaired, it is classified as a temporary total disability and the charge is only the actual number of calendar days lost.

For permanent impairments affecting more than one part of the body, the total charge is the sum of the scheduled charges for the individual body parts impaired. The total charge, however, shall not exceed 6000 days.

If an employee suffers a permanent partial injury to one part of the body and a temporary total injury to another part in one accident, whichever charge is greater is used and determines the injury classification.

The charge for a permanent injury not identified in the schedule of charges (such as damage to internal organs, lungs, or back, or loss of speech) is a percentage of 6000 days corresponding to the percentage of permanent total disability which results from the injury. This percentage is determined by the physician who treats the case.

## References

American National Standards Institute, 1430 Broadway, New York, N.Y. 10018.
  *Method of Recording and Measuring Work Injury Experience,* Z16.1-1967.
  *Method of Recording Basic Facts Relating to the Nature and Occurrence of Work Injuries,* Z16.2-1962.
  *Method of Recording and Measuring the Off-the-Job Disabling Accidental Injury Experience of Employees,* Z16.3-1973.
  *Method of Measuring and Recording Patron and Non-Employee Injury Statistics,* Z108.1-1971.
  *Uniform Recordkeeping for Occupational Injuries and Illnesses,* Z16.4-1977.

National Safety Council, 444 N. Michigan Ave., Chicago, Ill. 60611. *Accident Facts* (published annually).

Recht, J. L., "Bilevel Reporting," *Journal of Safety Research,* Vol. 2, No. 2 (June, 1970), pp. 51-54.

U.S. Dept. of Labor, Bureau of Labor Statistics, Washington, D.C. 20212. "What Every Employer Needs To Know about OSHA Recordkeeping," Report 412-3, 1978.

U.S. Dept. of Labor, Occupational Safety and Health Administration, Washington, D.C. 20212. "Recordkeeping Requirements under the Occupational Safety and Health Act of 1970." Rev. 1978.

Walker, Helen M., and Lev, Joseph. *Elementary Statistical Methods,* rev. ed. New York, N.Y., Holt, Rinehart and Winston, 1958.

# Accident
# Investigation,
# Analysis, and
# Costs

# Chapter
# 7

# 7—Accident Investigation, Analysis, and Costs

This chapter deals with the investigation of noninjury accidents as well as injury accidents. Therefore the term "accident" is used in its broadest sense to cover occurrences, and their causes, which may lead to property damage and work injuries.

Successful accident prevention requires a minimum of four fundamental activities:

1. A study of all working areas to detect and eliminate or control physical or environmental hazards that contribute to accidents.

2. A study of all operating methods and practices.

3. Education, instruction, training, and discipline to minimize human factors which contribute to accidents.

4. For causal analysis, a thorough investigation of at least every accident which results in OSHA lost workdays or a disabling injury (under ANSI Z16.1) to determine contributing circumstances. Accidents that do not result in personal injury (so-called "near-accidents" or "near-misses") are warnings. They should not be ignored.

This fourth activity, accident investigation and analysis, is a defense against hazards that are overlooked in the first three activities, those that are not obvious, or hazards that are the result of combinations of circumstances that are difficult to foresee.

## Accident Investigation and Analysis

Accident investigation and analysis is one of the means used to prevent accidents. As such, the investigation or analysis must produce information that leads to corrective actions that prevent or reduce the number of accidents. The more complete the information, the easier it will be for the safety professional to take effective corrective actions. For example, knowing that 40 percent of a plant's accidents involve ladders is not as useful as knowing that 80 percent of the plant's ladder accidents involve broken rungs.

A good recordkeeping system, as discussed in Chapter 6, is essential to accident investigation in that it allows the basic facts about an accident to be recorded quickly, efficiently, and uniformly. An investigation of at least every OSHA lost workday case or ANSI Z16.1 disabling injury should be made. Accidents resulting in no-lost-workday injuries, or no injuries, and also "near-

accidents," should be investigated if time and facilities permit, especially if there is frequent recurrence of certain types of injuries, or if the frequency of accidents is high in certain areas or operations.

For purposes of accident prevention, investigations must be for fact-finding, not fault-finding; otherwise, they may do more harm than good. This is not to say that responsibility may not be fixed where personal failure has caused injury, or that such persons should be excused from the consequences of their actions. It does mean that the investigation itself should be concerned only with facts. The investigating individual, board, or committee is best kept free from involvement with any punitive actions resulting from their investigation.

## Types of investigation and analysis

There are a variety of accident investigation and analysis techniques available to the investigator. Some of these techniques are more complicated than others. The choice of a particular method will depend upon the purpose and orientation of the investigation. The Hazard Mode and Effect approach discussed in Chapter 4, "Acquiring Hazard Information," could be very useful for investigating situations where large, complex, and interrelated machinery and procedures are involved, but may be of limited value in the investigation of accidents involving hand tools. If management procedures and communications and their relationship to accidents are of great interest, the Management Oversight and Risk Tree analysis (MORT, see references at the end of Chapter 4) could prove to be very helpful.

The accident investigation and analysis procedure outlined in the ANSI Z16.2 Standard focuses primarily on unsafe acts and unsafe conditions. Other similar techniques involve investigation within the framework of defects in man, machine, media, and management (the "4 M's"), or education, enforcement, and engineering (the "3 E's"). For analysis purposes, these techniques involve classifying the data about a group of accidents into various categories. This has been referred to as the statistical method of analysis. Corrective actions are designed on the basis of most frequent patterns of occurrence.

Other techniques discussed in Chapter 4 come under the systems approach to safety. Systems safety stresses an enlarged viewpoint that takes into account the interrelationships between the various events that could lead to an accident. As accidents will rarely have one cause, the systems approach to safety can point to more than one place in a system where effective corrective actions can be introduced. This allows the safety professional to choose the corrective actions that bests meet the criteria for effectiveness, speed of installment, cost/benefit, and the like. Systems safety techniques also have the advantage of application before accidents have occurred and can be applied to new procedures and operations.

## Persons making the investigation

Depending on the nature of the accident and other conditions, the investigation may be made by the supervisor, the safety professional, or inspector, the safety and health committee, the general safety committee, or an engineer from the insurance company. If the accident involves special features, consultation with an engineer from the state labor department or U.S. Bureau of Mines, or with a union representative, may be warranted.

**The supervisor or foreman.** The supervisor or foreman should make an immediate report of every injury requiring medical treatment and other accidents he may be directed to investigate. He is on the scene, he probably knows more about the accident than anyone else, and it is up to him, in most cases, to put into effect whatever measures may be adopted to prevent similar accidents. The Supervisor's Accident Report in the previous chapter illustrates one form that can be used to record the findings of an accident investigation.

**The safety professional.** A representative of the safety department should verify the findings of the supervisor and make an investigation of every important accident for his own information, and in most cases he should make a written report to the proper official or to the general safety committee.

Nowhere are the safety professional's value and ability better shown than in the investigation of an accident. His specialized training and analytical experience enable him to search for all the facts, apparent and hidden, and to submit a report free from bias or prejudice. He has no interest in the investigation other than to get information that can be used to prevent a similar accident.

**Special investigative committee.** In some companies, a special committee is set up to investigate and report on all serious accidents. This function is particularly important where a contributing factor was an unsafe act on the part of the worker.

If this committee, composed of the injured employee's fellow workers, investigates the accident immediately, finds that the injured person did contribute to the accident, and so reports to the general safety and health committee or to management, and if this report is then publicized, it will be more generally accepted among the workers than a similar report made by the supervisor or the safety professional.

On the other hand, many companies disagree strongly with this concept of the duties of the workers' safety committee, believing that the task of assigning responsibility for an accident is sometimes an unpleasant one and should not be foisted upon workers.

See the discussion of safety committees in Chapter 3, "Hazard Control Program Organization."

**The safety and health committee.** In many companies, especially those of small or moderate size, a number of safety activities are handled by a safety and health committee, one of whose activities is accident investigation. Ordinarily, such investigation would be handled in a routine manner, but in important cases the chairman might call an extra meeting of the committee to conduct a special investigation.

## Cases to be investigated

An accident that causes death or serious injury obviously should be thoroughly investigated. The "near-accident" that might have caused death or serious injury is equally important from the safety standpoint and should be investigated; for example, the breaking of a crane hook or a scaffold rope, or an explosion associated with a pressure vessel.

Each investigation should be made as soon after the accident as possible. A delay of only a few hours may permit important evidence to be destroyed or removed, intentionally or unintentionally. Also, the results of the inquiry should be made known quickly, inasmuch as their publicity value in the safety education of employees and supervisors is greatly increased by promptness.

Any epidemic of minor injuries demands study. A particle of emery in the eye or a scratch from handling sheet metal may be a very simple case; the immediate cause may be obvious, and the loss of time may not exceed a few minutes. However, if cases of this or any other type occur frequently in the plant, or in any one department, an investigation should be made to determine the underlying causes.

The chief value of such an investigation lies in uncovering contributing causes. The energetic safety professional or manager is constantly alive to the advantage of this kind of accident investigation, which may prove more valuable, though less spectacular, than the "inquest" following a fatal injury.

Fairness and impartiality are absolutely essential. The value of the investigation is largely destroyed if there is any suspicion that its purpose is to place the blame or pass the buck. No one should be assigned to investigation work unless he or she has earned a reputation for fairness and is experienced in gathering evidence. It should be made quite clear that accident investigations are conducted entirely for the purpose of obtaining information which will help to prevent recurrence of accidents.

In the early years of the safety movement, accident prevention usually was a hit-or-miss activity. This approach has been replaced by more scientific techniques—see Chapter 4, "Acquiring Hazard Information."

In the earlier years, a reduction in accident rates was prompted primarily by humanitarian appeal to management and workers. Although this appeal is still important, methods today are aimed at isolating and identifying accident causes in order to permit direct, positive action (corrective actions) to prevent their recurrence.

Like other phases of modern business management, accident prevention must be based on facts that clearly identify the problem. An approach to the accident prevention problem on this basis not only will result in more effective control over accidents, but will permit this objective to be accomplished with savings in time, effort, and money.

Accident analysis of individual cases will identify the plants, locations, or departments in which injuries occur most frequently, and will suggest corrective actions necessary to reduce accidents in those areas.

Sometimes an overall high rate is not identified with one or a few departments, but instead represents a high frequency of accidents through-

out the establishment. Under such circumstances, it is even more important that an analysis of the accidents be made.

Similar accidents may occur frequently but at widely seaparated locations, so that their high incidence is not always apparent. Accidents may be more numerous in the operation of some machines than in the operation of others, or in the performance of certain procedures. Some unsafe practices which cause accidents may be committed repeatedly but at different times and in different places, so that their importance as accident causes is not immediately recognized.

Analysis of the circumstances of accidents can produce these results:

1. Identify and locate the principal sources of accidents by determining, from actual experience, the materials, machines, and tools most frequently involved in accidents, and the jobs most likely to produce injuries.

2. Disclose the nature and size of the accident problem in departments and among occupations.

3. Indicate the need for engineering revision by identifying the principal hazards associated with various types of equipment and materials.

4. Disclose inefficiencies in operating processes and procedures where poor layout, for example, contributes to accidents, or where outdated methods or procedures that overtax the physical capacities of the workers can be avoided, for example by using mechanical handling methods.

5. Disclose the unsafe practices which necessitate training of employees.

6. Enable supervisors to use the time available for safety work to the greatest advantage by providing them with information about the principal hazards and unsafe practices in their departments.

7. Permit an objective evaluation of the progress of a safety program by noting in continuing analyses the effect of corrective actions, educational techniques, and other methods adopted to prevent injuries.

### The minimum data

The purpose of an accident investigation is to identify facts about each injury and the accident that produced it and to record those facts. These records, individually and collectively, serve as guides to the areas, conditions, and circumstances to which accident prevention efforts may be directed most profitably.

The paragraphs that follow describe the data elements that comprise the minimum amount of information that should be collected about each accident. The Supervisors Accident Report Form, Fig. 6–2 in the previous chapter, shows a "minimum data set" that was developed to improve the quality of accident investigation and analysis. The minimum data set tries to identify the "why" of some of the accident characteristics as well as the "who, what, when, and where." It acknowledges the existence of multiple causes of accidents by not restricting the investigator or analyst to selecting a single act or condition which "caused" the accident.

The investigation is also expanded from focusing solely on the injury and accident type to include the entire sequence of events which led to the injury, as far back in time as the investigator feels is relevant to the accident. This expanded view of the accident sequence allows an employer to identify and implement a wider variety of corrective actions.

• The first of the eight groups of data elements is *employer characteristics*. This includes the type of industry and the size of the establishment (number of full-time equivalent employees). It is needed when data from one establishment is compared with that of another.

• Second is *employee characteristics*: The victim's age and sex, the department and occupation in which he worked, and whether full time, part time, or seasonal. Questions about the victim's experience are also asked. How long he has been with the company? How long in his current occupation? and How often he repeats the activity in which he was engaged when the accident occurred?

• The third group is about the accident itself. A narrative description should be prepared; it should include what the person was doing, what objects or substances were involved, and actions or movements which led to the injury. This is elaborated into a detailed accident sequence that starts with the injuring event and works backward in time through all of the preceding events that directly contributed to the accident. The data also includes a description of any product or equipment that was directly involved with the accident sequence and the task being performed. Any other conditions such as temperature, light, noise, and weather, that pertain to the accident should also be noted here.

• The fourth group deals with the characteristics of the equipment associated with the accident. The description should include the type, brand, size, and any distinguishing features of the equipment, its condition, and the specific part involved.

• Fifth is the characteristics of the task being performed when the accident happened: The general task (such as repairing a conveyor) and the specific activity (such as using a wrench). The description should include the posture and location of the employee (for example, squatting under the conveyor) and whether he was working alone or with others.

• Time factors are the sixth group. The investigator should record the time of day and how that related to the shift the victim was working, whether first hour of the shift, second hour, or later. What type of shift—day, swing, straight, rotating, etc. And the phase of the employee's workday; performing work, rest period, meal period, overtime, entering or leaving plant.

• The seventh group, use and nature of preventive measures, includes the following questions: What personal protective equipment was being worn and did the employee's apparel affect the accident sequence? What kind of training did the employee have for the task he was performing? Did standards or procedures exist for the task? Were they written? Were they followed? If not followed, how did what happened differ from what should have happened? Were all guards in place and in use? What was the nature of supervision at the time of the accident? What immediate remedial actions were taken to prevent recurrence?

• The last group of questions concerns the severity of the injury. The nature of the injury or injuries and the parts of the body effected must be recorded as well as the OSHA severity class. If the accident resulted in some permanent impairment this should be noted.

The answers to the questions in these eight groups constitutes the *minimum* information needed to proceed with an analysis. The nature of a company's operations or the interests of the

## TABLE 7–A

### AREAS FOR CORRECTIVE ACTIONS

I. Machines.

    A. Hazardous conditions, construction, or design

    B. Equipment, tools, and objects

II. Environment.

    A. Location of equipment, tools, and objects in the work space.

    B. Location of employees in the work space.

III. Person.

    A. Action, task or activity

    B. Work procedures.

    C. Personal protective equipment

IV. Management.

    A. Supervision.

    B. Program evaluation.

---

analyst may suggest other questions to be answered in the investigation.

There are two kinds of analysis that may be done. First the individual accident may be examined to determine the corrective action or actions that will prevent future occurrences of this specific sequence of events. The other kind of analysis, the statistical analysis, examines a group of similar occurrences for patterns which may lend themselves to corrective actions. Over time this statistical analysis can show what corrective actions have been more effective than others.

### Corrective action selection

In any accident, there are many factors at work that permit the sequence of events leading to the injury to occur. The idea behind the corrective action selection procedure is to identify all of the factors for which a corrective action is possible and then to select from them the ones likely to be most effective, most cost/beneficial, and most acceptable, etc., and implement those.

Table 7–A lists the general areas in which corrective actions may be taken. Note that these areas correspond to the questions asked in the minimum data set.

The first step is to form a basic understanding of the events which took place; not just the injury or damage producing event, but all of the events in the accident sequence. Then at each step in the sequence of events the analyst can refer to the list in Table 7–A to see if a change in one *or more* of those areas would have prevented the sequence from continuing on to produce the injury.

After listing all of the possible corrective actions identified this way each candidate must be evaluated for practicality, cost, feasibility, reliability, acceptance, and any other factor deemed important, before deciding which ones to implement.

This systematic approach to selecting corrective actions ensures that all major types are considered, that the analyst does not stop with only his favorite corrective actions, and that each corrective action chosen for implementation is well thought out.

### Classifying accident data

Even in large company operations in which hundreds of accidents may occur annually, only rarely do two accidents occur in exactly the same way. Accidents do follow general patterns, however, and grouping them according to pattern is necessary for purposes of analysis.

Finding the patterns and common features of groups of cases is the statistical approach to accident analysis.

Setting up classifications. Before the actual analysis work is begun, classifications must be set up for grouping the various data. For each basic fact, general classifications should be established in which similar data may be grouped. Then, more specific classifications should be set up within each general classification to preserve as many of the details as possible.

For example, in ANSI Z16.2, among the general classifications recommended for the key fact "Hazardous condition" are the following:

1. Defects of agencies

2. Dress or apparel hazards

3. Environmental hazards

## Analysis of Ladder Accidents

| Code No. | Unsafe Conditions | | Total no. of cases |
|---|---|---|---|
| 1 | Slippery rungs | ⅣⅡ Ⅰ | 6 |
| 2 | Broken rungs | ⅢⅠ | 3 |
| 3 | Lack of hooks for fastening ladder at top | Ⅰ | 1 |
| 4 | Worn ladder shoes | Ⅰ | 1 |
| 5 | Weak, worn, cracked rails | Ⅱ | 2 |

### Unsafe Acts

| Code No. | Unsafe Acts | | Total no. of cases |
|---|---|---|---|
| 10 | Failure to secure ladder at top | ⅣⅡ ⅣⅡ ⅣⅡ ⅣⅡ ⅣⅡ ⅢⅠ | 29 |
| 20 | Failure to secure ladder at bottom | ⅣⅡ ⅣⅡ Ⅱ | 12 |
| 30 | Placing ladder unsafely | | 22 |
| 31 | On boxes or other equipment | ⅣⅡ ⅣⅡ ⅢⅠ | 14 |
| 32 | Near moving equipment | Ⅱ | 2 |
| 33 | On planking over opening | Ⅰ | 1 |
| 34 | On inclined or irregular surface | Ⅱ | 2 |
| 35 | At too great an angle | Ⅲ | 3 |
| 40 | Working in unsafe position | | 10 |
| 41 | Overreaching | ⅣⅡ Ⅰ | 6 |
| 42 | Improper stance while using leverage tools | Ⅱ | 2 |
| 43 | Straddling space between ladder and nearby object | Ⅱ | 2 |
| 50 | Ascending or descending improperly | | 35 |
| 51 | Improper or insecure grip | ⅣⅡ ⅢⅠ | 9 |
| 52 | With back to ladder | Ⅰ | 1 |
| 53 | Running up or down ladders | ⅣⅡ Ⅰ | 6 |
| 54 | Jumping from lower steps to ground | ⅣⅡ | 5 |
| 55 | Oily or wet shoes | Ⅲ | 3 |
| 56 | Carrying too heavy loads | ⅣⅡ ⅣⅡ Ⅰ | 11 |
| 60 | Using ladders known to be defective | ⅣⅡ Ⅲ | 8 |

Fig. 7–1.—Original tabulations of hazardous conditions and unsafe acts that contributed to ladder accidents. The safety professional (or his clerk) compiled the information from Supervisor's Accident Reports (shown in the previous chapter) and set up the classifications on the basis of actual experience, such as recorded in these reports.

4. Placement hazards

5. Inadequate guarding

6. Public hazards.

Within each one of these general classifications, more specific classifications are set up. Under "Defects of agencies," for example, are listed:

1. Composed of unsuitable materials

2. Dull

3. Improperly constructed, assembled, etc.

4. Improperly designed

5. Rough

6. Sharp

7. Slippery

8. Worn, cracked, broken, etc.

9. Other.

It is not always possible to set up classifications before the analysis is begun. In this case, classifications can be developed as reports are reviewed and situations are revealed.

For example, if an analysis is being made of ladder accidents and it is found that in a number of cases broken rungs caused the accidents, a specific group "Broken rungs" should be set up under the classification "Defects of agencies."

ANSI Z16.2 recommends general and specific classifications for all the key facts. These classifications are presented principally as *suggestions* to guide the analyst in setting up classifications to fit his own problems. The point must be emphasized that for an analysis to be of maximum usefulness, classifications must be set up to encompass the situations which are pertinent to the particular company.

Use of a numerical code. Regardless of the method which eventually will be used to sort and tabulate the various key facts, the work will be facilitated if code numbers are assigned to the different classifications. With this method, each case need be read only once, at which time code numbers are assigned to the different facts, and subsequent sorting of the various facts can be quickly completed merely by reference to the code numbers.

A numerical code is simply the assigning of numbers in sequence to a list of similar facts. For each basic fact (agency of accident, accident type, hazardous condition, etc.), there should be no duplication of numbers; but for the different facts, the numbering series may be repeated. Fig. 7-1 shows how code numbers were assigned for two key facts in an analysis of ladder accidents.

After the cases have been reviewed and code numbers have been assigned to the different key facts, the reports can be easily and quickly sorted or arranged by any of the facts to reveal the principal data concerning the accidents.

Numerical codes are already assigned to all the classifications which are included in ANSI Z16.2, and if an analyst uses this standard, he can use the code numbers, too. If he uses the standard as a starting point and adds other classifications to cover the specific accident experience of his own company, he can code the additional items to fit into the code of the standard.

## Making the analysis

Experience has proved that the most effective way to reduce accidents is to concentrate on one phase of the accident problem at a time rather than attempting to stop all accidents at once. There are different ways in which the problem can be approached on this basis, any one of which should prove effective.

The reports may be grouped by occupation of the injured person. Each group of reports, then, may be reviewed to determine what accident types, sources of injury, and agencies of accident are most prevalent among different occupations. Such information is particularly helpful in planning employee training and in developing educational materials and programs.

Injury incidence rates computed by departments may reveal that injuries occur at sharply higher rates in some departments than in others. If this is the case, an analysis should be made of the accidents in the highrate departments to find out the sources of the accidents and their causes. This method will permit concentration of effort in the locations in which accidents occur most frequently.

If injury incidence rates reveal that a high rate of occurrence is general throughout the plant, the accident reports might be grouped by agency of accident, source of injury, or accident type. Any one of the key facts may be used as a starting point for an analysis.

Steps to follow in an agency-of-accident anal-

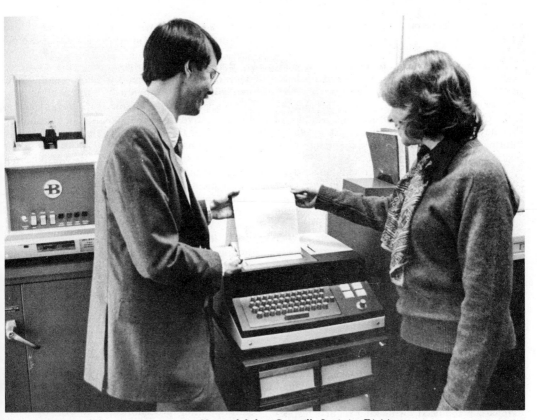

Fig. 7-2.—View of the computer room at National Safety Council's Statistics Division.

ysis. An analysis by agency of accident will always reveal information which can be used effectively in reducing accidents. In one large company, a grouping of accidents in this manner revealed a large number involving ladders, and because accidents of this type often resulted in serious injuries, these cases were analyzed as described below to obtain information that could be used to decrease their occurrence.

Since this was the first analysis of ladder accidents undertaken in this company, classifications for the various key facts had to be set up as the cases were reviewed. Separate sheets were used to list the classifications which were developed for each fact. Also shown on these sheets were the code numbers assigned these classifications, and a tally of occurrences.

Fig. 7-1 shows a listing of hazardous conditions and unsafe acts. The detailed classifications are not in order according to frequency of occur-

rence because they were set up on the sheets as they were observed. Each classification is specific, relating directly to the ladder accidents. Similar sheets were developed for accident type, unsafe act, and nature of injury.

After each accident report was reviewed, the proper code number was placed opposite each fact on the report. Subsequent groupings of the reports, then, merely required arranging them by the code numbers, rather than rereading each case.

Because the analysis of ladder accidents was relatively simple, single classifications of each fact revealed practically all the information necessary to permit correction of the situations which contributed to the accidents. In a more involved agency of accident analysis, cross classifications might be made, e.g., between hazardous conditions and accident type; but in this instance the majority of the accidents were falls, and it was

**207**

necessary to determine only their principal causes.

**Methods of tabulating.** In the preceding analysis, the tabulation was accomplished by hand sorting and tallying. For analyzing a small number of reports (up to about 100), this method is the most efficient. The principal advantage is that the original records are being used, and all the information is available should reference to it become necessary.

Other methods of tabulation may be used for larger numbers of cases. Punched cards and mechanical sorting equipment are satisfactory for a few hundred cases. Modern data processing equipment is best for very large collections of cases, and is useful for smaller data sets as well because it can sort and display cases very quickly allowing the investigator to concentrate on the accidents and test alternate hypotheses easily. Fig. 7–2 shows the computer room in the National Safety Council's Statistics Division.

## Using the analysis

Of course, merely obtaining the information will not prevent recurrence of the accidents. The conditions which contributed to the accidents must be corrected. As an example, the information obtained from the ladder analysis (Fig. 7–1) emphasizes the need for making regular inspections of ladders and for removing from service or repairing those ladders having defects.

The fact that most of the accidents resulted from improper use of the ladders indicates the even more important need for employee training in the use of this equipment. The very definite and specific causes shown in Fig. 7–1 indicate exactly what points must be stressed in a training program. The irrefutable statistical evidence also furnishes data for posters and other safety materials which the safety director will want to include in an all-out assault on ladder accidents.

The causes of the ladder accidents have been ascertained in terms so definite that guesswork can be completely supplanted by direct, positive action, which can have no other result than a marked decrease in the frequency of this kind of accident.

## Estimating Accident Costs

This discussion concerns the elements of cost most likely to result from a work accident and presents a method whereby an organization can obtain an accurate estimate of the total costs of its work accidents.[*]

Reliable cost information is one basis for decisions upon which efficiency and profit depend. Even in so obviously desirable an activity as accident prevention, some proposed measures or alternatives must be accepted or rejected on the basis of their probable effect on profits.

Although most executives want to make their company a safe place to work, they also have a responsibility to run their business profitably. Consequently, they may be reluctant to spend money for accident prevention unless they can see a prospect for saving at least as much as they spend. *Without information on the cost of accidents, it is practically impossible to estimate the savings which are effected through expenditures for accident prevention.*

Annual reports expressed in terms of dollar savings are as meaningful to higher management as those which use incidence rates. Facts about the costs of accidents may be used effectively in securing the active cooperation of supervisors. Supervisors are usually cost conscious because they are expected to run their departments profitably. Monthly reports showing the cost of accidents or the savings resulting from good accident records are an important motivation to achieve safe operating procedures.

## Definition of work accidents for cost analysis

Work accidents, for the purpose of cost analysis, are unintended occurrences arising in the work environment. These accidents fall into two general categories: (a) incidents resulting in work injuries or illnesses and (b) accidents that cause property damage or interfere with production in such a manner that personal injury might result.

The inclusion of the no-injury accidents makes "work accident" roughly synonymous with the type of occurrences a safety department strives to prevent.

---

[*]This procedure for estimating costs was developed by Rollin H. Simonds, Ph.D., Professor, Michigan State College, under the direction of the Statistics Division, National Safety Council.

## Method for estimating

To be of maximum usefulness, cost figures should represent as accurately as possible the specific experience of the company iteslf. A fixed ratio of indirect to direct costs developed from experience representing many different companies in many different industries does *not* serve such a purpose. Estimated costs of accidents in general do not take into account differences in hazards from one industry to another or the more important differences in safety performance from one company to another.

Since the distinctions between "direct" and "indirect" costs are difficult to maintain they have been abandoned in favor of the more precise terms "insured" and "uninsured" costs. Using these data, a company can estimate its accident cost with reasonable accuracy.

**Insured costs.** Every organization paying compensation insurance premiums recognizes such expense as part of the costs of accidents. In some cases, medical expenses, too, may be covered by insurance. These costs are definite, and they are known. They comprise the insured element of the total accident cost.

In addition to these costs, many other costs arise in connection with accidents. The cost of damaged equipment is easily identified. Others, such as wages paid to the injured employee for hours during which he is not producing, are hidden. These items comprise the uninsured element of the total accident cost.

**Uninsured (indirect) costs.** Insured costs can be determined easily from accounting records. The difficult part is determining uninsured (frequently called "indirect") costs, and the method described here will serve that purpose.

The first step is to make a pilot study to ascertain approximate averages of uninsured costs for each of the following four classes of accidents:

CLASS 1 — Cases involving lost workdays, if records are kept under OSHAct, or permanent partial disabilities and temporary total disabilities, if records are based on ANSI Z16.1.

CLASS 2 — Medical treatment cases requiring the attention of a physician outside the plant.

## TABLE 7–B

### PREDETERMINED AVERAGE COSTS

| Class of Accident | Number of Accidents Reported | Average Uninsured Cost |
|---|---|---|
| Class 1 | 20 | $ 90.00 |
| Class 2 | 30 | 28.95 |
| Class 3 | 50 | 5.60 |
| Class 4 | 20 | 181.75 |

CLASS 3 — Medical treatment cases requiring only first aid or local dispensary treatment and resulting in property damage of less than $20.00 or loss of less than 8 hours' working time.

CLASS 4 — Accidents which either cause no injury or cause minor injury not requiring the attention of a physician, and which result in property damage of $20.00 or more, or loss of 8 or more employee-hours.

Once average costs have been established for each accident class, they may be used as multipliers to obtain total uninsured costs in subsequent periods. These costs then may be added to known insurance premium costs to determine the total cost of accidents.

## Example of a cost estimate

An estimate of costs made by one company is given in the following example. First, a pilot study was made to get the average cost of each class of accident. Included in the study were 20 Class 1 accidents, 30 Class 2 accidents, 50 Class 3 accidents, and 20 Class 4 accidents. Costs were determined and averages developed as in Table 7–B.

During the entire year, the company had 34 Class 1 accidents, 148 Class 2 accidents, and 4000 Class 3 accidents. No record was kept of the Class 4 accidents after the pilot study was completed. Instead, the ratio of the number of Class 4 to Class 1 accidents found in the pilot study was used. This ratio was shown to be about 1 to 1, and since there were 34 Class 1 accidents during the year, it was assumed there were about 34 Class 4 accidents. (A separate record could be kept of the number of Class 4 accidents.)

**209**

# 7—Accident Investigation, Analysis, and Costs

DEPARTMENT SUPERVISOR'S ACCIDENT COST INVESTIGATION REPORT

Injury/Accident_____

Date_____ Name of Injured_____ Dept._____

| | TIME LOST |
|---|---|

1. How much time did other employees lose by talking, watching, or helping at accident? Number of employees _____ x hours =

2. How much productive time was lost because of damaged equipment or loss of reduced output by injured worker?
   Estimate Hours =

3. How much time did injured employee lose for which he was paid on the day of the injury?
   Estimate Hours =

4. Will overtime be necessary? Estimate Hours =

5. How much of the supervisors or other managements' time was lost as a result of this accident?
   Estimate Hours =

6. Were additional costs incurred due to hiring and training or replacement?
   Training Time Estimate Hours =

7. Describe the damage to material or equipment. _____
   _____

8. If machine and/or operations were idle, can loss of production be made up?
   Yes_____ No_____

9. Will overtime be necessary? Yes_____ No_____

10. Any demurrage or other cost involved? Yes_____ No_____

   ADDITIONAL ACCIDENT COSTS

   To compute the total costs of the accident, it is necessary to complete the following costs. Should the supervisor have access to this information it is advised he complete as much as possible. Safety Department will develop those costs not known by supervisor.

11. Estimate of demurrage or other costs.     $

12. Costs associated with giving medical attention, first-aid,
    ambulance costs, etc.     $

13. Workers Compensation costs.     $

14. Hospital medical costs.     $

15. Costs associated with placing injured on other work when
    unable to perform regular work.     $

16. Costs associated with questions 1 through 6.

                 16-1                  $
                 16-2                  $
                 16-3                  $
                 16-4                  $
                 16-5                  $
                 16-6                  $_____

17. Company dollars lost on accident:     TOTAL $

Stock No. 129.27

FIG. 7–3.—This cost form (8¹/₂ x 11 in.) should be prepared by the department supervisor as soon after the accident as information becomes available on the amount of time lost by all persons and the extent of damage to product and equipment. It is to be sent to the safety department not later than the day after the accident.

## TABLE 7-C

### ESTIMATE OF YEARLY ACCIDENT COSTS

| Class of Accident | Number of Accidents | Average Cost Per Accident (from pilot study) | Total Uninsured Cost |
|---|---|---|---|
| Class 1 | 34 | $ 90.00 | $ 3,060.00 |
| Class 2 | 148 | 28.95 | 4,284.60 |
| Class 3 | 4,000 | 5.60 | 22,400.00 |
| Class 4 | 34 | 181.75 | 6,179.50 |
| Total Uninusred Cost | | | $35,924.10 |
| Insurance Premiums | | | 19,500.00 |
| Total Accident Cost for the Period | | | $54,424.10 |

The average cost for each accident class was applied to these totals to secure the results shown in Table 7–C.

Since the final total is the sum of many estimates, it should not be implied that the total figure suggests absolute accuracy. Whether $54,000 or $55,000 is chosen as the final figure depends largely on the analyst's judgment of whether the various elements may have been overestimated or underestimated. In this case, the analyst judged that the pilot study represented conservative estimates of the average costs. So he reported to the plant manager, "During the past year, accidents cost this company about $55 thousand in compensation, medical expense, lost time, and property damage."

*The average costs determined in this pilot study represent the actual experience of this particular company. Until important changes*

INVESTIGATOR'S COST DATA SHEET

Class 1_____
(Permanent partial or temporary
total disability)

Class 2 _____
(Temporary partial disability or
medical treatment case requiring
outside physician's care)

Class 3 _____
(Medical treatment case requiring
local dispensary care)

Class 4 _____
(No injury)

Name _____

Date of injury _____    Its nature _____

Department _____    Operation _____Hourly wage _____

 Hourly wage of supervisor $_____

 Average hourly wage of workers in department where injury occurred $_____

1. Wage cost of time lost by workers who were not injured, if paid by employer $_____

   a. Number of workers who lost time because they were talking, watching, helping ___

      Average amount of time lost per worker _____ hours _____ minutes

   b. Number of workers who lost time because they lacked equipment damaged in

      accident or because they needed output or aid of injured worker _____.

      Average amount of time lost per worker _____ hours _____minutes.

2. Nature of damage to material or equipment _____

   _____

   Net cost to repair, replace, or put in order the above material or equipment $_____

3. Wage cost of time lost by injured worker while being paid by employer

   (other than workers compensation payments)                          $_____

   a. Time lost on day of injury for which worker was paid _____ hours _____ min.

   b. Number of subsequent days' absence for which worker was paid _____ days.

      (Other than workers' compensation payments) _____ hours per day.

   c. Number of additional trips for medical attention on employer's time on

      succeeding days after worker's return to work _____

      Average time per trip _____ hours. _____ min. Total trip time _____ hrs. _____

   d. Additional lost time by employee, for which he was paid by company _____ hrs.

      _____ min.

(over)

FIG. 7–4.—This 8½ x 11 in. form can be used to convert time losses into money losses. Initial time losses are obtained from the "Department Supervisor's Accident Cost Report" (Fig. 7–3), and subsequent time losses are obtained from first aid and other departments as

4. If lost production was made up by overtime work, how much more did the work cost than if it had been done in regular hours? (cost items: wage rate difference, extra supervision, light, heat, cleaning for overtime.)   $_____

5. Cost of supervisor's time required in connection with the accident   $_____
   a. Supervisor's time shown on Dept. Supervisor's Report _____ hrs. _____ min.
   b. Additional supervisor's time required later _____ hrs. _____ min.

6. Wage cost due to decreased output of worker after injury if paid old rate   $_____
   a. Total time on light work or at reduced output ____ days ____ hours per day
   b. Worker's average percentage of normal output during this period _____

7. If injured worker was replaced by new worker, wage cost of learning period   $_____
   a. Time new worker's output was below normal for his own wage ____ days _____ hours per day. His average percentage of normal output during time _____ His hourly wage $_____ .
   b. Time of supervisor or others for training _____ hrs. Cost per hour   $_____

8. Medical cost to company (not covered by workers' compensation insurance)   $_____

9. Cost of time spent by higher supervision on investigation, including local processing of worker's compensation application form. (No safety or prevention activities should be included.)   $_____

0. Other costs are not covered above (e.g., public liability claims; cost of renting replacement equipment; loss of profit on contracts cancelled or orders lost if accident causes net reduction in total sales; loss of bonuses by company; cost of hiring new employee if the additional hiring expense is significant; cost of excessive spoilage by new employee; demurrage).   $_____

Explain fully:

   Total uninsured cost ...........................................................$_____

Name of Company _____

Published by National Safety Council

444 North Michigan Avenue
Chicago, Illinois 60611

Stock No. 129.28

necessary. Wage rate information is obtained from the accounting department. The reverse side of the form, shown at the right, contains space for additional costs pertinent to the accident under study. See text discussion, under subsequent section Making a pilot study.

*take place in this company's safety program, in the kind of machinery used or persons employed, or in other aspects which affect costs, the same average costs may continue to be used.*

## Adjusting for inflation

The effects of inflation can quickly make obsolete the cost figures found in a pilot study. To account for this effect, the cost factors should be adjusted each year. The wage-related cost elements can be multiplied by the change in the general level of wages in the company. Other cost elements can be brought up to date by multiplying them by the general inflation rate as measured by the change in the Consumer Price Index. Because these adjustments are only approximate, the pilot study should be repeated at least every five years to establish new benchmarks.

## Items of uninsured (indirect) cost

Important to a pilot study is a careful investigation of each accident to determine all the costs arising from it. The following items of uninsured or indirect cost may clearly be shown to result from work accidents and are subject to reasonably reliable measurement. Less tangible losses, such as the effect of accidents on public relations, employee morale or on the wage rates necessary to secure and retain employees, are not included in this method of estimating costs but may be an important factor in some cases.

Information on some of the items is derived from the Department Supervisor's Accident Cost Report, National Safety Council's Form IS-7 (Fig. 7–3).

The items are discussed in the order in which they appear on the Investigator's Cost Data Sheet, Form IS-8 (Fig. 7–4, shown on the previous pages).

1. **Cost of wages paid for time lost by workers who were not injured.** These are employees who stopped work to watch or assist after the accident or to talk about it, or who lost time because they needed equipment damaged in the accident or because they needed the output or the aid of the injured worker.

2. **Cost of damage to material or equipment.** The validity of property damage as a cost can scarcely be questioned. Occasionally, there is no property damage, but a substantial cost is incurred in putting back in order material or equipment which has been thrown into a state of disorder. The charge should, however, be confined to the net cost of repairing or putting in order material or equipment that has been damaged or displaced, or to the current worth of the equipment less salvage value if it is damaged beyond repair.

An estimate of property damage should have the approval of the cost accountant, particularly if the current worth of the damaged property used in the cost estimate differs from the depreciated value established by the accounting department.

3. **Cost of wages paid for time lost by the injured worker,** other than workers' compensation payments. Payments made under workers' compensation laws for time lost after the waiting period are not included in this element of cost.

4. **Extra cost of overtime work necessitated by the accident.** The charge against an accident for overtime work necessitated by the accident is the difference between nromal wages and overtime wages for the time needed to make up lost production, and the cost of extra supervision, heat, light, cleaning, and other extra services.

5. **Cost of wages paid supervisors for time required for activities necessitated by the accident.** The most satisfactory way of estimating this cost is to charge the wages paid to the foreman for the time spent away from normal activities as a result of the accident.

6. **Wage cost caused by decreased output of injured worker after return to work.** If the injured worker's previous wage payments are continued despite a 40 percent reduction in his output, the accident should be charged with 40 percent of his wages during the period of such low output.

7. **Cost of learning period of new worker.** If a replacement worker produces only half as much in his first two weeks as the injured worker would have produced for the same pay, then half of the new worker's wages for the two weeks' period should be considered part of the cost of the accident that made it necessary to hire him.

A wage cost for time spent by supervisers or others in training the new worker also should be attributed to the accident.

8. **Uninsured medical cost borne by the company.** This cost is usually that of medical services provided at the plant dispensary. There is no great difficulty in estimating an average cost per visit for this medical attention.

The question may be raised, however, whether this expense may properly be considered a variable cost. That is, would a reduction in accidents result in lower expenses for operating the dispensary?

9. **Cost of time spent by higher supervision and clerical workers** on investigations or in the processing of compensation application forms. Time spent by supervision (other than the foreman or supervisor covered in Item 5) and by clerical employees in investigating an accident, or settling claims arising from it, is chargeable to the accident.

10. **Miscellaneous usual costs.** This category includes the less typical costs, the validity of which must be clearly shown by the investigator on individual accident reports. Among such possible costs are public liability claims, cost of renting equipment, loss of profit on contracts canceled or orders lost if the accident causes a net long-run reduction in total sales, loss of bonuses by the company, cost of hiring new employees if the additional hiring expense is significant, cost of *excess* spoilage (above normal) by new employees, and demurrage. These cost factors and any others not suggested above would need to be well substantiated.

Miscellaneous costs were found in less than 2 percent of the cases in a group of several hundred that were reviewed in connection with this study.

### Making a pilot study

The purpose of the pilot study is to develop for different classes of accidents average uninsured costs which can be applied to future accident totals. Therefore, it is desirable not to include the costs of deaths and permanent total disabilities. Such accidents occur so seldom that the costs should be calculated individually and not estimated on the basis of averages.

Some flexibility in the grouping of classes of cases is desirable. If no distinction is made in the records between medical-treatment cases requiring a physician's attention and those not requiring a physician's attention, the pilot study may combine Classes 2 and 3. (See Method for estimating earlier in this chapter.)

The following discussion assumes that the study of costs will be made with the injuries grouped in the recommended classes. The discussion covers Classes 1, 2, and 4. A different method must be applied to Class 3 injuries, and it will be discussed later.

**Classes 1, 2, and 4.** To analyze uninsured costs for accidents in Classes 1, 2, and 4, the supervisor in charge of the department where an accident occurs should secure for each accident the information indicated on the Department Supervisor's Accident Cost Report form (Fig. 7–3). These data can be obtained during the supervisor's regular investigation of the accident. As soon as each report form is completed, it should be sent to the safety department.

In the safety department, the information from the department supervisor's report will be transferred to the Investigator's Cost Data Sheet (Fig. 7–4). The safety department then assumes responsibility for securing the supplementary information from the accounting department, industrial relations department, and other departments where records on lost time and other necessary information are kept.

As an alternative, a member of the safety department could secure all information needed on the data sheet. In this case, the supervisor's report form is not used, and the supervisor is required only to report each accident in Classes 1, 2, or 4 to the safety department as soon as it occurs.

Before he computes averages, the investigator should be certain that the pilot study has covered a sufficient number of cases of Classes 1, 2, and 4 to be representative. This number will rarely be less than 20 cases. However, more cases should be studied if the costs of the cases in a particular class vary widely. Information should be secured on enough cases of each class so that the average cost per case in each class is fully representative of past experience and therefore, by inference, will be applicable to future experience.

Once a sufficient number of cases has been accumulated, the investigation of individual cases can be discontinued. For the data thus collected, separate averages should be calculated for the cases of each class. It is recognized that these costs are averages of the uninsured costs only.

**Class 3 injuries.** These injuries are the common first aid cases in which no significant property damage results from the accident. They are the most difficult to analyze from the standpoint of cost, because such loss of time is likely to occur repeatedly and for only short periods, and the injuries may occur so frequently as to place an undue burden on the supervisor and safety director if a complete report form and data sheet are filled out for each case.

The points of essential information needed are the average amount of working time lost per trip to the dispensary, the average dispensary cost per treatment, the average number of visits to the dispensary per case, and the average amount of supervisor's time required per case.

The following method of developing averages for each of these items is recommended:

1. Secure an estimate of average working time lost per trip to the dispensary for first aid. Departmental time records should be consulted as they may show the amount of time each worker is absent from his job for first aid. If so, a random sample of 50 to 100 records of persons known to have received first aid should be selected from different departments. The average time lost per dispensary visit is calculated by adding the absence time for all visits in the sample and dividing by the total number of visits.

   If departmental records do not contain this information, it will be necessary to assign an investigator to observe a random sample of 50 or more persons visiting the dispensary.

   As before, to secure the average time, all the estimated time intervals of absence are added and then divided by the total number of persons observed.

2. Make an estimate of the average cost of providing medical attention for each visit by dividing the total cost of operating the dispensary for a year by the total number of treatments given during the year.

3. Calculate the average number of visits to the dispensary per case by dividing the number of treatments of Class 3 injuries in a representative period, perhaps a month or six weeks, by the number of Class 3 injuries reported during the same period of time.

4. Calculate the average amount of supervisor's time required per case, where possible, by

observing the activities of representative supervisors in connection with first aid cases.

When a sufficient number of cases has been studied to be representative both of the activities of supervisors in different departments and of different types of first aid cases, the average time spent by a supervisor is computed by adding all the time intervals recorded and dividing by the number of cases.

If it is impossible to make a time study of the supervisor's activities in connection with first aid cases, the only alternative is to secure from each supervisor an estimate of the time he spends on the usual first aid case, and to average these estimates by adding them and dividing by the number of supervisors.

Determine the average value of this time by multiplying it by the average hourly wage of a supervisor.

The average total uninsured cost of a case in Class 3 is estimated from the data accumulated above as follows: the average amount of time lost for a trip to the dispensary (1, above) is multiplied by the plant's average wage rate, secured from the payroll department, to get the average cost per trip for the worker's time lost. To this figure is added the estimated cost of providing medical attention for a single visit (2). This figure is then multiplied by the average number of dispensary visits per medical treatment case (3), and to this result is added the average value of supervisor's time required (4).

This method of recording costs is designed to provide estimates of the average uninsured cost per case for accidents causing localized property damage or, at most, a few injuries.

The method of cost investigation for accidents resulting in deaths, permanent total disabilities, or extraordinarily extensive property damage is the same as for others, but the difference is that every one is investigated separately and should be included in the final cost estimate as a separate item. In estimating the cost of a fire, the investigator should bear in mind that the company's fire insurance may cover property damage that would appear as an uninsured cost in other work accidents.

## Development of final cost estimate

Once the average for each class of case has been established, costs for any period in which a sufficiently large number of accidents has occurred to be representative can be estimated with considerable accuracy by multiplying the average uninsured cost per case for each of the four classes by the number of cases occurring in that class during the period.

If any deaths, permanent total disabilities, or extraordinarily extensive property damage accidents have occurred, the specific uninsured costs of these should be added to the estimated costs of the four classes of accidents.

To these uninsured cost totals should be added the cost of workers' compensation and insured medical expense. For companies which are self-insured, this will be the total amount paid out in settlement of claims plus all expenses of adminis-tering the insurance. For companies not carrying their own insurance, it will be the amount of their insurance premiums.

The method will have to be modified in accordance with the recordkeeping systems of different companies. For example, most self-insurers will find it impossible to separate compensated medical expense from dispensary care. In that case, these items should be combined into one, and the dispensary cost omitted from the analysis of noncompensated costs on the data sheets.

For an illustration of the development of a final cost estimate, see the example in Tables 7–B and –C.

## References

American National Standards Institute, 1430 Broadway, New York, N.Y. 10018. *Standard Method of Recording Basic Facts Relating to the Nature and Occurrence of Work Injuries*, Z16.2-1969.

DeReamer, Russell. *Modern Safety and Health Technology*. New York, N.Y., John Wiley and Sons, Inc., 1980.

Kuhlman, Raymond. *Professional Accident Investigation*. Loganville, Ga., Institute Press, Div. of International Loss Control Institute, 1977.

Simonds, Rollin H., and Grimaldi, John V. *Safety Management—Accident Cost and Control*. Homewood, Ill., Richard D. Irwin, Inc., 1975.

# Workers' Compensation Insurance

## Chapter
# 8

# 8—Workers' Compensation Insurance

In the late 1970's, about 13,000 workers died each year from work-connected injuries or diseases, another 90,000 were permanently disabled, and more than 2,300,000 were temporarily disabled—and these deaths and disabilities were only one-fifth of the total accidental injuries from all causes. Injured workers and their families suffered substantial economic losses as well as bodily injuries. Their employers and society also suffered sizable economic losses.

When a worker dies, is disabled, or merely requires medical attention because of work-connected injury or disease, the economic consequences affect the worker, his family, his employer, and society.

## Economic Losses

The worker and his family may suffer two types of economic losses (a) a loss of earnings and (b) extra expenses.

If a worker dies because of work-related injury or sickness, his survivors lose the income he would otherwise have earned, less the amount that he would have spent to maintain himself during the remainder of his working career and his retirement years. This loss can be substantial.

Total and permanent disability cause an even greater earnings loss than death because the worker must be maintained.

Permanent partial disability causes some fraction of the permanent total disability loss, depending upon the proportion of the annual earnings lost. A worker who is totally disabled for a temporary period loses his income for a specific number of weeks or months. Loss of even a month's earnings is a serious loss for the typical worker. In addition to these earnings losses, the deceased or disabled worker may no longer provide valuable household services that must now be forgone or replaced at additional cost.

Not all injured workers are disabled but almost all require some form of medical attention. For all injuries combined, medical expenses are less than the total earnings loss; but for many workers, their medical expenses exceed their earning loss.

In addition to these losses, society loses the taxes that would have been paid by the injured employees and the products or services they would have produced. Some injured employees and families become public assistance beneficiaries and must be supported by other members of society.

## Cost details

It would be inappropriate to overlook the effect of increasing medical and hospital costs on costs of work injuries and illnesses. (More details are given later in this chapter under Cost Levels and Allocation.) For several years, these costs have increased at a rate somewhat in excess of inflation rates, and there are many reasons to believe that they will continue to do so. National Safety Council estimates, in its 1980 edition of *Accident Facts*, that the total cost of work accidents in 1979 was $27.3 billion. Cost categories that make up this loss are "Visible Costs," "Other Costs," and "Fire Losses." Total cost per worker is estimated at $280.

Visible costs are estimated at $12.6 billion and include wage losses, insurance administrative costs, and medical costs. Other costs are also estimated at $12.6 billion and include the money value of time lost by workers other than those with disabling injuries who are directly or indirectly involved in accidents. Also included would be the time required to investigate accidents, complete accident reports, etc.

Fire losses are estimated at $2.1 billion.

It is of interest that visible costs have a one-to-one ratio to other costs. Other costs are comparable to what have been called indirect, or uninsured, costs related to the direct, or insured, costs of work injuries and illnesses.

There is a much greater interest in the total costs related to incidents that may or may not result in work injuries or illnesses. Safety practitioners have a greater opportunity than has been the case in the past to influence managements toward the adoption of more effective safety measures—that interest being related to the more important place rapidly rising costs must be given in executive decision making.

## Workers' Compensation in the United States

This discussion elaborates on the History of the Safety Movement given in Chapter 1.

In the United States, efforts to implement a system of compensation for industrial injuries lagged far behind the countries of Europe. As work-related injuries and diseases and their consequences grew less and less tolerable towards the end of the 19th century, the situation became ripe for a radical change. The first evidence of interest in workers' compensation was seen in 1893 when legislators seized upon John Graham Brooks' account of the German system as a clue to the direction of efforts at reform. This interest was further stimulated by the passage of the British Compensation Act of 1897.

## Early laws

In 1902 Maryland passed an act providing for a cooperative accident insurance fund; this represented the first legislation embodying to any desgree the compensation principle. The scope of the act was restricted. Benefits, which were quite meager, were provided only for fatal accidents. Within three years, the courts declared the act unconstitutional. In 1908, a Massachusetts act authorized establishment of private plans of compensation upon approval of the state board of conciliation and arbitration. This law had no practical significance; it was a dead letter from the start.

By 1908, there was still no workers' compensation act in the United States. President Theodore Roosevelt, realizing the injustice, urged the passage of an act for federal employees in a message to Congress in January. He pointed out that the burden of an accident fell upon the helpless man, his wife, and children. The President declared that this was "an outrage." Later in 1908, Congress passed a compensation act covering certain federal employees. Though utterly inadequate, it was the first real compensation act passed in the United States.

During the next few years, agitation continued for state laws. A law passed in Montana in 1909, applying to miners and laborers in coal mines, was declared unconstitutional. Nevertheless, many states appointed commissions to investigate the feasibility of compensation acts and to propose specific legislation. The greater number of compensation acts were the result of these commissions' reports, all of which favored some form of compensation legislation, combined with recommendations from various private organizations. Widespread agreement on the need for compensation legislation unfortunately did not end all conflict over reform. Interest groups clashed over specific bills and over questions of coverage, waiting periods, and state versus commercial insurance.

In 1910, New York adopted a workers' compensation act of general application which was compulsory for certain especially hazardous jobs, and optional for others. None of the early state compensation acts expressly covered occupational diseases. Statutes which provided compensation for "injury" were frequently interpreted to include disability from disease, but those acts which limited compensability to "injury by accident" excluded occupational disease. All except Oregon's act required uncompensated waiting periods of one to two weeks; several states provided retroactive payments after a prescribed period.

The 1911 Wisconsin workers' compensation act was the first law to become and remain effective. The laws of four other states (Nevada, New Jersey, California, and Washington) also became effective that year. In 1916, the United States Supreme Court declared workers' compensation laws to be constitutional; see p. 5 for details. Although 24 jurisdictions had enacted such legislation by 1925, workers' compensation was not provided in every state until Mississippi enacted its law in 1948.

## Current acts

Today there are compensation acts in the 50 states, the District of Columbia, Guam, and Puerto Rico. In addition, the Federal Employees' Compensation Act covers the employees of the U.S. Government, and the Longshoremen's and Harbor Workers' Compensation Act covers maritime workers, other than seamen, and workers in certain other groups. The latter act provided compensation for workers in the "twilight zone" between ship and shore, since the U.S. Supreme Court had ruled they could not be covered under state compensation laws.

While economic changes and public policy have prompted increases in benefits and scope of the laws, the basic concepts have not undergone any radical changes. Employees and labor are both dissatisfied with certain aspects of workers' compensation. Labor attacks the system for inadequate benefits, coverage limitations, and exclusion of many injuries, illnesses, and disabilities that they consider job-related. Employers are critical because the system covers some injuries and diseases they do not consider job-related and is costly relative to its apparent benefits. Thus, while the early advocates of workers' compensation conceived it as a simple, speedy, efficient, equitable remedy that would reduce litigation over industrial injuries, some people have expressed doubt that their hopes have been realized.

# 8—Workers' Compensation Insurance

## Objectives of Workers' Compensation

Workers' compensation programs can be evaluated by the extent to which they satisfy the following commonly accepted objectives:

1. Income replacement

2. Restoration of earning capacity and return to productive employment

3. Industrial accident prevention and reduction

4. Proper allocation of costs

5. Achievement of the other four objectives in the most efficient manner possible

Not all of these objectives are equally important or accepted. The first two generally are considered most important. These objectives sometimes conflict with one another but in most ways they are linked by the design of the program.

### Income replacement

The first objective listed for workers' compensation is to replace the wages lost by workers disabled by a job-related injury or illness. According to this objective, the replacement should be adequate, equitable, prompt, and certain.

To be adequate, the program should replace lost earnings (present and projected, including fringe benefits), less those expenses such as taxes and job-related transportation costs that do not continue. The worker, however, should share a proportion of the loss in order to provide incentives for rehabilitation and accident prevention. The two-thirds replacement ratio that is found in most state statutes is generally considered acceptable, although recently the alternative of replacing 80 percent of "spendable earnings" has received favorable attention.

To be equitable the program must treat all workers fairly. According to one concept of fairness, most workers should have the same proportion of their wages replaced. However, a worker with a low wage may need a high proportion of his lost wage in order to sustain himself and his family. If a guaranteed minimum income plan existed, there would be less need to favor low-income workers. A high-income worker who can afford to purchase private individual protection may have his weekly benefit limited to some reasonable maximum. If workers' compensation insurance is regarded primarily as a wage replacement program however, relatively few persons should be affected by this maximum. An alternative philosophy would argue in favor of a more substantial welfare component with a higher minimum benefit, low maximum benefit, and extra benefits when there are dependents.

Ideally, workers would be treated the same regardless of the jurisdiction in which they are injured. This criterion, therefore, implies a minimization of interstate differences in statutory provisions and their administration.

The program should pay all disabled persons an income starting as soon after their disability commences as possible. Finally, workers should know in advance what benefits they will receive if they are injured on the job and that these benefits will be paid regardless of the continued solvency of the employers.

Under the whole-man theory, the system would be required to indemnify the worker or his family for the effect on all his personal activities, not his earning capacity alone.

### Restoration of disabled workers

The second listed objective is medical and vocational rehabilitation and return to productive employment. To achieve this objective, the worker should receive quality medical care at no cost to himself, care which will restore him as well as possible to his former physical condition. If complete restoration is impossible, he should receive vocational rehabilitation that will enable him to maximize his earning capacity. Finally the system should include incentives to disabled workers and prospective employers so the workers will return to productive employment as quickly as possible.

### Accident prevention and reduction

Occupational accident prevention and reduction is a third commonly accepted objective of workers' compensation. Those who consider this objective to be important believe that the system should and can provide significant financial and other incentives for employers to introduce measures that will decrease the frequency and severity of accidents. More specifically, the pricing of workers' compensation should reward good safety practices and penalize dangerous operations. Employees should also have some incentive to follow safe work practices by sharing some of the losses. Injured workers should have the opportunity and be encouraged to return to work as soon as they are physically able.

222

## Proper cost allocation

The fourth objective of workers' compensation, which has a narrower support than the first three, is to allocate the costs of the program among employers and industries according to the extent to which they are responsible for the losses to employees and other expenses. Such an allocation is considered equitable by supporters of this objective because each employer and industry pays its fair share of the cost. The economic effects are considered desirable because this allocation tends in the long run in a competitive economy to shift resources from hazardous industries to safe industries and from unsafe employers within an industry to safe employers. Higher workers' compensation costs will force employers with hazardous operations to consider raising their prices. To the extent that consumers will not accept the price increase, employer profits and their willingness to commit resources to this use will decline.

Critics of this objective argue that workers' compensation costs are such a small part of the cost of production that they have little, if any, effect on resource allocations. Consequently, they would avoid the complicated pricing practices necessary to achieve this objective.

## Major Characteristics

### Covered employment

While most of the state workers' compensation laws apply to both private and public employment, none of the laws covers all forms of employment. For various historical, political, economic, or administrative reasons, each of the laws has certain gaps. Laws that are elective rather than compulsory permit the employer to reject coverage; but in the event he does, he loses the customary common law defenses: assumed risk of the employment, negligence of a fellow servant, and contributory negligence.

A few states still restrict compulsory coverage to so-called hazardous occupations. Many laws exempt employers having fewer than a specified number of employees. The most common exception is for employers having fewer than three employees or less in eight states to fewer than four in three states. Most of the laws exclude farmwork, domestic service, and casual employment. Many laws also contain other exemptions, such as employment in charitable or religious institutions.

Two other major groups outside the coverage of the compensation laws are interstate railroad workers and maritime employees. Railroad workers, any part of whose duties involve the furtherance of interstate commerce, are covered by the Federal Employers' Liability Act (FELA). Maritime workers are subject to the Jones Act, which applies provisions of the FELA to seamen. The Federal Employers' Liability Act is not a workers' compensation law. It gives an employee an action in negligence against his employer and provides that the employer may not plead the common law defenses of fellow servant or assumption of risk; moreover, the principle of comparative negligence is substituted for the common law concept of contributory negligence.

As to the state and local employees, the actual number of these employees subject to workers' compensation or provided with such protection voluntarily is not available. All states (as well as Puerto Rico, Guam, and the District of Columbia) have some coverage of public employees but with marked variations. Some laws specify no exclusions or exclude only such groups as elected or appointed officials. Others limit coverage to employees of specified political subdivisions or to employees engaged in hazardous occupations. In still others, coverage is entirely optional with the state or with the city or political subdivision.

Certain other groups, such as the self-employed, unpaid family members, volunteers, and trainees, generally are not protected by workers' compensation.

Gradual extension of coverage over the years has been achieved by piecemeal actions: replacement of elective laws by compulsory provisions, elimination or reduction of numerical exemptions, and adoption of amendments granting protection to farm workers and other previously excluded groups. States still must strive for complete coverage.

### Covered injuries and diseases

Workers' compensation is presently intended to provide coverage only for certain work-related conditions, not all of the worker's health problems. Statutory definitions and tests have been adopted to provide the line of demarcation between those conditions which are compensable and those which are not. Because, in drafting workers' compensation laws, all jurisdictions relied to some extent on the English system (or other statutes that in turn relied upon the English model), their statutory language is remarkably similar. Nevertheless, as there are variations in language as well as differences in interpretation, a condition considered compensable in one state may be held non-compensable in others.

The statutes usually limit compensation benefits to personal injury caused by accident arising out of and in the course of the employment. Although this presents four distinct tests which must be met, in practice they are often considered in pairs: The "personal injury" and "by accident" requirements in one set, and the "arising out of" and "in the course of" requirements in the other.

**Personal injury and "by accident."** If interpreted narrowly, personal injury would deal solely with bodily harm, such as a broken leg or a cut, while the "by accident" test would refer to the cause, such as a blow to the body or an episode of excessive or improper lifting. In practice, however, the distinctions are blurred.

The "by accident" concept is a carry over from the English law. Early judicial interpretations of the English law made it quite clear that for their purposes the "by accident" requirement was intended to do little more than deny compensation to those who injured themselves intentionally. A number of U.S. jurisdictions, however, have applied the test so as to narrow the range of unintentional injuries which can be compensated.

One of the early victims of the "by accident" requirement was occupational disease coverage. As the typical judicial holding was that occupational disease and accidental injury were mutually exclusive, special legislation was required in order to provide disease coverage. At present occupational diseases are treated separately in about six states.

All jurisdictions how have full coverage of all occupational diseases. The injury "by accident" provisions in most occupational disease statutes can be and have been made for diseases, as injuries by accident, when there was (a) something particularly unusual about the cause of the disease and (b) the mode of conveyance was specific.

The injury "by accident" concept was also used in many jurisdictions to deny compensation unless the injury was caused by some sort of unusual, traumatic occurrence, generally requiring the application of outside agency. Obviously this would and did drastically limit the kinds of cases which would be compensated. At present, this use of the by accident test is limited to a few

narrow areas.

Impairment involving psychological difficulties has been the source of much controversy based on application of the personal injury requirement. In some cases, a mental stimulus such as fear can produce a physical lesion, such as a cerebral hemorrhage. In the event of a physical lesion, the courts have not encountered much difficulty in conceding personal injuries. Compensation is usually approved also if, as a result of a clear physical injury, the patient suffers psychological disorder.

As might be expected, disagreement is most likely when it is alleged that mental stimulation has resulted in a mental illness without obvious physical change. Although many jurisdictions award compensation in such cases, others are still reluctant to compensate work-related psychological disorders.

**Work-related impairment.** The term "arising out of and in the course of the employment," applied by almost every jurisdiction, is meant to define a certain level of relationship between the employment and injury of disease as a condition of eligibility for workers' compensation. The phrase obviously lacks certainty. Often it is quite difficult to determine whether a given set of facts will support an award of compensation.

The "course of the employment" aspect of this test refers primarily to the time frame of the injury. Virtually every jurisdiction holds that an employee is within the course of his employment, barring certain types of unusual circumstances or unreasonable conduct, from the moment he steps onto the employer's premises at the beginning of the work day to the moment he leaves the premises at the end of the day.

Although this test appears to be relatively simple to apply, it has not been so. One uncertain issue is, what are the premises? Injuries which clearly occur off premises but appear to deserve compensation lead to a search for exceptions and encourage courts to modify the basic rules. Many workers are not attached to particular premises. Even though an injury occurs off premises, as in travel to and from work, the employee may be compensated if a sufficient employment relationship can be found, such as payment for time or expense of travel or the provision of a company vehicle for transportation. In these circumstances, the period of travel time to and from home may be incidental in the course of employment.

The "arising out of" segment of the test is intended to provide a casual relationship between the employment and the injury. For example, it is not enough that an employee suffer a heart attack while at work. He must show that the heart attack arose out of the employment or, in other words, that it was causally related to the employment.

This means that at a minimum (some states have more stringent rules) it must be shown that it was the stress and strain or exertion of the employment that caused the heart attack, not merely a spontaneous breakdown of the cardiovascular system.

The degree of employment relationship necessary varies from state to state and has been modified as workers' compensation law has evolved. In earlier years, it was generally felt that the hazard-causing injury must be peculiar to the particular employment or be increased by the employment before the injury could be said to "arise out of the employment." This rather narrow view of compensability has been modified and to some extent abandoned in recent years.

Although it is difficult to place each jurisdiction in a particular category as to what it will hold sufficient to meet the "arising out of" test, two additional theories have been developed and followed. The first and more widespread is the "actual risk doctrine," which requires that the hazard resulting in injury be a risk of the particular employment, without regard to whether it was also a risk to which the general public is exposed. The second or "positional risk doctrine" could also be called the "but for" test. Here, if the employment places the worker in a position where he is injured ("but for" the employment the injury would not have occurred), the injury "arises out of the employment."

## Benefits

More than $8 billion in cash and medical benefits were received by workers in 1977 through the workers' compensation system. Benefits include medical service, cash benefit payments to the worker while totally disabled, payments for residual partial disability, burial allowances for work-related deaths and benefits to the worker's dependent survivors.

Some states provide special benefits also to cover attendants or prostheses; about three-fourths of the states provide maintenance and other services for rehabilitation. The largest pro-

portion of benefits are in cash, either as periodic payments or as lump sums in settlement of claims. More than $5.8 billion, almost two-thirds of the $8.5 billion 1977 benefit total, were paid to workers or their survivors in cash.

Benefits are paid through three channels: commercial insurance policies; publicly operated state insurance funds; and self-insured employers. In 1977, more than $4.6 billion in workers' compensation was paid by private insurers, $2.7 billion by state funds, and $1.2 billion by self-insurers.

## Income replacement

Of the $5.8 billion benefits paid in 1977 as cash income, almost 85 percent went to disabled workers and the other 15 percent to survivors of workers killed on the job. Although 70 percent or more of recent workers' compensation cases are for temporary total disablement, such cases have accounted roughly for only one-fourth of cash benefits. At the same time, income benefits in the last few years to workers for permanent partial disabilities accounted for almost two-thirds of the total dollar amount.

**Basic features.** In general, the cash benefits provided for temporary total disability, permanent total disability, permanent partial disability, and death are payable as a wage-related benefit—the weekly amount is computed as a percentage of the worker's wage. The benefit varies by state and by type of disability but most commonly is set at two-thirds of wages. In some states, the statutory percentage varies with the worker's marital status and the number of dependent children, especially for survivors' benefits, which in a majority of states pay 67 percent or less of the deceased worker's wage to surviving widows without dependent children.

The benefit rate is limited to less than two-thirds of wages for many beneficiaries by another statutory provision—the maximum ceiling on the weekly benefit payable. Disabled workers whose wages are at or above the statewide average receive benefits below the statutory benefit rate in almost all states because of this ceiling, although for such individuals benefits may exceed preinjury take-home pay because benefits are tax-free.

As inflation boosts wage levels, some states have attempted to prevent the deterioration in effective benefit-wage rates by providing for

**225**

future increases in the maximum without need for further legislation—40 automatically adjust the maximum (for new beneficiaries only) in relation to changes in the state's average weekly wage. Much less common but gaining more interest in the last few years are provisions that, as wage levels of workers rise, will raise benefits for beneficiaries already on the rolls—sixteen states plus the Federal Employees' Compensation Act and the Longshoremen's and Harbor Workers' Compensation Act provide such automatic increases.

Another type of limitation on benefits sets maximum time periods or aggregate dollar amounts. Such limitations in permanent total disability and death cases may cut off benefits even though the income need continues. Only fourteen states limit the duration of total dollar benefits to widows and orphans.

In order to reduce administrative costs and to discourage malingering, benefits in all states are payable only after a waiting period following the report of disability. This delay in payment applies to the cash indemnity payments, not to medical and hospital care. The waiting period ranges from three days to seven. In all states, workers who are disabled beyond a specified minimum period of time receive payment retroactively for the waiting period. In more than three-fourths of workers' compensation laws, the minimum period before retroactive payment of disability benefits begins in two weeks.

**Benefits by type of disability.** Most compensation cases concern workers who incur temporary disability but recover completely. The maximum weekly benefit for temporary total disability is at least $98, and the median is $197. In 31 jurisdictions, the percentage of the state's average weekly wage for temporary total disability is $100 or more.

For workers with dependents, about one-third of the states augment the weekly benefit for temporary disability, usually by some dollar amount for each dependent up to a specified total.

Benefits for permanent total disability are for disabilities that preclude any work or regular work in any well known branch of the labor market and that can be of indefinite duration. These are similar to benefits for temporary total disability benefits. In a few states, the weekly payment for permanent disability benefits is less than for temporary.

Six states restrict the duration of benefits for permanent disabilities, typically to from 6 to 10 years.

Residual limitations on earning capacity after recovery (that is after a permanent partial disability) are awarded compensatory benefits on a relatively complex basis. Partial disabilities are divided into two categories—"schedule" injuries, those listed in the law such as loss of specific bodily members; and "non-schedule" injuries, those which are of a more general nature, such as back and head injuries.

Weekly benefits for schedule injuries are a percentage of average weekly wages, usually the same as the benefit rate for permanent total disability. The maximum weekly benefit is for the most part the same as or lower than that for total disability.

Nonschedule injuries are paid at the same or similar rate but as a percentage of wage loss, the difference between wages before injury and the wages the worker is able to earn after injury.

The schedule benefits are paid for fixed periods varying according to the type and severity of the injury. For example, most state laws call for payments ranging from 200 to 300 weeks for loss of an arm and 20 to 40 weeks for loss of a great toe.

The maximum period for non-schedule injuries for each state is the same as or, more generally, less than the duration limits established for permanent total disability.

In the majority of states, compensation payable for permanent partial disability is in addition to that payable during the healing period or while the worker is temporarily and totally disabled.

Death benefits are intended to furnish income replacement for families dependent upon the earnings of an employee whose death is work-related. As is true for the other types of benefits, the amount of survivor benefits and the length of time they are paid vary considerably from state to state. Benefits computed as a percentage of the deceased worker's wage often are less than that for permanent total disability benefits if the survivor is a widow without dependents. If there are dependent children, the benefit in many states will be augmented. In most states, the duration of benefits is unlimited, although nine states retain duration limits in a range from 7 to 20 years. In 28 states, payments to widows continue usually as long as they do not remarry and to children until they are no longer dependent, usually to age 18. In many states, benefits to children continue to age

23 or 25 if in school. Benefits may be terminated earlier in the four states which also limit total dollar benefits.

In addition to benefits for widows, widowers, and children, some states pay survivor benefits to dependent invalid widowers, parents, or siblings of the dead worker. Burial expenses are payable in all states.

## Medical benefits

For many years, disbursements for medical services provided under workers' compensation have comprised about one-third of total outlay for benefits. Care includes first aid treatment, services of a physician, surgical and hospital services, nursing and drugs, supplies, and prosthetic devices. Some large employers, in addition to first aid facilities, employ staff physicians for workers. Most employers insure their medical care responsibility as they do the income benefits under workmen's compensation.

Every state law requires the employer to provide for medical care to the injured worker. In most jurisdictions, such treatment is provided without limit either through explicit statutory language or administrative interpretation. In the few states that limit the total medical care by specified maximum dollar amounts or maximum periods, the initial ceiling may be exceeded by administrative decision. Also, if specified types of injuries or disease are denied cash benefits, medical care also is denied.

A major issue concerning medical benefits for workers' compensation is the procedure for choosing the physician who is to furnish the care. Almost half of the states give the employer the right to designate the physician. In practice, the insurance company of the employer will ordinarily select the physician since it is the insurer that handles the claim for benefits. Where the doctor is chosen in this way, the medical care furnished may be more highly skilled and effective because of the selected physician's specialized experience. On the other hand, workers feel that a more important consideration is the emphasis that their personal family physician is likely to put on their health and well-being. They feel other considerations may influence a physician they do not select.

## Rehabilitation

Along with industrial safety, medical care, and cash compensation, rehabilitation of workers is recognized at least theoretically as one of the primary goals of the workers' compensation system. At present the most widespread benefits offered through workers' compensation laws to restore a worker to his fullest economic capacity are the special maintenance benefits authorized in more than half of the states. These benefits usually are paid (sometimes in addition to the regular disability compensation) for various training, education, testing, and other services designed to aid the injured person to return to work. In addition, some state programs provide for travel expenses and for books and equipment needed for the training.

Ohio, Oregon, Rhode Island, Washington, and Puerto Rico directly operate rehabilitation facilities under the workers' compensation program. Some insurance companies also have in-house facilities for rehabilitating workers.

Probably the main source of retraining and rehabilitation is the federal-state vocational program. The facilities operated by this program accept individuals with work-related disabilities as well as others. In all states, these institutions are directed by state vocational rehabilitation agencies. They provide medical care, counseling, training, and job placement. Unfortunately, not all workers' compensation cases referred for vocational rehabilitation can be accepted promptly. Many others are never brought to their attention.

One notable drawback preventing full utilization of available rehabilitation facilities is the often protracted, adversary proceedings for determining a worker's right to benefits. Because the determination of whether there should be an award for permanent partial or total disability (and how large an award should be for partial disability) is conditioned on the worker's lack of ability to work, the claim may be a strong disincentive for rehabilitation. Further, in the many compromise settlements, the employer's (or insurer's) motivation is to pay an agreed amount of money and foreclose future responsibility for medical, vocational, or other needs arising from the injury. Such settlements also work against a full-fledged effort to restore the worker to full health and productivity.

## Administration

The goal of workers' compensation is to provide for quick, simple, and inexpensive determination of all claims for benefits and to provide such medical care and rehabilitation services as

**227**

are necessary to restore the injured worker to employment. Nearly all of the states have agencies to carry out these administrative responsibilities. The agency is either in the labor department; a separate compensation board or commission, or other department; in four, administration is left to the courts. Several states have separate, independent appeals boards to review claims when agency decisions are appealed.

## Objectives

An agency's many correlated responsibilities include close supervision over the processing of cases. The primary objective is to assure compliance with the law and to guarantee an injured worker's rights under the statute. Administration by a division within the labor department or by a board or commission has been found to be more effective in achieving the full purpose of the law than administration by the courts. The courts are not organized and equipped to render the services needed.

One criticism of state agencies concerns the delays in the first payment of compensation to the disabled worker. Although in most states insurers mail the checks, the state administrative agency has the responsibility to see that payments commence promptly. Full and prompt payment is essential because few workers can afford to wait long for benefits due. In one state, perhaps the best, the claims are paid within 15 days; in most states, however, it appears that the first payment comes as much as 30 days late.

Another responsibility of the agency is to see that the injured worker gets the full benefit due. To do this, it is important to follow an injury from the first report to the final closing of the case. Some states not only check the accuracy of total payments, but also require signed receipts for every compensation payment. Some require the filing of a final receipt which itemizes the purpose of each element in the total outlay, to permit a complete audit of individual payments.

Frequently, however, the legislation itself requires a workers' compensation agency to operate on the assumption that each injured worker is responsible for securing his rights and that its primary function is to adjudicate contested claims. Even where the law does not favor this policy, lack of staff may force the agency to this restricted role.

Although it is known that many workers are not familiar with the provisions of their workers'

compensation act, in only a few states does the administrator (as soon as possible after the injury is reported) advise the worker of his rights to benefits, medical and rehabilitation services, and assistance available at the commission's office. Too many states fail to insist on prompt reporting of accidents by employers, on prompt payment of benefits, or on final reports which spell out the amounts paid and how these amounts were computed. Although prompt reporting is usually required, sometimes no penalty is imposed for violation.

## Handling cases

Workers' compensation claims may be either uncontested or contested.

**In uncontested cases,** the two main methods followed are the direct payment system and the agreement system.

Under the direct payment system, the employer or his insurer takes the initiative and begins the payment of compensation to the worker or his dependents. The injured worker does not need to enter into an agreement and is not required to sign any papers before compensation starts. The laws prescribe the amount of benefit. If the worker fails to receive this, the administrative agency can investigate and correct any error. Jurisdictions whose laws provide the direct payment system include Arkansas, Michigan, Mississippi, New Hampshire, Wisconsin, and the District of Columbia; it is also provided for in the Longshoremen's and Harbor Workers Compensation Act.

Under the agreement system, in effect in a majority of the states, the parties (that is, the employer or his insurer, and the worker) agree upon a settlement before payment is made. In some cases, the agreement must be approved by the administrative agency before payments start.

**In contested cases,** most workers' compensation laws provide for a hearing by a referee or hearing officer, with provisions for an appeal from the decision of the referees or hearing officer to the commission or appeals board and from there to the courts. As the administrative agency usually has exclusive jurisdiction over the determination of facts, appeals to the courts usually are limited to questions of law. In some states, however, the court is permitted to consider issues both of fact and law anew.

## Security Requirements

All states except Louisiana require their employers in private industry to demonstrate that they are able to pay the benefits required under the workers' compensation law. About two-thirds of the states have a similar provision for public employers.

These security provisions, in effect, require that active steps be taken by employers to guarantee that workers, when they are disabled, will receive the benefits called for by the law.

## Types of insurers

Most laws allow employers to satisfy the security requirement by insuring with private companies or to self-insure. As of January 1, 1972, only six states (Nevada, North Dakota, Ohio, Washington, West Virginia, Wyoming), Puerto Rico, and the Virgin Islands required employers to purchase protection from exclusive state operated funds. Three of these states (plus one that has no state fund) and Puerto Rico and the Virgin Islands also prohibit self-insurance. Besides the jurisdictions with exclusive state funds, 12 others have publicly operated programs in competition with private insurers. Regardless of the method of protection purchased, the same statutory benefits must be provided to the injured worker in that state.

## Compliance checks

In order to make sure that workers will receive benefits as intended, states need a method of checking that employers do in fact meet the security requirements. The workers' compensation agency ordinarily requires not only notice of insurance secured by employers but of cancellations of such insurance. In more than a fifth of the states, however, no formal procedures are in effect to make sure that all employers have given proper notice.

Generally, it is believed that most employers comply with security requirements. In part, a high degree of compliance may be expected because of sanctions available to the state for noncompliance. In almost four-fifths of the states, noncomplying employers become liable to worker suits with the employer's traditional common law defenses abrogated; in some states, the business may be stopped from operating. In addition some statutes call for fines against the employer or imprisonment or both.

## Regulation of insurers

Where employers are allowed to self-insure, they must generally demonstrate sound financial condition. An employer may have to make a deposit of a specified amount with the workers' compensation agency or post a surety bond. In at least a third of the states, all applicants for self-insurance must meet this requirement; in a similar proportion of states, at the discretion of the agency, this deposit may not be required. Other types of requirements imposed on self-insurers in various states are minimum payroll size, minimum number of employees, type of business, safety record, and proof of proper facilities for administering claims.

Besides restrictions imposed upon employers directly, activities of workers' compensation insurers also are regulated. Such regulation serves in part to assure that workers receive benefits when disabled. In order to write workmen's compensation insurance, insurers must conform to rules and regulations of both the state insurance department and the state agency administering the workers' compensation act (usually the industrial commission).

The insurance department primarily regulates the conditions for establishment of insurance companies in the state, their continuing solvency, and their business practices. Like self-insurers, insurance companies (in many states) must post bond or make a deposit with the state insurance department.

Generally the role of the industrial commissions in regulating insurers is limited. Few have either the authority concerning companies' rights to underwrite workers' compensation in their state or the information about financial status and operations of insurers. Further, although industrial commissions would seem to have a direct interest and concern in the claims-handling performance of insurers, few state agencies collect data on promptness of payment, amount of benefits paid, number of beneficiaries currently receiving benefits, and similar aspects of benefit operations. Generally, industrial commissions (to the extent they supervise claims operations) do so through review of individual cases, often only in the event of a dispute.

## Financing

The total cost of workers' compensation to employers has increased over the years and now is about two percent of covered payroll. Since insurance is the main vehicle for meeting the statutory requirements of the workers' compensation acts, the programs are financed mostly through insurance premiums.

## Financing insured benefits

For both public funds and commercial insurance, class premiums are established by an elaborate system of rates that take into account the general occupational classifications or industrial activities of the insured. About 15 percent of the employers, paying about 85 percent of the premiums, are experience-rated. That is, their premiums are modified to reflect their loss experience in the past relative to others in the same class. Also, the statistical reliability of that experience is taken into account; the larger the business, the more credible its experience. Since employers with a small number of workers are likely to experience volatile changes in injury rates from year to year, only employers of large numbers are experience rated.

Another factor in the premium setting procedure is that discounts are given according to the size of the risk; this is an advantage to large companies. Their rates thus reflect the economies of scale which result from spreading certain fixed costs over a larger amount of premium. Finally, large companies by retrospective rating may have their premiums adjusted at the end of a policy year to match their actual experience.

Most insurers use rates developed by a rating bureau. In some states, the rates developed by the bureau are mandatory; in others, advisory only. Almost half the premiums are written on a participating basis. Participating policyholders receive periodic dividends that reflect insurer experience and sometimes their own.

## Financing self-insured benefits

Firms that cover workers' compensation risks through private insurance companies or state funds pay a premium in advance. In contrast, self-insurers have several options for financing. They may simply pay for liabilities as they are experienced, directly from operating funds, or they may provide some advance funding in one or more ways. In those states requiring deposits of funds by self-insurers, part or all of the funding for outstanding liabilities is provided for in advance mandatorily. Even if not required, a self-insurer may set aside reserves, or even formally insure its

risk through a wholly owned subsidiary insurance company created for this purpose.

Such advance funding prevents severe disruptions in cash flow from unforeseen loss experience or accumulated liabilities.

## Insurer administrative costs

One of the recurring issues in evaluating workers' compensation is the financial efficiency of the insurance mechanism for providing benefits. A major part of the issue is the comparison between private and state fund insurance.

The premiums collected by private insurers are used not only to pay benefits but also for expenses associated with claims such as investigation and legal fees; for sales, supervision, and collection; for administration; for safety programs; and for taxes, licenses, and other mandatory fees as well as for earnings. In 1970, stock insurers that did not pay dividends to policyholders had expenses totaling 31 percent of premiums earned; their underwriting gain was 5 percent of premiums paid. For stock insurers that pay dividends to policyholders, the expense ratio was 25 percent; the underwriting gain, 14 percent. Mutual insurers had an expense ratio of 24 percent and underwriting gain of 13 percent. The dividend-paying stocks and mutuals returned part of their underwriting gain to their policyholders. In addition to their underwriting gains, these insurers had investment profits.

State funds have much the same costs as private insurers with these exceptions: lower (or no) taxes and fees to the state government, no margin for private profit, and lower sellling costs. Consequently, although the variation among individual funds is great, expenses have averaged less than 10 percent of total premiums paid, well below the ratio for private insurers. Some state funds incur smaller expenses for administrative and legal services, which may be financed from other government funds. On the other hand, state funds in some instances may insure greater proportions of high-risk companies than private carriers and incur proportionately heavier charges for benefits.

## Other administrative costs

Another aspect of financing workers' compensation relates to the cost of supporting the public agency that administers the program. The cost of operating the industrial commission (or other administering agency) is borne either by assessments upon insurers and self-insurers or through appropriations from public funds. In the former event, the cost of administering the program is simply one more expense item in the premium charge to the employer. Where funds for the industrial commission are obtained from legislative appropriations, this part of the program is paid out of general taxes. More than one-third of state agency administrative costs nationally are funded by legislative appropriations.

In addition to that part of administrative costs financed by state general revenues, other elements in the workers' compensation system may not be financed through insurance premiums paid for by employers. For example, many employers provide medical services at their establishment or by direct payments to medical facilities. Second- or subsequent-injury funds, which bear part of the cost of injuries to handicapped workers, are financed sometimes through assessments on insurers, reflected in premiums; in some states, as direct charges upon employers; as appropriations from state funds; in a few states, as joint employee and employer contributions to the fund; or by other means. Other special funds, paid for by general revenues, have been established for such purposes as supplementing benefits depreciated by inflation or paying benefits for specified occupational diseases.

## Occupational Safety

From the beginning, the workers' compensation movement in the United States has been associated with the movement to prevent occupational injury or disease. Although some interest in this work was manifested by various employers before the enactment of workers' compensation laws, the organized safety movement, as we know it, began shortly after the first compensation laws went into effect. This movement was due in large part to an assumption on the part of industrial leaders that one of the best ways to reduce compensation costs would be to reduce the number of accidents.

The first move toward an organized effort came at the convention of the Association of Iron and Steel Electrical Engineers at Milwaukee in 1912, as discussed in Chapter 1. A session devoted to safety set up a committee on organization, which called a meeting of all interested groups and individuals in New York City the following year. This meeting resulted in the formation of the National Council for Industrial Safety, which

since 1915 has been called the National Safety Council.

### Safety activities of insurers

Although the insurance business had been extended into the industrial accident field before the first workers' compensation act was passed in this country, industrial accident insurance received great impetus from this legislation. As specific schedules of payments for all work-connected injuries made the risk more definitely calculable, the business became more attractive to the underwriter.

From the first, insurance companies writing workers' compensation policies have had a large part in the movement to prevent accidents. They have developed or aided in the development of safety standards and safe practices and have contributed to the development of methods and techniques of accident prevention. Much of the basic data of safety engineering has been supplied by insurance engineers. An important motive for their accomplishment is, of course, the fact that their business thrives on a declining injury rate. Unduly large losses jeopardize the financial solvency of an insurance company. Progressively lower losses make it easier for the stock company to show a profit to its stockholders and for the mutual to pay dividends to its policyholders.

The effective work of insurers, however, has been confined mainly to large establishments. The cost of providing technical assistance in accident prevention makes it difficult for an insurer to provide service adequately to plants whose premiums are small. Owners of small plants, moreover, cannot expect to receive much reduction in premium rates either through dividends or experience rating, no matter how effective their safety program.

Precise statistics are not available showing the total amount of money invested by the insurance industry in safety. Data compiled by the National Council on Compensation Insurance show that private insurance companies reported about $37.8 million or 1.1 percent of net premiums earned were applied to safety in 1970. The data also show that selected state insurance funds spent about 1.4 percent of net premiums earned, or $3.9 million.

### Insurance price incentives

In addition to offering technical assistance, insurers have also tried, by various means, to make safety pay the policyholder in the form of immediately reduced premium rates. This monetary benefit for accident prevention is to some extent inherent in mutual insurance, since the surplus remaining after losses and expenses is distributed among the policyholders. To offer a similar inducement to policyholders in stock companies and to give further incentive to mutual policyholders, a system of merit rating was adopted to obtain reductions in premium rates for policyholders.

The first type of merit rating used was schedule rating, under which the reduction in premium rate was computed on the basis of the policyholder's performance in providing physical safeguards. This tactic proved unsatisfactory because safeguards, while vital, are only one part of prevention. The system now in general use is experience rating, described earlier in this chapter.

Historically, it has been assumed by many authorities that merit rating provided a powerful stimulus to the safety movement. However, safety professionals do not rely solely on the merit rating system to stimulate accident prevention efforts by industry. In fact, some recent studies have questioned the value of merit rating as a strong impetus to safety.

## Covered Employment

Although many controversies have divided students of workers' compensation, one point on which there is broad agreement is that coverage under the acts should be virtually if not completely universal. With few exceptions, employers and workers alike agree on the desirability of this basic protection. For the employer, it represents a relatively inexpensive way to protect himself against the possibility of lawsuits for injuries to his employees. For the worker it represents an important segment of his protection against income loss.

The principle of virtually universal coverage of all gainfully employed workers is basic. Yet, even today, none of the state laws meets this goal, though a few come close. Although it is believed generally that coverage has progressed and although the public has been educated on the justification for including all employment in the workers' compensation system, for the past 20 years the proportion of covered civilian wage and salary workers included has hovered around four-fifths of the potential. Recently, it has edged up to about 88 percent, largely as a result of a shift of workers to covered employment. In 1977, according to the Social Security Administration, average weekly coverage under state and federal workers' compensation totaled 71.8 to 72.4 million, out of the 81.8 million civilian wage and salaried workers in the country.

### Limitations on coverage

Most of the arguments originally brought against extension of coverage have lost their force. Nevertheless, in view of the persistence of some of the exemptions or exclusions in many state laws, a review of some of the reasons behind the original limitations may be helpful. Nearly all state acts were prepared and enacted in the face of constitutional challenges and outright opposition of certain interests. Thus, each act was the result of compromises rather than the outcome of a consistent, ideal program, even if, in some instances, much weight was given to a carefully studied plan.

### Other criteria

Workers' compensation was hailed as an innovation that would introduce a great deal of certainty in the calculation and payment of benefits, in contrast to the common law system. A worker could sue under common law. If he won, he might be assured of an adequate payment; those who lost would be left with nothing but debts. To reduce uncertainty, the workers' compensation law specified the benefits that would be paid to all regardless of fault. Although the outcome of workers' compensation cases is far more certain than the ordinary suit where negligence must be shown, the law is not "automatically" applied.

In part, this uncertainty stems from the variety of the permanent partial disability cases which the schedules do not cover satisfactorily. Two factors give rise to compensation litigation. One is the uncertainty as to whether an accident did or did not arise out of and in the course of employment; the other is the extent of disability. As workers' compensation comes to encompass more and more of the ailments to which the general population might be susceptible, it becomes difficult to separate impairments that are work-connected from those that are not. In addition, it requires an exercise of legal skills and medical judgment to assess the extent of disability in occupational diseases, injuries to the soft tissue of the back, heart conditions, or cases where the only evidence before the commission may be a subjective complaint.

## Conclusion

Workers' compensation permanent partial disability benefits are the least duplicated benefit of any paid to injured workers. There is a variety of benefit levels for temporary disability, permanent total disability, and death. Nowhere is the variety more apparent than in permanent partial disability. States differ in benefit levels, in relationships among benefits paid to the various types of disabilities, in minimums, in maximums, in weeks scheduled for particular losses, and above all in benefit payment philosophies. Not only are twice as many weeks allotted for loss of the use of a member in one jurisdiction than in another, but also what is normally and usually considered, say, a 50 percent loss of use of a member in one jurisdiction may be rated at 25 percent of loss of use in another. A particular residual impairment may rate 50 percent total disability in one state and go uncompensated in another because the employee has lost no wages. In a third jurisdiction, the award may be at a different percentage because of an administrative judgment about the estimated loss in wage-earning capacity. Such variety is in addition to the differences in statutory replacement ratios and minimums and maximums on a weekly or aggregate basis.

Because of the difficulty of predicting an award for a standard impairment and because of a lack of knowledge about the relationship between a given impairment and wage loss, we have no consistent and reliable estimates of the adequacy of permanent partial awards. Some estimates were presented on the basis of a 50 percent disability, but these estimates are possible only in states where aggregate limits or rating philosophies permit one to specify the number of weeks which will be paid.

Death benefits are payable to widows and other eligible survivors at a rate which usually is the same as that paid in the permanent disability cases. Although most jurisdictions provide for payments during widowhood and until children reach a specified age, some limit the duration of payments.

Adequacy comparisons were based on a hypothetical worker making the average wage in his jurisdiction. The percentage of wage loss replaced in each jurisdiction was shown in the analysis. Certainty of payment, a prime objective of early compensation laws, has not been attained because of the litigation which persists over issues of liability and extent of disability. Promptness of payment, also an early goal, has been attained in some jurisdictions but, for most states, data on this aspect of administration are not available.

In the compromise and release cases, certainty is attained but often at the expense of closing out all possibility of future recovery should a worker's condition worsen. As most states do not maintain records on postsettlement developments, it is difficult to know how much compromise and release settlements interfere with the basic objectives of the law. In the usual case, the workers' compensation benefit is paid in periodic installments as wages are paid so that, if the employee's condition changes, the case can be reopened within the period designated in the statute of limitations. The compromise and release settlements, of course, obviate this possibility.

### Rehabilitation

Most employees injured in work accidents return to their jobs after minor medical attention with little if any worktime lost. As the effects of the injury are transient, the incident usually fades from memory. Even those who suffer days or weeks of disability and possibly endure substantial medical treatment may find the injury is not permanent. Although the loss of income and the medical expenses are distressing, eventually, when workers resume their jobs, they recover economically, too.

A minority, unfortunately as much as 10 percent of the total injured, according to a California report (see References), suffer injuries that disrupt their lives. Even when these workers receive effective medical care so that eventually they return to productive jobs, their lives are physically and emotionally scarred. Injuries for some are so severe that prolonged medical treatment and convalescence fail to restore them completely. Residual handicaps prevent their acceptable performances in their former jobs. Only retraining and education combined with special treatment offer a prospect for future employment.

Some never return to work. If they do not die from their injuries, they live with such severe disabilities that they barely can manage for themselves. Often, the most that health services can do is to lighten the burden on those who take care of these persons.

The treatment for workers whose livelihood is threatened by work-related impairments consists of medical rehabilitation and vocational rehabilitation.

## Medical rehabilitation

It is easier to discuss individual programs than to review medical rehabilitation in the United States as a whole. Each program, whether set up by an insurance company or workers' compensation agency, contains its own requirements for treatment, qualifications for eligibility and definitions of service.

**The delivery system.** The worker who requires medical rehabilitation often receives it much as he receives other medical care. Workers' compensation laws obligate employers and insurers to pay costs of medical care for injured workers. The worker receives whatever medical care is needed to treat the impairment and restore lost function. He may report first to the plant nurse or physician for immediate attention. If the injury is serious, he may go to a hospital. Costs are covered by having health service workers on salary, by contractual arrangement with health personnel, or by payment of hospital and doctor bills. The insurer may or may not have much influence in the selection or course of treatment.

For injuries associated with chronic disabilities, the insurer usually attempts to control the selection of the rehabilitation services, frequently by directing the worker to a particular specialist or facility with a particular expertise. Often the insurer pays for transportation to the specialist or facility as well as for rooms during treatment.

Some insurance companies operate rehabilitation facilities, under individual or joint ownership, with medical personnel on salary, at least parttime.

When insurers contract to share rehabilitation programs or facilities, they may pay expenses case by case or through a rental agreement.

Some workers' compensation agencies may be isolated from and unaware of rehabilitation procedures. Others keep relatively close tabs on the services rendered.

When informed of the potential need for rehabilitation, some agencies do little more than notify the worker and insurer that medical rehabilitation is worth considering. Other agencies conduct formal evaluations of the need for further medical care and recommend action. They seek to convince disabled workers of the wisdom of rehabilitation. When the workers agree, the insurers can be required to finance the care.

**Rehabilitation in insurance.** In 1972, a questionnaire concerning rehabilitation programs in workers' compensation insurance was sent to 25 major insurance companies in the United States. The answers from 22 revealed a variety of policies and practices in rehabilitation under workers' compensation so that generalizations are difficult. The following comments on various rehabilitation programs, therefore, are not to be regarded as typical of the entire industry.

In the insurance industry, the concern some carriers have for both medical care and medical rehabilitation is termed "medical management." It is the attempt to minimize the total costs of compensation through emphasis on well-timed, high quality medical treatment. The concept tends to focus attention on the physical condition of the worker rather than on the monetary compensation due. The ultimate goal is to reduce the degree of disability. The insurer would like to see the worker's earning abilities fully restored rather than pay compensation indefinitely.

## Vocational rehabilitation

Vocational rehabilitation prepares the injured worker for a new occupation or for ways of continuing in his old one. Usually, vocational rehabilitation is assigned when medical treatment fails to restore the worker to the job he held when injured. The worker's injury may be so severe or his work requirements such that residual impairment prohibits effective performance. Workers with such impairment must be trained to surmount or by-pass the residual limitations. Many will enter new occupations. In practice, the more effective the medical rehabilitation, the less the need for vocational rehabilitation.

This definition of vocational rehabilitation distinguishes it from medical rehabilitation more than it should. While the difference in kind of treatment seems clear enough—retraining as opposed to medical care—the categories overlap. In the public vocational rehabilitation programs in each state, services include medical diagnosis and evaluation, surgery, psychological support, the fitting of prostheses, and other health services along with education, vocational training, on-the-job training, and job placement.

The two programs blend also on the record. Recordkeeping by workers' compensation insurers does not separate claimants who receive medical rehabilitation from those who receive vocational rehabilitation, although some distinguish between medical rehabilitation and acute medical care. In contrast, records kept by workers' compensation agencies usually separate vocational rehabilitation from other benefits.

**The delivery system.** The relatively few injured workers who need vocational rehabilitation are served by several means. An employer or insurer may channel the worker to whatever sources he thinks will provide satisfactory service. Some workers are referred to the public vocational rehabilitation program where services may be financed by taxes, although insurers may reimburse the public agency. Other insurers direct workers into private facilities where vocational training is conducted by technical schools or on the job. For such services, insurers always pay the costs.

As with medical rehabilitation, some workers' compensation agencies support vocational rehabilitation so that, if the insurer does not direct the worker into a program, the agency often will. Several jurisdictions select candidates either in conjunction with screening for medical rehabilitation or separately. Workers with serious injuries, permanent disabilities, or those who receive extended compensation payments are reviewed by the agency for referral to the state's public vocational rehabilitation agency or to the insurer.

Some workers obtain vocational rehabilitation through their own efforts. If no one refers them, they may go directly to the public vocational rehabilitation office. Since 1920, the federal government and the states have cooperated financially in supporting a vocational rehabilitation program, 80 percent federal and 20 percent state, which can be utilized by anyone with a vocational handicap. Rehabilitation counselors, who usually determine a referral's acceptability, simply look for a vocational handicap without regard to the source and consider the possibilities of overcoming the handicap. If the candidate shows relatively good prospects, a plan is designed for his restoration. For those who cannot return to a paying job, the objective of vocational restoration may be to

enable clients to care for themselves and to free other members of the family to earn wages.

The worker may be referred also by his physician, a friend, or a member of his family.

Once a worker is established in a vocational rehabilitation program, he is aided by whatever sources the counselors think best fit his needs. Generally, the sources are not owned and operated by the vocational rehabilitation agency but are private vendors or other public agencies. A worker may be sent to a private rehabilitation center or school or a sheltered workshop such as those run by Goodwill Industries of America, or he may be enrolled in a public institution.

## Degree of Disability

Determination of the extent of disability is perhaps responsible for more litigation than any other single issue in workers' compensation. It requires not only correct application of legal principles but also evaluation of facts, subjective complaints and opinions, and attempts to predict the future.

As a general proposition (some jurisdictions use different terminology and slightly different classifications), disability can be categorized in one of four classes: temporary total disability, temporary partial disabilty, permanent partial disability, and permanent total disability.

### Temporary disability

Temporary total disability occurs when an injured worker, incapable of gainful employment, has a possibility or probability of improvement to the degree he will be able to return to work with either no disability or merely partial disability. Temporary partial disability is similar to temporary total in that it assumes a physical condition which has not stabilized and is expected to improve. The difference lies in the worker's current abilities. When temporarily partially disabled, the worker is capable of some employment, such as light duties or part-time work, but is excepted to improve to the degree that he will attain much of his former capability.

Permanent partial disability is reached when the injured worker has attained maximum improvement without full recovery. That is, the worker has benefited from medical and rehabilitative services as much as possible and still suffers a partial disability.

Permanent total disability represents the same

physical situation except that the disability is total.

The determination of temporary disability, either total or partial, is least difficult as it requires merely a determination of the employee's present physical condition in comparison with the work opportunities available. In practice, evaluation of temporary disability is concerned only with the ability of the employee to return to work for his last employer. Assuming that an employee will be able at some point to return to work for his employer, and given the difficulties involved in obtaining employment for workers still under medical care, compounded by the probability that the new employment will be temporary, most adjudicators have either expressly or in practice adopted the proposition that unless the worker can return to his last job, or can be supplied with temporary light or part-time duties with his last employer, he remains temporarily totally disasbled, even though he might be able to perform another job involving duties within his temporary physical limitations.

## Permanent partial disability

The determination of the extent of permanent partial disability depends on what the jurisdiction chooses to label "permanent partial disability." Three basic theories have been discussed in conjunction with the payment of workers' compensation benefits for such disability. Their underlying philosophies differ somewhat, as do the factors to be considered in applying each to a specific situation.

The "whole-person" theory is concerned solely with functional limitations. Here, the only considerations are whether the worker has in fact sustained a permanent physical impairment and, if he has, to what extent does it interfere with his usual functions and abilities. Age, occupation, educational background, and other factors are not considered.

In the "wage loss" theory, the aim is to determine what wages the worker would have been able to earn had he not suffered a permanent impairment. When, owing to impairment, his earnings dip below the estimated wage figure, he is paid compensation equal to some percentage of the difference between the wages that he should have earned and those he is actually earning. Here the actual degree of physical impairment is of little or no importance. The only concern is the actual wage loss which has been sustained and whether it is due to the impairment.

The "loss of wage-earning capacity" theory requires a peek into the future. After the worker has reached his maximum physical improvement, many factors, such as impairment, occupational history, age, sex, educational background, and other elements which affect one's ability to obtain and retain employment are all considered in an effort to estimate, as a percentage, how much of the worker's eventual capacity to earn has been destroyed by his work-related impairment. The worker is awarded benefits on the basis of this computation. Benefits may be paid at the maximum weekly rate for a limited number of weeks or they may be based upon a percentage of the difference between wage-earning capacity before and after disability, to be paid until a dollar or time maximum has been reached.

Combinations. There three basic theories are capable of being used also in combination. For example, some states expressly or in practice provide for the use of either the "wage loss" theory or the "loss of wage-earning capacity" theory but also provide a benefit floor determined by the actual medical impairment. Thus, a worker who sustains impairment but no loss of wage or of wage-earning capacity would still receive some permanent disability benefits.

The tedious or controversial aspects of rating for a significant proportion of permanent partial disability cases have been relieved by the use of schedules. The typical schedule covers injuries to the eyes, ears, hands, arms, feet, and legs. It states that for 100 percent loss (or loss of use) of that member, compensation at the claimant's weekly rate will be paid for a specified number of weeks. If loss or loss of use is less than total, the maximum number of weeks is reduced in proportion to the percentage of loss or loss of use. Only physical impairment is considered and the effect of the injury on wages or wage-earning capacity is ignored. If an injury is confined to a scheduled member, the benefits provided by the schedule are exclusive, even though disability rating on a wage loss or loss of wage-earning capacity basis might result in greater benefits. Although this statement is true generally, some states provide additional benefits if use of one of the other theories does result in higher benefits being paid, if diminished wage-earning capacity continues after the scheduled amount is paid, if the scheduled injury results in permanent total disability, or if several scheduled injuries are sustained in the same accident.

Use of the schedule may be avoided also by showing that the effect of the scheduled injury, such as radiating pain, extends into other parts of the body. A few jurisdictions limit the use of schedules to amputation or 100 percent loss of use of a member, as opposed to partial loss of use. Another group not only makes the schedule exclusive for permanent disability awards but requires that the weeks for which benefits are paid during the healing period be deducted from the number of weeks authorized by the schedule before an award is made for permanent partial disability.

Despite commentary and statutory language to the contrary, the workers' compensation systems of the United States, with a few exceptions, operate primarily on the "loss of earning capacity" theory. Even where statutory language seems to indicate clearly that only functional impairment is to be considered, the courts have managed to hold that loss of earning capacity is the real consideration. Even the use of schedules has been justified on an earning capacity basis as merely a legislative determination of presumed wage loss resulting from the impairment listed in the schedule.

It is questionable that any legislative history would back up this rationale. A consideration of its practical day-to-day application shows that in individual cases the presumption is without basis in fact. When one considers that a concert pianist and a laborer who have both lost two fingers would receive exactly the same compensation under a schedule award, the justification for the use of schedules, that of administrative efficiency, is questionable by all who hold equity as a basic aim of workers' compensation.

## Permanent total disability

Permanent total disability evaluation is, in most respects, merely an extension of the determination of permanent partial disability. In fact, it is a part of the same process, since the factfinder's only additional task is to determine whether the worker's wage-earning capacity is so destroyed that he is unable to compete in the job market.

Two aspects of the permanent total disability question warrant special attention.

First, most states employ presumptions that make the factfinder's job much easier. For example, it may be presumed that the loss of sight of both eyes or the loss of any two limbs will constitute permanent total disability and thereby relieve the factfinder of the difficult task of evaluating all the factors previously mentioned. These presumptions in some cases may be rebutted by evidence of an established wage-earning capacity or may only apply for a limited period of time.

Second is the concept of what permanent total disability actually means. The injured employee need not be completely helpless nor unable to earn a single dollar at a job. His limitations need only prevent him from competing in a practical way in the open job market and are such that no stable job market exists for him.

## The 'exclusive remedy' doctrine and third party liability

Before workers' compensation laws were enacted in the states, an employee, in order to recover damages for a work-connected injury, always was required to show some degree of fault on the part of his employer. Under what is now known as the "quid pro quo of workers' compensation law," employers accepted, or were required to accept, responsibility for injuries arising out of and in the course of employment without regard to fault. In exchange, employees gave up the right to sue employers for unlimited damages. These agreements are usually referred to in the state acts as "exclusive remedy" provisions, a term that is quite misleading. In no state are workers' compensation benefits necessarily the only remedy available to an injured worker. Depending upon the working of the applicable statute, the worker may bring a negligence action against a fellow worker, another contractor on the same job, or some other entity or individual who caused the compensable injury. From the employer's viewpoint, it is best to refer to the doctrine as the "exclusive liability rule." As the employee sees the rule, it remains an "exclusive remedy" for obtaining compensation from the employer. But neither liability nor remedy are perfectly exclusive.

## Private Insurer Programs

Private insurers dominate the coverage. The ten leading groups wrote almost half the business;

**237**

the top twenty about 68 percent, up from 62 percent in 1950, although the share of the top ten has changed little. The ten leaders wrote as much as 88 percent of the coverage in Hawaii to as little as 51 percent in Kansas and Nebraska. In four states, one insurer wrote one-fourth of the business.

Only 36 of the 383 insurers earned workers' compensation premiums of $20 million or more, but these 36 cornered more than 78 percent of the total. Companies with nation-wide operations accounted for 83 percent. Insurers licensed in only one state, more than 20 percent of all insurance companies, wrote less than 4 percent of the premiums.

Workers' compensation is the second largest property-liability insurance line; it is topped only by automobile insurance. Workers' compensation premiums are about 11 percent of the total premium income. Among the ten leading private insurance groups, four derive at least one-third of their business from workers' compensation.

## Classifications of insurers

Private insurers can be classified according to their legal form of organization, their marketing methods, and their pricing policies.

Legally, insurers may be classified as proprietary or cooperative insurers. Proprietary insurers have owners who bear the risks of the insurer and whose representatives manage the operations. The leading example by far is the stock insurer owned by stockholders who elect the board of directors. In 1970 of the 383 private groups in workers' compensation insurance, about 68 percent were stock companies, with about 70 percent of the total premium volume.

Cooperative insurers have no owners other than their policyholders. The leading example is the advance premium mutual whose board of directors is elected by those policyholders who exercise their right to vote.

Unlike stock insurers, these insurers have no capital stock. Instead, retained earnings serve as a cushion against adverse experience. In 1970, mutual insurers, about 32 percent of the private workers' compensation insurers, wrote 30 percent of the premiums earned.

Almost all of the 1970 workers' compensation insurance premiums not written by stock or mutual insurers were written by reciprocal exchanges which, in their modern form, closely resemble advance premium mutuals.

The relative importance of stock, mutuals, and reciprocal exchanges varies among states. In several states, stock insurers write over 75 percent of the business. In a few states, mutual insurers dominate the private insurance field.

Since 1951, when their share was 59 percent, stock insurers have steadily increased their proportion of the business.

## Self-insurers

In all jurisdictions (except Nevada, North Dakato, Puetro Rico, Texas, the Virgin Islands, and Wyoming), employers are permitted under certain conditions to self-insure workers' compensation. Although most jurisdictions reported 200 or fewer self-insurers, self-insured employers in 1977 paid 14.1 percent of the workers' compensation benefits.

Self-insurance is becoming popular among those who qualify. In 1960 self-insurers paid only 12.4 percent of the benefits. Most states report an increase also in the number of self-insurers. Possible explanations are increasing cost consciousness, sales activities of agencies who seek to manage self-insurance programs, and the business merger movement which increases the size of firms and their ability to self-insure.

Self-insurance is attractive primarily because it may be less costly than insurance. An insurance premium is designed to pay the losses and expenses of the insurer and provide a margin of profit for contingencies. The self-insurer hopes to save money on the loss or the expense and profit components of the premium.

The loss component equals the average loss the insurer expects the employer and others like him to experience. If the employer is so much better than the average employer in his class that his expected loss may be less, he would save money by self-insuring. In the short run, however, the loss experience may differ substantially from the expected loss. Indeed the loss in a single year might be catastrophic. The larger the number of employees, the less the risk of fluctuation in annual losses. For most employers, the risk is such that self-insurance is out of the question. For others, the comparison bewteen actual and expected loss is an important consideration.

By self-insuring, the employer can save that part of the premium charged to cover selling expenses, some general administration expenses, and profits. There may also be savings on loss prevention and loss adjustment services even though these services must still be performed.

Other considerations include the relative quality of the safety and claims services provided by insurers, by management service organizations, and by employers themselves; by tax factors; and by the opportunity cost of paying an insurer a premium instead of paying losses and expenses as they occur.

## Cost Levels and Allocation

Workers' compensation costs and other costs of industrial accidents impose a burden on industry, workers, and society generally. The magnitude of these costs and their distribution have important economic implications and pose several critical issues of policy.

### Cost levels

Workers' compensation in 1970 cost employers almost $5 billion, or more than $1.13 per $100 of payroll. These costs include the premiums paid to private insurers on state funds and the benefits and administrative costs paid by self-insurers. Other employer costs of industrial accidents or the losses to employees not covered by workers' compensation are not available.

**Variation over time.** Costs per $100 of payroll were less in 1970 than in 1940, but have increased since the late fifties. The 1970 dollar costs were 11.6 times the 1940 costs, 4.8 times the 1950 costs, and 2.4 times the 1960 costs.

**Variation among industries.** In its 1980 sample survey of employee benefits, the Chamber of Commerce of the United States found that workers' compensation costs were 1.5 percent of gross payroll. In manufacturing industries, the costs were 1.9 percent; in nonmanufacturing industries 0.7 percent. These rates changed from 0.2 percent for banks and financial institutions, to 3.0 percent for the manufacture of glass, stone, and quarry products.

A 1970 sample survey by the Bureau of Labor Statistics found workers' compensation costs equal to 0.9 percent of gross payroll plus employer payments for legally required insurance programs and employee benefit plans. In manufacturing, compensation costs were 0.8 percent, in nonmanufacturing, 0.9 percent. The percentage for office workers was 0.3; for nonoffice or production workers, 1.3 percent.

### Workers' compensation incentives for safety

The asserted safety incentive of workers' compensation is based on the merit-rated pricing policy. "Merit rating" includes both the experience rating and retrospective rating systems. All state funds use merit rating of some sort. In most states, although private insurers are not required to rate employers on merit, they are permitted to. Under this procedure, the firm is charged a premium that is related to the dollar amount of claims for which it is liable. Consequently a merit-rated firm has an incentive to reduce the amount of its claims through loss preventive measures.

The strength of this incentive has been challenged. Only about one-fourth of insured firms, usually large ones, are eligible for merit rating. The yearly accident record of firms with only a few employees is not a sufficiently reliable indication of their characteristic experience to be considered in establishing premium rates. On the other hand, merit-rated firms account for 85 percent of the dollar volume of premiums paid. In addition, self-insured firms which pay approximately 14 percent of all benefits are implicitly merit rated. Nevertheless, if incentive effects are inherent in experience rating, they are not available to a large number of small firms and their employees.

Firms not eligible for merit rating are class rated. Under this procedure, all employers engaged in similar business operations within a state pay the same rate per $100 of payroll. These employers have strong incentives to reduce the rates paid by their industry and may therefore exert efforts to reduce accidents within the industry. The only accident prevention incentive generated for individual employers within an industry is that as poor risks, they may land in an assigned risk pool.

Other problems, even under merit rating, moderate the incentive for safety. As benefit levels do not reflect the full costs of accidents, the premiums paid are less than adequate; consequently, any savings from safety programs are proportionally minimized. A saving in premium costs could be a significant reward for success in accident prevention if benefits were higher because premiums would then more truly measure the cost of accidents at work. The higher the benefit levels, the larger the premium costs to be avoided and the larger the incentive for prevention.

Even for the merit-rated firm, the functional relationship between injury rates and premium levels is not as direct as might be desirable. The sensitivity of premium to accident experience is dependent on the firm's payroll. As firms increase in size, the premium rate more nearly reflects the individual firm's experience. It has been suggested that more credibility be assigned to the experience of smaller merit-rated companies to increase their safety incentives.

The premium rate for firms of all sizes is more dependent on the frequency rate than the severity rate on the assumption that loss frequency is more within the control of the employer. Thus, firms are encouraged to be more concerned with the number of accidents than with the consequences of accidents. Some critics, however, believe too much emphasis has been placed on loss frequency.

Merit rating suffers the further criticism that, since premiums are related to the level of claims paid, some firms may try to reduce costs by fighting claims rather than by preventing accidents.

Finally, workers' compensation safety incentives have been questioned because the costs usually amount to little more than 1 percent of payroll and many feel that a firm is insensitive to any cost that small. Other costs of worker accidents that are not insurable provide even stronger incentives. In evaluating this criticism, it should be remembered that the costs of workers' compensation for employers in hazardous industries or with unsafe operations are much greater than 1 percent of payroll.

Unfortunately, there has been little research on this question, but there is little evidence to indicate that any substantial connection exists between merit rating and accident prevention in most states. Conceptually, however, workers' compensation should impel firms to operate at an optimal level of accident prevention activities in a least-cost fashion.

An improvement in functioning is what is needed.

## References

California Department of Education, San Francisco, Calif. *The Vocational Rehabilitation of Industrially Injured Workers.* A report to the California Legislature, 1961.

Chamber of Commerce of the United States, Washington, D.C. *Analysis of Workers' Compensation Laws,* 1980.

Clifford, Joseph A. *Workmen's Compensation—New York.* Binghamton, N.Y., Gould Publications, 1979.

Gaunt, Larry, D., and McDonald, Maurice E. *Examining Employers' Financial Capacity to Self-Insure Under Workmen's Compensation.* Atlanta, Ga., Georgia State University, College of Business Administration, 1977.

Manuele, Fred A. "Economics of Work Injuries and Illnesses," *Transactions of the 1975 Safety Congress,* Fertilizer Section. Chicago, Ill. National Safety Council.

Martin, Roland A. *Occupational Disability—Causes, Prediction, Prevention.* Springfield, Ill., Charles C. Thomas, 1975.

National Commission on State Workers' Compensation Laws,° Washington, D.C. Available through Government Printing Office, Washington, D.C. 20402.
*Compendium on Workmen's Compensation,* 1973.
*Supplemental Studies* (3 vols.), 1973.

National Council on Compensation Insurance, 200 E. 42nd St., New York, N.Y. 10017. Rate and rating plan manuals.

National Safety Council, 444 N. Michigan Ave., Chicago, Ill. 60611. *Accident Facts* (annually).

---

°The National Commission was disbanded in 1972. The Employment Standards Administration of the U.S. Department of Labor is responsible for tracking the progress of states' workers' compensation laws in comparison with the 19 essential recommendations of the Commission.

# Safety
# Training

# Chapter
# 9

# 9—Safety Training

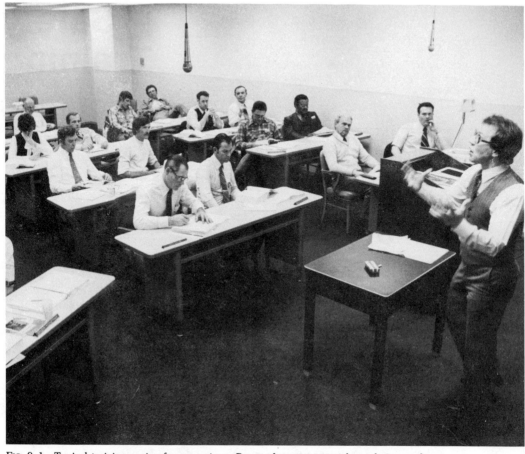

FIG. 9–1.—Typical training session for supervisors. Prepared course materials are being used.

An effective accident prevention and occupational health hazard control program is based on proper job performance. When people are trained to do their jobs properly, they will do them safely. This, in turn, means that supervisors must (a) know how to train an employee in the safe, proper way of doing a job, as well as (b) understand company (plant) policies and procedures, (c) know how to detect and control hazards, investigate accidents, and handle emergencies, and (d) know how to supervise. It also means the safety professional should be familiar with sound training techniques. He may, or may not, become directly involved in the training effort, but he should be able to recognize the elements of a sound training program.

This chapter is devoted to safety training.

Although training and education cannot be separated completely, safety education is broader in scope and usually covers a number of subjects not normally included in a training program. The "human relations" value of education will be covered in the section on Learning in Chapter 11, "Human Behavior and Safety."

Training is only one way to influence human behavior. Safe performance is encouraged by the example of an employer who spares no effort to create safe working conditions. Safe performance is encouraged by developing safe work procedures, by teaching the procedures effectively, and by insisting that they be followed. Safe performance is also encouraged by teaching prople the facts about accident causes and preventive measures.

**242**

A well-planned training program will not only train employees, but will also help change these other influences so they will complement the effect of the training. Firms that conduct intensive safety activities, including training, for all employees make the greatest progress in safety. Supervisors and managers, as well as unskilled and skilled workers, benefit from safety training.

## Developing the Training Program

When developing a training program, consider the training needs, program objectives, course outlines and materials, and training methods. Safety training must be integrated with job training.

### Training needs

A training program is needed (a) for new and reassigned employees, (b) when new equipment or processes are introduced, (c) procedures have been revised or updated, (d) when new information must be made available, and (e) when employee performance needs to be improved. Unless a training program is needed however, there is little justification for spending time and money just to have one.

Here are some indications of a need for a good training program:

1. Proportionately more accidents and injuries, or insurance rates higher than other companies in the same type of work, or a rate that is on the upswing.

2. High labor turnover.

3. Excessive waste and scrap.

4. Company expansion of plant and equipment.

### Program objectives

Training programs should be based on clearly defined objectives that determine the scope of the training and guide the selection and preparation of the training materials. Objectives should be planned carefully and written down. They should indicate what the trainee is to know or do by the end of the training period.

To make sure the objectives really cover the needs of those to be trained, the duties and responsibilities of the trainees should be determined. Job descriptions and job analyses (including job hazards) should be reviewed. (See the discussion in Chapter 5 and later in this chapter.)

These, along with personal observations and performance tests will reveal where training is needed. For example, if a job description (or list of duties) for supervisors includes training workers, then supervisors should be trained to train. This now becomes one of the objectives of a supervisory training program.

A total safety training program is complicated; it has many different kinds of activity. Thus, a statement of safety training objectives is equally complex, and it will cover activity that may not be obvious from a quick reading of the statement. While any program must have management approval, of course, and full acceptance by the supervisors, in many companies the key level that must be reached is the group of people one level above the supervisors. All these groups must give both approval and acceptance.

There is no set of objectives that will serve all companies and all situations. Each must be developed to meet its own circumstances and its own situation. All objectives must be adapted to the needs of the company, and above all, it must be so phrased that management will fully and completely accept it. (The Council publication *Communications for the Safety Professional* gives examples of a statement of policy; training objectives are given later in this chapter.)

All recommendations must be included in a statement of corporate policy, such as those discussed in Chapter 3, "Organization of Hazard Control Programs." Funds for its implementation must be included in the corporate budget, under the control of the safety director.

### Course outlines and materials

After defining the training program objectives, the next step is developing the outline of what is to be covered. Often, an outline can meet the program objectives by using existing texts and course materials, or by combining parts of several texts or courses already in use. (A later section in this chapter, A Basic Course for Supervisors, describes the National Safety Council's 12-session safety course outline for supervisors.)

Sometimes, a completely new program must be designed. Either way, the outline must be developed in detail. Major topics and subtopics should be arranged logically and the time allotted to each should be in proportion to the importance of each. So arranged, the course outline is the framework that determines the method of training.

# 9—Safety Training

## Training methods

At this stage in planning a training program, a decision must be made as to the training method that will best reach the stated objective. For job (of skill) training, the best method is the four-step method called "job instruction training," or JIT.

Full details of this system—ideal for training new workers or upgrading more experienced ones—are given under this section On-the-job Training, later in this chapter.

## The lesson plan

The safety professional and others who must often teach safety subject should be familiar with lesson plans. They are the blueprint for presenting material contained in a course outline. In addition to standardizing training, lesson plans help the instructor:

1. Present material in proper order

2. Emphasize material in relation to its importance

3. Avoid omission of essential material

4. Run the classes on schedule

5. Provide for trainee (student) participation

6. Increase his confidence, especially if he is new

Names for the parts of a lesson plan may vary, even the order may not always be the same. The following is a good example of arrangement for a lesson plan:

1. **Title:** Must indicate clearly and concisely subject matter to be taught.

2. **Objectives:**
   a) Should state what the trainee should know or be able to do at the end of the training period.
   b) Should limit the subject matter.
   c) Should be specific.
   d) Should stimulate thinking on the subject.

3. **Training aids:** Should include such items as actual equipment or tools to be used, and charts, slides, films, etc.

4. **Introduction:**
   a) Should give the scope of the subject.
   b) Should tell the value of the subject.
   c) Should stimulate thinking on the subject.

5. **Presentation:**
   a) Should give the plan of action.
   b) Should indicate the method of teaching to be used (lecture, demonstration, class discussion, or a combination of these).
   c) Should contain suggested directions for instructor activity (show chart, write key words on chalkboard).

6. **Application:** Should indicate, by example, how trainees will apply this material immediately (problems may be worked; a job may be performed; trainees may be questioned on understanding and procedures).

7. **Summary:**
   a) Should restate main points.
   b) Should tie up loose ends.
   c) Should strengthen weak spots in instruction.

8. **Test:** Tests help determine if objectives have been reached. They should be announced to the class at the beginning of the session.

9. **Assignment:** Should give references to be checked or indicate materials to be prepared for future lessons.

The self-checklist shown in Fig. 9–2 will aid the instructor in improving his teaching techniques.

## Safety Training for Supervisors

The immediate job of preventing accidents and controlling work health hazards falls upon the supervisor, not because it has been arbitrarily assigned there, but because safety and production are part of the same supervisory function.

### Responsibilities of the supervisor

Whether or not a company has a safety program, the supervisor has these principal responsibilities:

1. Establish work methods

2. Give job instruction

3. Assign people to jobs

4. Supervise people at work

5. Maintain equipment and the workplace

## SELF-CHECK TEST FOR INSTRUCTORS

A good instructor should be able to answer "Yes" to at least 18 of these questions. Under 15 would be below average.

| | Yes | No |
|---|---|---|
| 1. Do you check your classroom for ventilation, lighting, seating arrangement? | ☐ | ☐ |
| 2. Do you prepare a lesson plan? | ☐ | ☐ |
| 3. Do you use training aids when possible? | ☐ | ☐ |
| 4. Do you preview all films before showing them? | ☐ | ☐ |
| 5. Do you use test results to find weak points in your teaching? | ☐ | ☐ |
| 6. Do you vary your type of presentation according to the material? | ☐ | ☐ |
| 7. Do you stay on the subject? | ☐ | ☐ |
| 8. Do you cover the material in each lesson? | ☐ | ☐ |
| 9. Do you make any attempt to know your students and to learn their names? | ☐ | ☐ |
| 10. Do you introduce yourself to each class? | ☐ | ☐ |
| 11. Do you make clear the objectives of the lesson? | ☐ | ☐ |
| 12. Do you summarize each lesson? | ☐ | ☐ |
| 13. Do you introduce each new subject and explain its importance? | ☐ | ☐ |
| 14. Do you refrain from using sarcasm in your class? | ☐ | ☐ |
| 15. Do you start and dismiss your class on time? | ☐ | ☐ |
| 16. Do you have all your equipment ready and tested at class time? | ☐ | ☐ |
| 17. Do you talk directly to the class and avoid such practices as staring at the floor, pacing the floor, juggling a piece of chalk? | ☐ | ☐ |
| 18. Do you keep your meeting place orderly? | ☐ | ☐ |
| 19. Do you use words that are easily understood by the class? | ☐ | ☐ |
| 20. Do you make assignments, and are they clear? | ☐ | ☐ |

FIG. 9-2.—A self-check test can help a supervisor rate his own training methods.

These principal responsibilities of the supervisor are the very activities through which the work of preventing accidents is carried out. A brief examination of these jobs and their relation to safety will make this fact apparent.

**Establishing work methods** that are well understood and consistently followed is essential to orderly and safe operation. Many injuries and health hazards have been reported to result from "unsafe method of procedure," when later investigation disclosed that no standard method or procedure had been set up for those jobs. The method was declared hazardous only after it resulted in an accident. Making sure that safe procedures are established is a supervisory responsibility.

**Giving job instruction,** with necessary emphasis on safety aspects of the job, will help eliminate one of the most frequent causes of accidents—lack of knowledge or skill. If employees are expected to do their work safely, supervisors must show them exactly how to do the work and must make sure that the employees have the knowledge and skill to do it in exactly that manner.

**Assigning people to jobs** is closely related to job instruction. Whenever a supervisor makes a work assignment, safety, as well as good job performance, requires that he makes sure the worker is qualified to do the job and thoroughly understands the work method. Even an experienced worker needs some direction.

**Supervising people at work** is necessary even after a safe work method has been established and workers have been instructed according to that method. People deviate from established safe practices and injuries result. Usually, it is then found that the injured employees have been neglecting safe practices. In order to prevent injuries from this cause, supervisors must watch for unsafe work methods and correct them as soon as they are observed.

**Maintaining equipment and workplace** in safe condition is no different from maintaining them in efficient condition. Accidents results from tools and equipment in poor condition, from a disorderly workplace, or from makeshift tools used because the right tools are not available. The supervisor who keeps his department and equipment in top condition helps to prevent accidents while improving efficiency.

## Supervisors must accept their duties

Not only are these five functions a normal part of the supervisor's job but, unless lines of organization and authority are seriously disregarded, nobody else but the supervisor can perform them. Sometimes this fact is overlooked. Since all these functions are closely allied with safety, it is only natural that safety should be integrated into the duties of the supervisor. If however, management wants to be sure that supervisors accept this role, it should be included in a policy statement and lines of authority should be established.

A clear and positive executive order defining the safety duties of all persons and departments should be issued. A careful program of education should be instituted to help supervisors understand and accept their role and to give them specific help in their work of preventing accidents.

Many supervisors have acquired their present positions in organizations where some sort of safety program was already in existence, and their understanding of the program as it has existed is firmly established. However, a safety professional undertaking the safety training of supervisors will almost invariably find that the first major job is to get supervisors of all levels to understand and accept their role in accident prevention. This job cannot be done in a single meeting or by a single communication.

Simply getting supervisors to agree in theory that safety is one of their duties is not enough. They must come to understand the many ways in which they can prevent accidents, and they must become interested in improving their safety performance.

## Objectives of supervisor safety training

Before the safety training of supervisors is undertaken, the objectives of that training must be understood and stated specifically. Determining objectives for supervisory training is so important and involves so many kinds of activity that it should be made the subject of careful study and consultation. Members of the safety department should not attempt to set up objectives alone, but should confer with representative supervisors and members of higher management.

The following statement of objectives should be used only as a guide to be studied and modified to fit specific situations and should be accepted only to the extent that the management persons concerned agree to it. Stated in general terms, the objectives of safety training for supervisors may be any or all of the following:

1. To involve supervisors in the company's accident prevention program

2. To establish the supervisor as being the key person in preventing accidents

3. To get supervisors to understand the nature of their safety responsibilities

4. To provide supervisors with information on causes of accidents and occupational health hazards and methods of prevention

5. To give supervisors an opportunity to consider current problems of accident prevention and to develop solutions based on their own and others' experience

6. To help supervisors gain skill in accident prevention activities

7. To help supervisors do the safety job in their own departments.

## A Basic Course for Supervisors

The knowledge and philosophy of accident prevention is not "just common sense," as some slogans proclaim. It is a specialized body of information accumulated over a period of many years. It is the job of the safety professional to help supervisors gain whatever information is available that will make their safety efforts more productive.

The most direct way to develop the desired attitudes and to impart the necessary information about safety to supervisors is to provide a course of instructions. Courses in safety and other management subjects, conducted for supervisors by many companies, follow a fairly well-established pattern.

## Subject outline of course

The following outline based on the National Safety Council's 12-hour "Supervisors Development Program" shows the subjects that should usually be included in a safety course for supervisors. Visual aids are available on all the subjects and should be used at every meeting. Titles of films and other aids are not included here because new ones are being produced constantly. The person conducting a course should secure and use those best suited to his needs. (See the latest "General Materials Catalog" published by the National Safety Council.)

### Session 1
#### SAFETY AND THE SUPERVISOR
Safety and efficient production go together. Accidents affect morale and public relations. The duties of a supervisor under OSHA.

### Session 2
#### KNOW YOUR ACCIDENT PROBLEMS
Elements of an accident. Unsafe acts, unsafe conditions, accident investigations, measurements of safety performance. Accident costs.

### Session 3
#### HUMAN RELATIONS
Motivation. Basic needs of workers. The supervisor as a leader. The alcohol and drug problem.

### Session 4
#### MAINTAINING INTEREST IN SAFETY
Committee functions, maintaining good employee relations. The supervisor's role in off-the-job safety.

### Session 5
#### INSTRUCTING FOR SAFETY
Importance of job instruction. Making a job safety analysis (JSA). Job instruction training (JIT).

### Session 6
#### INDUSTRIAL HYGIENE
Environmental health hazards. Skin diseases. Lighting, noise, ventilation, temperature effects.

### Session 7
#### PERSONAL PROTECTIVE EQUIPMENT
Eye protection, face protection, foot and leg protection, hand protection. Respiratory protective equipment. Protection against ionizing radiation. OSHA requirements.

### Session 8
#### INDUSTRIAL HOUSEKEEPING
Results of good housekeeping. The responsibility of the supervisor. OSHA requirements.

### Session 9
#### MATERIAL HANDLING AND STORAGE
Lifting and carrying, handling specific shapes. Hand tools for material handling. Motorized equipment. Hazardous liquids and compressed gases.

### Session 10
#### GUARDING MACHINES AND MECHANISMS
Principles of guarding. Benefits of good guarding. Types of guards. Standards and codes. OSHA regulations.

### Session 11
#### HAND AND PORTABLE POWER TOOLS
Selection and storage. Training in the safe care and use of hand tools and power tools.

# 9—Safety Training

Session 12

FIRE PROTECTION

Determining fire hazards. Understanding fire chemistry. Fire brigades. The supervisor's role in fire safety.

## Tips on running a course

All supervisors should be given a basic course of the type just outlined. It should be repeated from time to time for new supervisors and prospective supervisors.

It should be given with considerable formality. Attendance records should be kept, and certificates or diplomas issued upon completion. Some companies give a diploma that may be framed and displayed; others favor a pocket-size card. Both may well be given.

It adds to the dignity of the training program if, at the beginning of a course, a company executive meets with the group and explains the importance of the supervisor's role in the safety program and the value of the training. At the end of the course, a formal graduation ceremony is often held.

Some large companies with wide-spread operations have made up their own courses to be given throughout the organization. The preparation of such a course is, however, a major and costly project. It is not recommended except for very large organizations with proportionately large safety and training staffs.

Prepared courses, such as the National Safety Council's "Supervisor's Development" course, are available, complete with text book, the "Supervisors Safety Manual," "Instructors' Guide," student kit, certificate of completion, and visual aids. Courses can be adapted to local needs. They have been thoroughly tested by use in hundreds of companies and many kinds of operations. Use of a prepared course saves a great deal of preparation time and effort. Let the instructor give it the company slant.

## Providing instructors

One problem in giving a basic in-house safety course to supervisors is providing qualified instructors. A considerable burden is placed on the safety personnel if they must conduct every class. Many companies have found that the best instructors are general supervisors or division managers. In addition to serving usefully as instructors, these people also learn a great deal about safety in the process of teaching.

It is well for those who are to serve as instructors to take a short course on how to instruct or, at least, hold two or three meetings on the subject of how best to give the instruction. After preparing his own lesson plan for each meeting by following the format outlined in this chapter and by using company situations and problems as examples, each instructor then takes charge of one class.

Safety professionals may feel that there is some risk of not getting good instruction by this method, but those who have tried it have found that the experience and understanding of those who are themselves supervisors more than offsets a lack of formal teaching experience.

In addition, acceptance by the group is improved because the members know that the instructor is a person who has done the things he is talking about. In the case of a general supervisor who is teaching a group of his own supervisors, the meetings can become planning sessions in which agreement is reached as to how the group is to handle situations in the future. Training linked with actual operation can be most effective.

Courses conducted locally should be planned and instructed by safety professionals experienced in training and in the subject to be covered. Criteria for such instructors might include:

- Professional member or member of the American Society of Safety Engineers, or

- Certified Safety Professional (CSP), or

- Holder of the National Safety Council's "Advanced Safety Certificate," or

- Two years' recent experience in safety training, or equivalent experience.

Regardless of the experience of the person selected to do the teaching, each instructor should make a self-evaluation of his own teaching methods. A self-check test for instructors is an ideal guide for such evaluation.

## Conducting the "in-house" course

Training sessions should not be longer than one hour. Longer sessions are likely to become tiresome, and supervisors will become apprehensive about their work during a prolonged absence.

It is desirable to hold sessions during working hours, if possible. Regular attendance and freedom from interruptions are of great importance and should be required by management.

If courses are held after working hours or

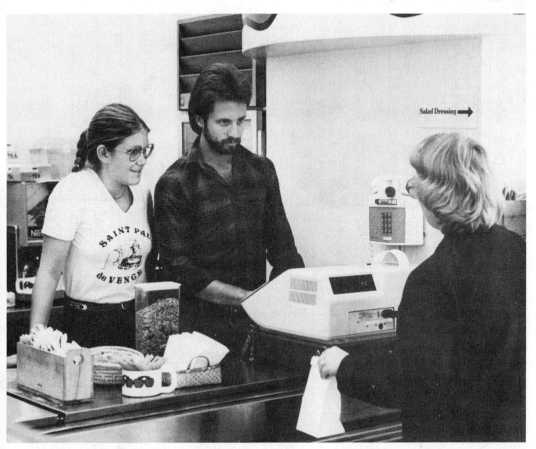

FIG. 9–3.—Over-the-shoulder coaching. The trainee is expected to develop and apply skills in the work situation under the guidance of a qualified person.

between shifts, sessions are usually two hours; occasionally dinner or refreshments are provided. In any event, courses should be conducted in a professional, businesslike manner.

A supervisors safety course can produce many benefits—an increased understanding of safety, acceptance of responsibility for the prevention of accidents, and greater interest in all supervisory duties.

### Special Training for Supervisors

Success in supervision requires skill as much as it requires knowledge and understanding. Basic training in the elements of a safety program is aimed toward imparting knowledge about safety and creating a proper attitude toward safety.

Many accidents, however, result from unskillful handling by supervisors of some of the important tasks of supervision—giving orders, assigning jobs, correcting workers for wrong performance, and the like.

If training in accident investigation has been given, remedial measures will have been assigned for specific accidents, but no detailed consideration may have been given as to how remedies should be applied.

To be able to do a good safety job, supervisors also need training in supervisory skills.

Among the most important of these skills are giving job instruction, supervising workers at work, determining accident causes, and building safety attitudes among workers. Special courses may be given in these subjects.

**249**

Date March 1
Supervison L.O.
Department Office

| Employee | CASHIER | | | | | CLERICAL | | | | | | | | Notes |
|---|---|---|---|---|---|---|---|---|---|---|---|---|---|---|
| Tasks | KNOW CUSTOMERS | CUSTOMER RELATIONS | ACCURACY IN CASH | MAKE UP DEPOSIT | BANK DEPOSIT | TAKE DICTATION | STENO | COMP. OPERATOR | STENCILS | FILE | MAIL TELEGRAMS | PLANT ORDERS | TELE PHONE BOARD | |
| 1. Mrs A.M. | X | X | X | X | X | | | | ⊗ | | ? | | | FREQUENTLY ABSENT. MISS B.C. HAS TO TAKE OVER WORK |
| 2. Miss B.C. | X | X | | | X | NQ | X | X | ⊗ | | | | ✓ | |
| 3. Miss W.E. | X | | X | X | X | X | X | X | X | | | X | | TRAIN HER IN CASH AND DISBURSEMENT JOURNALS |
| 4. John D. | | | X | X | X | | | X | X | X | X | | | CAUTION ON MORE CARE IN CHECK WRITING ON PLANT PAYROLL |
| 5. Mrs W.C. | ⊗ | ⊗ | ⊗ | ⊗ | ⊗ | | | | | | | | | TRAIN HER TO HELP ON FREIGHT BILLS |
| 6. Miss E.M. | | | | | | ⊗ | ⊗ | ⊗ | ⊗ | ⊗ | ⊗ | ⊗ | | START HER ON CHECKING BANK STATEMENT—ASK W.E. TO HELP |
| 7. Miss J.O. | | | ? | | ? | | | | | | | 3/5 | | GET HER STARTED TO HELP ON TELEPHONE BOARD |
| 8. Miss M.O. | | | | | | X | | X | ⊗ | X | | | | TRAIN ON STENCILS |
| 9. Miss K.B. | | | | | | | | | X | X | X | | | GOOD PERSON'TY—HOW ABOUT WORKING TOWARD CASHIER AIDE |
| 10. Miss L.B. | | | | | | | | | X | X | X | | | |
| 11. Bill K. | | | | | ⊗ | | | ⊗ | ⊗ | B/W | X | | | WORK WITH HIM ON MAIL—RE-ARRANGE—FIND BETTER WAY |

CODE
NQ – Not qualified
X – Can do
B/W – Better way?
? – Check it can do
⊗ – Regular Job OK
% – Target date

FIG. 9-4.—Training chart keeps track of who needs (and who has) what training.

## On-the-Job Training

On-the-job training (OJT) is widely used because the trainee can be producing while he is being trained. Whether the supervisor does the instructing himself or has someone else do it, the training should be carefully planned and organized. Again the safety professional should be familiar with his organization's training program so that appropriate and correct safety training is integrated into it.

In too many cases, on-the-job training is a hit-or-miss procedure where the trainee is told to follow another worker around and learn his job. In situations of this type, the worker may be too busy to do any training, or may not know good training procedures. He may even be reluctant to train another to do his work.

Remember, it is the supervisor's responsibility to make sure the person doing the training can, in fact, train. On-the-job training includes many techniques and approaches and there is no one method that will fit all situations. Job safety analysis (JSA, discussed in the next section and in Chapter 5, "Removing the Hazard from the Job") is one method, job instruction training (JIT) is another, and over-the-shoulder coaching is still another widely used method. These methods may be used separately or in combination depending upon the complexity of the job and the time element.

### Over-the-shoulder coaching

Over-the-shoulder coaching is perhaps the most flexible and direct of the three training methods. In coaching, the trainee is expected to develop and apply his skills in typical work situations under the guidance of a qualified person. The person to whom the trainee has been assigned should be one who knows the job thoroughly, is a safe operator, and has the patience, time, and desire to help others. (See Fig. (9–3.)

The advantages of training of this type are:

1. The worker is more likely to be highly motivated because the guidance is personal.

2. The instructor can identify specific performance deficiencies and take immediate and proper corrective action.

3. Results of the training are readily apparent since real equipment is being used and finished work can be judged by existing standards.

4. The training is practical and realistic and can be applied at the proper time.

Timing is important; not only do the trainees like to get help when needed, but also the instructor can judge the trainee's progress continually so he can present the next unit or phase of instruction when the trainee is ready.

To help keep track of the progress of each individual, a training chart is valuable. On the top of the chart are listed the various tasks required of a person in a particular job classification. By observation and direct discussions, the instructor can determine whether the employee is qualified to perform the tasks necessary to fill the job. The instructor determines the degree of skill and knowledge of the trainee and estimates his training needs. Notes and comments can be made on the chart. Such a chart prevents neglecting training that is important; it also prevents unnecessary training. (See Fig. 9–4.)

### Job safety analysis

A job safety analysis (JSA) is a procedure to make a job safe by:

1. Identifying the hazards or potential accidents associated with each step of a job, and

2. Developing a solution for each hazard that will either eliminate or control the exposure.

**Benefits of JSA.** The principal benefits that arise from job safety analysis are these phases of a supervisor's work:

• Giving individual training in safe, efficient procedures

• Making employee safety contacts

• Instructing the new person on the job

• Preparing for planned safety observations

• Giving pre-job instructions on irregular jobs

• Reviewing job procedures after accidents occur

• Studying jobs for possible improvement in job methods

For further discussion and application of job safety analysis, see Chapter 5, "Removing the Hazard from the Job."

### Job instruction training

The job instruction training (JIT) method described here is often called the Four-Point

**251**

---

# JOB INSTRUCTION TRAINING (JIT)

## HOW TO GET READY TO INSTRUCT

**Have a Timetable—**
How much skill you expect the operator to have, by what date

**Break Down the Job—***
List important steps, pick out the key points. (Safety is always a key point.)

**Have Everything Ready—**
The right equipment, materials and supplies.

**Have the Workplace Properly Arranged—**
Just as the trainee will be expected to keep it.

*Use JSA, Job Safety Analysis, breakdown to locate hazards.

**SAFETY TRAINING INSTITUTE
NATIONAL SAFETY COUNCIL**

## HOW TO INSTRUCT

**1. Prepare**
Put trainee at ease.
Define the job and find out what he or she already knows about it.
Get the employee interested in learning the job.
Place in correct position.

**2. Present**
Tell, show, and illustrate one IMPORTANT STEP at a time.
Stress each KEY POINT.*

**3. Try Out Performance**
Have the employee do the job—coach him or her.
Have the employee explain each key point to you during the process.
Make sure the worker understands.
Continue until YOU know the worker knows.

**4. Follow Up**
Let the employee work independently.
Designate whom to go to for help.
Check frequently. Encourage questions.
Taper off extra coaching and close followup.

*Safety is always a key point.

---

FIG. 9–5.—Every supervisor should follow the JIT format when teaching job skills.

Method, because the instructing job is broken into four parts, each of which is shown in detail in Fig. 9–5:

1. Preparation
2. Presentation
3. Application
4. Testing.

Selection of the trainer in JIT is an important consideration. The supervisor can do the training or may choose to delegate that responsibility to a skilled person within the department. In either case, the instructor should have the following qualifications:

- Know the subject thoroughly
- Have a desire to teach
- Be friendly and cooperative
- Be a good leader
- Have a professional attitude.

The four-point method is intended to help an instructor teach a learner to do a specific job. It aims at faster learning and better learning. When combined with JSA, it becomes an excellent method for teaching safety along with job skills. (The reader will be relieved to know that it takes longer to describe some of these steps than it does to do them.)

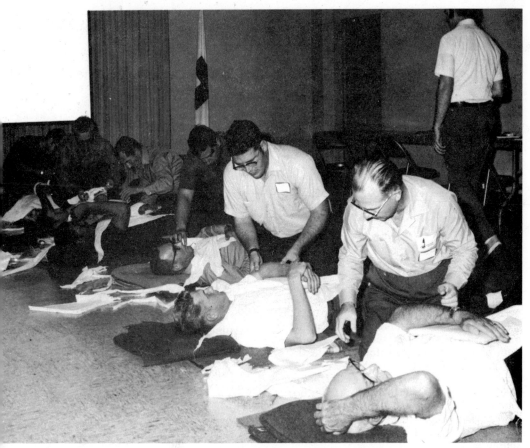

FɪG. 9–6.—First aid course teaches knowledge and skills necessary for emergency care and transport of victims. Both simulation and role playing are used as group techniques.

*Shell Pipeline Corporation, Rocky Mountain Division.*

## Conference Method of Teaching

To aid understanding and stimulate participation in instruction courses, industrial educators many years ago developed the conference method of teaching. This method is widely used in teaching management subjects to people in business and industry.

The conference leader should be skilled in this method of teaching. He should know how to draw out information and opinions from the conferees, and sum up their conclusions. As is desirable in a participation class, the number of people in a conference group should be small enough that free discussion can occur.

The leader's part is mainly that of asking questions that will provoke thinking and discussion. Learning can take place in a conference if the conferees have a background of experience that enables them to discuss the subject intelligently.

### Problem-solving conferences

Since a conference is a device for getting a job done, it is particularly useful in an area like safety where many people are involved. A conference yields big returns in education for all who participate, even though its immediate purpose is to solve a current problem, not merely a hypothetical one.

**253**

# 9—Safety Training

Frequently, the safety professional has problems relating to the operation of the safety program which needs to be discussed with production supervisors. The problem may have to do with the occurrence of a number of similar accidents, with some new feature of the safety program, with a new type of work to be undertaken, with a method of operation or plan to be worked out, or with any other subject in which both the supervisor and the safety department are interested. To find a solution to the problem, the safety professional may call a conference with a group of supervisors.

The conference leader should be familiar with the relationships of the members of the conference and with the general area of the subject matter.

It is of the utmost importance that the leader and members of the conference know the scope and limitations of what they are expected to do. If, for example, a conference is called to decide how to put into practice a policy or a directive that has been issued, the members should understand that it is not within their authority to have the policy or directive changed. If they meet to discuss improvement of procedures for the elimination of a hazard, they should know whether or not they may consider extensive alterations of buildings and installation of new machinery. If they do not know the limitations within which they must work, then the conference becomes a source of dissatisfaction and frustration or is regarded as simply play-acting.

If the job of a conference group is to recommend action and they do recommend action, they should, of course, know what becomes of their recommendation.

Often, however, a conference group will discuss a matter that affects only the members, in which case their conclusions are drawn for their own guidance. This is probably the most usual and most satisfactory kind of conference.

## Conference leading

Every safety professional and supervisor should attempt to become a skillful conference leader. Since such skill comes mainly from practice, opportunities for holding conferences should be accepted, even if he has not had a great deal of experience. The application of good sense and an understanding of what a conference is supposed to accomplish will go far toward making the conference successful.

The sequence of conference leading is as follows:

1. State the problem.

2. Break the problem into segments to keep the discussion orderly.

3. Encourage free discussion.

4. Make sure that members have given adequate consideration to all the significant points raised.

5. Note any conclusions that are reached.

6. State the final conclusion in such a way that it truly represents the findings of the group.

A person who attends many conferences has opportunities to observe examples of successful and unsuccessful conference leading. This should help him when he assumes the role of conference leader. The new leader should also seek help from training people and others who may give sound advice that can lead to productive conferences.

## Misuse of the conference method

If a conference leader, in his eagerness to get across his ideas or in order to cover ground quickly, departs from true conference procedures and steers the discussion in the way he wants it to go, then a meeting becomes a "conference" in name only.

Such a closely guided or controlled "conference" is not an effective teaching method. Worse still, because it is called a conference, it may establish in the minds of conferees and the leader a pattern of conduct that makes it difficult for them to serve usefully as members of a true conference. Conferences are almost indispensable in business, and any process that tends to make them unproductive should be avoided.

## Other Methods of Supervisory Training

Many methods of instruction and many teaching aids are available for training supervisors in accident prevention. Using a variety of methods in a single course or even in a single session makes for interest and understanding, so long as the methods chosen are appropriate for both the subject and the learners. Each training technique has its strengths and weaknesses, and each must be analyzed according to these criteria.

The economic factor can also be important. Taking the information that follows at its face value, one might conclude that "simulation" is a technique that can almost always be used. But simulators are expensive, and simulation games are time-consuming. This may not turn out to be the best choice. For example, with a small number of trainees and with many problems to be covered, the optimum selection may be a good instructor with a good understanding of the laws of learning and an ability to use good training techniques. On the other hand, if there is a large training load and relatively stable material, the best investment might be some sort of simulation.

All techniques have value as educational methods if they encourage participation.

Training techniques fall into three major categories: working with groups, working with individuals, and programmed instruction.

## Group techniques

Group training techniques encourage participants to share ideas, to evaluate information, to support each other in mutual development, and to participate in life-like situations that help in making decisions. When there are a large number of people to be trained quickly, some sort of group approach is called for.

**Brainstorming.** A form of creative thinking usually resulting from group interaction; technique of obtaining new ideas by the free association of ideas within a group. The technique is based on four groundrules:

1. Ideas that are presented should not be criticized.

2. "Free wheeling," or the building of new ideas on ideas just presented, is encouraged.

3. As many ideas as possible should be presented quickly.

4. The combination of ideas and improvement of those already before the group are encouraged.

The function of the moderator is to cut off negative comments quickly and to encourage full participation. A recorder is responsible for jotting down the ideas as the group presents them.

Brainstorming is good for developing ideas quickly, for stirring the imagination, and for involving timid persons. For best effectiveness, it is limited to five to ten people of fairly similar background.

**Buzz sessions.** A group is divided into smaller groups of four to six people. A question is presented and each group discusses it for a few minutes; the group selects one of its members to chair the discussion and another to record it. At the end of the time, the recorders summarize their group's thinking for the entire audience.

This technique permits wide participation, yet furnishes a screen for impractical ideas. A good briefing session should be held before the groups begin so that they can start quickly and accomplish something positive.

**Case study.** A report of a real situation that has occurred, or a structured situation—both are designed to develop basic concepts and principles. The study describes what has happened in a particular case and the events leading up to the situation, but it leaves to the group the task of deciding the nature of the problem or problems, their significance, and the probable solution.

This technique encourages participation, develops insight and ability to use problem-solving methods, and develops power of discrimination in drawing generalizations and conclusions. It is difficult, however, to evaluate either group or individual progress or results.

**Incident process.** A mini case study. This is a method of learning where an incident is presented to a group in written form. The individuals ask questions concerning relevant facts, clues, and details. The instructor supplies the answers to these questions, and the group assembles the facts, learns what happened and arrives at a decision.

Although the technique requires less reading and preparation than the case study, the discussion can easily turn into an argument unless it is properly controlled; the discussion may be limited to a few unless all are prepared.

**Discussion.** A procedure involving an exchanging of ideas and the standardizing of procedures and techniques. A discussion allows students to pool their knowledge and become active participants in a controlled program.

This procedure is very effective with small groups because the leader can fit the discussion to the backgrounds and needs of individuals. The direction of the discussion is difficult to control and can be time-consuming unless the leader is skillful.

**Role playing.** An instructional method in which incidents based on real-life situations are re-enacted by selected members of the class playing roles and making their own decisions. The decisions are discussed by the entire class and the instructor to bring out and highlight behavior patterns.

This technique is excellent for developing an understanding of how people behave in specific situations; it leads to good discussions. However, it needs careful planning, it must be kept democratic with the instructor not giving the answers, and it is not effective for solving problems.

**Lecture.** A discourse or talk to impart knowledge or to present new materials to a group; supplementary or background material is often passed out.

It works well with large groups with limited time. It is useful in motivating, developing attitudes, and summarizing. Students must be able to hear the lecturer.

**Panel.** A planned session consisting of two or more qualified persons, each discussing an assigned topic or subject.

Like the lecture, this technique permits a great deal of information to be imparted quickly; it is also nuidirectional in flow of information, unless a question-and-answer session follows.

**Question-and-answer sessions** can follow a lecture or a panel or be part of a discussion group.

Sessions are an excellent way to bring a group to understand new procedures or methods when they are familiar with old ones. It requires some preparation by the participants or only a few persons will be ready to ask questions.

**Simulation.** Simulation often involves a simulator, such as those used for driver trianing and pilot training. Railroads have also developed simulators for training engineers. Simulation can also be achieved by the use of various types of management games, such as the "in basket technique," "war games" developed by the military, and, more recently, simulation techniques for the training of astronauts in the proper operation of space capsules. Simulation is a good method for paralleling real-life or actual conditions, thus affording opportunities for decision making without risk. (See Fig. 9–6.)

It attains intense involvement among the participants. Careful planning and attention to details are required. Participants must be carefully selected and briefed for a meaningful learning experience. Initial cost is high. (It is discussed under Programmed Instruction later in this section.)

## Individual techniques

**Drill.** Repetition and guided practice to develop skill. Drills are used primarily for the most important and fundamental skills of a trade, job, or task.

**Demonstration.** A method widely used to teach skills. The operation is demonstrated by the instructor and then performed by the student as in job instruction training (JIT), discussed earlier in this chapter.

**Quizzes.** Usually given in written form and often of the objective, or multiple-choice, type. This technique is good for determining achievement of objectives; it is also used as a review procedure and as a check on individual comprehension.

**Television.** Educational TV and closed circuit TV (CCTV) are widely used for skill and other types of training.

Videotape training uses television's "instant replay" techniques. The basic technique is to record the visual procedure and the directions on a videotape and then play it back instantly by means of a monitor. Processes or manual skills, once recorded, can be replayed many times. This technique is good for training employees as well as supervisors.

Because it is also thought of as being an audiovisual, TV is discussed in Chapter 14, "Audiovisual Media."

**Reading material.** Companies should provide supervisors with reading material—safety newsletters, safety magazines, magazines on supervision, booklets, and reprints. Many companies subscribe to the National Safety Council's 16-page monthly magazine *Industrial Supervisor*, and some also issue a monthly bulletin devoted to safety which is distributed to all supervisors.

In addition to periodical material made available to supervisors, it is desirable to have a management library from which supervisors may borrow books on safety and related subjects and which can furnish information about books that are worth reading.

## Programmed instruction

Programmed instruction may be used as a substitute or supplement for classroom and textbook methods of supervisory training.

Programmed instruction, often called *PI*, is a self-teaching system that can be offered in a self-contained book or through some kind of a mechanical or electronic teaching machine. In both situations, the key to the value of the system is in the program or *software*. This is the term generally adopted for the developed material, in contrast with the machinery and equipment which are termed *hardware*.

The program is presented to the learner in a series of small, sequential steps, carefully planned to progress from the simple to the complex. The student is guided through the program according to the nature of his response. At intervals, he must make an active response that tests his comprehension of the material. He writes in an answer, fills in a missing word or phrase, chooses a correct statement or picture. He then gets an immediate response of some kind.

The nature of his response will determine what happens next. In general, he will be told to advance if his answer is correct or to reread the preceding statement if his answer is wrong. Or he may be directed to a related problem, depending on the nature of his incorrect response.

This may be done through the physical structure of a book, which directs the student to a specific page for each answer, correct or incorrect. A computer also can be programmed to present the desired material according to which answer has just been selected. The teaching machine may, for example, include a filmstrip that will not advance until the correct answer has been indicated to the question just presented. A computer can be programmed to bring up what is most appropriate according to the instructions written into its program.

The responses of a machine to those of the student can be very complex. A good example of this is the simulator, described earlier, which has been developed to train automobile and bus drivers, airline pilots, and locomotive engineers. The trainee is placed in a realistic replica of his working position. Through his windows or on a TV screen, he sees a projection of a scene. He operates his controls in response to what he sees in the constantly changing projection. His instruments respond, and the projection changes to give him the feeling of moving through reality. In some simulators, the instructor can introduce stimuli to which the student must respond. Many of the computer-based systems have the capacity to record student responses, both in their degree of accuracy and in time taken.

PI guides the progress of the learner by means of immediate confirmation of the correctness of his responses, and controls the learner's orderly process in much the same way as a tutor. It permits each student to progress at the rate that he selects.

It has many of the advantages of a human tutor, although it lacks the ability of a human to adapt to new situations. It knows whether the student has selected the right response or not, but it does not know his reasons for the selection. Was it a knowledgeable answer, or simply a lucky guess? What flaw in reasoning led the student to a wrong answer? A good instructor, on a one-to-one basis, can often determine this through observation and experience, characteristics that are difficult to build into a computer program.

Writing a programmed instructional course is a time-consuming process. The writer must make sure that each step is clear, and the reason for selecting each of the responses represents, as much as possible, a single kind of misunderstanding or lack of understanding. This is essential if the right kind of correctional material is to be presented. Obviously, this is an expensive operation and can be justified only if the number of trainees is large or if other training techniques are more expensive.

Additional details of PI methods and examples of programs are given in the Council's book *Communications for the Safety Professional* (see References).

## School courses

**Independent study.** Courses offered through correspondence are often called home study courses or independent study courses. These have some advantages over other methods described—the student can set his own pace, and he can study on his own time (which makes home study an ideal training method where a company's operations are scattered).

The National Safety Council offers two courses of this type for training supervisors—"Supervising for Safety," and "Human Relations for Supervisors."

See listings of many courses in Chapter 24, "Sources of Help."

**Seminars and short courses.** A number of seminars and short courses are offered by colleges and universities on all phases of supervisory know-how. Insurance companies and private organizations also offer supervisory training courses. Check locally for what is available.

## Personal instruction and coaching

Often overlooked as a method of instruction is personal discussion with individual supervisors. When the safety professional and the supervisor meet and talk about the job, there can be a complete and free interchange of ideas that is not possible in a group. In private conversation, the supervisor will often express reservations or doubts that he would not voice in a meeting, and the safety professional will have the opportunity to clear up misunderstandings.

The safety professional who meets with the individual supervisor not only instructs and coaches, but also learns many things he needs to know. Supervisors appreciate his interest in their work and are usually eager to teach him about the processes of their departments. The safety professional can learn much from them about the mechanical processes and also about problems of supervision. Possibly most important is that he becomes personally acquainted with the supervisors. Every safety professional ought to allot a part of his time to these personal contacts.

## Policies and Attitudes in Supervisory Training

The person conducting a training program for supervisors should remember a number of facts which experienced educators know.

## Teaching at the adult level

Supervisors are adults; they must be treated accordingly. The smart supervisor is aware that a portion of his job is to get out production and do it safely. Safety is not a separate job to be done when other responsibilities permit time to do it. Rather, the supervisor should be thinking in terms of *producing safely.*

In this regard, the supervisor very likely reflects the attitude of the immediate superior as to what is important. If the superior lets it be known that the supervisor will be measured in terms of the safety job to be done, the proper attention will be given to that portion of the overall job. This fact is a strong argument for starting safety education at the upper levels of supervision.

## Integrating safety into all training

In a company that has a formal training program, safety training should fit into that program; the director of training and the safety professional should work together in the planning of various kinds of safety training activity.

In the training of supervisors—usually the first concern of a training department—practically everything that is taught about good supervision helps to promote safety. Likewise, anything taught specifically for the purpose of promoting safety generally improves supervision in other ways.

In the arrangement of formal courses, safety subjects may be integrated with other instruction on general problems of supervision, or one or two safety meetings may be included in the course.

The number of participants in a class of supervisors should be small enough to allow free discussion; fifteen is about the upper limit. The leader uses carefully planned questions when he wants to get people to talk. There is no limit to the visual aids and demonstrations and other devices that are available to make the material interesting and educational, and the discussions easy to follow.

## Continuing programs get best results

Safety training for supervisors needs to be a continuing program if it is to accomplish the best results. The program should cover many subjects, presented interestingly and in different ways. A limited effort, such as holding a few meetings, may cause supervisors to do a better job for a short time, but interest will lag if the initial effort is not followed up.

Industrial management must be dynamic because change is continually taking place. New methods and new ideas get attention. To hold its own in this atmosphere of change and progress, safety, too, must not be allowed to become static.

The safety professional who strives constantly to help line supervisors take over direct responsibility for safety in their operations finds the results of those efforts multiplied many fold. He becomes a true leader who gets the job done better, not by extending the scope of his own activities, but by helping supervisors assume their natural safety responsibilities.

## Training New Employees

Safety training begins at the time of employment, before the employee starts work. An effective safety training program will include a carefully prepared and presented introduction to the company.

When a new employee comes to work, many new things are learned immediately. Attitudes are formed about the company, the job, the boss, and fellow employees. This happens whether or not the employer makes an effort to train the person. In order for the new employee to learn the things necessary to do a safe, productive job and to develop proper attitudes toward safety, the employer will want to provide the right kind of start.

### Indoctrination

At the beginning of his employment, each employee should know the company's safety policy, but the amount he can learn during the induction procedure is limited. Unfamiliarity with his surroundings, interest in many matters of seemingly more immediate concern, the detailed procedure of getting onto the payroll—all make it difficult for the employee to absorb and retain much safety instruction. It is necessary, therefore, to consider what safety information must be given first, and then the best way to present it.

Each employee needs to learn the following things if he is to have a good start in safety training:

1. Management is sincerely interested in preventing accidents.

2. Accidents may occur, but it is possible to prevent them.

3. Safeguarding equipment and the workplace has been thoroughly done, and management is willing to go further as needs and methods are discovered.

4. Each employee is expected to report to his supervisor unsafe conditions which he encounters in his work.

5. The supervisor will give job instructions. No employee is expected to undertake a job until he has learned how to do it and is authorized to do it by his supervisor.

6. No employee should undertake a job that appears to him to be unsafe.

7. If an employee suffers an injury, even a slight one, it must be reported at once.

In addition to these points, any safety rules which are a condition of employment, such as wearing of eye protection or safety hats, should be understood and enforced at once.

### Preliminary instruction

This preliminary safety instruction is most often given to individuals or small groups by the personnel department. Sometimes the safety professional or a management executive gives the safety instruction. This method may add force and interest, but it has the practical disadvantage that safety professionals and executives are busy people and may not always be available or may be so pressed with other duties that they skimp on the introduction job or delegate it to subordinates less able to handle it.

More important than who gives the talk is how it is given. The talk should be prepared and presented with the utmost regard for the effect it will have on the new employees. Verbal instruction should be given earnestly and with an attitude of good will and friendly cooperation.

A safety film may do a good job of interesting and instructing new employees. It changes the pace and relieves the monotony of much talking. The film should be brief and should be limited to such essential points as those previously mentioned.

Some companies produce their own films. Although the production of a film may seem costly, if it is shown to all new employees, the cost per employee showing may be only a few cents. Films for the purpose may also be purchased. Other companies have had good results with sound-slide shows. (See Chapter 14, "Audiovisual Media," for comparisons.)

One important advantage of an induction film is that it can present a carefully planned message in a consistent and effective manner. Management can be sure that its safety message is going to be told in exactly the same way to every new employee.

Charts illustrating points presented in the induction talk add interest and aid both understanding and conviction. Charts should be large enough and simple enough to be seen and understood easily by every member of the group.

If a company has preplacement physical examinations, the doctor or nurse should establish good relations with each new employee at the time of the examination. The doctor or nurse should tell about the work of the medical department as it relates to the employees and should encourage them to make use of its services. Medical or nursing personnel, as well as the person who gives general safety information, should emphasize the importance of reporting all injuries.

The final step in the personnel office safety procedure should be to emphasize the importance of the position of the supervisor in the safety program. The employee must understand that the supervisor is responsible for job training, and that such training will include safe work procedures.

In order that there will be no gap and no contradiction between the information given in the employment office and that given later, the supervisor should know what has been covered in the induction talks.

## Make rule books logical, enforceable

The use of rule books or manuals° has long been a part of the early training given to new employees. Such rule books should be prepared so the rules are presented in terms that are easily understood. Only logical and enforceable rules should be included. Employees cannot be expected to respect and follow rules that are illogical, unfair, or unrealistic.

Rules that supervisors have had a chance to review are likely to be more effective than those they have had no part in formulating.

Rule books or manuals should contain general instructions as to the employee's responsibility in safety. The rules should cover such items as first aid, personal protective equipment, work clothing, firefighting, electrical equipment, and housekeeping.

Rule books alone cannot be counted upon to accomplish much in the way of influencing attitudes. Well-prepared, illustrated booklets or cards, however, can add much to the start of a good training program if the contents are briefly reviewed and discussed when the booklets are presented and if the employee is not loaded with a great mass of printed matter. (See Fig. 9–7.)

## Departmental induction and training

When a new employee reaches his own department, his supervisor should give him additional safety instruction. This may cover some of the points made in the employment office interview, but now applied specifically to the kind of work the employee is going to do.

The supervisor may repeat the earlier instruction about reporting unsafe conditions, not undertaking a job without instruction and authorization, and other matters of policy. The supervisor should tell the new employee about the safety record and the safety program of the department.

The supervisor will explain general safety regulations of the department and will see that the new employee is provided with the personal protective equipment furnished by the company for the job. The supervisor will also make provisions for training in safe work procedures. He will make certain to follow up to make sure that safe procedures are achieved.

Some safety departments have followup interviews with employees from one week to one month after employment. At this time, the safety professional reviews the points discussed at the time of employment and encourages the employee to talk about his experiences on the job.

Companies following this plan report that discussion with an employee after a few days on the job is more profitable than information given before the employee starts work. The new person has overcome his feeling of strangeness and uneasiness and can relate the discussion to what he has already experienced. If the personnel department handles the initial safety instruction, it is especially desirable for a representative of the safety department to talk with the employee a few days later.

Of course, any direct contact by the safety department with an employee should be with the knowledge and approval of the employee's

---

°The development, approval, and distribution of printed safety rules by industrial concerns are discussed in National Safety Council Data Sheet 664, *Writing and Publishing Employee Safety Regulations*. The Council also publishes a number of rule booklets and leaflets on both general and specific subjects, aimed at employees.

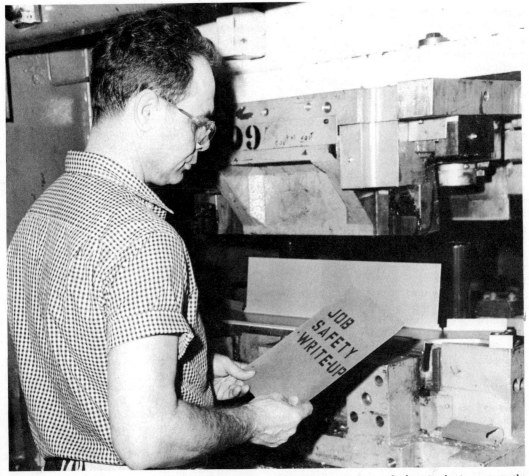

FIG. 9–7.—A job safety analysis, called a "job safety write-up" by some companies, can be kept in plastic case near the equipment so that the operator can review it at any time, especially when he starts a different job. Also, it is readily available for the supervisor to use for training a new operator on the job.

*Courtesy* Automotive, Tooling, Metalworking, and Associated Industries Newsletter.

supervisor.

This induction procedure is the least a new employee should receive if he is to get a real feeling that safety is important to his job, and if he is to understand the company's attitude toward safety.

Some companies have more elaborate induction programs. These may include a plant tour, discussion of the company's products, viewing a film, and listening to talks by representatives of various departments. The program may take one-half to a full day.

Companies having formal induction training programs are convinced that they pay off in lower labor turnover, in good employee relations, and in prevention of accidents.

In these programs, it is the job of the safety department to make sure that safety is presented as interestingly and effectively as any part of the program. Safety must not be submerged in a mass of information so that it will be remembered only vaguely, if at all. *The employee must carry away a deep conviction that safety is important to himself and his company.*

# 9—Safety Training

## Good supervision—consistent instruction and "discipline"

A consistent training program should include the supervisory function as a part of job instruction.

If the supervisor observes workers taking short cuts or otherwise departing from safe methods, he should correct them at once. If he does not correct them, the unsafe method soon becomes standard practice.

Much has been said about "discipline" for violations of safe practices. "Discipline" in this connection means penalties, usually following an oral or written warning and in the form of time off without pay. Probably every employer recognizes the theoretical necessity for penalties to punish willful misconduct, whether the offense has to do with safety rules or other company regulations. Actually, such penalties are rarely assessed and many companies never use them at all.

Too often, violations of safety rules are overlooked until an accident occurs. If employees are corrected for every infraction of a safety rule or safe practice as soon as it is observed, there will be few occasions which require "discipline." In any event, if a penalty is to be assessed, it should be for the act and not for the accident.

## First aid courses

First aid courses for employees have been conducted in some industries for many years. The American National Red Cross or the Mine Safety and Health Administration have excellent courses. The need for personnel trained in first aid is spelled out in OSHA requirements if there is no infirmary, clinic, hospital, or physician in proximity or reasonably accessible.

The direct value of first aid training is greatest in companies that have night shifts, or skeleton crews working, when medical facilities are closed or where field crews are working at points far removed from professional medical help. Public utilities, mines, oil-well drilling, and logging are a few operations where employees have become proficient in caring for seriously injured persons and in transporting them to the hospital. Providing instruction in first aid is a necessity in these industries. (See Fig. 9–6.)

Even in companies with complete medical departments, trained first-aiders are a potential asset because they can stop dangerous bleeding, administer artificial respiration, and transport injured workers safely. Not only can they render these services, which may be needed at any time, but their value in a disaster would be great.

In addition to its possible direct benefit on the job, first aid training has inherent interest for employees. On the theory that first aid students learn something about the causes of accidents and acquire an accident awareness that makes them cautious, some companies that sponsor courses believe that instruction in first aid makes an employee less likely to have accidents.

Companies sponsoring first aid courses usually arrange for a qualified instructor, provide a meeting place, pay for textbooks and supplies, and often reward the graduates with a dinner or other celebration.

## The so-called "accident-prone" individual

Probably no phrase in safety causes so much disagreement as to what it exactly means that does "accident proneness." Most definitions hinge upon the idea that a person with certain personality traits is very likely to have accidents. When a person is said to be "accident-prone," it is generally meant that some psychological characteristics he has predisposes him toward having accidents.

Too often the term is loosely applied to anyone who has more accidents than others who do the same type work. A person could, however, have more than his share of accidents because he never was trained properly, or because he needs new glasses, or simply because he is working in cramped quarters or where he can be jostled. Behavior of this type may also be due to poor supervision or the attitude of management toward accident prevention. A language barrier may be a factor in other cases.

It is true that a small group of people often account for more than their expected share of accidents during a given period, but over a long time period, the composition of the group changes—the accident repeaters of one time period do not usually show up during the next time period. Much more research has to be done in this field before any person can be positively identified as being accident prone. Above all, such a label should not be placed in the personnel file of any individual.

See the Council's book *Supervisors Guide to Human Relations* for a detailed discussion of "accident-" and "safety-prone" persons.

## OSHA and MSHA Training Requirements

The continued importance of training is evidenced by the significance placed upon it by the requirements of both the Occupational Safety and Health Administration and the Mine Safety and Health Administration.

### OSHA requirements

Listed next are the major parts of the OSHA regulations (Title 29—Labor, *Code of Federal Regulations*) that include training requirements and a convenient index indicating the type of hazard and the parts of the regulations requiring training to protect against the hazard.

Part 1910, Safety and Health Training Requirements for General Industry

Part 1915-18, Safety and Health Training Requirements for Maritime Employment

Part 1926, Safety and Health Training Requirements for Construction

Part 1928, Occupational Safety and Health Requirements for Agriculture.

An index of OSHA training requirements is given in Table 9–A.

TABLE 9–A
INDEX TO OSHA TRAINING REQUIREMENTS

| Hazard | Part | Subpart | Section |
|--------|------|---------|---------|
| Blasting or Explosives | 1910.109 | H | (d)(3)(i)(iii) |
| | 1926.901 | U | (c) |
| | 1926.902 | U | (i) |
| | 1915.10 | B | (a) thru (b) |
| | 1916.10 | B | (a) thru (b) |
| | 1917.10 | B | (a) thru (b) |
| Carcinogens | | | |
| 4-Nitrobiphenyl | 1910.1003 | Z | (e)(5)(i) thru (ii) |
| alpha-Naphthylamine | 1910.1004 | Z | (e)(5)(i) thru (ii) |
| 4,4'-Methylene bis (2-chloroaniline) | 1910.1005 | Z | (e)(5)(i) thru (ii) |
| Methyl chloromethyl ether | 1910.1006 | Z | (e)(5)(i) thru (ii) |
| 3,3'-Dichlorobenzidine (and its salts) | 1910.1007 | Z | (e)(5)(i) thru (ii) |
| bis-Chloromethyl ether | 1910.1008 | Z | (e)(5)(i) thru (ii) |
| beta-Naphthylamine | 1910.1009 | Z | (e)(5)(i) thru (ii) |
| Benzidine | 1910.1010 | Z | (e)(5)(i) thru (ii) |
| 4-Aminodiphenyl | 1910.1011 | Z | (e)(5)(i) thru (ii) |
| Ethyleneimine | 1910.1012 | Z | (e)(5)(i) thru (ii) |
| beta-Propiolactone | 1910.1013 | Z | (e)(5)(i) thru (ii) |
| 2-Acetylaminofluorene | 1910.1014 | Z | (e)(5)(i) thru (ii) |
| 4-Dimethylamino-azobenzene | 1910.1015 | Z | (e)(5)(i) thru (ii) |
| N-Nitrosodi-methylamine | 1910.1016 | Z | (e)(5)(i) thru (ii) |
| Vinyl chloride | 1910.1017 | Z | (j)(1)(i) thru (ix) |
| Cranes and Derricks | 1910.179 | N | (m)(3)(ix) |
| | 1910.180 | N | (h)(3)(xii) |
| Decompression or Compression | 1926.803 | S | (a)(2) |
| | 1926.803 | S | (b)(10)(xii) |
| | 1926.803 | S | (e)(1) |
| Employee Responsibility | 1910.109 | H | (g)(3)(iii)(a) |
| | 1926.609 | U | (a) |

*(Table concluded on next page.)*

## TABLE 9-A (Concluded). INDEX TO OSHA TRAINING REQUIREMENTS

| Hazard | Part | Subpart | Section |
|---|---|---|---|
| Equipment Operations | 1910.217 | O | (f)(2) |
| | 1926.20 | C | (b)(4) |
| | 1926.53 | D | (b) |
| | 1926.54 | D | (a) |
| | 1910.252 | Q | (c)(6) |
| Fire Protection | 1916.32 | D | (e) |
| | 1917.32 | D | (b) |
| | 1926.150 | F | (a)(5) |
| | 1926.155 | F | (e) |
| | 1926.351 | J | (d)(1) thru (5) |
| | 1926.901 | U | (c) |
| Forging | 1910.218 | O | (a)(2)(i) thru (iv) |
| Gases, Fuel, Toxic Material, Explosives | 1910.109 | H | (d)(3)(i) and (iii) |
| | 1910.111 | H | (b)(13)(ii) |
| | 1910.266 | R | (c)(5)(i) thru (xi) |
| | 1910.106 | H | (b)(5)(vi)(v)(3) |
| | 1916.35 | D | (d)(1) thru (6) |
| | 1926.21 | C | (a) and (b)(2) thru (6) |
| | 1926.350 | J | (d)(1) thru (6) |
| General | 1926.21 | C | (a) |
| Hazardous Material | 1915.57 | F | (d) |
| | 1916.57 | F | (d) |
| | 1917.57 | F | (d) |
| Medical and First Aid | 1910.94 | G | (d)(9)(i) and (vi) |
| | 1910.151 | K | (a) and (b) |
| | 1915.58 | K | (a) |
| | 1917.58 | F | (a) |
| | 1926.50 | D | (c) |
| Personal Protective Equipment | 1910.94 | G | (d)(11)(v) |
| | 1910.134 | I | (a)(3) |
| | 1910.134 | I | (b)(1), (2) and (3) |
| | 1910.134 | I | (e)(2), (3) and (5) |
| | 1910.161 | K | (a)(2) |
| | 1915.82 | I | (a)(4) |
| | 1915.82 | I | (b)(4) |
| | 1916.57 | F | (f) |
| | 1916.58 | F | (a) |
| | 1916.82 | I | (a)(4) |
| | 1916.82 | I | (b)(4) |
| | 1917.57 | F | (f) |
| | 1918.102 | J | (a)(4) |
| | 1926.21 | C | (b)(2) thru (6) |
| | 1926.103 | E | (c)(1) |
| | 1926.800 | S | (e)(xii) |
| Pulpwood Logging | 1910.266 | R | (c)(5)(i) thru (xi) |
| | 1910.266 | R | (c)(6)(i) thru (xxi) |
| | 1910.266 | R | (c)(7) |
| | 1910.266 | R | (e)(2)(i) and (ii) |
| | 1910.266 | R | (e)(9) |
| | 1910.266 | R | (e)(1)(iii) thru (vii) |
| Powder-Actuated Tools | 1915.75 | H | (b)(1) thru (6) |
| | 1916.75 | H | (b)(1) thru (6) |
| Power Press | 1910.217 | O | (e)(3) |
| Power Trucks, Motor Vehicles, or Agricultural Tractors | 1910.109 | H | (d)(3)(iii) |
| | 1910.109 | H | (g)(3)(iii)(a) |
| | 1910.178 | N | (1) |
| | 1910.266 | R | (e)(9) |
| | 1910.266 | R | (e)(6)(viii) |
| | 1928.51 | C | (d) |
| Radioactive Material | 1916.37 | D | (b) |
| Signs—Danger, Warning, Instruction | 1910.96 | G | (f)(3)(viii) |
| | 1910.145 | J | (c)(1)(ii) |
| | 1910.145 | J | (c)(2)(ii) |
| | 1910.145 | J | (c)(3) |
| | 1910.264 | R | (d)(1)(v) |
| Tunnels and Shafts | 1926.800 | S | (e)(xiii) |
| Welding | 1910.252 | Q | (b)(1)(iii) |
| | 1910.252 | Q | (c)(1)(iii) |
| | 1915.35 | D | (d)(1) thru (6) |
| | 1915.36 | D | (d)(1) thru (4) |
| | 1916.35 | D | (d)(1) thru (6) |
| | 1917. | D | (d)(1) thru (6) |

## MSHA regulations

The following is a summary of the training requirements under the MSHA Regulations, published in the *Federal Register*, Vol. 43, No. 199, October 13, 1978.

### Subpart B—Training and Retraining Miners Working at Surface Mines and Surface Areas of Underground Mines

#### §48.21 SCOPE.

Subpart B sets forth the mandatory requirements for submitting and obtaining approval of programs for training and retraining miners at surface mines and surface areas of underground mines. It also includes requirements for compensation for training and retraining.

#### §48.22 DEFINITIONS.

(a) "Miner"—Any person working in a surface mine or surface area of an underground mine and who is engaged in the extraction and production process, or is *regularly* exposed to mine hazards, or who is a maintenance or service worker (whether employed by operator or contractor) working at the mine for frequent or extended periods.

Short-term, specialized contract workers (drillers, blasters, etc.) who have received training under §48.26 (training of newly employed experienced miners) may be trained under §48.31 (hazard training) in lieu of other subsequent training.

Excluded from definition

   (i)    Construction, shaft and slope workers covered in Subpart C, Part 48.

   (ii)   Supervisory personnel (covered under MSHA-approved state certification requirements).

   (iii)  Delivery, office or scientific or short-term maintenance workers and any student engaged in *academic* projects.

(b) "Experienced miner." A person currently employed as a miner; or a person who received training *acceptable* to MSHA from an *appropriate* state agency within the preceding one month; a person with 12 months experience working in surface operations during the preceding 3 years; a person who received new miner training (§48.25) within the past 12 months.

(c) "New miner." Not experienced.

(d) "Normal working hours." Regularly scheduled work hours.

(e) "Operator." Owner, lessee, person that controls or supervises the operation; or any contractor performing similar function.

(f) "Task." Regular work assignment which requires physical abilities and job knowledge.

(g) "Act." The Federal Mine Safety and Health Act of 1977.

#### §48.23 TRAINING PLANS

(a) Each operator shall have a MSHA-approved plan for training:
New miners.
Newly employed experienced miners
Miners for new tasks

## 9—Safety Training

For annual refresher
For hazard.

(1) Existing mines shall submit the training plan to MSHA for approval within 150 days of the effective date (October 13, 1978). The plans must be filed by March 11, 1979.

(2) Unless extended, MSHA shall approve the operator's plan within 60 days.

(3) New mines—reopened mines. Must have an approved plan prior to (re)opening.

(b) Training plan shall be filed with the Chief of Training Center, MSHA, for the area in which the mine is located.

(c) Information to be filed:

(1) Company name
Mine name
MSHA I.D. number.

(2) Name and position of person responsible for health and safety training.

(3) List of MSHA-approved instructors along with the courses they are qualified to teach.

(4) Location of training site.

(5) Description of teaching methods and course materials which are to be used.

(6) Number of miners. Maximum number of miners to attend each session.

(7) Refresher training—a schedule of time or period of time when such training will be given. To include titles of courses, total number of instruction hours for each course, and predicted time and length of each session.

(8) New task training for miners.

(i) Submit complete list of task assignments to correspond with the definition of "task."

(ii) Titles of the instructors.

(iii) Outline training procedure for each work assignment.

(iv) The evaluation procedures used to determine the effectiveness of training.

(d) Two weeks prior to plan submission, a copy of the plan shall be given to the employees' representatives.

Should there be no employee representative, the plan shall be posted on the mine bulletin board two weeks prior to submission.

All written comments from employees must be delivered to MSHA. Miners may deliver such comments directly to MSHA.

(e) The training plan is subject to review and evaluation by MSHA. Course materials, including visual aids, handouts, etc., must be available to MSHA. At the request of MSHA, the operator must alter, change or modify the plan.

A schedule of upcoming training must be given to MSHA.

(f) A copy of the APPROVED plan must be available at the mine for MSHA, miners, and miners' representatives.

(g) All courses shall be conducted by MSHA-approved instructors except as provided for in the "New Task Training of Miners" and "Hazard Training" sections.

(h) Instructors are approved in the following ways:

    (1) Receive instructor training from MSHA or from a person designated qualified by MSHA.

    (2) Instructors may be approved by MSHA to teach specific courses based on written evidence of qualifications and teaching experience.

    (3) MSHA may approve instructors based on the performance of the instructors while teaching classes are monitors by MSHA. This program must be approved in advance by MSHA.

    (4) Cooperative instructors, designated by MSHA to teach approved courses within the past 24 months, shall be considered approved.

(i) MSHA can revoke the approval of an instructor for good cause. There is a specific appeal procedure provided.

(j) MSHA shall notify the operator and miners' representative in writing the statue of the MSHA approval within 60 days from the date the plan is submitted.

    (1) Any revision to the plan required by MSHA in order to gain approval shall be given to the operator and employees' representative. The operator and the employees' representative have the right to discuss alternative revisions or changes with MSHA—within a specified period of time.

    (2) MSHA can approve portions of a plan and withhold approval on the balance.

(k) Training shall begin within 60 days after approval of the plan.

(l) The operator shall submit any proposed changes or modifications to an approved plan to the employees' representative and MSHA prior to making such changes. MSHA must approve such changes prior to implementation.

(m) MSHA must notify, in writing, the operator and employee representative of the disapproval or recommended changes to the submitted plan. Such notification will include:

    (1) State specific changes or deficiency.

    (2) Action needed to bring plan into compliance.

    (3) MSHA will take punitive action against the operator should remedial action to effect compliance be delayed or ignored.

(n) All MSHA-recommended changes shall be posted on the bulletin board and a copy of same delivered to the employees' representative.

## §48.24 Cooperative Training Program

(a) Training programs may be conducted by the operator, MSHA, MSHA-approved programs conducted by state or other federal agencies, or associations of operators or miners' representatives, private associations, or educational institutions.

(b) Instructors and courses shall be approved by MSHA.

## §48.25 Training of New Miners. Minimum courses of instruction; hours of instruction.

(a) Each new miner shall receive not less than 24 hours of training. Unless otherwise stated, this training shall take place before they start work duties. At the discretion of MSHA, a new miner may receive a portion of this training after he starts his work duties. Provided, that not less than 8 hours of training shall be given before the employee starts work. This first 8 hour training shall include:

    (1) Introduction to work environment

(2) Hazard recognition

(3) Health and safety aspects of the tasks assigned.

The remainder of the 24 hours training or up to 16 hours will be given within 60 days. This program must be approved by MSHA. Certain conditions at a mine, such as employee turnover, mine size or safety record may cause MSHA to require the full 24 hour training prior to the start of work.

(b) New miner training program shall include:

(1) Instruction in the statutory rights of miners and their representatives.

Authority and responsibility of supervisors

A review and description of the line of authority of supervisors and miners' representatives.

Introduction to mine rules and procedures for reporting hazards.

(2) Self-rescue and respiratory devices—instruction and demonstration in the use, care, and maintenance (where applicable).

(3) Transportation controls and communication systems—instruction on the procedures in effect for riding on and in mine conveyances where applicable; the controls for the transportation of miners and materials; use of mine communication systems, warning signals, and directional signs.

(4) Introduction to work environment. Includes tour of mine and a description of the entire operation.

(5) Escape and emergency evacuation plans, fire warning and firefighting. Review mine escape system and emergency evacuation plans and instructions in fire warning signals and firefighting procedures.

(6) Ground control; working in areas of high walls, water hazards, pits and spoil banks; illumination and night work.

(7) Health—instruction includes the purpose of taking dust measurements and noise and other health measurements, and any health control plan at the mine shall be explained. The operator shall explain the health provisions of the act and warning labels.

(8) Hazard recognition—course includes recognition and avoidance of hazards present in the mine.

(9) Electrical hazards—includes recognition and avoidance of electrical hazards.

(10) First Aid—must be a MSHA-approved course.

(11) Explosives—includes a review and instruction on the hazards related to explosives. This course can be omitted if no explosives are used or stored at the mine.

(12) Health and safety aspects of the tasks to which the new miner will be assigned. The course includes instruction in the health and safety aspects of the work, the safe work procedures, and the mandatory health and safety standards pertinent to the work.

(13) Any other courses deemed necessary by MSHA based on special circumstances and conditions at the mine.

(c) The training plan shall include oral, written or practical demonstration methods to determine successful completion of the training. These methods shall be administered to the miner prior to assignment to work duties.

(d) A newly employed miner who has received the full 24 hours training within the 12 months preceding employment need not go through the operator's new miner training program. However, the miner will have to receive and complete the instruction for the "newly employed experienced miner" and "new task training of miners before commencing."

§48.26 Training of Newly Employed Experienced Miners, Minimum Courses of Instruction

(a) The newly employed experienced miner shall receive and complete the training listed below before being assigned to work duties.

(b) The training program includes the following:

(1) Introduction to work environment. Includes a tour of the operation and a description of the total operation.

(2) Mandatory health and safety standards. Includes those standards pertinent to the tasks assigned.

(3) Authority and responsibility of supervisors and miners' representatives. Includes a review of supervisors and miners' representatives line of authority, and the responsibility of such persons. Also, an introduction to the operator's rules and procedures for reporting hazards.

(4) Transportation controls and communication system. Includes instruction on the procedures for riding on and in mine conveyances; controls for the transportation of miners and materials; and use of the mine communication system, warning signal, and directional signs.

(5) Escape and emergency evacuation plans; fire warning and firefighting. Includes review of the mine escape system; escape and emergency evacuation plans and instruction in the fire warning signals and firefighting procedures.

(6) Ground controls; working in areas of high walls, water hazards, pits and spoil banks; illumination and night work. Includes introduction and instruction on the high wall and ground control plans; procedures for working near high walls, water hazards, pits and spoil banks, illuminated work areas, and procedures for working during hours of darkness.

(7) Hazard recognition. Includes recognition and avoidance of hazards, particularly any hazards related to explosives where explosives are used or stored at the mine.

(8) Any other courses MSHA deems necessary based on special mine circumstances and conditions.

§48.27 Training of Miners Assigned to a Task in Which They Have Had No Previous Experience; Minimum Courses of Instruction

(a) A miner shall be trained to safely perform any new work task prior to starting such work. The exceptions to this rule are:

(1) If the miner received such training within the preceding 12 months and can demonstrate knowledge of the safe procedures.

(2) If the miner performed the work within the preceding 12 months and can demonstrate knowledge of the safe procedures.

The training program shall include the following:

(i) Health and safety aspects and safe operating procedures for work tasks, equipment or machinery. Includes instruction in the health and safety aspects and safe operating procedures and given on-the-job.

(ii) Supervised practice during nonproduction. Practice training in the work task will be conducted at times or places where production is not the primary objective.

Supervised operation during production. Training will be conducted while under supervision and during production in the operation of equipment and performance of work task.

(iii) NEW or MODIFIED machines and equipment. Where new or different operating procedures are required as a result of new or modified equipment, the miner will be fully trained in the new procedures.

(iv) Any additional courses MSHA may deem necessary as a result of special conditions or circumstances at the mine.

(b) Miners shall not operate equipment or engage in blasting operations without direction and immediate supervision until the miner has demonstrated safe operating procedures for equipment or blasting operation.

(c) Miners assigned to a new task not covered in the paragraph shall be instructed in the safety and health aspects and safe procedures of the task prior to starting such task.

(d) All training and supervised practice shall be given by qualified trainers or experienced supervisor or other person experienced in the new task.

§48.28 ANNUAL REFRESHER. Training of miners.

(a) Required—8 hours of annual refresher.

(b) Refresher shall include the following:

(1) Mandatory health and safety standards. The standards relating to the miner's task.

(2) Transportation controls and communication system. (Same as paragraph 48.26, b, 4.)

(3) Escape and emergency evacuation plans; fire warning and fire fighting. (Same as paragraph 48.26, b, 5.)

(4) Ground control; working in areas of high walls, water hazards, pits and spoil banks; illumination and night work. (Same as paragraph 48.26, b, 6.)

(5) First aid—method acceptable to MSHA.

(6) Electrical Hazards—recognition and avoidance of electrical hazards.

(7) Prevention of accidents—review of accidents and their causes and instruction in accident prevention in the work environment.

(8) Health—explain purpose for taking dust, noise and other health measurements, and any health control plan in effect at the mine. Further, explain warning labels and health provisions of act.

(9) Explosives—review and instruct on the hazards related to explosives: This course is not needed when explosives are not used or stored at the mine.

(10) Self-rescue and respiratory devices. Instruct and demonstrate the use, care and maintenance of self-rescue and respiratory devices.

(11) Any additional courses MSHA may deem necessary.

(c) All experienced miners will receive refresher training within 90 days after the training plan is approved by MSHA.

(d) Annual refresher training sessions shall not be less than 30 minutes of actual instruction time and miners shall be notified that the session is part of annual refresher training.

§48.29 RECORDS OF TRAINING

(a) Upon completion of the MSHA-approved training, the operator shall record and certify on MSHA form 5000-23 that the miner has received the specified training. A copy of the training certificate is given to the miner. A copy of the certificate is filed at the mine site to be available to the various government agencies and the miners.

(b) False certification that training was given is punishable under Section 110 (a) and (f) of the Act.

(c) Copies of training certificates for current employees shall be retained at the mine site for two years and for 60 days after a miner terminates.

## §48.30 COMPENSATION FOR TRAINING.

(a) Training shall take place during normal working hours and the miner receives the rate of pay as though working at the work task.

(b) Should the training be given at a location other than the normal workplace, miners shall be paid for additional costs, such as mileage, meals, and lodging, they may incur in attending the training.

## §48.31 HAZARD TRAINING

(a) All miners shall receive hazard training before starting work duties. Such training shall include the following:

(1) Hazard recognition and avoidance;

(2) Emergency and evacuation procedures;

(3) Health and safety standards, safety rules, and safe working procedures;

(4) Self-rescue and respiratory devices; and,

(5) (i) Any additional courses MSHA may deem necessary.

(ii) Miners will receive training at least once every 12 months.

(iii) The hazard training program will be submitted to MSHA along with the other training programs.

(iv) Recordkeeping and completion certification shall be maintained in the same manner as the other training plans

## §48.32 APPEALS PROCEDURES.

The operator, miner, and miners' representative can appeal any decision of the MSHA Training Chief.

(a) Appeals to MSHA shall be in writing to:

Director of Education & Training
MSHA
4015 Wilson Blvd.
Arlington, Va. 22203

The appeal must be within 30 days after notification of a MSHA decision.

(b) The Director can request additional information from all parties.

(c) The Director shall render a decision on the appeal within 30 days after receipt of the appeal.

## Conclusion

The emphasis on job instruction in this chapter may seem to indicate disregard of many mental and emotional states that lead to unsafe acts. Lack of knowledge or skill is, of course, but one cause. Some of the other causes of unsafe acts are:

| | |
|---|---|
| Physical or mental handicap or inability | Overconfidence |
| | Absent-mindedness |
| | Undue haste |
| Disregard of danger | Distraction |
| Resentment of authority | Anger |
| | Impatience |
| Inattention to instruction | Playfulness |
| | Fatigue |
| Indifference | Boredom |

General estimates as to which of these factors most frequently cause accidents are unreliable. The original report in any given case has to be made by an investigator who makes a judgment about why other people acted as they did. Often the investigator's judgment is influenced by his own feelings or his past experiences. Often, too, he tries to select one cause for the unsafe act when there may have been two or more causes, all interrelated.

For example, a worker who lacks skill at a job of loading heavy parts into a car may become fatigued from his clumsy efforts to do what a more skilled worker would do easily. He may fall behind and then try to hurry in order to catch up. Encountering a minor difficulty, he may lose patience and throw his weight heedlessly into the work, with the result that he falls or suffers a back sprain.

It is easy to see that one cause of the unsafe act was anger or impatience. Another was undue haste. Still another was fatigue and, back of that, lack of skill. It is unlikely that any two investigators would report the same causes. Even the injured person often does not know what caused the unsafe act.

There seems to be no specific training aimed at such human failings as impatience, boredom, distraction, and so on. Good job instruction, however, will prevent many of the harmful acts that could arise from these mental or emotional states. A sufficiently skilled worker does not break the pattern of good work performance even when he is seriously disturbed, at least not as readily as a person less skilled.

Good job instruction not only produces more skilled workers; it also impresses the person receiving the instruction with the high value the employer places on safety. Frequent follow up and attention on the part of the supervisor to correct work practices also help to create understanding and to eliminate resentment, which is a source of some of the undesirable attitudes.

## References

### Programmed instruction

"A Bibliography of Programs and Presentation Devices." Carl Hendershot, 4114 Ridgewood Dr., Bay City, Mich. 48706.
> A listing of programmed instructional materials and devices with quarterly supplements.

"Library of Programmed Instruction Courses." E.I. du Pont de Nemours and Co., Inc., Education and Applied Technology Division, Wilmington, Del. 19898.
> A listing of vocational training courses. Also available on request is a list of safety training courses.

National Society for Programmed Instruction, P.O. Box 137, Cardinal Station, Washington, D.C. 20017.

### Management games

"Accident Case Studies Kit." National Safety Council, 444 N. Michigan Ave., Chicago, Ill. 60611
> A kit containing a series of six incidents following the format of the Paul Pigors' incident method.

"A Catalog of Ideas for Action Oriented Training." Didactic Systems, Inc., P.O. Box 4, Cranford, N.J. 07016.
> A listing of simulation games of all types, programmed instruction materials, and a listing of books on effective training.

Carlson, Elliot. *Learning Through Games: A New Approach to Problem Solving.* Washington, D.C., Public Affairs Press. 1969.

Duke, Richard D. *Gaming: The Future Language*. New York, N.Y., Halsted Press Div. of John Wiley & Sons, Inc. 1974.

"The In-Basket Method." Bureau of Industrial Relations, Department of Training Materials for Industry, The University of Michigan, Graduate School of Business Administration, Ann Arbor, Mich. 48104. A series of packaged courses, each set consisting of letters, notes, memos, and reports.

"The In-Basket Kit." Allan A. Zoll, Addison-Wesley Publishing Co. Inc., Reading, Mass. 01867. A kit of materials covering management practices that involve the learner.

"Simulation Series for Business and Industry." Science Research Associates, Inc., Department of Management Services, 259 East Erie St., Chicago, Ill. 60611.
This series includes Decision Making, Collective Bargaining, Equipment Evaluation, Supervisory Skills, Purchasing, Production, Control Inventory, and Interviewing.

## Books

Anderson, C. Richard. *OSHA and Accident Control Through Training*. New York, N.Y., Industrial Press, Inc. 1975.

Brilhart, John K. *Effective Group Discussion*. Dubuque, Iowa, William C. Brown Co. 1974.

Craig, Robert L., and Bittel, Lester R., eds. *Training and Development Handbook*. New York, N.Y., McGraw-Hill Book Co. 1967.

Hamblin, A.C. *Evaluation and Control of Training*. Maidenhead, Berkshire, England, McGraw-Hill Book Co. (UK). 1974.

Hannaford, Earle S. *Supervisors Guide to Human Relations*, 2nd ed. Chicago, National Safety Council, 1976.

Konikow, Robert B., and McElroy, Frank E. *Communications for the Safety Professional*. National Safety Council, 444 N. Michigan Ave., Chicago, Ill. 60611. 1975.

Lateiner, Alfred, and Heinrich, H.W. *Management and Controlling Employee Performance*. West New York, N.J., Lateiner Publishing. 1968.

Mager, Robert F. *Preparing Instructional Objectives*. Palo Alto, Calif., Fearon Publishers. 1962.

Mager, Robert F., and Beach, Kenneth M., Jr. *Developing Vocational Instruction*. Palo Alto, Calif., Fearon Publishers. 1967.

Mager, Robert F., and Pipe, Peter. *Analyzing Performance Problems of 'You Really Oughta Wanna.'* Belmont, Calif., Lear Siegler, Inc./Fearon Publishers. 1970.

ReVelle, Jack B. *Safety Training Methods*. New York, John Wiley and Sons, 1980.

Rose, Homer C. *The Instructor and His Job*, 2nd ed. Chicago, Ill., American Technical Society. 1966.

*Supervisors Safety Manual*, 5th ed. National Safety Council, 444 N. Michigan Ave., Chicago, Ill. 60611. 1978.

"Training Requirements of OSHA Standards," OSHA No. 2254. U.S. Department of Labor. Available from U.S. Government Printing Office, Washington, D.C. 20402, or local OSHA regional office.

Wittich, Walter A., and Schuller, Charles F. *Instructional Technology: Its Nature and Use*, 5th ed. New York, N.Y., Harper & Row. 1973.

# Human Factors Engineering

# Chapter 10

# 10—Human Factors Engineering

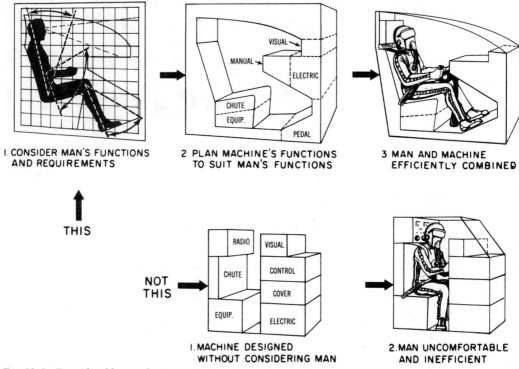

1. CONSIDER MAN'S FUNCTIONS AND REQUIREMENTS

2 PLAN MACHINE'S FUNCTIONS TO SUIT MAN'S FUNCTIONS

3 MAN AND MACHINE EFFICIENTLY COMBINED

THIS

NOT THIS

1. MACHINE DESIGNED WITHOUT CONSIDERING MAN

2. MAN UNCOMFORTABLE AND INEFFICIENT

FIG. 10-1.—Example of human factors engineering in equipment design.

*From* Human Engineering Guide to Equipment Design *by C. T. Morgan. Copyright by McGraw-Hill Book Co. Used with permission.*

Designing-in safety—*in* the job, *in* the machine, and *in* the environment—and not trying to make man perform other than by "hat comes naturally" is a major goal of human factors engineering. This chapter tells how controls, machines, and workplaces can be made more convenient and more comfortable and less confusing, less exasperating, and less fatiguing to the user.

Human factors engineering is vital to system analysis—a technology aimed at optimizing system performance (see Chapter 4, "Acquiring Hazard Information").

The five main factors with which human factors engineers work are:

- Selection of workers
- Training of workers
- Operating rules, procedures, and instructions
- The design of equipment
- Design of the environment.

They treat these five ingredients as elements of system design, and they deal with them as a system (Chapanis, 1980).

By definition, a system is an orderly arrangement of interrelated components that act and interact to perform some task in a given environment. Not mutually exclusive, components interact with each other. And this interaction is always carried out in some environment.

For example, when one can select highly trained workers, training requirements may be reduced, somewhat more complex operating rules and procedures can be tolerated, and the equipment itself can be, and very often should be, designed differently. On the other hand, if one cannot select workers, or if selection standards have to be very low, then training requirements usually have to be increased, operating rules and procedures must be simplified, and equipment itself has to be designed accordingly (Chapanis, 1980).

It is easy to see that the vast majority of systems are composed of men and machines. Human factors engineering, since its inception during World War II, has been concerned with the interaction (or interface) between man and machine—and man and his environment.

Although human factors engineering was originally limited to applications in the aviation and aerospace fields, it has since been applied to the problem of safety in industrial environments. Figure 10-1 demonstrates the difference between an engineering solution which includes and omits human factors in the case of an equipment design problem.

**Definitions.** The discipline has various names. In the United Kingdom, it is called "ergonomics." Others call it biomechanics, biotechnology, biophysics, human engineering, human factors, and engineering psychology; however, each of these are specific fields with their own definitions. Despite the variety of names, there is general agreement that human factors engineering is concerned with the interaction of a number of disciplines including psychology, physiology, anthropometry, and engineering.

There are several definitions of human factors engineering, but the three following simplified ones will serve the purpose here:

1. Engineering something for the population that will use it.

2. Designing a system so that machines, human tasks, and the environment are compatible with the capabilities and limitations of people—to minimize error.

3. Designing the system to fit the characteristics of people rather than retrofitting people into the system.

Definitions for other closely related fields are:

Engineering anthropometry concerns itself primarily with body dimensions and mobility

Biomechanics concerns itself primarily with the mechanical structure and stress behavior of the body

Work physiology concerns itself primarily with the physiological capabilities for the performance of work tasks

Psychology and sociology describe respectively the mental attitudes and capabilities of people concerning their tasks and the relationship among people at work.

Some general principles of human factors engineering, applicable to a wide variety of industrial tasks, will be presented in the remainder of the chapter.

Before this can be done, however, it is necessary to examine a system in detail.

### Man–Machine Systems

Fig. 10-2 is a schematic of a man–machine system. A number of things should be noted about it.

First, input can enter the system at any point (as depicted by the arrow entering the circle at "machine operation").

The subsystem "machine" has displays and controls. Reading the displays (which may be of any variety—visual, audible, tactual), the "man" component decides how he should use the controls. When an adjustment is required, it is done by the human muscle (effector) system—with such adjustments serving as new input.

The entire man–machine system operates in an environment of heat, stress, humidity, noise, and the like. The environment, to one degree or another, affects the performance of the system's components.

The system illustrated is called a "closed-loop" system, one that allows the operator to correct the system's performance. An "open-loop" system does not allow for corrective action; once activated, no further control is possible. Firing a rifle is an example of an "open-loop" system.

Fig. 10-2 also shows that in any man–machine system, man serves three functions—sensor, information processor, and controller—and interacts with the machine at two points—displays and controls. Each of these three functions will be discussed separately.

Here is the crux of the matter: *The purpose of human factors engineering is to minimize errors in using displays and controls by designing systems that will be compatible with both the "man" and "machine" components, while considering man as fulfilling one or all three of his functions—sensing, processing information, controlling. Human factors engineering, then, is concerned with the interaction (or interface) between*

**277**

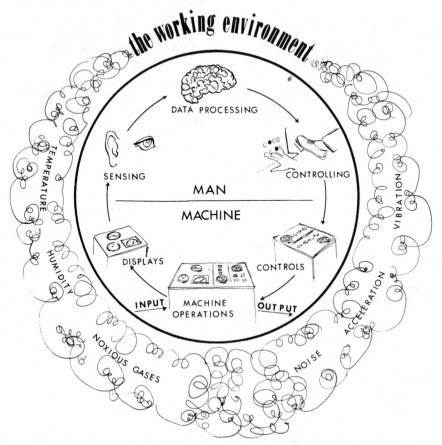

FIG. 10–2.—In any man-machine system, man serves three functions—sensor, information processor, or controller. Man interacts with the machine at two points—displays and controls. The purpose of human factors engineering is to minimize errors made at these two points.

*man and machine—and man and his environment.*

Additionally, much of human factors engineering is concerned with the environment within which the man works. Thus, concern must be directed to such elements as:

• The atmospheric environment (including the effects of altitude, temperature, humidity, and toxicants).

• The mechanical environment (including the effects of acceleration, vibration, and noise).

In this "Occupational Safety and Health Series," specific consideration to a number of common environmental conditions, which affect human performance, is given in *Fundamentals of Industrial Hygiene.*

### Errors and accidents

Human factors engineering is not an exact science—getting good, dependable data is very difficult when one deals with people. It is, however, a scientific approach to problems of designing and constructing things, which people are expected to use—so the user will be more efficient, comfortable, and less likely to make errors resulting in accidents. Those design features that make for easy, comfortable, and convenient human use also make for safe use at the same time.

Chapanis (1980) emphasizes that human factors engineers are not solely or even primarily concerned with safety. Some of the major goals of their work are:

- Increasing the efficiency of human work

- Reducing fatigue and boredom in human work

- Increasing human comfort

- Increasing the convenience with which things can be used

- Increasing the reliability of man–machine systems

- Reducing training requirements

- Reducing maintainability requirements

- Reducing manpower requirements in systems

- Decreasing errors and increasing safety.

The one goal of human factors that is of most concern to the safety professional is the reduction of errors and accidents. Errors are so numerous in man–machine systems that examples could be cited almost endlessly. At the very least, errors are disruptive of normal routines and result in inefficiency. At the worst, errors may result in accidents, injuries, and fatalities.

Most human factors engineers do not worry much about the distinction between errors and accidents for a good reason. For purposes of man–machine system design there is often no essential difference between an error and an accident. The important thing is that both an error and an accident identify a troublesome, or potentially dangerous, situation.

This in no way implies that errors and accidents are equivalent in terms of their human consequences, because they are not. In their noninjurious forms, accidents are simply errors. However, the reverse is not true. Many errors, even in their most extreme forms, never result in accidents. It is difficult to imagine, for example, how simple typing errors, or errors in using a minicomputer could ever be called accidents. Errors of this kind might be annoying, distracting, and even costly, but they would never by themselves be referred to as "accidents."

Another characteristic of errors and accidents is that the former are much more common than the latter. From a scientific, or design standpoint, one difficulty with accidents is that they are rare,

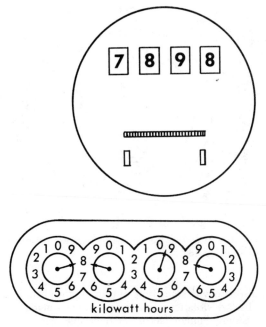

FIG. 10–3.—Application of HFE to meter reading. Reading on top meter requires no special knowledge for interpretation.

and even when one looks at any reasonable collection of accidents, they all seem to be unique. It is hard to find among them sufficient common factors of the kind that suggest countermeasures, or design changes. Errors, on the other hand, are much more common than accidents. That means that the human factors engineer can usually collect within a reasonable period of time enough error data to yield information about specific man–machine mismatches for which countermeasures, or alternative designs, can be devised.

## HFE and training

Much of the effort in occupational safety has been directed toward altering the man by training. The approach to the machine has been to guard the obvious hazards—many of which are simply products of engineering design that did not take man's limitations into consideration.

There are at least three limitations to altering the man by means of training:

- The long-term, high cost of training in terms of dollars and time. Obviously, it is not possible to

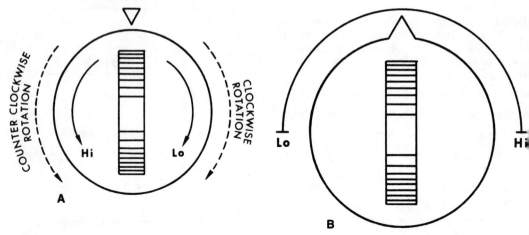

FIG. 10–4.—Control B is designed to eliminate errors in the information-processing and machine controlling functions. (See also Fig. 10–16.)

dispense with some type of training for virtually all work situations. But in certain man–machine systems, human factors engineering principles applied in the design of the machine will significantly reduce training requirements.

• Training sometimes fails as a solution. No amount of training will make some man–machine systems function more effectively. For example, attempting to retrain an operator to read correctly a poorly designed display will not solve the problem.

• Training will not overcome poor or disrupted performance arising out of undue stress caused by machine design—where the limits of the operator have been exceeded.

The problem, from a human engineering point of view, is simply that training is often not the most efficient technique for dealing with the man–machine interface. Indeed both the machine and the environment in industry can be largely structured to suit both the needs and abilities of man. Then, training can be used to increase the probability of successfully reducing human error and increasing system effectiveness.

## Applications of HFE

A couple of examples help to clarify the possibilities of applying human factors engineering to displays, controls, and workplaces.

Fig. 10–3 shows two electric meters. To read the meter on the bottom (an old, but still-used meter), a person relies heavily on previous knowledge of such meters. But the meter at the right has been redesigned to read out directly, which requires no special knowledge or interpretation to record.

Two heat-regulation controls are shown in Fig. 10–4. Control A is not designed with the human operator in mind; Control B, on the other hand, is designed to eliminate errors in the information-processing and machine-controlling functions.

Although these two illustrations are elementary, they present the possibilities that human factors engineering holds.

## Allocation of tasks

In any man–machine system, there are tasks that are better performed by man than by machine—and, conversely, tasks that are better handled by machines. See Fig. 10–5.

In general, machines can usually perform more efficiently on those tasks that must be performed routinely and rapidly with a high degree of accuracy. Man performs better the tasks calling for responsibility and flexibility (adaptability), in addition to tasks that cannot be anticipated.

Man is generally *excluded* from tasks that are likely to result in a high probability of error. Such tasks are:

| MAN VS. MACHINE | |
|---|---|
| *Man Excels in* | *Machine Excels in* |
| Detecting certain stimuli of low-energy levels | Monitoring (both man and machines) |
| Sensing an extremely wide variety of stimuli | Performing routine, repetitive, or very precise operations |
| Perceiving patterns and making generalizations about them | Responding very quickly to control signals |
| Detecting signals in high-noise levels | Exerting great force, smoothly and with precision |
| Storing large amounts of information for long periods—and recalling relevant facts at appropriate moments | Storing and recalling large amounts of information in short time-periods |
| Exercising judgment when events cannot be completely defined | Performing complex and rapid computation with high accuracy |
| Selecting own inputs | Sensitivity to stimuli beyond the range of human sensitivity (such as infrared, radio waves) |
| Improvising and adopting flexible procedures | |
| Reacting to unexpected low-probability events | Doing many different things at one time |
| Applying originality in solving problems: i.e., coming up with alternate solutions | Computing deductively—going from general to specifics |
| Profiting from experience and altering the course of action | Being insensitive to extraneous factors |
| Performing fine manipulation, especially where misalignment appears unexpectedly | Operating very rapidly, continuously, and precisely the same way over a long period |
| Continuing to perform even when overloaded | Operating in environments which are hostile to man or beyond human tolerance. |
| Reasoning inductively—specifics to general | |

FIG. 10-5.

*Source:* W. E. Woodson, Human Engineering Guide for Equipment Designers.

• Perceptual requirements near or beyond the physiological limits or that conflict with established perceptual patterns.

• Response requirements that are physically difficult, conflict with established patterns, or cannot be readily checked or monitored for adequacy.

• Decisions that require undue reliance on short-term memory or must be accomplished within too short a time interval in view of other necessary tasks.

• Tasks that overload the human, resulting in an imbalanced workload/time distribution, or do not permit adequate or timely monitoring of the system.

• Communication requirements that conflict

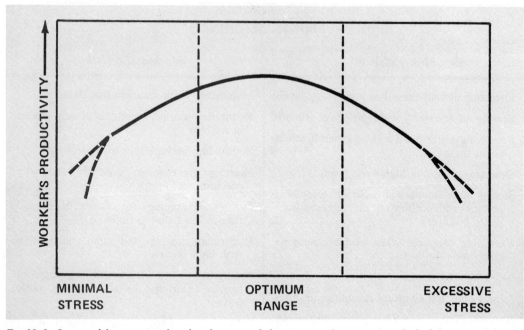

Fig. 10–6.—In general, long continued work under extremely low stress conditions produces lack of alertness; work under high stress conditions produces fatigue. Both factors are known to play a leading role in causing accidents.

with other activities.

Often, man's contribution to a system is to provide a counter-measure in the event of system malfunction or component failure. To do this he must know that a failure has occurred (or is about to occur) and what to do about it.

Generally, displays provide the failure information and, therefore, must be designed to communicate such information to the operator. The operator must then perform the proper response with the controls provided with a minimum of error—yet it is at this point that breakdowns in the system frequently occur.

### Task analysis

Just as equipment can be designed to fit human limitations and capabilities, so, too, can jobs (or tasks) be designed for humans.

Human factors engineering research has shown that man needs to be challenged but not overburdened. If a job is too easy and too routine it is possible that monotony, boredom, and eventually errors (and accidents) will occur.

Machines have a built-in upper tolerance limit. If an electrical circuit, for example, is overloaded, the fuse will blow and no harm to the system will result.

Man, on the other hand, does not have a "safety fuse box." He can work for short periods under overload conditions, for example, high production demands; however, when such an overload reaches some undefinable point, the human may completely break down. Such stress overloading may account for the employee who suddenly "flies off the handle."

The task of the job designer, then, is to find the happy blend between "easy" and "difficult" jobs. With very low levels of psychological stress (boring jobs) performance is also low; as stress increases, however, performance also increases—to a point.

The task is to design jobs that will be centered around optimum performance. (See Fig. 10–6.)

How to predict task requirements. Human tasks are predicted from the design of the equipment and from the tentative organizational and procedural setup. A breakdown of the task requirements can be used for determining training requirements, modification of hardware, and

# CHECKLIST
## HUMAN FACTORS ENGINEERING EVALUATION

**Task:**

CONTROL DESIGN
Compatibility of movement with display
Movement required:
(push, pull, turn, move left, move right, move up, move down, combination)
Critical controls coded
Critical controls labeled
Controls coded
Controls labeled
Coding used (size, color, shape, movement)
Location of controls (accessibility to operator, frequency of use, critical to the system)
Control resistance
Anthropometric requirements

DISPLAY DESIGN
Type of displays (visual, auditory, other)
Control/display ratio
Control/display movement compatible

TASK DESIGN
Monitoring (vigilance)                   Receive communications
Information processing                    Memory
Decision making                          Recording
Relay information                        Overload
Transmit communications                  Underload
                                         Anthropometric requirements

SIZE DESIGN
Operator (seated, standing, both)
Control size
Display size
Accessibility for movement
Accessibility for maintenance
Work space allocation

ENVIRONMENTAL FACTORS
Atmospheric pressure                     Space limitation
Heat                                     Noise
Cold                                     Vibration
Acceleration                             Light
Deceleration                             Glare

NOTE: This is not intended to be a comprehensive checklist for all systems. Other items, equally important, should be added depending on the system.

FIG. 10–7.

### TABLE 10–A
### SELECTED STRUCTURAL BODY DIMENSIONS AND WEIGHTS OF ADULTS
#### (Ages 18 To 79)

| Body feature (See accompanying diagrams) | Dimensions (inches) | | | | | | Dimensions (centimeters)† | | | | | |
| --- | --- | --- | --- | --- | --- | --- | --- | --- | --- | --- | --- | --- |
| | Male, percentile | | | Female, percentile | | | Male, percentile | | | Female, percentile | | |
| | 5th | 50th | 95th | 5th | 50th | 95th | 5th | 50th | 95th | 5th | 50th | 95th |
| 1 Height | 63.6 | 68.3 | 72.8 | 59.0 | 62.9 | 67.1 | 162 | 173 | 185 | 150 | 160 | 170 |
| 2 Sitting height, erect | 33.2 | 35.7 | 38.0 | 30.9 | 33.4 | 35.7 | 84 | 91 | 97 | 79 | 85 | 91 |
| 3 Sitting height, normal | 31.6 | 34.1 | 36.6 | 29.6 | 32.3 | 34.7 | 80 | 87 | 93 | 75 | 82 | 88 |
| 4 Knee height | 19.3 | 21.4 | 23.4 | 17.9 | 19.6 | 21.5 | 49 | 54 | 59 | 46 | 50 | 55 |
| 5 Popliteal height | 15.5 | 17.3 | 19.3 | 14.0 | 15.7 | 17.5 | 39 | 44 | 49 | 36 | 40 | 45 |
| 6 Elbow-rest height | 7.4 | 9.5 | 11.6 | 7.1 | 9.2 | 11.0 | 19 | 24 | 30 | 18 | 23 | 28 |
| 7 Thigh-clearance height | 4.3 | 5.7 | 6.9 | 4.1 | 5.4 | 6.9 | 11 | 15 | 18 | 10 | 14 | 18 |
| 8 Buttock-knee length | 21.3 | 23.3 | 25.2 | 20.4 | 22.4 | 24.6 | 54 | 59 | 64 | 52 | 57 | 63 |
| 9 Buttock-popliteal length | 17.3 | 19.5 | 21.6 | 17.0 | 18.9 | 21.0 | 44 | 50 | 55 | 43 | 48 | 55 |
| 10 Elbow-to-elbow breadth | 13.7 | 16.5 | 19.9 | 12.3 | 15.1 | 19.3 | 35 | 42 | 51 | 31 | 38 | 49 |
| 11 Seat breadth | 12.2 | 14.0 | 15.9 | 12.3 | 14.3 | 17.1 | 31 | 36 | 40 | 31 | 36 | 43 |
| 12 Weight* | 120 | 166 | 217 | 104 | 137 | 199 | 58 | 75 | 98 | 47 | 62 | 90 |

*Weight given in pounds (first six columns) and kilograms (last six columns).
†Centimeter values rounded in whole numbers.

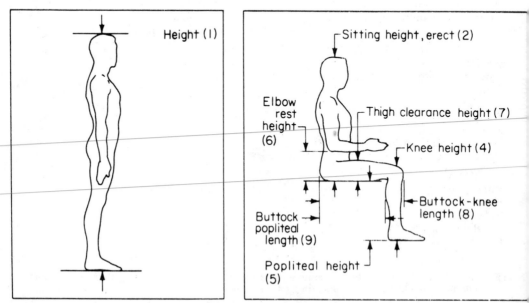

*From* Weight, Height, and Selected Body Dimensions of Adults: 1960-1962. *Data from National Health Survey, USPH. Publication 1000, series 11, no. 8, June, 1965.*

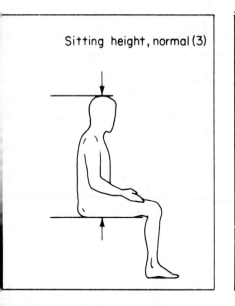

Sitting height, normal (3)

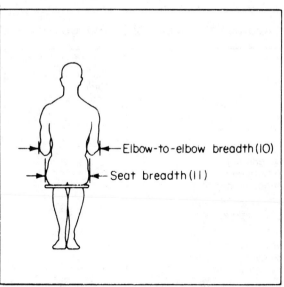

Elbow-to-elbow breadth (10)

Seat breadth (11)

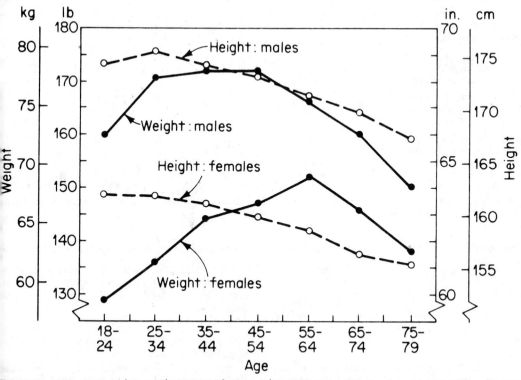

FIG. 10–8.—Average weight (left scale) and height (right scale) of 6672 adults, showing changes by age. Other physical characteristics also are related somewhat to age. (Based on data from National Health Survey. See Table 10–A.)

## TABLE 10-B
## ADDITIONAL DIMENSIONS THAT CLOTHING ADDS TO NUDE BODY MEASUREMENTS

| Measurement | Civilian clothing: Underwear, shirt, trousers, and tie (or dress). Jacket and shoes.[1] | Army uniform: Underwear, khakis or fatigues, combat suit, overcoat, socks, shoes, gloves, wool cap, helmet and liner.[2] | Air Force WW- heavy winter flying clothes jacket, trouser helmet, boots and gloves.[3] |
|---|---|---|---|
| Weight (lb.) | 4–6[a] | 22.9 | 20.0 |
| Stature (in.) | 1.0[b,c] | 2.75 | 1.9 |
| Abdomen depth (in.) | 1.2 | 2.54 | 1.4 |
| Arm reach, anterior (in.) | | .37 | 0.4 |
| Buttock-knee length (in.) | 0.3 | .70 | 0.5 |
| Chest breadth (in.) | | | 0.6 |
| Chest depth (in.) | | 1.54 | 1.4 |
| Elbow breadth (in.) | 1.0 | 2.12 | 4.4 |
| Eye height sitting (in.) | 0.1 | | 0.4 |
| Foot breadth (in.) | 0.2–0.3 | .22 | 1.2 |
| Foot length (in.) | 1.2–1.6 | .20 | 2.7 |
| Hand breadth (in.) | | 1.60 | 0.4 |
| Hand length (in.) | | .30 | 0.4 |
| Head breadth (in.) | | 2.8 | 0.4 |
| Head length (in.) | | 3.5 | 0.4 |
| Head height (in.) | | 1.45 | 0.2 |
| Hip breadth (in.) | | 1.40 | 1.3 |
| Hip breadth sitting (in.) | 0.8 | 1.40 | 1.7 |
| Knee breadth (both) (in.) | | 1.68 | 2.5 |
| Knee height, sitting (in.) | 1.0[b] | 1.44 | 1.8 |
| Shoulder breadth (in.) | | 1.16 | 0.7 |
| Shoulder-elbow length (in.) | | .62 | 0.3 |
| Shoulder height sitting (in.) | | .80 | 0.6 |
| Sitting height (in.) | 0.1[c] | 1.67 | 0.6 |

[a] for women, 3 to 4.   [b] for women, 0.5 to 3.0.   [c] add another 1.0 ± for headgear

*Data reported in* The Human Body in Equipment Design, *by A. Damon, H. W. Stoudt, and R. A. McFarland. Cambridge, Mass., Harvard University Press. 1966.*

for qualitative and quantitative personnel estimates.

The general steps of task analysis are:

• Identification of the broad functions that the human will perform in the system (for example, detection, processing data, decision making, and maintenance).

• Selection of the types of information and control that the human will require in order to perform the function (for example, information to make a decision and the response requirements).

• Detailed specification of the controls, displays and auxiliary equipment (for example, layout, size, lighting, display brightness, and control movements).

A human factors engineering checklist for system or product design considerations will be found in Fig. 10-7.

Some of this, however, cannot be done in the design phase, but must wait until mockup development.

However, in any system or product development, management's constraints are cost, schedule, and performance of the system. Design engineers will also be concerned with reliability, quality, maintainability, and like factors. It must be recognized that management constraints and other design requirements may, unfortunately, take precedence over human factors engineering.

## Anthropometric considerations

Including anthropometric measurements in system design is another approach to assist in making man and the machine more compatable with each other. Physical facilities should "fit" people!

This means considering and applying dynamic and static body measurements as design criteria to improve the ease, efficiency, and safety of the human in the system. Such data is abundant.

Tables 10–A and –B present representative anthropometric information on structural body dimensions in fixed positions and weight for adult civilian populations. Measurements, particularly weight and height, can vary with age (Fig. 10–8).

Anthropometric data is useful for deriving optimum and limiting dimensions for a wide variety of operator positions. (See Fig. 10–9.) Most often design engineers attempt to meet the requirements within the 5 percent to 95 percent range. That is, 10 percent of the population will lie outside of this range. These are considered rare cases and are not normally accounted for.

Unfortunately, the idea that the "average person" is a "misleading and illusionary concept as a basis for designing criteria" has been accepted only very slowly. It is not surprising, then, that designs for the average person do not fit, in reality, anybody. (See VanCott and Kinkade, 1972, for details.) Designs must be fitted to a given user population. (See Chapter 20, "The Handicapped Worker," for special design factors for people in wheelchairs.)

A checklist for relating design of the work place and equipment to body dimensions and to posture, strength, and movement is given in Fig. 10–10.

## Function 1—Man as Sensor

Previously, it was pointed out that one of the functions man serves in a man–machine system is that of sensor, or information seeker. Contrary to the popular notion, man has something like 12 to

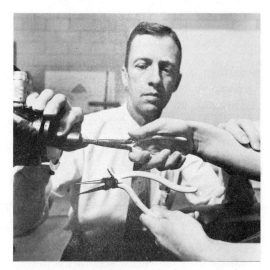

Fig. 10–9a.—Conventional pliers (top) require the wrist to be bent. Redesigned tool (bottom) has contour handles, spring, and thumb stop to reduce worker fatigue.

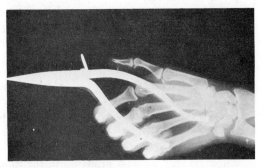

Fig. 10–9b.—X ray shows how contour handles fit easily into a natural hand position.

*Courtesy Western Electric Company, Inc.*

13 senses—not just five. (Some of these are given in Fig. 10–11, along with the sensing organ and physical energy of various stimuli).

As the senses are used as communications channels, they can all be used as signaling or communicating inputs, even though one generally thinks of communication only by means of sight or sound. Of importance to the safety practitioner is protecting all of the operator's senses by holding energy levels within a safe range.

**287**

## THE HUMAN BODY IN WORK PLACE DESIGN

### Design in Relation to Body Dimensions

The design of the work place and work equipment shall take into account constraints imposed by body dimensions, with due regard to the work process.

The work area shall be adapted to the operator. In particular:

*The height of the working surface* shall be adapted to the body dimensions of the operator and the *kind of work performed;*

*The seating arrangements* shall be adjusted to the anatomic and physiological features of the individual;

*Sufficient space shall be provided for body movements,* in particular for the head, arms, hands, legs, and feet;

*Controls shall be within functional reach* of the hand or foot;

*Grips and handles shall be fitted* to the functional anatomy of the hand.

### Design in Relation to Body Posture, Muscular Strength, and Body Movements

The design of the work shall be such as to avoid unnecessary or excessive strain on muscles, joints, ligaments, and on the respiratory and circulatory systems. Strength requirements shall be within physiologically desirable limits. Body movements should follow natural rhythms. Body posture, strength exertion, and body movement should be in harmony with each other.

1. *Body posture*

Attention shall be paid primarily to the following:

The operator should be able to alternate between sitting and standing. If one of these postures must be chosen, sitting is normally preferable to standing; standing may be permissible if necessitated by the work process.

If high muscle strength must be exerted, the chain of force or torque vectors through the body should be kept short and simple by allowing suitable body posture and providing appropriate body support.

Body postures should not cause static muscular fatigue. Alternations in body postures shall be possible.

2. *Muscular strength*

Attention shall be paid primarily to the following:

Strength demands shall be compatible with the physical capacities of the operator.

Muscle groups involved must be strong enough to meet the strength demands. If strength demands are excessive, auxiliary sources of energy shall be introduced into the work system.

Maintainance of uninterrupted tension in the same muscle for a long time (static muscle tension) shall be avoided.

3. *Body Movement*

Attention shall be paid primarily to the following:

A good balance shall be established among body movements; motions shall be preferred to prolonged immobility.

Amplitude, strength, speed, and pace of movements shall be mutually adjustable.

Fig. 10–10.

*Adapted from the International Standards Organization, "Ergonomic Principles of the Design of Work Systems," Draft International Standard ISO/DIS 6385. Geneva, Switzerland, 1978.*

| Man's Senses and the Physical Energies that Stimulate Them | | | |
|---|---|---|---|
| **Sensation** | **Sense Organ** | **Stimulated by** | **Originating** |
| Sight | Eye | Some electromagnetic waves | Externally |
| | | Mechanical pressure | Externally or internally |
| Hearing | Ear | Some amplitude and frequency variations of the pressure of surrounding media | Externally |
| Rotation | Semi-circular canals | Change of fluid pressures in inner ear | Internally |
| | Muscle receptors | Muscle stretching | Internally |
| Falling and rectilinear movement | Semi-circular canals | Position changes of small, bony bodies in the inner ear | Internally |
| Taste | Specialized cells in tongue and mouth | Chemical substances dissolvable in saliva | Externally on contact |
| Smell | Specialized cells in mucous membrane at top of nasal cavity | Vaporized chemical substances | Externally |
| Touch | Skin mainly | Surface deformation | On contact |
| Vibration | None specific | Amplitude and frequency variations of mechanical pressure | On contact |
| Pressure | Skin and underlying tissue | Deformation | On contact |
| Temperature | Skin and underlying tissue | Temperature changes of surrounding media or of objects contacted | Externally and on contact |
| | | Mechanical movement Some chemicals | |
| Cutaneous pain | Unknown but thought to be free nerve endings | Intense pressure, heat, cold, shock, chemicals | Externally on contact |
| Subcutaneous pain | Thought to be free nerve endings | Extreme pressure and heat | Externally and on contact |

FIG. 10–11.

*Source: H. W. Sinaiko,* Selected Papers on Human Factors in the Design and Use of Control Systems.

## Information displays

An information display is a device used to gather needed information and to translate such information into inputs that the human brain can perceive.

• Two general classes of information displays—pictorial and symbolic—are utilized.

IN PICTORIAL DISPLAYS, the geometrical and spa-

FIG. 10–12.—Proposed set of pictorial symbols designed to enable firefighters to quickly find (from upper left) automatic sprinkler control valve, electric service equipment (or other main disconnecting means), standpipe connection, and fire extinguisher.

*Courtesy NFPA Fireafety Symbols Committee.*

tial relationships are shown as they exist. Maps, pictures, and TV are examples of pictorial displays. (See Fig. 10–12.)

SYMBOLIC DISPLAYS present the information in a form that has no resemblance to what is being measured. Some examples are a speedometer, a thermometer, a pressure gage, and an altimeter.

The two most common types of symbolic displays are the visual and auditory. See Fig. 10–13 for a comparison of the advantages of one over the other. Much study has been given to the design characteristics of these types of displays and some general principles have emerged.

• Displays can also be described as being either static or dynamic.

STATIC DISPLAYS are those that are fixed over time, such as signs, graphs, charts, labels, and other forms of printed or written material.

DYNAMIC DISPLAYS change through time and include these types: (*a*) Displays that show the status or condition of a variable, such as temperature and pressure gages, tachometers, clocks, and altimeters. (*b*) Certain cathode ray tube (CRT)

displays, such as radar, sonar, and television. (*c*) Displays that present intentionally transmitted information, such as record players, television, and motion pictures. And (*d*) those that aid the user to control or set some variable, such as the temperature control of an oven.

Some devices do double duty as both displays and controls; this is especially true with devices used for making settings, such as oven controls.

## Visual displays

**Principles of parsimony.** Visual displays are used for one of three purposes:

• QUANTITATIVE READINGS—to determine the exact quantity involved, such as a scale.

• QUALITATIVE READING—to determine the state or condition at which the machine or system is functioning—usually three conditions, such as above, within, or below tolerance.

• DICHOTOMOUS (check) READINGS—to check operations or to identify one or two levels, such as OFF or ON.

The purpose for which the display is to be read will dictate its design. But as a general principle, the simplest design is the best.

Fig. 10–14 shows three types of dials appropriate for the three purposes just stated. The dial on the left is suitable for check readings; the one in the center, for qualitative readings; and the one on the right, for quantitative readings.

**Principle of compatibility.** The principle of compatibility holds that the motion of the display should be compatible with (or in the same direction as) the motion of the machine and its control mechanism.

For example, a display increasing in numerical value should indicate that the variable being measured is also increasing.

Furthermore, a pointer that moves to the right, up, or clockwise to show an increase should have its corresponding control mechanism designed so that a rightward, upward, or clockwise movement of the control will increase the machine value and the corresponding display output value.

**Principle of arrangement.** As the design of the display is important, so too is its location or arrangement with other displays. A poor arrangement of displays can be the source of error. Displays should be grouped according to their

| RELATIVE MERITS OF AUDITORY AND VISUAL PRESENTATIONS | |
|---|---|
| **Use Auditory Presentation if:** | **Use Visual Presentation if:** |
| Message is simple | Message is complex |
| Message is short | Message is long |
| Message will not be referred to later | Message will be referred to later |
| Message deals with events in time | Message deals with location in space |
| Message calls for immediate action | Message does not call for immediate action |
| Receiving location is too bright | Receiving location is too noisy |
| Person's job requires him to move continually | Person's job allows him to remain in one position |
| Visual system of person is overburdened | Auditory system of person is overburdened |

FIG. 10–13.

function and/or their sequence of use.

Sometimes dials must be arranged in groups on a large control panel. If all the dials must be read at the same time, they should be pointing the same direction when in the desired range. This will reduce check-reading time and increase accuracy.

**Principle of coding.** All displays should be coded (or labeled) so that the operator can tell immediately just what variable the display refers to, what units are being used, and what the critical range is.

Labeling is especially important if operators are unfamiliar with the equipment.

The effectiveness of labels is greatly affected by the environment. If the equipment is being used in a dimly lighted area, illumination must be provided. Glare, of course, may be a problem in a brightly lighted room.

Other problems may be caused by vibration, acceleration, and, in the case of auditory displays (described next), noise.

## Auditory displays

Auditory displays should follow the principles outlined for visual displays.

In addition, special problems are posed by auditory displays.

The most immediate problem the system designer faces is whether an auditory or visual display should be used. Fig. 10–13 compares the relative advantages of auditory and visual displays.

Other considerations, though, are equally important. The following principles can act as a guide:

• SITUATIONALITY. The designer of auditory dis-

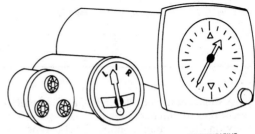

CHECK   DIRECTIONAL   QUANTITATIVE

FIG. 10–14.—Three dials illustrate the principles of parsimony: Check readings (for one- or two-level operations), directional readings (qualitative reading, usually of three conditions), and quantitative readings (show exact quantity involved).

**291**

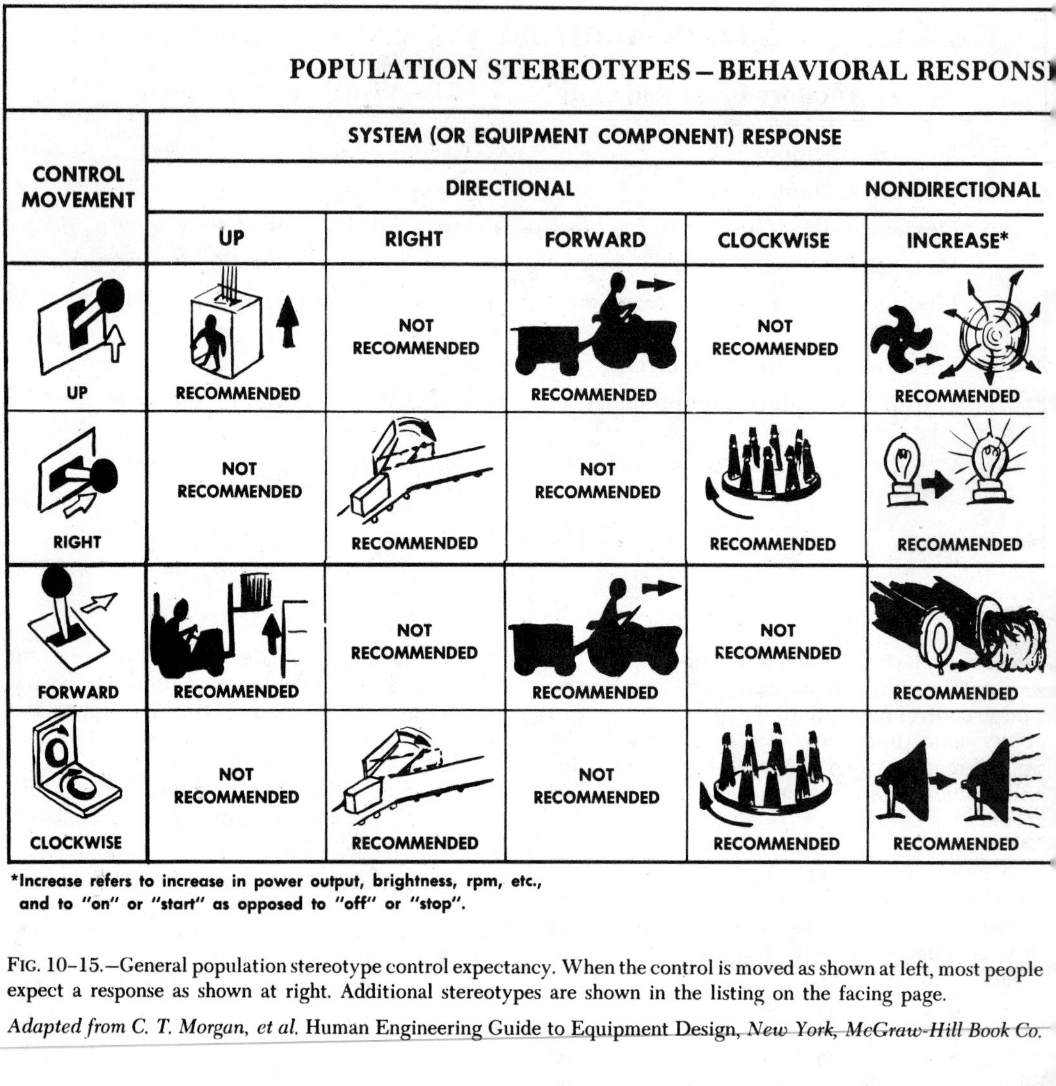

## POPULATION STEREOTYPES – BEHAVIORAL RESPONSE

| CONTROL MOVEMENT | SYSTEM (OR EQUIPMENT COMPONENT) RESPONSE | | | | |
| --- | --- | --- | --- | --- | --- |
| | DIRECTIONAL | | | | NONDIRECTIONAL |
| | UP | RIGHT | FORWARD | CLOCKWISE | INCREASE* |
| UP | RECOMMENDED | NOT RECOMMENDED | RECOMMENDED | NOT RECOMMENDED | RECOMMENDED |
| RIGHT | NOT RECOMMENDED | RECOMMENDED | NOT RECOMMENDED | RECOMMENDED | RECOMMENDED |
| FORWARD | RECOMMENDED | NOT RECOMMENDED | RECOMMENDED | NOT RECOMMENDED | RECOMMENDED |
| CLOCKWISE | NOT RECOMMENDED | RECOMMENDED | NOT RECOMMENDED | RECOMMENDED | RECOMMENDED |

*Increase refers to increase in power output, brightness, rpm, etc., and to "on" or "start" as opposed to "off" or "stop".

Fig. 10–15.—General population stereotype control expectancy. When the control is moved as shown at left, most people expect a response as shown at right. Additional stereotypes are shown in the listing on the facing page.

*Adapted from C. T. Morgan, et al.* Human Engineering Guide to Equipment Design, New York, McGraw-Hill Book Co.

plays should consider other relevant characteristics of the environment in which the system is to function (for example, noise levels, types of responses controlled by the auditory signal).

● COMPATIBILITY. Where feasible, signals should "explain" and exploit learned or natural relationships on the part of the users, such as high frequencies being associated with "up" or "high"

and wailing signals indicating emergency.

● APPROXIMATION. Two-stage signals should be considered when complex information is to be displayed and a verbal signal is not feasible. The two stages should consist of (a) attention-demanding signals to attract attention and identify a general category of information, and (b) designation signals to follow the attention-demanding

- Handles used for controlling liquids are expected to turn clockwise for off and counter-clockwise for on.

- Knobs on electrical equipment are expected to turn clockwise for on, to increase current, and counter-clockwise for off or to decrease current. (Note this is opposite to the stereotype for liquid.)

- Toggle switches are expected to turn "on" when flipped up, "off" when flipped down.

- Certain colors are associated with traffic, operation of vehicles, and safety.

- For control of vehicles in which the operator is riding, the operator expects a control motion to the right or clockwise to result in a similar motion of his vehicle, and vice versa.

- Sky-earth impressions carry over into colors and shadings. Light shades and bluish colors are related to the sky or up, whereas dark shades and greenish or brownish colors are related to the ground or down.

- Things which are further away are expected to look smaller.

- Coolness is associated with blue and blue-green colors, warmth with yellows and reds.

- Very loud sounds or sounds repeated in rapid succession, and visual displays that move rapidly or are very bright, imply urgency and excitement.

- Very large objects or dark objects imply heaviness. Small objects or light-colored objects appear light in weight. Large, heavy objects are expected to be at the bottom. Small, light objects are expected at the top.

- People expect normal speech sounds to be in front of them and approximately head height.

- Seat heights are expected to be at a certain level when a person sits down.

*Source: Woodson and Conover (1964).*

signals to designate the precise information within the general category.

- DISSOCIABILITY. Auditory signals should be easily discernible from other sounds (be they meaningful or noise).

- PARSIMONY. Input signals to an operator should not provide more information than is necessary to carry out the proper response.

- FORCED ENTRY. When more than one kind of information is to be presented, the signal must prevent the receiver from listening to just one aspect of the total signal.

- INVARIANCE. The same signal should designate the same information at all times.

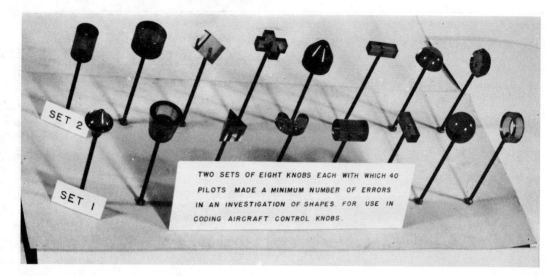

TWO SETS OF EIGHT KNOBS EACH WITH WHICH 40 PILOTS MADE A MINIMUM NUMBER OF ERRORS IN AN INVESTIGATION OF SHAPES FOR USE IN CODING AIRCRAFT CONTROL KNOBS.

### HFE display evaluation

When designing a display, a number of human factors should be considered. But a few questions about any existing displays quickly evaluates them:

• Has the threshold level for that sense been reached by the display? (Because each sense has its own threshold level, energy intensities below it cannot be perceived.)

• Is the sense overloaded? What other demands are made on this sense at the time the display in question is to be read?

• Is the display compatible with similar displays, controls, and machine movements?

• What environment factors, if any, will mask the display?

### Function 2—
### Man as Information Processor

Much research is presently being performed to learn more about man as an information processor (McCormick, 1976).

Human judgements may be classified as either relative or absolute. A relative judgement is one that is made when an opportunity to compare two or more objects presents itself.

An absolute judgement is made in the absence of any standard or comparison. For example, it has been estimated that most people can differentiate as many as 10,000 to 300,000 different colors on a relative basis—but only 11 to 15 on an absolute basis. In general, therefore, a system should have more relative than absolute judgements.

### Function 3—Man as Controller

The third function man serves in the man–machine system is that of controller. Just as principles exist for designing displays for man to use more readily, so, too, can controls be designed to eliminate error.

The control function in the man–machine system can be considered as the response to a given stimulus.

For many situations, a generalized response is given. Most Americans, for example, expect a light switch to be turned ON by flipping the switch "up." A clockwise motion generally refers to an increase. Conversely, people expect the reverse kinds of movements to turn a system OFF or to decrease a function.

Such responses are called "population stereotypes," a behavioral response common to nearly everyone in the population. Some examples are given in Fig. 10–15, on the previous page.

In occupational safety, population stereotypes are particularly important from the point of view of hazard identification and recognition through various warning systems. Ideally, a visual

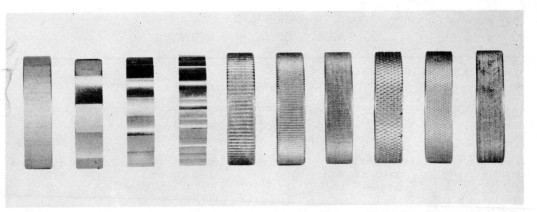

Fig. 10–16.—*Left:* Shape coding. Two sets of knobs for levers that are distinguishable by touch alone. *Above:* Texture coding. Ten texture codings that can be distinguished.

*Courtesy Department of the Air Force, Wright-Patterson AFB.* Left: W. O. Jenkins, *"Psychological Research on Equipment Design," Research Report 19, 1947.* Above: J. V. Bradley, *"Tactual Coding of Cylindrical Knobs," Tech. Report 59-182.*

or auditory warning system should make use of known associations for words (danger, caution, warning) and colors (red, yellow, green, blue) in specifying the degree of hazard associated with a specific industrial condition. For example, research on accident prevention signs as specified in American National Standard *Specifications for Accident Prevention Signs*, Z35.1 (Bryk and Bresnahan, 1971), has demonstrated that workers do associate different degrees of hazard with various visual hazard alert cues. Thus, DANGER signs (color-coded red) elicit higher amounts of hazard association than CAUTION signs (color-coded yellow). Likewise, THINK signs (color-coded green) elicit higher amounts of hazard association than NOTICE signs (color-coded blue).

Any display–response that calls for a movement contrary to the established stereotype is likely to produce errors. The designer is calling for errors by asking the operator to change, in this or that unique situation, a behavior pattern that can be described as habit.

If an operator misreads a poorly designed display and operates the wrong control or the right control in the wrong direction, safety may be jeopardized, and the system effectiveness degraded, if not lost entirely.

Despite the fact that many accident reports would classify this as an "unsafe act" or human error, it is, in fact, a design error. Retraining of the operator would not prevent reoccurrence of the series of events that lead to the accident.

A great many stereotypes, or natural expectancies, have been studied and tabulated in human engineering textbooks and guides (see, for example, Chapanis, 1965; McCormick, 1976; and Morgan, 1963). It can be concluded that a system should never require an operator to do things that are unnatural, or unexpected.

**Design principles**

Through research, these principles of control design have emerged:

**Compatibility.** Just as in the design of displays, control movement should be designed to be compatible with the display and machine movement. A lift truck, for example, that has the lift controls move right to left to raise or lower the lift is bound to have a number of errors associated with its operation. The correct movement would be up and down.

**Coding.** Whenever possible, all controls should be coded in some way. A good coding system can reduce many errors by shape and texture, location, color, and operation. A summary and comparison of various visual coding methods is presented in Table 10–C.

• SHAPE AND TEXTURE. Controls can be coded by their shape or their texture (see Fig. 10–16). The

TABLE 10–C

COMPARISON OF CODING METHODS

| Code | Maximum number of items * | Evaluation | Comment |
|---|---|---|---|
| Color | 11 | Good | Little space required<br>Location time short |
| Numerals and letters | Unlimited for combinations of symbols | Good | Little space required if contrast and resolution is good<br>Location time longer than for color |
| Geometric shapes | ~15 | Good | Little space required if resolution is good |
| Size | 5 | Fair | Considerable space required<br>Location time longer than for color or shapes |
| Number of dots | 6 | Fair | Considerable space required<br>Easily confused with other coded items |
| Orientation of line | 12 | Fair | For special purposes |
| Length of line | 4 | Fair | Will clutter display with many signals |
| Brightness | 4 | Poor | Poor contrast effects will reduce visibility of weaker signals |
| Flash rate | 4 | Poor | Interacts poorly with other codes |
| Stereoscopic depth | Unknown | Fair | Requires complex electronic displays and special viewing equipment |

* That generally will give overall accuracies of 95 percent or better.

*From C. T. Morgan, et al.* Human Engineering Guide to Equipment Design. *New York, McGraw-Hill Book Co. Used with permission of the publisher.*

1. Useful where illumination is low or where device may be identified and operated by feel only

2. Supplement to visual identification

3. Useful in standardizing controls for identification purposes.

Some undesirable features are:

1. Limited number of controls that can be identified

2. Use of glove reduces sensitivity of hand.

• LOCATION. Controls can be identified by their location. For example, all brakes on forklift trucks can be placed on the left side regardless of model. Location coding can also be achieved by providing a minimum distance between controls.

The advantages of coding by location are the same as those for shape and texture. Disadvantages include:

1. Limited number of controls that can be identified

2. Increased space requirements

3. Identification not as certain as with other types of coding.

• COLOR. Color may also be used as a coding technique for various controls. Color codes can:

1. Be useful for visual identification

2. Be useful for standardizing controls for identification purposes

3. Offer a moderate number of coding categories.

On the other hand the undesirable features associated with the use of color as a code are:

1. Controls must be viewed directly

2. Illumination cannot be poor or restricted

3. People must have adequate color vision.

• LABELS. Controls can be coded by the use of labels. The desirable features of labeling include:

1. Can identify a large number

2. Does not require much learning.

The undesirable features of labeling include:

1. They must be viewed directly

2. Need good illumination.

• OPERATION. Some controls make use of an operational method of coding; that is, the mode of operation will be different for different controls—for example, automobile windshield wiper controls could require lifting a lever upward to activate, while the headlight control must be pulled. The desirable features associated with such a system are:

1. Usually controls cannot be operated incorrectly

2. System designers can usually capitalize on compatible relationships.

With such a system, the following undesirable features are associated:

1. The control must be activated before the operator knows if the correct control has been selected

2. Specific design might have to incorporate incompatible relationships.

Regardless of the type of coding used, all controls and displays should be labeled. Labeling is crucial where the operators change often or equipment is shared. The use of labels may also reduce operator training time.

## Arrangement

Remember that a system is task-oriented and that its components act and interact with each other to perform this task. Consequently, the various elements and components of the system need to be arranged with these considerations in mind:

• OPTIMUM-LOCATION PRINCIPLE. This principle provides for the arrangement of items so that each one is in its "optimum" location in terms of some criterion of usage (convenience, accuracy, speed, strength to be applied, etc.).

• FUNCTIONAL PRINCIPLE. This principle provides for the grouping of elements or components according to their function—those having related functions are grouped together.

• IMPORTANCE PRINCIPLE. Components can be arranged by their importance. Items of some type (displays, controls, components) should be grouped in terms of how critical they are in carrying out a set of operations. The important controls should be positioned in the best locations for rapid and easy use.

Relative importance, of course, is largely a matter of judgement. So, to apply this principle one must be in a position to obtain judgements from persons who are knowledgeable about the equipment. This can be done by either interview or questionnaire.

• SEQUENCE-OF-USE PRINCIPLE. In using controls, sequences or patterns of relationship typically or frequently occur. In applying this principle, then, items can be so arranged as to take advantage of such patterns; thus, items used in sequence typically would be in close physical relationship with each other.

• FREQUENCY-OF-USE PRINCIPLE. To arrange items in terms of frequency of use, first obtain information about how often different items might be expected to be used. Then place the less frequently used items in more distant locations.

In the event there is conflict among principles some trading-off must be done. Although no one principle should be held rigorously, frequency of use and sequence of use should be given major consideration.

Seek to avoid arrangements on which frequent transfers (of the entire body, or of the eye, hand, or other body member) from place to place would be required.

## Control evaluations

The following questions should be considered in assessing the human element in the design of controls:

• What bodily limbs are involved? Is any one muscle overloaded?

• Where are the controls placed? Can they be reached? Are they spaced far enough apart? Are they labeled and coded?

• What type of control is used? Is it compatible?

• Do the controls themselves present a hazard?

• Are similar control operations similar in design and function? How standardized are the controls?

## Conclusions

Every organization is obliged to improve its safety performance where it can. The safety professional and his management are evading the issue if either ignores the smaller accident problems and continually harps upon the total accident problem that cannot be solved by a single action.

Most occupational safety countermeasures deal with a bit of the entire occupational safety problem. Slowly, but surely, the improvement that results from solving bits of the whole problem will be significant. If solutions to small bits of the total are ignored, then nothing will be accomplished.

Human factors engineering will help solve a bit of the whole problem. The lack of response to the human factors engineering approach is one of the outstanding failures in occupational and product safety efforts. Human factors engineering considerations have not been explored as at least a partial answer to safety problems. This neglect is partially due to lack of understanding the role of human factors engineering in occupational and product safety.

The examination of human factors engineering, combined with the traditional approach, clearly establishes its role in the safety movement. Among benefits that may be expected are:

• Greater system effectiveness.

• Fewer performance errors.

• Fewer accidents resulting in injury or damage to property.

• Minimizing redesign and retrofit after the system is operational—if applied at the design phase.

• Reduced training time and cost.

• More effective use of personnel with less restrictive selection requirements.

The role of human factors engineering will become more significant as systems become more and more complex and automated. The application of human factors engineering is indispensable as a basic consideration in the design of future systems if optimum safety and system effectiveness are to be achieved.

## References

Bennett, E., et al. (eds.) *Human Factors in Technology.* New York, N.Y., McGraw-Hill Book Co., 1963.

Bryk, J. A., and Bresnahan, T. "Safety Uses of Signs, Colors, and Other Visuals." Chicago, Ill., Alliance of American Insurers.

Chapanis, A., *Man–Machine Engineering.* Belmont, Calif., Wadsworth Publishing Co., 1965.

————(ed.). *Ethnic Variables in Human Factors Engineering.* Baltimore, Md., Johns Hopkins University Press, 1975.

————"Human Factors Engineering for Safety," *Professional Safety,* Vol. 25, No. 7 (July 1980).

Christensen, J. M. "An Overview of Human Factors Engineering," *National Safety Congress Transactions,* 1967.

Davis, H. L. (ed.) "Human Factors in Industry," *Human Factors* (Special Issue), Vol. 15, 1973.

Grandjean, E. *Fitting the Task to the Man,* 2nd ed. London, England, Taylor & Francis Ltd., 1969.

Haddon, W. "Energy Damage and the Ten Counter-measure Strategies," *Human Factors,* Vol. 15, 1973.

Hertig, Bruce A. "Ergonomics." *Fundamentals of Industrial Hygiene,* 2nd ed., Chicago, Ill., National Safety Council, 1979.

Human Factors Society, P.O. Box 1369, Santa Monica, Calif. 90406. *Human Factors* (journal).

Jones, D. F. *Human Factors—Occupational Safety.* Toronto, Ontario Department of Labour, 1969.

Kroemer, K. H. E. *Material Handling: Loss Control Through Ergonomics.* Chicago, Ill., Alliance of American Insurers, 1979.

McCormick, Ernest J. *Human Factors in Engineering and Design,* 4th ed., New York, N.Y., McGraw-Hill Book Co., 1976.

McFarland, R. A., "Application of Human Factors Engineering to Safety Engineering Problems," *National Safety Congress Transactions,* 1967.

Meister, D., and Rabideau, G. F. *Human Factors Evaluation in System Development,* New York, N.Y., John Wiley & Sons, Inc., 1965.

Morgan, C. T  et al. *Human Engineering Guide to Equipment Design.* New York, N.Y., McGraw-Hill Book Co., 1963.

Murrell, K. F. H. *Human Performance in Industry.* New York, N.Y., Reinhold Publishing Corp., 1965.

National Safety Council. "Safety Performance Measurement in Industry," *Journal of Safety Research* (Special Issue), Vol. 2, 1970.

Olishifski, J. B. *Fundamentals of Industrial Hygiene,* 2nd ed. Chicago, Ill., National Safety Council, 1979.

Poulton, E. *Environment and Human Efficiency.* Springfield, Ill., Charles C. Thomas, 1970.

Powell, P. I., *et al. 2000 Accidents: A Shop Floor Study of Their Causes.* London, National Institute of Industrial Psychology, 1971.

Sinaiko, H. W. (ed.) *Selected Papers on Human Factors in the Design and Use of Control Systems.* New York, N.Y., Dover Publications, Inc., 1961.

Surry, J. *Industrial Accident Research: A Human Engineering Appraisal.* Toronto, University of Toronto, Department of Industrial Engineering, 1969.

Tarrants, W. E. "The Role of Human Factors Engineering in the Control of Industrial Accidents," *Journal of the American Society of Safety Engineers,* Vol. 8, 1963.

Tichaurer, E. R. *The Biochemical Basis of Ergonomics: Anatomy Applied to the Design of Work Situations.* New York, N.Y., John Wiley & Sons, Inc., 1978.

Van Cott, H. P., and Kinkade, R. G. *Human Engineering Guide to Equipment Designers,* rev. ed. Washington, D.C., U.S. Government Printing Office, 1972.

Woodson, W. F., and Conover, D. W., *Human Engineering Guide for Equipment Designers,* 2nd ed. Berkeley, Calif., University of California Press, 1964.

Yoder, T. A., and Botzum, G. D. The Long-Day Short-Week in Shift Work: A Human Factors Study. Indianapolis, Ind., Eli Lilly and Company, 1971.

# Human Behavior and Safety

# Chapter
# 11

The function of a safety professional in industry is to assist line management in achieving maximum production by preventing or mitigating work-related fatal or injury accidents. As discussed in the previous chapter, the occupational environment is composed of various interacting components, such as the worker, materials, and equipment. A comprehensive safety program addresses all aspects of the work environment and recognizes that each component interrelates in the work place. Consequently, a major responsibility of a safety professional is directed toward changing worker behavior in order to facilitate safe working conditions.

This does not reduce the importance of the other facets of a sound safety program—the safety professional is also concerned with safe design and plant layouts, safety devices on machines and use of such devices by employees, the wearing of safe clothing and use of protective equipment—all of which contribute to the reduction of disabling accidents.

When, however, in spite of every precaution on the part of the manufacturer of equipment, the supplier of materials, the supervisor, and the safety professional, accidents still occur, the human element emerges as an important factor. It takes working with supervisors and other line management, as well as individual employees, if accidents are to be reduced.

This chapter is designed to promote understanding of human behavior in the work environment. It complements the previous chapter, which emphasized designing equipment, controls, and jobs to fit the limitations of the human being.

## Psychological Factors in Safety

Many topics that the industrial psychologist is concerned with are too detailed to be covered in this chapter. Some of them play a direct part in the success or failure of sound personnel procedures in industry, but they are not all directly related to safety, or they do not fall within the assigned duties of the safety professional. They may, as part of the regular personnel procedures, contribute indirectly to safety in the shop.

Psychological factors that influence safety program success are described in the following paragraphs.

• **Individual differences.** Individual differences are one of the ever-existent problems within industry. These differences are seen constantly. Yet, within the framework of differences in people are factors that are common to all, and therefore useful in dealing with work groups.

• **Motivation.** Understanding the motivations of people is important. To want something is motivation, but not to want something also requires motivation. To use a safety device to protect one's fingers from a saw is, perhaps, indicative of motivation for safe practices, but the desire to ignore a safety device because it might decrease production is also motivated. Conflicting motivations should also be considered in any attempt to understand human relations.

• **Emotion.** Humans frequently respond to their emotions. While emotions can be constructive at times, they can also be destructive—working to the detriment of both the individual and the safety program. Emotion can also interfere with the thought processes, resulting in behavior on the part of the individual that conflicts with a rational approach.

• **Attitudes and attitude change.** Industry has recognized the effect that attitudes can have on production, plant morale, turnover, absenteeism, plant safety, and the like. As a result, management has spent much time and money in determining workers' attitudes. Measuring, developing, and changing attitudes constitute a major problem for the personnel staff and psychologists—one of extreme importance to the safety professional.

• **Learning processes.** Finally, there should be concern with learning processes. Learning starts on the first day of birth, and in all of the topics previously mentioned, it plays a major role. One cannot understand motivation, attitudes, emotions, or even individual differences without some consideration of the learning process involved in bringing them about.

Much of the success of a safety program depends upon its acceptance by those to whom it is directed. Program acceptance in turn is dependent upon an understanding of the psychological factors which influence program success.

An effective exploration must find factors common to the group and upon which the safety professional and the supervisor can use to promote safe conduct on the part of all workers. The basic question is, "What factors associated with human behavior can be utilized to increase the effectiveness of safety programs?"

Each of the five psychological factors previously listed are important enough to discuss separately.

## Individual Differences

When a chemist analyzes a chemical compound, he can accurately specify its exact nature and composition. When he uses this compound, he knows exactly what behavior he can expect. The action and reaction of this sample is usually the same as other samples of the compound he has analyzed.

When the psychologist studies human behavior, however, he is not dealing with the same degree of certitude as is the chemist. The psychologist does not know the composition of the agent he is dealing with—in many instances, he has very little knowledge of his subject's past history.

In addition, the behavior of one person is not the same as the behavior of another person. Person A in the sample is not equivalent to Person B, in the way one cubic centimeter of distilled water equals all other cubic centimeters of distilled water.

The known fact that people differ has been referred to as the "personal equation" or, more commonly, "individual differences." The personal equation presents many problems for both the safety professional and supervisor. The case is not hopeless, for within the framework of individual differences, certain general patterns common to a group do exist.

For example, human behavior is typically motivated. Regardless of what the individual does, there is usually some purpose underlying the behavior. The purpose, for example, may be to reduce some basic tension which must be resolved. The degree and nature of this tension depends in part upon the individual's values and perceptions. More about motivation later.

Here is another example. Even though each child develops at his own rate and to different levels of efficiency, each crawls before he walks, forms words before forming sentences, etc.

The general model used to describe such modes of development is the following:

$$B = f(S,E).$$

Behavior (B) is a function (f) of the present situation (S) and all previous experiences (E).

Whether or not an employee works safely

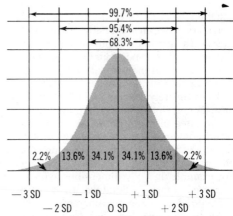

FIG. 11-1.—Many human characteristics are assumed to be distributed according to the normal curve shown here. Because the normal curve has a known shape, it is possible to state the percentage that lies between +1 and −1 standard deviation, or between any other two points expressed in SD units. Thus, it is easy to describe a normal distribution of data using the simple statistics—the mean (average) and the standard deviation, SD. For example, about 68 percent of all the measured values lies within ±1 standard deviation about the mean, 95% are within ±2 SD, and so on. Given the mean and standard deviation, therefore, the complete distribution of items in a normal distribution can be known.

depends (a) upon his present situation—is he rushed? fatigued? in poor health?—and (b) his past experiences—did he avoid accidents in the past? What amount of training does he have? Under this general model, the E variable and the S variable comprise individual personality (Tyler, 1965).

### The average-person fallacy

In the previous paragraphs, the point was stressed that each person differs from each other person (although there are certain common characteristics). The fact that individual differences exist should not be news. What is important is how one deals with individual differences.

Fig. 11-1 presents the distribution of scores in a normal curve. Many human characteristics (for example, anthropometric characteristics or IQ) are assumed to be distributed according to the normal distribution (often referred to as the "normal curve"). Note that in such a distribution, half of the persons are below the mean (the arithmetical average) and half of the persons are above it.

**303**

# 11—Human Behavior and Safety

Often the manager of an enterprise or director of a safety program realizes that individual differences exist and that it is physically impossible to handle every one individually. The manager or director may erroneously attempt the next best thing—appeal to the "average person."

Unfortunately, inept usage of the mean as the primary descriptive value of a population sample has resulted in misinterpretation and misuse of anthropometric data, culminating in the misconception of the so-called "average person." People, in reality, are highly unlikely to be "average." For example, in body dimensions, which can be measured more accurately than emotional, behaviorial, or intellectual characteristics (see the previous chapter), less than four percent of a group that was studied had three common average dimensions, and less than one percent was average in five or more dimensions at the same time. Therefore, when an appeal is aimed at the average, by definition it misses much of the population.

A better approach is the use of percentiles. When designing the system, instead of setting the standards to fit the average, design it to fit all but the upper 5 percent and the lower 5 percent. Then the system will fit 90 percent of the population.

The use of percentiles (for example, between the 5th and 95th percentile), rather than averages, has long been the technique for relating individual test scores to a group as a whole, and also a guiding rule in the design of man-machine relations.

## Fitting the person to the job

Very often when managers are replacing or relocating personnel, they strive to find the individual possessing most of the characteristics deemed necessary. Job specifications and employee requirements are given in terms of a minimum, but very seldom are psychological factors expressed within a minimum and maximum; see the previous chapter.

When looking for someone, often the best qualified is considered to be the one who is most intelligent, most loyal, biggest, or whatever. In other words, they look for the perfect rather than the right person. For example, a person with a below-average IQ might be more desirable for a monotonous job than will a person with an average or above-average IQ. The amount of boredom, monotony, etc., may be less for the less bright, thereby eliminating carelessness, or other factors associated with poor productivity.

As an additional example, the person who comes to work under any condition, whether ill or not, may be as undesirable as the one who uses every excuse to take off. The worker with a high fever, bad cold, or sore back is a potential hazard, especially if he is under heavy medication.

**Physical characteristics of the individual.** Reaction time, psychomotor skills (for example, manual dexterity), and visual abilities seem to have at least some bearing on safe performance. While the extent to which they are directly responsible for accidents is neither clear nor constant, it appears that a certain minimum degree of physical competence is required for successful, accident-free performance. Some types of jobs demand superior physical abilities while others do not. It is not possible to redesign a job to allow a person with certain physical handicaps to perform efficiently and safely.

Most of the research to date has considered these factors individually. More recently a few studies have examined the connection between combinations of physical shortcomings and accidents. Such studies were initiated because investigators realized that physical and psychological abilities operate not as single, discrete items, but rather in interacting combination. For example, one study investigates the general perceptual skills and accidents, and not with just the separate abilities that contribute to perception.

**Individual personality.** It is the function of personnel people in industry to screen candidates on the basis of relevant characteristics required by the specific job for which application is made. In many cases, both (a) physical characteristics, such as size, visual acuity, and steadiness, and (b) personality characteristics are important, so many individuals will not be considered because they do not have all the necessary qualifications.

In the design of equipment, human engineering experts take into consideration physical limitations as well as other human characteristics in an effort to make machines as nearly perfect as possible. See Chapter 10 for a discussion of human factors engineering in relation to occupational safety.

Where hazards cannot be eliminated, guarding provides protection against potential failure of people to utilize equipment correctly. Both safe design and guarding minimize the effect of individual differences on accident frequency and severity.

## Methods of measuring characteristics

Regardless of what technique is used to screen, place, and motivate employees, a method of measuring program effectiveness is necessary. Techniques used to obtain feedback range from the across-company accident rates, to the within-company approach of safety sampling, or critical incident technique, described on pp. 67-68, Examining accident causation, and in the next column.

Measuring techniques can be assessed by determining reliability and validity.

**Reliability** refers to consistency of measurement. The reliability of a given measurement, such as by a test or instrument, can be estimated in various ways. In general, however, the concept of reliability refers to measurement stability, whether it is (a) assessed across time or between settings, or (b) assessed using the same or different group of individuals, or (c) assessed for internal consistency or consistency between alternate forms of the same test or instrument.

Underlying the concept of reliability is that of measurement error. Any gauge used to assess performance will have, to varying degrees, associated measurement error. Measurement error refers to the estimated fluctuations likely to occur in performance by an individual or group as a result of irrelevant or chance factors.

The degree of reliability associated with an instrument or test is typically estimated statistically by a correlation coefficient. The sign of this coefficient refers to direction (either positive or negative) of the relationship; the value (e.g., $r = 0.89$) is an index of the magnitude of the relationship. Therefore, the greater the magnitude of the reliability coefficient is (and thus the less the measurement error), the more stable or consistent the results obtained by the instrument will tend to be (Anastasi, 1976).

**Validity** refers to the degree to which the test or instrument measures what it is thought or is purported to measure. The validity of a test or instrument can be assessed in various ways, such as (a) the relevance or plausibility of items (or the overall instrument) with regard to the given behavior (face validity), (b) whether all aspects within the rubrics of a given concept are adequately covered (content validity), (c) the extent to which the test or instrument may be said to measure a specific construct or trait (construct validity), and (d) a demonstrable relationship between the performance as measured by the given test or instrument and some other related behavior (e.g., IQ and school aptitude) (Anastasi, 1976).

Once again validity is expressed as a correlation coefficient. A negative sign, however, is as useful as a positive coefficient. An illustration might be testing for a job that requires very little mental ability—it may be negatively correlated with an IQ test so that the desirable workers for the job are those with the lower test scores.

A measurement may be reliable without being valid, but a valid measurement must also be reliable. To illustrate that a reliable measure may not also be valid, consider a yardstick. A yardstick is very reliable—it gives a consistent measurement every time it is used. It is also valid for measuring the length of a table. But if a yardstick is used for weighing the table, it is no longer valid for measuring.

In addition to reliability and validity, a measuring technique must be practical. A technique may possess high validity but be so cumbersome and intricate that it can only be used in special situations, and then only by highly skilled technicians. In spite of its statistical value, such a technique is almost worthless.

**Two sampling techniques** used for evaluating potential accident-producing behavior are (a) the critical incident technique, described in Chapter 4, and (b) behavior sampling.

- *The critical incident technique* involves the following. A random sample of employees is interviewed in order to collect accident information concerning near misses, difficulties in operations, and conditions that could have resulted in death, injury, or property loss. Those participating are asked to describe any of these incidents that has come to their attention; see Fig. 3–3 on p. 67. This technique can be useful in investigating worker-equipment relationships in past or existing systems, modifications to existing systems, or in the development of new systems (Hammer, 1972).

- *The behavior sampling* or activity sampling technique involves the observation of worker behaviors at random intervals and the instantaneous classification of these behaviors according to whether they are safe or unsafe. Calculations are then made to determine either *(a)* the percent of time the workers are involved in unsafe acts or *(b)* the percent of workers involved in unsafe acts during the observation period. Various components of a safety program (such as safety lectures, posters, brief safety talks, safety inspections, motion picture films, supervisory training) can be applied and an immediate indication of their influence on unsafe behavior can be obtained.

It is important that the safety professional approach any psychological evaluation with caution. Texts and references in industrial, social, and personnel psychology will provide guidelines for the development and use of test batteries for measuring individual differences. These tests or evaluative instruments are best developed and administered by competent professionals who specialize in this work.

With respect to the problem of screening employees or potential employees in regard to their accident potential, caution must be exercised. To date, no systematic screening procedures have been developed that meet both reliability and validity criteria and that are adequate for use in all industries or even in a specific industry. While in theory such a screening procedure is possible, the state of scientific knowledge in occupational safety research is too limited to support the development of such screening measures.

## Motivation

Through the interaction of hereditary and environmental factors, each worker is an individual personality. The safety professional must be continually aware of individualities when dealing with human beings.

There are instruments by which various aspects of human behavior can be evaluated, many of which are already in use in industry. Through psychological tests, interviews, rating scales, and allied aids and techniques, personnel departments have for a long time been evaluating individual differences. Insofar as they are doing adequate jobs, personnel departments are working with safety programs to eliminate job candidates who obviously would be unsatisfactory.

Each day millions of men and women work in the manufacture and distribution of industrial products. It hardly seems logical that if all these people were individual personalities they could

work together in harmony. Individual differences alone are not all there is to human behavior. There are some factors operating in all people which allow supervisors, safety professionals, and plant managers to obtain work and cooperation for a common cause. The psychologists, when they try to predict and control human behavior, are also concerned with these factors that all individuals have in common.

To have all personnel in a company from the president down to the lowest-paid employees working together productively and safely is one of the goals of a safety program. Such cooperative effort must be motivated as an appeal to achieve a common goal, or as a means to another goal which is of greater importance to the individual. In either case, the result is of value to the safety program.

It is understandable, therefore, that the question most asked by safety professionals and supervisors alike is, "How do we best motivate our workers?"

## Complexity of motivation

Many theories contained in the psychological literature, to varying degrees, attempt to unify the concept of human motivation. Although not all of the hypothetical concepts associated with a given theory (nor all of the theories) are equally testable on an empirical level, several general concepts associated with human motivation are suggested.

The motivational problem is perhaps the most complex one in the field of human behavior. It is not possible at the present stage of development to give clear-cut, concise answers to all the questions that might be asked about other people's motivations. Rather, attempts are made to set forth some basic factors and point out where the complexities exist. Hierarchical motivation, multiple motivation, continuing psychosocial need, and conflicting motives must be considered.

**Hierarchical motivation** means simply that some needs take a higher priority—there is a hierarchy of motivational factors. It has been pointed out that the psychosocial needs (for example, recognition, affection, social approval) take precedence over the biological ones (for example, hunger, thirst, sex) when the latter are relatively well satisfied. This is but one aspect of the hierarchy of needs concept (Maslow, 1970).

The safety professional who plans carefully

and takes each detail of his program to his boss for approval may be exhibiting an overwhelming desire for achievement and recognition, a desire much stronger than his need for affection. This is true particularly if human relations skills in dealing with workers are concomitantly ignored. He may be so concerned with personal achievement, and perhaps the recognition given for it, that plans are forced upon workers that they would not accept if they had the choice.

Another example is the worker who considers recognition as the major need that must be satisfied. This individual, perhaps, would go all out to become a strong militant leader of the union if he were to lose a promotion in the company. The safety director may actually be in conflict with this individual who may not care about the safety director's disapproval and instead values the affection and recognition of his fellow workers. This hierarchy can change over the years.

What is desired more early in life may assume less importance later. For example, the need for achievement and recognition perhaps is greatest in youth, thus giving a drive toward accomplishment.

Later in life the warm affection of friends or the security of belonging to groups may assume major importance if one has already had recognition for past work.

**Multiple motivation** is the second facet that complicates the analysis of behavior. People are seldom motivated by just one need—many forces operate at any single moment. For example at lunch time, one may eat because he is in need of food, or just because it is the usual time. However, an individual might delay his lunch in order to be joined by several friends. Thus the individual combined the satisfaction of a psychosocial need and a biological need.

In another case, an employee could desire recognition from his fellow workers and so engage in practical jokes and harmful horseplay. At the same time, he may be seeking recognition from his supervisor by working hard on the safety committee. The need is the same but the means of satisfaction are in direct conflict.

This is multiple motivation. It would be to the safety professional's advantage, in the second case, to recognize what the need is that the worker is trying to satisfy, and find ways to channel the behavior so he can achieve recognition from fellow employees and the supervisor.

**Continuing psychosocial need** is akin to biological need. However, people often assume that in the psychosocial needs, satisfaction at one time should suffice for the future and thus they need not be concerned any longer with giving recognition, or affection, or social approval.

For all people, these needs continue throughout life. Satisfaction is always sought for these needs, but not always attained. It should be apparent also that the satisfactions sought by individuals will not necessarily be for the same needs. At one time, the motivation may be for social approval while at another time the need most requiring satisfaction might be affection. Thus, in dealing with people, one must recognize that what was effective yesterday may not work today, although the satisfaction-seeking behavior is to some degree similar.

Being aware that these needs continually want satisfaction makes it somewhat easier for the safety professional or anyone else to deal effectively with people in the work situation. There may be variance from day to day so the safety professional must therefore cultivate his own ability, and the ability of supervisors, to work with people so that he can sense which needs require satisfaction at a given time.

Since they spend so much time together and with workers, the safety professional and foreman (or supervisor) come to know each other and the workers very well. This should provide the key to determining what a worker's behavior at the moment means in terms of need satisfaction. This key is based on little cues in the individual's behavior which they have learned over the years to recognize, if they have taken the time and made the effort to know their people.

Careful observation is required. Safety professionals should make certain that any supervisory training program includes methods of effective observation of workers.

**Conflicting motives** constitute another major problem in motivation—needs themselves can be in conflict with one another. Seeking affection could lead to behavior that might be different with fellow workers than with supervisors. It may be necessary to determine which source of affection is the most important to an employee before doing anything.

People can internalize these problems to such a degree that the resultant physical stress or even behavior is completely inconsistent with that typically expected of them. For example, an individual who is assistant safety director in a given company may strongly desire to become the safety director and yet at the same time be fearful of the duties, the responsibilities, and obligations of the job. The promotion would mean more prestige, more money—in all, a better way of life. Here then is a serious conflict. This individual's answer will depend greatly on his background experiences. One of the things he might do would be to quit his job and seek employment elsewhere. He might, on the other hand, seek training to better qualify for the position. He has many choices available.

The same applies to the worker on the line. He may strongly desire the approval of his supervisor and at the same time desire to remain an accepted member of his work group. If the work group minimizes the importance of the safety program, this worker now is in conflict. He may follow the group or he may seek the approval of the management. He may do one or the other, or he may do something entirely inconsistent with either.

Some conflicts can be solved rather simply, for the alternatives lead to positive need satisfactions regardless of which way the individual goes. These are really no problem. Others may have at one pole a positive satisfaction and at the other a negative or unwanted result. This is no problem either for the obvious choice is the one which is satisfying to the individual. Those choices that *cause* the problems are those that put an individual in a dilemma.

The solution depends upon how the individual has learned to work out such situations. Whether he runs away or faces up to the problem will give the safety professional or supervisor a clue as to what will occur in the future in a similar situation.

### Job satisfaction

In the interest of further understanding of motivation in the work environment, many studies have been conducted to determine what constitutes job satisfaction in the workforce. Generally, these studies have sought to assess what workers claim to be the elements of their jobs that contribute to their satisfaction (or dissatisfaction) with their jobs. The results of these investigations suggest that the satisfaction of psychosocial needs rather than physiological needs may be the major motivational aspect of job satisfaction.

Table 11–A presents the results of a number of different surveys of job satisfaction. The numbers represent the rankings of the factors which were considered in each study. While different language and alternatives were used in each survey, the factors have been paraphrased to represent the elements covered in the surveys.

The results of these surveys suggest that high pay is not in itself a primary job motivator. Although workers expect a just and equitable income, they appear to expect only what others would be paid for comparable work. While the worker might feel dissatisfied if he were underpaid, higher pay alone does not guarantee job satisfaction (Clark, 1958; Adams, 1965).

On the other hand, steady work or job security does appear to be a primary job motivator. Workers want the security of knowing that on the basis of their performing their job well, they will have a job in the future. Job security, as a component of job satisfaction, may explain the willingness of a worker to maintain a low-paying, stable job instead of accepting a higher-paying, less-stable job.

Other factors which appear important as job satisfiers include—type of work, opportunities for advancement, and good working companions. Note that all of these factors seem related to the psychosocial needs of feeling important and belonging to a peer group which is acceptable to the worker. Likewise, comfortable working conditions (rated high by a number of employees) are probably associated with a desire of the worker to be treated humanely by the employer.

The results of these numerous surveys on job satisfaction are important when considering the safety program within the context of personnel policy. Inasmuch as the safety program is designed to ensure the well-being of the employee, it helps to maintain the employee's continued ability to do the work (which, in turn, gives job security).

Likewise, the safety program represents management's interest in the working companions and working conditions of the employee. All of these aspects of safety programming should be anticipated and incorporated into the approach which is taken with both supervisory staff and the employees. Honest and sincere positioning of the safety program within the context of the employee's welfare makes practical sense in light of our current knowledge regarding job satisfaction.

## TABLE 11-A

## SUMMARY OF DIFFERENT SURVEYS ON JOB SATISFACTION
In Order of Importance of Different Factors

| | Women Factory Workers | Union Workers | Nonunion Workers | Men | Women | Employees of Five Factories |
|---|---|---|---|---|---|---|
| Steady work | 1 | 1 | 1 | 1 | 3 | 1 |
| Type of work | | | | 3 | 1 | 3 |
| Opportunity for advancement | 5 | 4 | 4 | 2 | 2 | 4 |
| Good working companions | 4 | | | 4 | 5 | |
| High pay | 6 | 2½ | 2 | 5½ | 8 | 2 |
| Good boss | 3 | 5½ | 5 | 5½ | 4 | 6 |
| Comfortable working conditions | 2 | 2½ | 3 | 8½ | 6 | 7 |
| Benefits | | 5½ | 6 | 8½ | 9 | 5 |
| Opportunity to learn a job | 8 | | | | | |
| Good hours | 9 | 7½ | 7 | 7 | 7 | |
| Opportunity to use one's ideas | 7 | 7½ | 8 | | | |
| Easy work | 10 | | | | | |

## Management theories of motivation

As previously mentioned, there are many theories in the psychological literature that address human motivation. Within this literature, specific theories have evolved with special reference to management as it exists in industrial organizations. Two such theories are presented here, although other equally cogent points of view could be discussed.

Because theories of human motivation lack sufficient data to support all their tenets, they might best be viewed as philosophies of management. They are important to the safety professional because, if accepted, they can influence the direction in which management seeks to develop and implement a safety program.

## Theory X and Theory Y

In an attempt to analyze how management personnel view human motivation, McGregor (1960) has evolved the notion that there are two basic ways in which management can view the worker. According to which view management accepts, essentially different management practices will be observed.

Theory X, according to McGregor, assumes that the worker is essentially uninterested and unmotivated to work. In order to resolve this condition, the motivation must be instilled into the worker by the adoption of a variety of external motivation agents. In effect, the worker becomes motivated to work by virtue of the external rewards and punishments which are offered to him.

For example, in order to create motivation, a Theory X manager might use any and all of the following—introduction of rules to constrict the worker's behavior, pay incentives based on production, and threats to job security associated with performance failure.

Thus, under Theory X policy, management uses control and direction as the means of worker motivation.

Theory Y, according to McGregor, assumes that the worker is basically interested and motivated to work. In fact, work is assumed to be as natural and desirable as other forms of human activity, such as sleep and recreation. Under such circumstances, management is confronted with the role or organizing work so that the worker's job coincides with the goals and objectives of the organization. Thus, a Theory Y manager views the task as constructively using the worker's self-control and self-direction as the instrumentality for accomplishing the work to be done.

By emphasizing responsibility and goal orientation, management capitalizes upon the inherent motivation already present within the worker. If conflicts occur between the worker's goals and management's goals, they are resolved through mutual exploration and discussion. Always, under Theory Y policy, it is assumed that the worker's inherent motivation is essential to the completion of the organization's goals.

Both Theory X and Theory Y proponents exist, and apparently management systems operating on the basis of each of these theories can be found throughout American industry. What seems important is that whichever system is operating within an organization, it is necessary to recognize that safety programming can be initiated and implemented. While the technique of implementation may differ, Theory X and Theory Y approaches to human motivation can both be amenable to enhancing a worker's motivation to safe behavior.

### Job-enrichment theory

Another analysis of human motivation in occupational environments has been developed by Herzberg (1966). While being quite comparable to the Theory X and Theory Y distinction, Herzberg has been explicit in both the detail and philosophy which he has evolved. His concept of job enrichment, in many ways an extension of Theory Y, is a major current force in management theory.

The classic approach to motivation concerns itself with changing the environment in which a person works—the circumstances that surround the individual while working (good or poor lighting, an agreeable or offensive supervisor), and the

| Hygiene Approach | Job-Enrichment Approach |
| --- | --- |
| Company policies and administration | Achievement |
| Supervision | Recognition |
| Working conditions | Work itself |
| Interpersonal relations | Responsibility |
| Money, status, security | Professional growth |

Fig. 11-2.—Contrast of the hygiene approach to motivation and the job-enrichment approach.

incentives given in exchange for work (money, a pat on the back, a writeup in the company bulletin, to name a few).

Herzberg believes that the concern for environment is important—but not all-important. He says that it is not sufficient in itself for effective motivation. That, he contends, requires experiences that are inherent in the work itself.

Herzberg holds that there is no conflict between the classic (environmental) approach to motivation and his approach to motivation through work itself. He regards both as important. The classic approach is called hygiene whereas Herzberg's approach is called "job enrichment."

The hygiene approach may be understood by the following analogy—a person is provided with pure drinking water and waste disposal; both are necessary to keep this person healthy, but neither makes him any healthier. By extension, environmental factors always need replenishment. Good rapport may enhance an individual's job satisfaction, but job satisfaction alone will not necessarily result in safe work habits.

Fig. 11-2 presents a contrast of the classic hygiene approach to motivation and the job-enrichment approach.

Further, treating a person better does not enrich his job, although the individual may be unhappy if not treated well. Again, a salary increase may keep an employee from becoming dissatisfied for a time, but sooner or later another increase will be required.

Although there may be inherent hazards associated with a work environment, such as coal mining or bridge building, the worker has a right to expect controls to prevent the environment from becoming unreasonably unsafe, for example testing and removal of explosive gases, or safety nets and life lines. Such protection might not motivate him because it makes the job safer, but he might be very unhappy if he knew no effort was made to protect him.

Herzberg's idea that work itself can be a motivator represents an important behavioral science breakthrough. Traditionally, work has been regarded as an unpleasant necessity but it has not been thought of as a potential motivator.

Although automation is helping to phase out the unstimulating aspect of many jobs, a job should provide an opportunity for personal satisfaction or growth. When it does, it becomes a powerful motivating force.

People, Herzberg further theorizes, must be given the opportunity to do work that they think is meaningful. Merely telling an individual who is doing a routine job that he is happy and that he is doing something meaningful accomplishes nothing. But job rotation is not the answer, either; it does not enrich a job—it only makes it bigger.

Another point. Herzberg observes, "Resurrection is more difficult than giving birth." Obsolescence must, therefore, be eliminated by continued retraining—not just a once-in-a-while effort. Jobs should be kept up-to-date, and people doing the jobs must be kept up-to-date.

Even though a company may provide the hygiene factors, they must also provide a task that has challenge, meaning, and significance. If an unchallenged individual does not quit, he stays on—but with poor morale. That, says Herzberg, is the price a company pays for not motivating people.

In summary, seven principles of job enrichment can be itemized.

• Organize the job to give each worker a complete natural unit of work

• Provide new and more difficult tasks to each worker

• Allow the worker to perform specialized tasks in order to provide a unique contribution

• Increase the authority of the worker in his job

• Eliminate unneeded controls on the worker while maintaining accountability

• Require increased accountability of the worker

for his own work

• Provide direct feedback through periodic reports to the worker himself

## Frustration and Conflict

A motivated individual is one who is attempting to reach a goal. Often, however, a barrier is placed between the goal and the one who is seeking it. When this occurs, the individual becomes frustrated. This differs from mere *lack of satisfaction* of a need, which is called deprivation. Theoretically, the *thwarting of behavior* directed toward a goal results in frustration (Miller, 1959).

The barrier may come from within the individual himself. The person who sets impossible goals for himself may become frustrated when he is unable to reach the goals because he cannot work that fast. The "way out" may be an accident.

The barrier may also arise from the environment. An example—if the person mentioned above (who set a very high production output goal for himself) is unable to reach such limits because of faulty equipment.

A third type of frustration is caused by conflict. If two motives somehow conflict, the satisfaction of one means the frustration of the other. For example, the worker who sets high production and safety standards for himself, but is unable to meet both under the present system, must satisfy one and sacrifice the other.

It is to the conflict-caused frustration that we will now address ourselves. Basically, there are three types of conflicts—called "approach-approach," "avoidance-avoidance," and "approach-avoidance."

### Approach-approach

As the label implies the "approach-approach" conflict arises when an individual is faced with two goals which are equally attractive, but only one of which is obtainable at the time. An example is the college student who has been asked to go both to a dance and to a swimming party on the same evening.

The approach-approach conflict is the easiest to resolve. No matter what goal the individual selects, a need will be satisfied, without much loss to another need. Usually the individual will resolve such a conflict by satisfying one need first and then satisfying the other. If the person is both hungry and sleepy, for example, he might eat first and then retire.

**311**

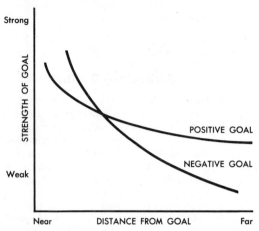

FIG. 11-3.—The approach-avoidance conflict is complicated by the different goal gradients for positive and negative goals.

## Avoidance-avoidance

A second type of conflict is the "avoidance-avoidance" or double-negative conflict. This conflict may arise when an employee is told to wear heavy fire-retardant outer clothing in the summer heat or else risk the possibility of catching his clothes on fire. This employee is, as the saying goes, caught "between the devil and the deep blue sea."

Two kinds of behavior generally result from such a conflict—vacillation and flight.

In vacillation, the individual approaches one goal; retreats, approaches the other, retreats, and so on. As he approaches a goal, the unpleasant portions of the goal increase, so he withdraws. In the example, the worker may stall off doing the job requiring wearing the heavy clothing until the quitting bell sounds.

Another result from the avoidance-avoidance conflict is flight. The athlete may leave the field or the worker may quit his job. Quitting a job, of course, has serious consequences in lost prestige and lost income.

A more common type of fleeing, therefore, is in a figurative sense—like daydreaming, fantasy, etc. The worker faced with an unpleasant task may repress the reality by daydreaming.

The avoidance-avoidance conflict is not as easy to resolve as the approach-approach, nor is it as difficult as this next conflict type.

## Approach-avoidance

The "approach-avoidance" conflict is the most difficult to resolve. The individual is both attracted and repelled by the same goal (Fig. 11-3). The worker who is striving for top production may be forced to take unnecessary risks to achieve that goal. One way out of such a conflict is by erasing or weakening one of the signs, thereby altering the individual's internal motivational system.

Approach-avoidance conflict refers to a single goal having both positive and negative attributes associated with it. Other things being equal, the strength of the approach or avoidance tendency will depend upon the proximity of the individual to the goal. At point A, for example, the tendency to avoid (or retreat) will be greater than the tendency to approach (since, as shown, the slope of the negative goal gradient is steeper than the positive goal gradient at point A). At point B, however, the tendency to approach the goal will be greater than the tendency to avoid. According to this theory, conflict will lead to retreat, vacillation, or indecision. Theoretically, the approach-avoidance conflict, and more complex double approach-avoidance conflict situations (that is, two goals, each mutually exclusive, having positive and negative attributes associated with each), are thought to be common situations (Miller, 1959).

## Reaction to frustration

In most cases, the conflicts described will lead to frustration. This frustration may often lead to positive, constructive resolution of the situation. For example, the individual who is facing the conflict of top production, but at increased risk, may develop a new system for processing the product at a faster *and* safer rate.

On the other hand the frustration often leads to some negative form of behavior, a few examples of which are listed next. This is by no means an exhaustive list, nor are they mutually exclusive; one may appear in combination with another (Dollard & Miller, 1950; Miller & Dollard, 1941).

**Aggression.** This form of behavior is characterized by some type of attack toward another person or object. The four-year-old boy who beats his playmate over the head with a baseball bat is obviously exhibiting aggressive behavior. The forms of aggression of adults can be overt, physical, or verbal. They can also be disguised; the tidbit of shop gossip, or the subtle comment by an aspirant for a promotion about one of his possible competitors, could be just as devastating to the victim as the baseball bat.

**Regression.** Regression is the tendency for an individual who finds himself in a frustrating circumstance to revert to an earlier form of behavior, such as putting on a temper tantrum or pouting. Such behavior most likely would occur in the case of an individual who, during his formative years, found that such behavior worked; in other words, he got his way by a display of temper.

**Fixation.** In fixated behavior, the individual persists in a particular kind of nonconstructive behavior even though it is clear that the behavior is inadequate to resolve the problem. Thus, a mechanic may persist in trying to fit a bolt in place, even though he realizes that it is the wrong size.

**Resignation.** Resignation is the tendency for an individual to give up—to withhold any sense of emotion or personal involvement in the situation. Failing to achieve some goal, this person loses any positive concern about his job and adopts an apathetic attitude toward the situation.

**Negativism.** In this form of behavior, the individual adopts a negative, resistive position with respect to the situation. A person whose suggestions have not been accepted may take a dim view of any other ideas.

**Repression.** This behavior is characterized by blocking out from consciousness those cognitive associations that are disturbing. It is an unrealistic form of behavior because it implies that the problem will simply go away if one does not think about it.

**Withdrawal.** In this type of behavior, the frustrated individual simply removes himself from the situation in question—either physically or psychologically. A person who is not able to cope with a business adversary may avoid situations which would put him in contact with the individual. An individual who is the butt of jibes and jokes may become a loner.

## Emotion and frustration

Negative emotions can have a disturbing influence upon a person's behavior. Anxiety is one emotional reaction which, because of its distracting influence, its stimulus to heightened reaction, and its generally upsetting effect, can make an individual more susceptible to accidents. This general upsetting feeling can be spread to others working in the same situation and create an atmosphere not conducive to safe procedures.

Anxiety, however, is but one kind of emotional pattern shown by individuals in the face of frustration. The anxious individual is worried, circular in his thinking, and fearful in such a way as to make his behavior inadequate to reach his goal. Even though the individual himself may realize that his behavior is getting him nowhere, he is unable to find a method that will solve his problem.

In frustration, some people become angry, some fearful, and some accept frustration as a challenge and attempt to solve the problem. Most people who react emotionally to frustration and threat find it extremely difficult to cope with life situations. It is not necessary to discuss the physiological pattern which develops in emotion for everyone is familiar with the feelings experienced during fear, anxiety, anger, shame, and other emotions. Rather, one needs to recognize that over the years people have developed accepted social expressions for emotions. To some degree, one individual can be aware of how another is feeling. This is not to say that one cannot be fooled or that the outward expression always truly indicates the feelings of the individual. Many people learn to mask their real feelings.

However, after day-to-day interaction over a long period of time, one may learn to tell the difference between internal feelings and those expressed. This is useful to the supervisor and the safety professional in his dealings with individuals in the shop. As they go about the plant carrying out their normal duties, they may discover those individuals having difficulties and take some extra precautions to avoid accidents.

It seems important to make note of the problem of behavior disorders within the context of employee problems. Individuals whose normal behavior is seriously disrupted or whose ability to react to frustration is seriously impaired may require professional services beyond the scope of the normal supervisory-employee relationship. Although a supervisor should assist in directing the employee to inplant services or outside agencies, he should avoid attempting to deal directly with psychological problems requiring professional care. While the current movement toward company-sponsored psychological services may grow, it is unlikely to be the standard in all industries in the near future. For a detailed discussion of industry programs for drug abuse and alcoholism, see Chapter 21, "Occupational Health Services."

### Non-directive counseling

Although no attempt can be made here to train safety professionals or supervisors to become personnel counselors, they can do much to help reduce the immediate result of strong emotion. The supervisor is in the best position to evaluate the emotional level of an individual worker and to do something about it.

Everyone is familiar with the emotional outbursts of people who have had a trying and upsetting experience. Such expression of emotion may take many forms from an outburst of bad language, a torrent of tears, to physical assault on inanimate objects which cannot strike back. The end result is the same—relief from the intolerable tension, and emotional relaxation.

The supervisor can sometimes alleviate work-related tension by providing an employee with an opportunity to talk about whatever is bothering him or her. This may be especially helpful if the problem is work-related or concerns a minor personal problem. The freedom to say what the individual pleases, without the evaluation of the supervisor, can reduce tension and open communication channels.

The stresses which cause emotional upset can occur within the work environment or away from it, but each kind has its effect on the other. A simple statement, such as "How are you today?" or "What's bothering you?," may well be sufficient to set off the verbalization of pent-up emotion. Ater the discussion, the employee can often evaluate more clearly and realistically the things that upset him in the first place.

To attack the problem at the roots calls for permissive listening on the part of the employee's immediate supervisor. In his normal routine every supervisor has an opportunity to talk with individual employees. Through the use of open-ended questions (those that do not allow for a simple yes-or-no answer) an employee is encouraged to discuss his problems. The supervisor needs to listen not only to words but the

feelings they carry. He must give his attention to the unspoken language of facial expressions, gestures, bodily postures, and the like. This will bring him closer to understanding the attitudes and strength of feeling attached to them.

In such face-to-face discussions or interviews, it is inappropriate for the supervisor to argue, caution, evaluate, or cajole the employee, but rather he should try to reverbalize and reflect the expressions of feelings and attitudes. Having ventilated the emotion, this reflection will give the employee a chance to reevaluate without emotion his own position. He will thereby come to make a new appraisal of the situation more in line with the requirements of objectivity.

Frequently it is impossible to discuss such matters at length in the work area, so the supervisor should set a time and a place away from other employees to allow the individual freedom of expression. Even though the supervisor may not have a completely private office in which to engage in such kinds of interviewing, some place can be found for a quiet face-to-face discussion.

This relationship between the supervisor and the worker must be one of the supervisor's normal everyday functions. Diligent observation and effective and sensitive listening should be tools of every supervisor.

### Attitude and Attitude Change

Although many existent psychological theories address attitude and attitude change, many basic concepts are still controversial. For example, whether or not attitudes are a precursor (or antecedent condition) of behavior is largely an unresolved theoretical issue in social psychology. Many theories on attitude formation and change assume an active behavioral role, that is, attitudes consist of three components, knowing-feeling-acting. Thus, such a theoretical approach distinguishes, yet integrates, such concepts as knowledge, emotions, and behavior or behavioral tendencies. Other theories regard attitudes as the delineation of values toward something or someone. Most of these theories agree, however, that attitudes (at least in part) are a disposition to evaluate objects, persons, or situations favorably or unfavorably (McGuire, 1969; Insko & Schopler, 1972).

What an individual's response can be is dependent, in part, upon the previous experiences of the individual. For example, if an individual sees a

TABLE 11-B

## FACTORS ASSOCIATED WITH PERSUASIVE COMMUNICATION

| Attitude-Change: Situation Types | Communication Process | Attitude Change: Behavioral Step |
|---|---|---|
| 1. Suggestive | 1. Source | 1. Attention |
| 2. Conformity | 2. Message factors | 2. Comprehension |
| 3. Group discussion | 3. Channel factors | 3. Yielding |
| 4. Persuasive messages | 4. Receiver factors | 4. Retention |
| 5. Intensive doctrination | 5. Destination factors | 5. Action |

*Source: McGuire (1969).*

person on the street who resembles a friend, he immediately may smile, make friendly gestures, and have a warm quality in his voice. When that person is perceived to be a stranger, there is an immediate change to another facial expression, gesture, voice quality, and so on. Anticipated reaction can be set off by a certain look from another person, a manner of speaking, a mustache or the lack of one, the color of hair, or kind of handshake. All individuals have certain feelings about these and may act in accordance to their attitudes, as these have been formed over the years.

Some of these attitudes are latent. The predisposition to respond will lie dormant within the individual until called forth. Given the appropriate stimulus, the attitude shows itself and the behavior exhibited is in accordance with the feelings of the individual. A certain word, for example, connotes different responses in different people. The words "union," "management," "labor," and even "safety" carry with them certain connotations that touch off different attitudinal reactions in individuals, depending upon the kinds of experiences they have had with the subject.

Because attitudes play such an important role in everyday relationships, consideration should be given to their development, their effects on individuals, and what can be done to change them.

### Determination of attitudes

Direct personal experience is thought to be one determinant of attitudes. In other words, expe-

riences that individuals have had in the past, especially those involving strong associative emotions, determine attitudes. For example, the attitude of a worker toward management or his supervisor may be fearful and hostile if the worker has lost jobs for no apparent reason, as he sees it. There may have been sound reasons for his dismissals or layoffs, but to admit this to himself would be a threat to his own pride, and so he puts the blame elsewhere. Because of the effects that these dismissals have had on him and his family, such as causing financial stress, he may become very angry. Management to him now is a menacing thing, and thus the cause of his present hostile and fearful attitude.

Many people have had experiences that were associated with fear, sorrow, pain, or happiness. All of these will tend to make them react the same way to anything that is similar to the original emotion-provoking situation. Although there is only one positive emotion listed among those just mentioned, it is not to be concluded that most attitudes are negative, for there are many positive ones.

### Attitude change

Factors associated with communication-induced attitude change are numerous. In summarizing the large body of psychological literature on attitude formation and change, McGuire (1969) suggested three components of attitude change (see Table 11-B). These include: types of attitude-change situations (column 1), variables associated with the communication process (column 2), and communication outcome (column 3).

• Relevant situational factors include: suggestive situations (where the desired attitude is repeatedly presented), conformity (where social or peer pressure is used to elicit the desired response), group discussion, persuasive messages and intensive doctrination. Each situation is associated with varying degrees of attitude change. Also, distinctive implications of each is dependent upon the type of communication variables involved.

• Source variables refer to characteristics associated with the person or represented organization presenting the message. The effect of the message on subsequent attitudes can vary as a function of the perceived credibility, attractiveness (for example, liking, familiarity), and power of the message (that is, inclusion or exclusion of basic pro and con issues), the order in which specific issues are presented, and dissimilarities between the presenter and recipient of the message. Channel factors consist of the mode of presentation, for example, direct personal experience, mass media. Receiver factors include active participation, and degree of influenceability of the audience. Destination factors refer to the degree of post-communication message decay across time, and time latency associated with delayed-action.

• According to McGuire (1969), the receiver (or audience) must proceed through the following steps in order for attitude change to occur. These are: attention, comprehension, yielding, retention, and action. According to this model, each step depends on the occurrence of the preceding one.

To add to the complexity, the communication variables, especially in daily situations, can interact with one another. And too, the sequential step process may have more intuitive than empirical support. Nevertheless, this conceptual framework should highlight the implications (e.g., difficulties or dangers) associated with oversimplifying or making broad unsubstantiated generalizations about the process of attitude change.

**Organization development.** Concern for the amount and rate of change within our technological society has focused on the industrial environment and its ability to withstand such change. Behavioral scientists have evolved an approach,

| Mechanical Systems | Organic Systems |
|---|---|
| Emphasis upon individual performance | Emphasis on relationships in group |
| Chain of command concepts | Confidence and trust among everyone |
| Adherence to delegated responsibility | Adherence to shared responsibility |
| Division of labor and management | Participation in multi-member teams |
| Centralized management control | De-centralized sharing of control |
| Resolution of conflict through grievance procedures | Resolution of conflict through problem solving |

FIG. 11–4.—Organization development seeks to implement organic systems in place of mechanical systems within organizations.

called "organizational development," which attempts to assess a corporation's ability to adjust to such conditions as rapid and unexpected change, growth in size, increasing diversity, and management system problems. Organizational development, which generally has as its goal the implementation of an educational strategy, is designed to alter the attitude and structure of organizations so that they can better adapt to a changing technology.

Generally, organizational development uses initial feedback of the employees and management to determine the climate and capacity of the organization to adapt its objectives to the technological environment. Based upon such feedback, an attempt is made to develop organic systems to replace mechanical systems within the organization. Organic systems are characterized by a preoccupation with people as they operate together whereas mechanical systems are characterized by a preoccupation with the structure that operates within a system. Fig. 11–4 presents a summary of the differences between mechanical and organic systems. In the final analysis, organizational development rejects bureaucracy as an organizational model and substitutes a model based on interpersonal competence.

In order to implement the ideas represented by organizational development, a number of procedures are used to effect changes in the organization. Since the changes are typically people-oriented, due consideration is given to the need to motivate acceptance of the changes within both management and work groups. Typically, such techniques as sensitivity training, confrontation groups, and transactional analysis are used to effect reorientations within the organization's staff. These techniques have merit in implementing change only so long as top management concurs with the changes and provides incentives within the organization for their adoption.

Ultimately, organizational development seems to provide the necessary means for preparing an organization for orderly planning for the future. Included in such an effort should be the recognition of how changes in an organization will affect the current safety program. By adopting widespread involvement of all elements of the organization in safety programming, it is likely that safety programs will be able to meet the future needs of modern organizations.

## Structural change

In the previous discussion of attitude formation and attitude change, no direct relationship between attitude change and behavioral change was assumed. In practice, however, safety personnel are interested, for example, in changing an employee's attitude regarding the wearing of protective equipment only so long as such an attitude change ultimately results in the employee's actually wearing the equipment. While the research literature indicates that a variety of influence efforts (training and counseling for example) can change attitudes, there is much less support for a direct relationship between attitude changes and subsequent behavior changes.

In effect, it is incumbent upon the safety professional to consider techniques other than attitude change when considering changes in the employees' behavior. Evidence suggests that it is possible to change behavior by the introduction of structural changes within the work environment. Structural changes are procedures designed to change the organizational constraints which operate within work groups. Examples include: changing job contents, modifying the physical arrangements of work, changing worker interaction patterns, and rearranging work procedures.

In each case, other than an appropriate introduction of the change, it is not necessary to expend the time and effort to change attitudes prior to changing behavior directly. Rather, the introduction of the structural change can modify behavior directly and possibly, in turn, attitudes may change.

While there has not been an extensive attempt to apply the structural change model in occupational safety, it warrants consideration in the future. Human behavior can be changed by eliciting the change through the very circumstances under which the individual works. Unsafe acts, for example, cannot occur where the conditions of the work and work groups preclude their occurrence.

## Learning

Learning underlies much of what makes for differences and similarities among people. Through learning, people have developed certain kinds of psychosocial needs, habitual patterns of behavior, ways of reacting to emotion, and the attitudes which they bring with them to industry. It is important to consider learning and the laws that affect it. This is especially vital in any discussion of safety, because training is a major consideration in safety programs.

Often, to change behavior, one must substitute new learning for old habits (Hulse, Deese, and Egeth, 1975). To change behavior in need-satisfaction sequences, one must teach better ways by which the goal can be achieved. In each case, some new learning must be substituted for old.

### Motivational requirements

Repeatedly in everyday living, people recall many things which they did not set out to learn. While unintentional learning does occur, it is the intentional kind of learning in which the safety professional is primarily interested.

In educational systems, great emphasis is placed upon making the individual want the knowledge which is available to him. Materials are designed to relate to practical situations. Teachers attempt to make the individual interested in the material as such. To teach a student something about angles or distances, the teacher may use a baseball diamond as an example. Teachers try to tap motivation to increase the possibility that learning will take place.

The safety professional must recognize that if

his workers are going to learn safe procedures, his workers must be motivated. To merely point out that accidents cost the company money will not motivate them. Rather, point out the hazards that are risked when using unsafe work procedures—the probability of serious and painful injury, the possible loss of earning power and the effect on his loved ones. The cost, not only in dollars but also psychologically to both the worker and his family, is of paramount importance to him and will motivate him to learn safe work methods.

It is not wise to assume that, because management sees the value of safe procedures, the worker will also. Management may be motivated to start a safety program because it will reduce insurance costs, reduce the amount of waste, and increase the number of units produced. Workers cannot be expected to desire it for the same reasons. In selling a safety program to the employees, one must capitalize on the things which will motivate them. Here the safety professional can capitalize on the needs discussed previously, and he probably can find many more which are consistent with the aims of the safety program. Everything that will motivate the worker to learn the right procedures should be used. (The next chapter discusses this in more detail.)

## Principles of learning

Some consideration of basic principles is valid whether the learning is to be done in a college classroom or in a work area. When training procedures utilize these principles, learning is more efficient and thorough.

**Reinforcement.** Through experimentation, psychologists have found that reinforcement can often facilitate learning. In practice, reinforcement can, for example, make work more efficient and more productive. When a worker's pay increases because of more units of production, he is receiving reward for his learning. This can have negative aspects as well—the worker who figures out a hazardous short cut, which produces more units, may be rewarded for an unsafe act, as was mentioned earlier in this chapter.

It is apparent that the employee must be rewarded only for safe work methods. Higher productivity because of safe work methods satisfies the need for achievement and recognition. This in itself reinforces the learning of the employee, but also spreads its effect to other employees who see this take place. A supervisor by recognizing the same needs, however, can reinforce this learning through praise for greater productivity and telling the worker how much better he is doing, for example.

The publicity given to a safety record, a bonus, a promotion, or anything which satisfies individual needs would serve as a reward to reinforce whatever learning has brought about the desired behavior.

Reinforcement tends to be more effective if it closely follows the desired behavior. Praise, for example, should be given at the time the desired behavior occurs, or if delayed, associated verbally with the desired behavior. This does not mean it must be instantaneous, but it should be within a reasonable length of time. If delay is necessary, certainly recall to the individual the reason for the reward.

Reinforcement will often increase the likelihood of a reoccurrence of the desired behavior. Shortcut hazardous methods or any deliberate unsafe acts must not be rewarded. In fact, in such situations reprimands or punishment may be more appropriate. In short, unsafe methods should be corrected by full and complete explanation and demonstration of safe work procedures. Such being the case, it also follows that there should be reinforcement of the new correct work pattern as soon as feasible.

This principle also applies to participation by employees in a safety program whether it be through suggestion systems, safety committees, discussion groups or training sessions. In all these areas an individual gains personal worth if his opinions are asked for and graciously received.

A safety program that gathers the ideas of all, either individually or by representation, satisfies the need people have for being "in the know." In this way, the safety professional may create a positive atmosphere about the program and a sense of obligation and responsibility for its success. Research has demonstrated that when employees feel that programs come from all, there is more chance for success.

Research on the effectiveness of punishment suggests that punishment can have diverse consequences. Punishment generally is thought to be less effective than reinforcement, perhaps because punishment provides indirect cues or information, i.e., what not to do; as opposed to positive reinforcement (i.e., reward) that provides direct information about the desired behavior

(Church, 1963).

The rewarding of correct procedures will lead to a more positive attitudinal response on the part of the worker than any punishment. A positive attitude toward training procedures is much to be desired. Both the positive and the negative aspects of reinforcement may generalize over the whole work situation. The supervisor's praise for a particular thing well done may spread over other aspects of the total situation, including training procedures, safety devices, and the safety program. The proper use of rewards thus can lead to efficient methods.

Much of the practice underlying programmed instruction (see Chapter 9, "Safety Training") is based upon the reinforcement concept as well as the other principles of learning which follow.

**Knowledge of results.** Closely allied to reward—in fact, one aspect of reward—is knowledge of results. Everyone likes to know how he is doing on a particular job. Letting the individual employee know how well he is getting along in his training program will likely motivate him to continue training and do a better job. To train a worker and not inform him of any improvement is defeating one's own purpose. It cannot be contended that the only one who needs to know about the effects of training is the supervisor or the safety professional. When the worker knows that this new procedure is helping him get greater production, he is getting reinforced for his learning and effort.

One of the factors which appears in some kinds of learning is a plateau at which learning levels off for some time before again showing an increase. Often some individuals become discouraged and learning can be retarded. If the trainer understands this phenomenon and indicates to the individual that a leveling off had been expected and that an increase will come later, the discouraging aspect of such a plateau may be avoided, with learning then proceeding more easily and efficiently. Demonstrating to the worker the achievements he is making through production curves, which are in effect learning curves, gives the worker knowledge of results, and this is a motivating factor for future learning.

**Practice.** The safety professional is interested in developing in an individual safe habit patterns which will become almost automatic in his work methods. Merely putting a worker through suffi-cient training sessions is not enough. Despite his apparent mastery, the next time through the work he may make one or more mistakes. To make sure that habit patterns are firmly entrenched, the worker must practice. The Job Instruction Training programs include one of the important aspects of training, namely, followup by the foreman. This is for no other purpose than to ensure mastery. Within a reasonable time, depending on the job complexity, this followup may become unnecessary.

Take, for example, a simple task such as bicycle riding. A youngster, in learning to ride a bicycle, needs to know how to balance, how to get on, how to get off, and how to stop, and he must learn all of these things as part of the total process. Perhaps he begins with balancing, then the start and stop, and then how to get on and off. Once he has accomplished all of these, he is not immediately left to himself. He needs several more sessions to make sure that he is doing it correctly. This, in effect, is reinforcement by practice. Furthermore, the youngster himself keeps practicing each time he goes out to ride. So it is also with the individual on the job.

**Whole vs. part learning.** Whole or part learning has been a knotty problem for industrial trainers for many years. Whether trainers should teach the procedure as a whole or break it down and teach it part-by-part is the question. There is no best answer. Both methods have advantages and disadvantages depending upon: job complexity, the trainee, and the kind of job breakdown used. Perhaps a combination of the two is best, using the whole method, but with sufficient flexibility to emphasize meaningful parts of the task wherever necessary.

**Meaningfulness.** Studies in verbal learning have demonstrated the importance of the meaningfulness of the material to be learned. Meaningfulness is important in safety education because the worker needs to understand why a certain procedure is better than another. Adequate explanation of a given movement or change in position, in terms of the hazards eliminated, with no decrease in production, gives meaningfulness to the procedure. With this understanding, the worker will be motivated to learn the safe procedure. Without it, he will be inclined to utilize his own method until he learns, perhaps by an accident, the inadequacy of it.

# 11—Human Behavior and Safety

The safety professional and line supervisor in safety programs should not forget the advantage of workers' understanding the reason for protective clothing, safety devices, safety meetings, and discussions, as well as the need for full and complete accident reports.

Meaningfulness to management and workers is understanding the value of a reduction of accidents, fewer disabilities, and retention of earning power.

**Selective learning.** Out of each day's many experiences, people select those which they desire to retain. This probably is related to motivation more than to anything else, and for that reason motivational aspects of a training program need to be considered. Safety trainers must be sure that the workers retain the most important facts. Relating subject matter to individual needs will ensure the proper selection.

**Frequency.** Everyone does best those things that he practices the most. This principle is certainly important to the safety professional for it emphasizes the necessity of frequent applications of safety rules and regulations in the training program. Frequent reference to the various kinds of problems, hazards, and procedures to eliminate accidents ensures greater effect than just a one-exposure routine. Giving the worker a copy of the safety rules and regulations in hopes that these will be learned and used is not enough. Means should be adopted which will bring them to his attention frequently and regularly.

A major railroad practiced this when its supervisors discussed with their employees a safety regulation each day before work began. Thus, each day, the staff was responsible for knowing, understanding, and applying this regulation, when appropriate or when asked by the supervisor. This company combined the principles of learning, reinforcement, and followup in one program activity.

A trainer must insist not only on frequent practice, but on the trainee's following the correct method. Day-after-day use of safe methods will create safe habit patterns that will later be followed almost automatically. The supervisor and safety director must make sure that the work method practiced is the safe one.

**Recency.** Closely allied to the principle of frequency is that of recency. That which is learned last can usually be most easily recalled. As has been indicated, handing a worker a set of safety rules and regulations does not ensure learning. Those who received printed instructions or a few training demonstrations a long time ago may not be able to recall now what the rules and regulations are. Safety professionals must devise means by which workers have constant contacts with these regulations through such continuing activities as contests, reviews of safety regulations, and committee work.

**Primacy.** The law of primacy must be taken into consideration in two aspects of the safety program. The worker's initial contact with procedures should be one of major importance. If this initial contact is of a negative nature—such as being tossed a book of rules, accompanied by a shouted, "Make sure you learn 'em"—the worker is left with the impression that safety is unimportant. From the very beginning of employment, the worker must get the impression that not only the rules but the whole program is of great importance. This will help assure the positive response desired.

Second, in the training program, habit patterns utilizing safe methods should assume primary importance. The supervisor must be certain that the worker does not have an opportunity to work by any other than the safe method. It becomes harder to establish good patterns after having first learned the poor ones. This principle applies to the golfer who has picked up bad techniques and then has to unlearn them as well as to the worker on the job. His training must be *right* from the very beginning. Old habits are hard to break and, to the safety professional, expensive in training costs and accident costs.

**Intensity.** Those things which are made most vivid to the worker will be retained the longest. Safety programs already utilize this principle in safety publicity with eye-catching posters and the like.

It is part of the safety professional's responsibility to enhance the worker's interest in the program. In this way, it will be a long-remembered experience. Under other conditions, it might well be forgotten minutes after it is over. To some degree, this is in effect positioning the safety program in the same way that advertisers position their commercials to catch the public's attention.

**Transfer of training.** All new learning occurs within the context of previous learning experiences. The fact that current learning (or performance) can be influenced by previous learning is known as transfer of training. Positive transfer of training occurs when the previous learning facilitates the current learning or enhances current performance. Negative transfer of training occurs when the previous learning makes the current learning experience more difficult or in some way inhibits current performance.

Inasmuch as the safety professional desires to facilitate the learning of correct responses in new situations, he should attempt to maximize the positive transfer which occurs within the industrial environment.

Generally, learning to make identical responses to new stimuli results in positive transfer. For example, learning to drive in a new (or different) automobile is facilitated by the fact that identical responses (such as accelerating or steering) are required to the new stimuli (accelerator, steering wheel). If the new stimuli are very similar to previous cars (for example, the location of the controls, their texture, and their direction of movement), positive transfer should be high. In such situations, positive transfer increases as a function of increased similarity of the stimuli in the two situations.

Learning to make new responses to identical stimuli results in negative transfer. For example, if the controls of the cars appear identical but each car requires a different response in order to be operated correctly, negative transfer can be expected. After driving a car in which the "park" position appears on the extreme right of the indicator panel, much difficulty (negative transfer) can be anticipated when driving a car in which the "park" position appears on the extreme left of the indicator panel. Or, if the "off" position of one toggle switch is the same as the "on" position of another, the potential for accidents is serious.

Such negative transfer can take the form of errors, delayed reactions, and generally inefficient performance on the new task. In such situations the amount of negative transfer increases as a function of increases in the similarity of the stimuli in the two situations.

With an understanding of transfer phenomena, it is possible to maximize the opportunities for positive transfer and minimize those for negative transfer within the industrial environment. This requires careful planning of machine purchases and work procedures to make sure that the new tasks required of a worker make use of (and do not conflict with) his previous learning experiences.

## Forgetting

This discussion of learning would not be complete without some consideration of the process of forgetting, which goes on as learning takes place. Never assume that learning and forgetting are mutually exclusive, for such is not the case. As one learns, one also forgets what has been previously learned. Curves of forgetting indicate that most is lost immediately after learning has taken place. Depending on the complexity of the job, the amount of learning lost will vary after each day's training session. There should be less forgetfulness or initial mistakes in successive days of training, and more need for patient reteaching.

Consideration of the various principles of learning and the motivational aspects of the problem are essential if one is to retard this process of forgetting. The safety professional needs to consider all of them from the initial stages of employment right on through to the everyday work situations in the company.

## Summary

The human factor operates at all levels in industry, and is perhaps the most potent factor for success or failure of a safety program. It makes a difference whether the president of a company approves or drags his feet, whether the safety professional works hard or coasts along, whether the supervisor emphasizes safety or subordinates it to production, whether the janitor cleans well or does only the minimum. Attitudes *are* important to safety in the company. Safety can be achieved only by working through all these people. The human factor must be dealt with in every area of industry.

To achieve some mark of success in dealing with people, individuals can best be considered within the framework established in this discussion. Each person is an individual, to some degree different from every other one. The differences are for the most part obvious, but there are subtle ones too, which must be recognized, if only to the extent that their existence is acknowledged.

Despite great differences in people, reasons for their activities are common to all. Many needs are the same, particularly at the biological level and to a large degree at the psychosocial level. It is upon these needs that the safety professional and others in positions of leadership in industry can capitalize to most effectively promote safety.

People become frustrated when their goals cannot be achieved. There are many ways of reacting to such frustrations, but the emotional reactions are of great concern to the safety professional. These reactions, as well as the attitudes formed during the reactions, can be highly disruptive to safety precautions and procedures.

Training programs are established to teach safe work methods. These learning situations, if they are to operate efficiently, call for knowledge of the basic principles of learning that cause people to learn and act as they do. These princi-ples should be used to make new learning more efficient.

In no way is this chapter intended to minimize or ignore the work already being carried on to reduce accidents. Safety devices, safer machines, safe work layout, and many other aids and measures all are a part of the total program. The human factor is one more aspect of the whole system.

Workers, machines, and materials are still the three components of industry that can contribute to safety.

Machines and materials can be controlled, but the human factor must be guided in the interests of accident prevention.

## References

Adams, J. S. "Inequity in Social Exchange." In L. Berkowitz (Ed.), *Advances in Experimental Social Psychology*, Vol. III. New York, N.Y., Academic Press, 1965.

Anastasi, A. *Psychological Testing*, 4th ed. Toronto, Canada, Macmillan, 1976.

Church, R. M. "The Varied Effects of Punishment on Behavior." *Psychological Review*, 70, 369-342, 1963.

Clark, J. V. *A Preliminary Investigation of Some Unconscious Assumptions Affecting Labor Efficiency in Eight Supermarkets*. Unpublished doctoral dissertation, Graduate School of Business Administration, Harvard University, 1958.

Dollard, J., and Miller, N. W. *Personality and Psychotherapy: An Analysis in Terms of Learning, Thinking, and Culture*. New York, N.Y., McGraw-Hill Book Co., 1950.

Hammer, R. W. *Handbook of System and Product Safety*. Englewood Cliffs, N.J., Prentice-Hall, 1972.

Herzberg, F. *Work and the Nature of Man*. Cleveland, Ohio, World Publishing Co., 1966.

Hulse, S. H., Deese, J., and Egeth, H. *The Psychology of Learning*, 4th ed. New York, N.Y., McGraw-Hill Book Co., 1975.

Insko, C. A., and Schopler, J. *Experimental Social Psychology*. New York, N.Y., Academic Press, 1972.

Maslow, A. H. *Motivation and Personality*, 2nd ed. New York, N.Y., Harper & Row, 1970.

McGregor, D. *The Human Side of Enterprise*. New York, N.Y., McGraw-Hill Book Co., 1960.

McGuire, W. J. "The Nature of Attitudes and Attitude Change." In G. Lindzey & E. Aronson (Eds.), *The Handbook of Social Psychology*, 2nd ed., Vol. 3. Reading, Mass., Addison-Wesley, 1968.

Miller, N. E., and Dollard, J. *Social Learning and Imitation*. New Haven, Conn., Yale University Press, 1941.

Miller, N. E. "Liberalization of Basic S-R Concepts: Extensions to Conflict Behavior, Motivation, and Social Learning." In S. Koch (Ed.), *Psychology: A Study of a Science*, Vol. 2. New York, N.Y., McGraw-Hill Book Co., 1959.

Tyler, L. E. *The Psychology of Human Differences*, 3rd ed. New York, N.Y., Appleton-Century-Crofts, 1965.

## Suggested Readings

Argyris, C. *Management and Organizational Development*. New York, N.Y., McGraw-Hill Book Co., 1971.

Bennis, W. G. *Organization Development: Its Nature, Origins, and Prospects*. Reading, Mass., Addison-Wesley Publishing Company, 1969.

Drucker, P. F. "New Templates for Today's Organizations." *Harvard Business Review*, Jan.-Feb. 1974.

Fishbein, M. and Ajzen, I. "Attitudes and Opinions." *Annual Review of Psychology*, Vol. 23, 1972.

Gausch, J. P. *Balanced Involvement: Safety, Production, Motivation,* Monograph No. 3. Park Ridge, Ill., American Society of Safety Engineers, 1973.

Hale, A. R. and Hale, M. *A Review of the Industrial Accident Research Literature.* London, Her Majesty's Stationery Office, 1972.

Hannaford, E. S. *Supervisors Guide to Human Relations.* Chicago, Ill., National Safety Council, 1976. (Course materials are available.)

Herzberg, F. "One More Time: How Do You Motivate Employees?" *Harvard Business Review,* Jan.-Feb. 1968.

Hinricks, J. R. "Psychology of Men at Work." *Annual Review of Psychology.* Vol. 21, 1970.

National Institute for Occupational Safety and Health. *The Present Status and Requirements for Occupational Safety Research.* Rockville, Md., U.S. Department of Health, Education, and Welfare, 1972.

Ruch, F. L. *Psychology and Life,* 7th ed. Glenview, Ill., Scott, Foresman and Company, 1967.

Shafai-Sahrai, Y. *Determinants of Occupational Injury Experience: A Study of Matched Pairs of Companies.* East Lansing, Mich., Michigan State University (Business Studies), 1973.

Zaleznick, A. *The Human Dilemmas of Leadership.* New York, Harper & Row, 1966.

# Maintaining
# Interest
# in Safety

# Chapter
# 12

# 12—Maintaining Interest in Safety

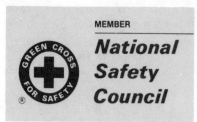

MEMBER

*National
Safety
Council*

GREEN CROSS
FOR SAFETY
®

FIG. 12–1.—A sticker like this one (actual size is shown here) can be placed on safety hats to remind everyone of a company's continuous efforts to work safely.

This chapter deals primarily with promoting and maintaining interest in safety on the part of supervisors and employees—but first, top management's interest must be assured. The safety professional should be certain that management is sincerely interested in the program and provide key executives and managers with details of the program; see Meetings of executives on p. 334. Any apparent lack of interest by top management should not be construed as indifference or even opposition to safety, because it usually can be traced to lack of awareness of the basic benefits of an organized safety program.

Top management must demonstrate its interest and actively support a solid safety program. Then, and only then, can activities to promote employees' interest be undertaken.

## Reasons for Maintaining Interest

Maintaining interest in safety is necessary (a) even if the work place has been designed for safety, (b) even when work procedures have been made as safe as possible, and (c) even after supervisors train their crews thoroughly and continue to enforce safe work procedures. Why is it still necessary to maintain interest? Because even with these optimum work conditions, accident prevention basically depends upon the *desire* of people to work safely.

Because all possible hazardous conditions, unsafe acts, and loss-control problems cannot be anticipated, each employee must frequently use his own imagination, common sense, and self-discipline to protect himself. Each employee must be stimulated to think *beyond* his immediate work procedures in order to act safely in questionable situations when he is "on his own."

The techniques used in modern advertising and merchandising have much in common with those used to "sell" safety. Just as most products and services require steady and imaginative sales promotion, safety likewise requires constant and skillful promotion.

Workers are accustomed to the modern techniques of advertising and sales promotion, so the basic elements of accident prevention can be made more understandable and acceptable if they are presented in a similarly interesting fashion.

### Indications of need for a program

Various yardsticks can indicate the attitude of supervisors and employees toward accident prevention. These can be used to point out areas of greatest need for a program to create and maintain interest in safety.

● Increased frequency of injuries, accidents, and near accidents may be one indication that a program is needed. If no explanation for such an increase can be found in engineering methods, training, or supervision, the reason is likely to be that employees are forgetting or ignoring work rules, failing to stay alert, or taking chances. A program to develop and maintain their interest will help reverse this trend.

● If housekeeping is deteriorating, protective equipment is not being used, and guards are not being replaced, it is time to tighten up on supervision and to promote more interest in safety on the part of supervisors.

● Incomplete or missing accident reports also indicate a slackening of interest on the part of supervisors and, perhaps, even the failure of employees to report minor accidents and injuries. Motivation to assure better reporting is then in order.

### Program objectives and benefits

A well-planned program can create and maintain interest in safety, although it cannot be expected to do *everything*. For example, it can:

1. Help develop safe work habits and safe attitudes, but it cannot compensate for unsafe conditions and unsafe procedures.

2. Focus attention on specific causes of accidents, although by itself it cannot eliminate them.

3. Supplement safety training, yet it cannot be

considered a substitute for a good training program.

4. Give employees a chance to participate in accident prevention activities, such as suggesting safety improvements in job procedures.

5. Provide a channel of communication between workers and management, because accident prevention is certainly a common meeting ground.

6. Improve employee, customer, and public relations, because it is evidence of management's sincerity with regard to accident prevention. (See Fig. 12–1.)

The ultimate objective of a program to maintain interest in safety is to prevent accidents. Usually, though, it is as difficult to determine the degree of success achieved by an interest-maintaining program as it is to isolate the effectiveness of an advertising campaign separate from the entire marketing program. The reason is that, generally, companies with such programs also have sound basic safety programs: working conditions are safe, employees are well trained and safety minded, and supervision is of a high caliber.

However, one prominent company that already had a good basic program attributed a reduction in its work injury rate to a stepped-up program to maintain interest. The program was based on an idea submitted by an employee: Each month candy bars were distributed to injury-free employees. Wrapped with some of the candy bars were slips that could be traded for free pairs of safety shoes.

Another company gave each employee who had an injury during the month a package of gum with the slogan "Something to chew on" and a friendly safety message and wishes for an injury-free future.

A meat-packing firm also was able to assess the value of its program to maintain interest. Several safety bulletin boards were installed, and posters and safety contest reports were displayed on them. These displays were credited with an impressive cut in the number of injuries and with a workers' compensation insurance refund of more than $1200.

## Selection of Program Activities

Safety directors frequently undertake promotional activities with no preliminary planning or determining of objectives. Some of them may use, for example, films or posters for no other reason than that they happen to be available at low cost.

All too often, safety professionals spend a disproportionate amount of time on committee work, contests, or "homemade" visual aids because of their bosses' or their own personal interests. Sometimes these activities are substituted for a sound, well-rounded program based on supervisory responsibility.

### Basis for the program

To be effective, a program for maintaining interest in safety must be based on needs. Select activities so they yield the desired results, not just because they will be popular. To develop suitable activities and promotional material, the needs of supervisors and employees must be known.

To find out what their employees really thought of the safety program and just how interested they were, one company inaugurated a safety inventory plan. Each year after the regular *stock inventory* had been taken, *safety inventory* cards were distributed to all employees—salaried workers as well as hourly.

The cards were distributed by supervisors who asked each employee to take stock of his job and environment with regard to safety. The following year's safety program was planned on the basis of the questionnaire returns, which ran better than 90 percent. Many suggestions for improvement of the safety program were received and subsequently put into practice.

### Factors to be considered

**Company policy and experience.** If a company ordinarily uses activities, such as committees, mass meetings, and contests in areas other than safety, then the safety director can consider them for his own program. He would be unwise to spend much time on activities that are foreign to company policy and experience, unless he was convinced the new "sales pitch" was justified.

On the other hand, if supervisors and employees are over-involved in committee work and such activities as sales promotion, quality control, and tool damage programs so that similar activities for safety would be lost or burdensome, then other approaches often prove more effective.

Once a promotional program is under way, it should not be permitted to unbalance other aspects of the accident prevention program or other company activities. For example, safety meetings should not take a great deal more time than meetings for quality control, sales, or industrial relations.

**Budget and facilities.** Plans for a safety promotion program will be affected by budget considerations. At first the program will require extra effort, time, and money, but this expenditure is justified because it is an investment that will produce direct as well as indirect benefits. If the program is to be successful, the budget will have to be sufficient to carry it out.

In the selection of program activities, consider the facilities available. Sound films, for instance, require not only a sound projector and screen, but also a darkened room free of background noise.

In many companies, facilities, publications, or services may be available from the industrial or public relations department, which also may be a valuable source of help in the planning of promotional activities.

The National Safety Council publishes a lot of motivational material; check the latest Council catalog.

**Types of operations.** The nature and organization of company operations affect the choice of activities and materials for maintaining interest in safety. When operations are widely scattered and diversified, as in the construction, railroad, marine, motor transport, and air transport industries, the job of selecting and disseminating safety information becomes more complicated.

When operations are decentralized, the safety director must rely upon materials that can be used readily in the field, such as publications and films. He should then depend on local supervisors to conduct meetings, present material, and handle posters.

The needs of employees doing widely different kinds of work at far-flung locations also must be considered. Where a poster program is used as one means for maintaining interest in safety at each outlying location, a trustworthy employee may be designated by the local supervisor to receive posters and take care of their distribution and posting. He should see to it that poster boards and display cases are kept clean, attractive, and free of extraneous paper.

Another method is to use a trailer equipped with permanent displays to carry the company

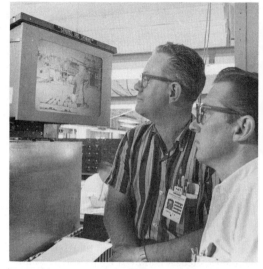

Fig. 12-2.—Rear-screen projector is used to show film strips at company's many diverse locations.

*Courtesy North American Aviation, Inc.*

safety story to far-flung locations. Self-contained rear-screen projectors are also well suited for use in scattered locations and in the field. (See Fig. 12-2.)

In the same organization, the types of educational materials used for different groups of employees may vary considerably. For instance, a movie scheduled for a day shift because a large number of employees could be taken off the job would not be suitable for a small night shift because no one could leave his job.

However, when activities are planned, night crews and maintenance employees should not be overlooked. Their work is as vital as that of other employees to the overall accident prevention effort. Programs for them will have to tie in to their specific requirements.

**Types of employees.** The types and backgrounds of employees have a bearing on the choice of safety promotion activities. For example, migrant workers frequently do not receive sufficient job training, particularly those who do not understand English. Material for these employees should present basic safe practices for their jobs in brief and easy-to-understand form. A similar approach should be used with temporary workers or those assigned from union halls.

| MISSABE DIV. | Jan. | Feb. | Mar. | Apr. | May | June | July | Aug. | Sept. | Oct. | Nov. | Dec. | Extra Balls | TOTAL |
|---|---|---|---|---|---|---|---|---|---|---|---|---|---|---|
| 1 NORTH END | 19 | 38 | 53 | 58 | 65 | 69 | 69 | 77 | 81 | 101 | 121 | 131 | | 131 |
| 2 ROAD | 20 | 50 | 78 | 96 | 104 | 124 | 143 | 163 | 180 | 187 | 203 | 209 | | 209 |
| 3 PROCTOR | 18 | 26 | 46 | 66 | 83 | 102 | 121 | 135 | 139 | 145 | 164 | 173 | | 173 |
| 4 STEELTON – M.J. | 7 | 26 | 45 | 62 | 69 | 75 | 95 | 110 | 115 | 135 | 153 | 161 | | 161 |
| 5 DOCKS | 19 | 39 | 59 | 79 | 93 | 97 | 115 | 133 | 151 | 171 | 191 | 201 | | 201 |

| IRON RANGE DIV. | Jan. | Feb. | Mar. | Apr. | May | June | July | Aug. | Sept. | Oct. | Nov. | Dec. | Extra Balls | TOTAL |
|---|---|---|---|---|---|---|---|---|---|---|---|---|---|---|
| | 4 / 5 | 8 / 12 | 14 / 17 | 19 / 22 | 21 / 24 | 23 / 27 | 27 / 31 | 33 / 34 | 36 / 39 | 41 / 43 | 44 / 48 | 52 | | 875 / 945 |
| 1 NORTH END | 20 | 37 | 44 | 64 | 78 | 82 | 102 | 122 | 142 | 172 | 192 | 202 | | 202 |
| 2 ROAD | 20 | 40 | 60 | 75 | 80 | 100 | 112 | 114 | 126 | 128 | 135 | 145 | | 145 |
| 3 TWO HARBORS | 28 | 48 | 66 | 84 | 102 | 120 | 137 | 144 | 162 | 180 | 196 | 202 | | 202 |
| 4 ELY-ENDION | 20 | 40 | 60 | 76 | 82 | 102 | 122 | 142 | 162 | 182 | 202 | 212 | | 212 |
| 5 DOCKS | 30 | 58 | 78 | 88 | 88 | 90 | 94 | 114 | 134 | 154 | 174 | 184 | | 184 |

FIG. 12-3.—This Safety Bowling Sweepstakes is based on the safety performance of a railroad's transportation department. Two divisions of the department form the teams; there are five areas within each division. "Strikes" are scored for each frame (month) that an area has no personal injury. "Spares" are marked when an area goes through a month with some personal, but no disabling injuries. Disabling injuries reduce the monthly (frame) points according to a system of handicapping that offsets the varying manhour exposures of the different divisional areas.

*Courtesy Duluth, Missabe & Iron Range Railway Company*

Employees who have difficulty understanding English need visual material. Material in Spanish is available from the Inter-American Safety Council. (See Chapter 24, "Source of Help.")

**Basic human interest.** If employees seem bored or uninterested in safety activities, an extra push must be given to pep up pallid programs. One approach is to base promotional activities on interests, such as bowling or fishing, that are shared by a large number of the workers. (See Fig. 12-3.)

Wise choice of promotional activities depends upon an understanding of basic human needs and emotions. The basic interest factors listed in Fig. 12-4 are forms of motivation common to all employees. The activities suggested, therefore, should be of general appeal.

**Other considerations.** Tasteful use of sex appeal, material featuring children and animals (human interest), and activities and contests based on a moderate amount of competition play a big part in the safety promotion programs of many companies. These elements are as effective in safety promotion as they are in sales and advertising promotion. Many successful safety directors capitalize on them without compromising company policy or offending anyone.

An Ohio company capitalized on the interest of most people on wagering. Employees in carpools were urged to participate in a little wager in which the rider who forgot to buckle his safety belt had to pay for lunch or dinner. The idea proved so popular the company decided to spread the word by means of a campaign featuring posters and announcements.

Ideas for maintaining interest often use humor with telling effect. The "light touch" is essential, and should be good-natured. Ridicule should not be used; it is likely to arouse only resentment.

A positive, constructive approach is generally better than a negative approach. However, the latter sometimes is preferable if it is more dramatic. A picture showing the consequences of an accident, such as a fall on a slippery floor, will have a greater impact than one depicting the safe act that could have prevented the accident.

---

### BASIC HUMAN INTERESTS AND CORRESPONDING ACTIVITIES

| Basic Interest Factors | Ways To Use These Factors |
|---|---|
| **Fear** of painful injury, death, loss of income, family hardship, group disapproval or ridicule, supervisory criticism. | **Visual material:** emotional or shocker posters, dramatic films, pictures and reports of serious injuries on bulletin boards, in company papers. |
| **Pride** in safe workmanship, in good records, both individual and group. | **Recognition** for individual and group achievement; trophies, personal awards, letters of appreciation. |
| **Recognition:** desire for approval of others in group and family, for praise from supervisors. | **Publicity:** photos and stories in company and community papers, on bulletin boards. |
| **Participation:** desire to be "one of the gang," "to get in the act." | **Group and individual activities:** safety committees, suggestion plans, safety stunts, campaigns. |
| **Competition:** desire to win over others, such as shown in sports. | **Contests** with attractive awards. |
| **Financial gain** through increased departmental or company profits. | **Monetary awards** through suggestion systems, profit-sharing plans, promotions, increased responsibility. |

---

Fig. 12–4.—Ways to put six basic human interest factors to effective use in promoting safety. Basic needs and desires that motivate people are left; right column lists direct appeals safety promotional programs can make.

Variety is essential. Often a simple change, such as a different type contest, redesign of a bulletin board, or revising the format of safety meetings, can result in renewed interest. The activity itself may not be more effective, but its new form stimulates thought, discussion, and interest. Although safe practices should become routine, their presentations should not.

Activities that require participation generate more interest than do those that involve only seeing and hearing. Companies that have allowed the National Safety Council to make movies in their plants report an upsurge in interest in safety because some of their employees got a chance to act in a film that emphasized the importance of what to them might have seemed routine.

Employees who are asked to submit suggestions for equipment guards or to help in the selection of personal protective equipment are more inclined to use the guards and the personal equipment than they would be if they had no opportunity to make their opinions known.

For the same reasons, helping to draft the safety rules encourages compliance on the part of those workers who participate in the project, and serving on a safety committee leads to increased awareness of safety responsibilities.

### Staff Functions

The job of creating and maintaining employee interest places certain demands upon the safety director, who has the basic responsibility for planning the safety program, and upon the supervisors, who have the responsibility for carrying it out.

### Role of the safety professional

The safety professional should be a well-informed specialist if he is to maintain interest in safety. He coordinates the program and supplies the ideas and inspiration, while enlisting the wholehearted support of management, supervision, and employees. He may work with local

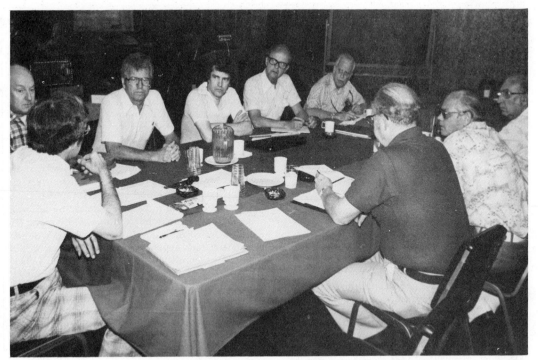

Fɪɢ. 12–5.—Council Industrial Division, Electronic and Electrical Equipment Section Subcommittee meets to work on "Electrically Related Industrial Accidents Study." Volunteers are the life blood of the Council and are responsible for producing many of its publications which, in turn, help the cause of safety throughout the world.

safety councils, chapters of the American Society of Safety Engineers, and other civic or technical groups interested in accident prevention.

The safety professional can gain much by attending the National Safety Congress and regional safety conferences. He can learn of the ideas and programs of thousands of other companies. He can translate many of those ideas into practical activities that will be useful to his own organization. After participating in round-table discussions (Fig. 12–5), listening to speakers, and meeting many people with similar interests, he should return with renewed enthusiasm.

Because the safety professional often may be called upon to address groups, he should be able to present his ideas clearly, effectively, and convincingly. He should cultivate his ability to speak because this will help his ability to deal with people.

The safety professional should be well versed in the use of visual aids and familiar with the techniques of advertising, sales, and publicity, particularly those used in his own organization. Ideas picked up from these sources often can be applied in the safety program.

Showmanship tactics, however, should be used with discretion. They should not consist of questionable activities which could reflect unfavorably on the safety professional, the company, or the safety program. Showmanship tactics can do more harm than good if they are insincere or if the basic safety program is weak or unsound.

Feel free to submit interesting data, difficult problems, or "gimmicks" of any nature to the National Safety Council. Through this clearing-house, problems can be solved or given to others for solution. The Council has information on every phase of safety, gleaned from the experience of members in various industries. One company's solution to a problem may be of real help to many others.

A vast amount of program material of use to

the safety professional is available in National Safety Council publications. For example, many of the illustrations in this chapter were selected from Sectional *Newsletters* and the monthly feature "Ideas That Worked" in the Council's *National Safety News*. Each month a committee of Council staff members judges the entries to this feature and selects the best one. Every individual submitting a winning entry receives a pen and pencil set. For information, contact the Industrial Department, National Safety Council.

### Role of the supervisor

The supervisor is the key person in any program to create and maintain interest in safety because he is responsible for translating management's policies into action and for promoting safety activities directly among the employees. How well he meets this responsibility will determine to a large extent how favorably the employees receive the safety activities.

The supervisor's attitude toward safety is a significant factor in the success, not only of specific promotional activities, but also of the entire safety program, because his views will be reflected by the employees in his department.

The supervisor who is sincere and enthusiastic about accident prevention can actually do more than the safety director to maintain interest. Conversely, if the supervisor pays only lip service to the program or ridicules any part of it, his attitude offsets any good that might be done by the safety professional.

Many supervisors are reluctant to change their mode of operation or to accept new safety engineering ideas, much less to regard with enthusiasm contests, safety stunts, committee projects, and other activities used to promote and maintain interest in safety. It is the safety director's task to sell these supervisors on the benefits of accident prevention, to convince them that promotional activities are not "frills," but rather projects that can help prevent injuries, and to persuade them that their wholehearted cooperation is essential to the success of the entire program. A supervisor's safety meeting can stimulate cooperation.

Setting a good example, for instance, wearing safety glasses and other personal protective equipment whenever they are required, is one of the most effective ways in which the supervisor can promote safety.

Teaching safety is an important function of the supervisor. He cannot depend upon safety posters, a few warning signs, or even general rules to do his job of training and supervision. A good balance of basic training and supervision and judicious use of promotional material proves effective. However, the supervisor himself must first be trained if he is to be competent. (See Chapter 9, "Safety Training," for details on training courses and techniques.)

The safety professional should help educate the supervisor so that he sees that working conditions are kept as safe as possible and insists that his workers follow safe procedures consistently, simply as a part of good job performance. The supervisor should not have to suddenly adopt a "get tough" approach to enforce safety rules. He should be consistently firm and fair. If workers have the impression that the supervisor either cannot recognize unsafe conditions and unsafe acts or does not care whether or not they exist, they too will become lax.

The supervisor is entitled to all the help the safety department can give through correspondence, supplies of educational material for distribution, and through as frequent visits as circumstances permit. He should also receive adequate recognition for independent and original activity.

Supervisors can be most effective in giving facts and personal reminders on safety to employees. This procedure is particularly necessary in the transportation and utility industries, where crews are on their own from terminal to terminal.

In any case, supervisors should be encouraged to take every opportunity to exchange ideas on accident prevention with workers, to commend them for their efforts to do the job safely, and to invite them to submit safety suggestions.

### Safety Committees and Observers

There are many different types of safety and health committees having many different functions. (For further details, see the Council publication, "You are the Safety and Health Committee.") However, *the basic function of every safety committee is to create and maintain interest in safety and health and thereby help reduce accidents.*

In some cases, other types of employee participation are preferred over formal safety committees. Some companies report that safety committees require a disproportionate amount of administrative time, that they generally tend to

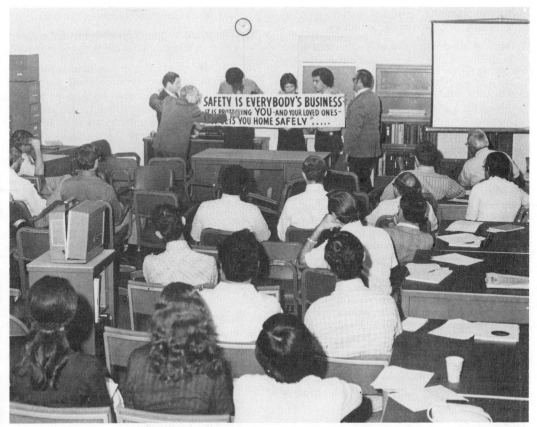

Fig. 12-6.—Bill Leonard, (pointing), retired training director from Southland Corp., talks on accident prevention throughout the country. He holds six citations and awards from the National Safety Council for his tireless efforts.

pass the buck, that they sometimes stir up more trouble than they are worth, and that some supervisors try to unload their responsibilities onto the safety committee.

The answer to these objections is not to abolish the committees but rather to reexamine their duties, responsibilities, and methods of operation. Such analysis often can lead to constructive changes that will enable a committee to fulfill its original objective—that of stimulating and maintaining interest in safety.

Involving employees in safety inspections, either alone, as observers, or as part of a formal safety and health committee has the same basic objective: to get more employees actively involved and interested in the safety and health program. Planning, publicizing, and following definite procedures will streamline the work of

both committees and observers and help ensure effective results.

## Meetings

Safety meetings may be conducted for supervisors, employees, or other groups, but in every case the purpose is to stimulate and maintain interest. If meetings fail to achieve this, they should be dropped, or their format or content should be changed sufficiently to make them effective.

### Types of meetings

Among the various types of safety meetings commonly held to arouse and maintain interest in accident prevention are the following. (Also see Chapter 9.)

1. Meetings of operating executives and supervi-

sors to formulate policies, initiate a safety program, or plan special activities.

2. Mass meetings of all employees, sometimes including families, or even the entire community to serve special purposes.

3. Departmental meetings to discuss special problems, plan campaigns, or analyze accidents.

4. Small group meetings to plan the day's work so that it can be done safely, to discuss specific accidents, or to review safety instructions.

**Meetings of executives.** When a safety program is to be inaugurated, it is especially important that the top executive officer of the company or plant should call a meeting to announce the general accident prevention plans and policies to all his foremen, supervisors, superintendents, and other operating executives.

If these persons meet at regular intervals to discuss operating problems, this announcement can be made at one of these regular meetings. Otherwise, the manager should call a special meeting for this purpose.

After this first meeting, the group may hold sessions periodically to evaluate the safety program, to check on the progress being made in accident prevention, and to appraise proposed activities.

**Departmental meetings** have many safety uses. Their purpose may be to discuss the company safety program so that employees will better understand what is going on. They may be held to provide information about accident causes and accident types. They may be purely inspirational (Fig. 12–6) to create an awareness of hazards and a desire to prevent accidents.

In many company programs, departmental safety meetings are held monthly. The trend is toward meetings conducted by the supervisor, who may receive assistance in planning as well as materials, such as visual aids, from the safety department.

The program for a departmental meeting may include the following:

1. Report of injuries in the department since the past meeting; report of a safety inspection in the department; and report of the department's standing in a contest. (The total time spent on reports must not be so great that this part of the meeting becomes tiresome.)

2. Discussion by the supervisor of where observance of safe practices needs to be improved.

3. Talk, demonstration, or audiovisual presentation on an appropriate accident prevention subject. The speaker may be the supervisor, a member of the department, the company safety director, an outside expert, or an executive of the company.

Departmental meetings give the supervisor an opportunity to point out the dangers of certain unsafe practices. By condemning those practices, he practically binds himself to set a good example for his workers. In addition, most workers welcome an opportunity to "get off their chests" whatever safety ideas they have.

At the conclusion of departmental meetings, the supervisor should be required to prepare written reports for presentation to the plant (or company) safety committees and review by the managers.

**Small group meetings** with people doing similar kinds of work can be held at or near the work place. (See Fig. 12–7.) The supervisor may discuss the causes of an accident of which the workers have personal knowledge or in which they have personal interest. Employees should be encouraged to join in the discussion, and a conclusion should be reached as to how the accident might have been prevented.

The supervisor may present a problem that has developed because of new work or new equipment. Again, all should participate and offer their views.

At times the supervisor may present a film or chart talk on a subject related to the work of the group members. Other audiovisuals such as models or exhibits may be used. Safety devices or pieces of equipment or material may be shown and discussed.

"Production huddles" are instruction sessions about a specific job being done that includes safety. Such meetings are particularly useful with maintenance crews when an unusual job is about to start. The plans for doing the job safely and efficiently are gone over and a procedure is agreed upon. Public utility line crews use this type of meeting and call it a tail board conference. Before starting a job, the crew gathers around the truck and discusses the job, laying out the tools and materials they will need and agreeing upon

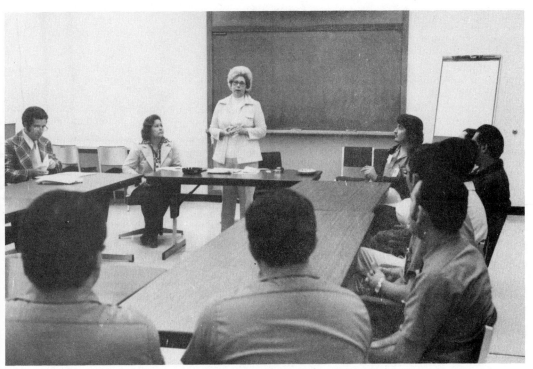

Fig. 12–7.—Safety meetings are held monthly to alert workers to possible work hazards and to review past accidents in order to prevent recurrence.

*Courtesy Abbott Laboratories.*

the part each person is to do.

A particular advantage of small group meetings is that they provide excellent opportunities for presenting all types of information, including safety information, directly to employees and stimulate exchange of ideas that can benefit the accident prevention program. To be successful, the same safety meeting must include a tangible message, originality of presentation, opportunity for audience participation, and a conclusion that spurs action toward an attainable goal.

**Mass meetings.** Large mass meetings are held for special purposes, such as the launching of a contest, the presentation of awards, the introduction of interesting new equipment, the explanation of a change in company policy, or the celebration of an exceptionally fine safety record, or an event such as "safety day" (Fig. 12–8).

In companies with plants in different cities, a top executive may call a meeting of employees when he visits a plant. His talk may cover safety as well as other subjects. One company president makes an annual round of plants with the safety director and speaks at a safety rally of all employees at each plant.

Under certain conditions, particularly in smaller communities, large meetings can be held in a local theater or public hall. It then is necessary to make fairly elaborate arrangements and to give the meetings considerable publicity to assure good attendance.

A mass meeting in a public hall naturally has one advantage over a plant meeting. It makes possible the attendance not only of employees, but also of their wives or husbands, families, and friends.

"Family safety nights" of this sort are very popular in the railroad industry. A considerable number may be held during a year at several

**335**

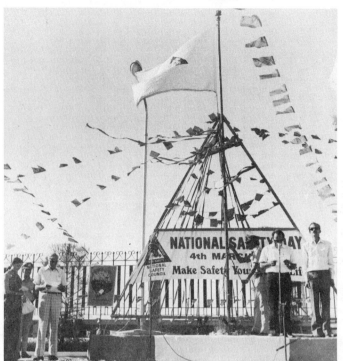

FIG. 12–8.—National Safety Day, celebrated in Kandla, India, by the Indian Farmers Fertilizer Cooperative, Ltd., involved employees, their families, and the community in many activities—such as a safety poster contest, essay competition, safety quizzes, exhibits, entertainment, and a bazaar. Photo at left shows the safety flag and (to left of sign) the green safety triangle of the Indian National Safety Council. Photo below shows the bazaar and safety exhibits.

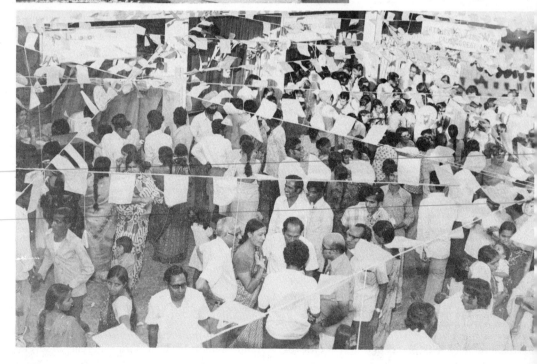

different cities and towns served by the railroad.

In addition to the address or two around which the program is centered, there should be some worthwhile entertainment. Often good talent can be found right in the plant or shop.

This type of meeting affords an excellent opportunity for using an outside speaker who can talk authoritatively and convincingly on general accident prevention work. Such a speaker can be obtained from a nearby plant, an insurance company, the city administration, an automobile club, or a community safety council.

If movies relating to accident prevention are desired, a suitable selection can be made from films available through the National Safety Council, or through regional film service organizations, whose locations may be obtained from the Council.

## Planning programs

Making the safety meeting interesting is of the utmost importance. There should be no complaining or scolding. Talks should be definitely limited in time and they should start and end on time. The subject matter of a talk should be considered in advance to make sure that it is pertinent and does not repeat other talks recently presented.

Large occasional meetings need even more careful planning and timing than do small meetings. People who are to speak, including company executives, should review what they intend to say with the person planning the meeting to assure that their remarks will serve the desired purpose. Films and other visual aids should be checked in advance.

Persons responsible for employee meetings should observe them critically to see whether or not they are accomplishing the purpose for which they are run. When meetings are held periodically, there is always danger that they will become dull routine. Only continual effort and planning will prevent this.

A plan of action to develop a successful safety meeting includes these points:

PREPARE IN ADVANCE. The preliminary arrangement determines the results. Do not conduct a meeting without preparation.

SELECT A MAJOR TOPIC. Make it timely and practical—one that the group can discuss.

OBTAIN FACTS AND FIGURES. Be sure they are cor-

rect and complete. Make a visual, such as a simple chart or table, whenever possible. An example of a statistical handout is given in Fig. 12–9.

MAP THE PRESENTATION. Decide on the best way to present the subject of the meeting. Try to anticipate the group's reaction and questions. Outline results you hope to accomplish.

SET A TIMETABLE. Allow adequate time, but set a reasonable limit.

BE SINCERE. Your sincerity and your interest in the employees' welfare must be unmistakable.

INTRODUCE THE TOPIC. Tell in simple terms what the meeting is all about. Use a punch line or other good lead-in.

PRESENT FACTS, AROUSE INTEREST. State highly pertinent facts in an interesting manner.

PROMOTE GROUP DISCUSSION. Ask questions that cannot be answered "Yes" or "No." Prompt members of the group to think individually and collectively. Let *them* talk.

AGREE ON DOING SOMETHING. Try for group agreement on methods of correction and improvement. Write these down.

SUMMARIZE THE MEETING. Review briefly what has been discussed and decided . . . follow up in the various departments.

## Contests Stimulate Interest

Many safety professionals say that contests (such as housekeeping contests, interdepartment contests, and many other types) are not substitutes for management interest, safe procedures, and "built in" safety. They will also agree that while a good accident prevention program is one and the same with good management, good training, and efficient operation, some *special* effort may be needed to maintain interest in good housekeeping, reporting hazards, and the like. Moreover, the interest value of contests (such as maintaining a high level of good housekeeping and efficiency) has direct bonus values in good publicity and improved employee morale.

A competition usually is held, therefore, only after the basic steps in a safety program have been taken—a policy statement made, a record system adopted, equipment safeguarded, a first aid department installed. Such substantial demonstration of management's interest, sincerity, and

**337**

## MONTHLY "FALLS" PROFILE
### MONTH OF MAY 19_____

Number of falls reported by Unusual Incident Reports    56

I. Age Group:

| 0 - 44 | 12 | 45 - 54 | 6 | 55 - 64 | 13 |
|---|---|---|---|---|---|
| 65 - 74 | 15 | Over 75 | 10 | | |

II. Sex:   Male  20   Female  36

III. Condition Before Incident:
   Normal  37   Disoriented  9   Senile  3   Not Shown  7

IV. Time:
   6AM-12N  22   12N-4PM  8   4PM-9PM  14   9PM-6AM  12

V. Activity Orders:
   Up with Assist  24   Bedrest  4
   Up without Assist  19   Restraint  1   Not Shown  8

VI. Bed Rails:
   Ordered  5   Not Ordered  14   Not Shown  37

VII. Bed Rails:
   Up  7   Down  11   Not Shown  38

VIII. Bed Position:
   High  5   Low  15   Not Shown  36

IX. Location - Unit

| 5W | 2 | 6E | 3 | 9W | 0 | 11E | 0 | 15W | 4 |
|---|---|---|---|---|---|---|---|---|---|
| 5NW | 2 | 7W | 0 | 9E | 3 | 12W | 0 | 15NW | 0 |
| 5NE | 3 | 7E | 1 | 10W | 2 | 12E | 2 | 15E | 1 |
| 5E | 1 | 8W | 10 | 10E | 5 | 14W | 0 | 16 | 1 |
| 6W | 3 | 8E | 3 | 11W | 1 | 14E | 0 | X-Ray | 5 |
| | | | | | | | | Other | 3 |

X. Location - Specific Location
   Patient Room  42   Washroom  5   Corridor  1
   Ancillary Dept.  8   Other  0

   Type of Fall:

| Bed | 20 | Walking Device | 1 | Dizzy | 3 |
|---|---|---|---|---|---|
| Chair | 5 | Footstool | 0 | Bath | 1 |
| Toilet | 3 | Wheelchair | 5 | Other | 7 |
| | | Walking | 11 | | |

XI. When Fall Occurred, Patient Was:
   Lying Down  7   Sitting  4   Walking  15
   Standing  7   Getting on or off  20   Other  1

---

## REVIEW OF INCIDENTS FOR THE MONTH OF MAY 19_____

| | | Number or Total Patients Days | Ratio of Incidents to 1,000 Patient Days |
|---|---|---|---|
| Male - 34 | 47* | | |
| Female - 69 | 60* | 16,981   16,982* | 6.1   6.3* |
| Total - 103 | 107* | | |

I. Type of Incident (Patients Only)

| Falls | 56 | 63* | Medications | 25 | 16* |
|---|---|---|---|---|---|
| Burns | 2 | 3* | Treatment | 1 | 3* |
| Other | 6 | 14* | Procedure | 13 | 8* |

II. Location of Incident

| 5W | 3 | 3* | 7E | 1 | 3* | 11W | 1 | 1* | 15NW | 2 | 2* |
|---|---|---|---|---|---|---|---|---|---|---|---|
| 5NW | 3 | 7* | 8W | 13 | 9* | 11E | 2 | 5* | 15E | 1 | 4* |
| 5NE | 4 | 5* | 8E | 3 | 4* | 12W | 2 | 3* | 16 | 3 | 6* |
| 5E | 4 | 2* | 9W | 7 | 3* | 12E | 3 | 4* | X-Ray | 5 | 1* |
| 6W | 6 | 7* | 9E | 7 | 8* | 14W | 2 | 0* | Other | 11 | 5* |
| 6E | 4 | 5* | 10W | 3 | 5* | 14E | 0 | 1* | | | |
| 7W | 1 | 3* | 10E | 7 | 6* | 15W | 9 | 5* | | | |

III. Apparent Reason for Incident

| Patient did not call for assistance | 19 | 28* |
|---|---|---|
| Assistance provided - more was needed | 11 | 8* |
| Defective equipment | 0 | 2* |
| Patient identification not properly checked | 3 | 2* |
| Improper review or recording of medicine order | 19 | 13* |
| Material on floor | 0 | 0* |
| Patient dizziness or fainting | 7 | 6* |
| Patient action - no deficiency | 26 | 29* |
| Misunderstanding of verbal orders | 1 | 1* |
| Other | 17 | 18* |

IV. Result of Incident

| No apparent injury | 81 | 81* |
|---|---|---|
| Known or suspected injury | 11 | 21* |
| Not shown | 11 | 5* |

V. Incidents Other Than Patients
   Visitor got dizzy and fell.  Taken to E.R. for minor treatment.
   Visitor apparently slipped on an ice cube in the Cafeteria. Taken to E.R. for minor treatment.
   Visitor fell while assisting his wife.  Refused to go to E.R.
   Visitor apparently sprained her ankle when she got up from couch in waiting area.  Taken to E.R.
   Wrench fell from the top of a door and hit a visitor on the head.  He did not go to E.R.
   A volunteer tripped over a cart in the Staff Room.  Taken to E.R. for minor treatment.

FIG. 12-9.—One way to get across accident prevention statistics to a safety committee is to use factual handouts. Here are two examples used in a hospital that summarize accidents to patients. *Left*—A profile of falls. *Right*—A description of incidents.

responsibility greatly helps to obtain the active participation of supervisors and workers in a contest.

## Purpose and principles

Safety contests are operated purely for their interest-creating value. A contest that creates favorable interest is valuable; one that does not create interest is worthless. In the usual type of contest, the competing groups are departments of the same plant or divisions of the same company. Generally, contests are based on accident experience and are operated over a stated period, with a prize for the group with the best record according to the contest rules.

Contests have been important almost from the time of the first safety programs, and a fairly well-established group of operating principles has been developed:

1. A contest should be planned and conducted by a committe representative of the competing groups.

2. Competing groups should be natural units, not arbitrary divisions.

3. Methods of grading must be simple and easily understood.

4. The grading system must be fair to all groups.

5. Awards must be worth winning and of the sort that create interest.

6. Good publicity and enthusiasm are important.

Contests may run for various periods—from a few months to a year. Those who recommend longer periods believe that if workers are kept on their toes for a longer time, safe working is more likely to become a habit. Some safety professionals, however, believe that greater interest can be aroused and maintained during a short period and therefore prefer short and frequent competitions. Contests of different duration can be tried to see which is most effective.

**A safety contest stock certificate idea** was developed by the Maxwell House Division of General Foods Corp. and ran for one year.

For each week a department works without a disabling work injury, the department receives a stock certificate worth 50 cents. Dividends are paid on this stock at the rate of: ten cents for the first 1000 consecutive safe hours worked; twenty-five cents for the first 10,000 consecutive safe hours worked; fifty cents for the first 50,000 consecutive safe hours worked; and one dollar for the first 100,000 consecutive safe hours worked. This means that if a department works 100,000 consecutive workhours without a disabling injury it receives a total of $1.84 in dividends for each share of stock held.

There are penalties, however. If a disabling injury occurs in a department, that department will be penalized one month's stock earnings. This means that during that particular month the department could not be awarded any stock or dividends. It would also mean that if an accident should occur in the latter few days of the month the department would lose all dividends and stock certificates previously issued for that month.

## Injury rate contests

In a contest based on injury rates, the measure of safety performance is the OSHA incidence rate, which was described in detail in Chapter 6, "Accident Records and Incidence Rates."

Contests should not be based upon severity, because severity data cannot be determined promptly and because severity frequently is a matter of luck and contributes little to knowing how to prevent the accident in the future. Using a combination of frequency and severity is not good for the same reason. Contests should not be based upon reduction of reported first aid cases because people, therefore, may fail to report such injuries.

If in-plant contests are to create interest, they must have variety and originality. The most effective contests generally do not run continuously, with a new one beginning as the old one ends. They are more in the nature of special campaigns to run for a specified time and are launched with advance publicity and fanfare. Often the president or other high official makes the original announcement, presents awards, and otherwise lends his prestige to the contest.

Competition, if properly organized, can do much to develop teamwork. Some workers who apparently give no thought to their own work habits can be influenced to cooperate with their fellow workers if they know that their unsafe acts and resulting accidents will descredit their department or "team."

**Council contests and awards.** National Safety Council members firmly believe in the value of contests for maintaining interest. The Council has

---

### RULES FOR THE 'XYZ COMPANY' SAFETY CONTEST

**Rule 1.** The contest shall begin January 1, and end December 31, 19 . . . .

**Rule 2.** The contest shall consist of two divisions.
- a. Fabricating units shall participate in Division I.
- b. Field erection departments under the direction of a superintendent shall participate as separate units in Division II, which shall be divided on the basis of size into two groups: Group A shall consist of the five erection units working the largest number of man-hours, and Group B shall consist of all other units. Units shall be tentatively grouped by size during the first three months, and the final classification shall be made on the basis of total man-hours worked at the end of four months. No further changes in size groups will be made after April 30, 19 . . . .

**Rule 3.** Recognition awards shall be:
- a. Trophies to the winners in Division I and Groups A and B of Division II.
- b. Engraved certificates to plants and erection units ranking second and third in Division I and in Groups A and B of Division II.

**Rule 4.** a. The winners shall be the contestants having the lowest weighted frequency rates.
- b. In the event that two or more contestants in any classification have had no chargeable injuries during the contest period, the winner shall be the contestant who has worked the largest number of man-hours since the last chargeable injury.

**Rule 5.** All injuries resulting in death, permanent total, permanent partial, or temporary total disabilities shall be counted, as defined by ASI Standard Z16.1, *Method of Recording and Measuring Work Injury Experience.*

**Rule 6.** A sum of $50.00 shall be presented to the units that have had no disabling injuries during the first six months of the contest or have reduced their average frequency rates for the first six months 50 per cent in comparison with the average rate for the preceding six months' period. The award shall be divided into prizes of $12, 10, 8, 6, 4, 2, and eight $1 prizes and raffled to employees. No employee may win more than one prize.

**Rule 7.** Standings shall be compiled monthly and published in a bulletin that will be distributed to all managers, superintendents, and foremen.

**Rule 8.** All questions pertaining to the definitions of injuries and rules shall be referred to the Contest Committee, whose decisions shall be final.

**Rule 9.** Awards shall be presented at an appropriate ceremony to be announced at the end of the contest.

---

Fig. 12–10.—A typical set of rules for a safety contest. (See text for a point-by-point discussion.)

## STANDINGS IN THE 'XYZ COMPANY' SAFETY CONTEST
### JANUARY–JUNE

Oakland leads at the halfway mark!

Tulsa moved into second place.

Chicago slipped from second to third place in June.

Corbin, in last place, had no disabling injuries during June. Good work!

Tulsa still leads for the President's Award for largest improvement over the previous year's record.

| Plant | Rank | January–June Frequency rates° | % Increase + or decrease – over last year |
|---|---|---|---|
| Oakland | 1 | 14.1 | –30% |
| Tulsa | 2 | 14.6 | –40% |
| Chicago | 3 | 17.5 | + 5% |
| Cincinnati | 4 | 21.9 | –20% |
| Corbin | 5 | 24.8 | +22% |

*Frequency rate is number of disabling injuries per 1,000,000 hours worked.

**Tips on How to Win, No. 6**

One-sixth of our disabling injuries occur in the use of cranes and hoists. Have foremen hold a safety meeting on safe practices in hitching loads and other crane operations for shop men. We'll furnish a film. Use posters on the subject. Require safe methods. See the enclosed bulletin for suggestions on how to solve this major accident problem.

FIG. 12–11.—Simple monthly contest bulletin gives essential information about current standings and also includes a suggestion for improvement in "Tips on How To Win."

about two dozen Industrial Section contests. All are open to Council members, and several include nonmember participants through specially arranged contests cosponsored with trade associations.

In the Council contests, companies are grouped according to size and operation so that competing units will be comparable with one another. The definitions and rules are established by the Council. OSHA incidence rates are compared.

Many Council members consider the sectional contest to be one of the most important features of Council service. Awards are presented at sectional meetings, local safety council meetings, and occasionally at trade association conventions.

Most of the Council's sectional contests are integrated with the Council's Award Plan. Under this plan, four levels of awards are set up to provide some recognition for every good safety record of a member company or unit. In order of importance, the awards are:

AWARD OF HONOR

AWARD OF MERIT

CERTIFICATE OF COMMENDATION

PRESIDENT'S LETTER

The Award Plan recognizes perfect records (no disabling injuries) covering an entire calendar year.

**Associate contests.** A number of associations conduct their own contests. Statistics from association contests are submitted to the National Safety Council, which uses them to give the corresponding industries' injury rates in its *Accident Facts* booklet. In addition to stimulating the interest of the associations' members, such contests give the Council a broad and reliable accident reporting base.

### The 'XYZ Company' contest explained

The "XYZ Company" is engaged in steel fabrication and erection. Rules for one of its safety contests are given in Fig. 12–10, p. 340, but some explanation is needed.

RULE 1. Although contests can run for any period of time, the company chose a one year period to allow development of safe working habits—the useful objective of the contest—and, since some of the departments were relatively small, to eliminate random (chance) factors from influencing an individual department's experience record.

RULE 2a. Hazards in steel fabrication and erection vary greatly; therefore, fabricating units compete in one division and erection units in another. Operations are similar enough to have a common basis for determining standings—see Rule 4.

Other companies may find that hazards differ sharply from one plant or operation to another, and the similar units may be too few to group. Such plants or operations may compete on an equitable basis in several ways.

• The participant achieving the largest percentage reduction in its frequency rate in comparison with a base period, such as the previous year, may be the winner. Since each unit competes against its past record as par, this method provides a fair basis for comparison of rates.

• The compensation insurance rates for different types of units in the same state have been used to establish a handicap factor to compensate for differences in hazards. If the rates per $100 payroll are $3.00 for Plant A, $2.00 for Plant B, and $1.50 for Plant C, factors for the units are 3, 2, and 1.5, respectively. The frequency rate of each plant is adjusted by dividing the rate by its factor. Plants are ranked from the lowest to the highest on the basis of the adjusted rates.

• The national average rates for different types of units may be used similarly for determining standings. If Plant A achieved a frequency rate of 10.0 and the national average for units in this industry was 12.0, Plant A's rate is 0.83 of the national average. Plant B's rate in comparison with its national average rate is 0.75. Therefore, Plant B would rank nearer the top than Plant A. Average rates for most industries are published annually in the National Safety Council's booklet *Accident Facts*.

RULE 2b. Separation of large and small units is essential because a small unit finds it easier to go through an entire contest period without a disabling injury than does a larger unit. If the number of units is sufficient, three size classifications may be set up. Unequal size groups can be competitive if they include units that can attain no-injury records. For this reason, the erection departments of the company in this example werre divided into Group A—the five largest departments—and Group B—the remaining units. Five contestants in a group are usually considered minimum.

RULE 3. Awards should be specified. "XYZ Company" follows the general practice of giving first, second, and third place awards.

RULE 4a. The frequency rate is most often used as the basis for determining standings as it can be computed promptly and easily.

RULE 4b. There should be a satisfactory method of determining the winner between two or more units having perfect records in order to give the smallest contestant a fair chance. Selecting the winner on the basis of the largest number of man-hours worked since the last chargeable injury is fair to all units, regardless of size.

RULE 5. A standard method of counting injuries is essential in order to avoid controversies and maintain confidence in standards. Use the incident rate described in Chapter 6, "Accident

Records and Incidence Rates."

First aid and other minor injuries generally are excluded because, if they are counted, workers may fail to obtain treatment so that cases will not be put on the record. The result could be an increase in infections.

RULE 6. Various "special rules" may be used in a contest that runs six or more months' duration in order to stimulate and maintain employee interest.

RULE 7. Frequent contest bulletins keep everyone informed about standings. Bulletins can be posted and standings discussed at safety meetings. Contest results can be announced in plant publications and in other ways to build and maintain interest.

RULE 8. Questions about rule interpretation will arise and must be settled fairly. This is an important function of the contest committee, which, in turn, may refer decisions about disputable injuries to outside judges. A committee of the American National Standards Institute has been set up to interpret standard definitions.

RULE 9. (See section Awards Should Be Meaningful, later in this chapter, for award ideas.)

## Interdepartmental contests

Interdepartmental competitions get "close to home" and place responsibility for a good showing on supervisors. Since workers have a greater personal interest in the standing of their department than in the record of the entire plant or other unit, this type of competition has proved popular for creating interest among both supervisors and workers.

An interplant contest plan often may be adapted to an interdepartmental competition. A company operating a number of similar plants may take advantage of workers' interest in their departmental records by conducting a competition among the same departments in various plants. Public utilities may conduct a contest among districts, and other nonmanufacturing companies may follow a similar plan. Since hazards in similar operating units are about the same, the basis of standings may be the frequency rate. Departments or other units may be grouped according to size. (A contest between divisional areas of a railroad is illustrated in Fig. 12–3.)

Most departmental contests, however, are conducted among dissimilar departments in one plant, and the departments often differ greatly in size. The difficulties due to variations in hazards and number of employees from one department to another may be overcome in the same manner as with similar differences between plants, just discussed.

One plan that produced excellent results was aimed particularly at foremen and supervisors in charge of departments having five to sixty employees. The principal rules were:

1. This contest will cover the period from July 1 to December 31.

2. Each department will compete against its own previous six months' accident record. Only disabling injuries are counted.

3. The department's accident experience will be judged by the frequency rate developed during the contest as compared with its frequency rate of the previous six months.

4. A suitable prize will be given each supervisor who reduces his department's frequency rate in the contest months by 50 percent or more over his frequency rate in the previous six months.

5. If a supervisor had no disabling injuries in his department during the previous six months, the prize will be given if he meets his previous six months' record.

A bronze trophy was given to each supervisor and department head who met the requirements for an award, and a dinner party was held. When the rates of the contest period were compared with the rates of the previous six months, the results were reductions of 30 percent in frequency and 62 percent in severity.

It is important that competing plants or groups be kept posted on the latest standings—Fig. 12–11, p. 341, shows a typical contest bulletin.

## Intergroup competitions

Intergroup contests are particularly suitable for units that employ fewer than 400 people and have small departments in which hazards vary sharply. Employees are divided into teams of from 20 to 50 workers. To equalize factors of size and difference in hazards, each team has a proportionate number of employees from the most and least hazardous occupations. Each group is led by a captain, whose principal duty is to contact members of the team and create interest in win-

# 12—Maintaining Interest in Safety

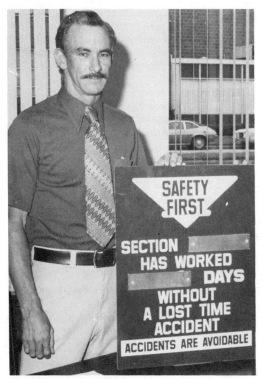

FIG. 12-12.—Signs like these can be up-dated easily to keep competing departments and sections up-to-date on how each is progressing in the plant-wide contest.

*Courtesy Baker Oil Tools, Houston, Texas.*

particular emphasis on the responsibilities of supervision and employees for avoiding accidents. These standards are often no-injury records for varying periods, achievement of lower injury rates in comparison with a previous period, and improvement over the average injury rates of similar units or of the industry. In this type of contest, units of an organization do not compete with one another; rather, each unit attempts to match or surpass established standards. (See Fig. 12-13.)

## Personalized contests

Some plants single out for acknowledgement employees who have safe records. Certificates are given to those who have worked one, two, five, and ten years without an injury. Holders of certificates have found them useful in obtaining promotion and even in seeking employment with other organizations.

Periodic raffles of merchandise or cash, or the use of a new car for three or four months, regardless of the injury record of a department or plant, also have been used successfully to encourage and acknowledge the efforts of safety-

ning. Team members may be members of contest committees.

Interest is promoted by naming teams after prominent baseball, football, or other outstanding sports teams, and the entire competition may be named after a league or other sports organization. Team names can be drawn from a hat and membership can be shown by colored pin-on buttons. Signs are placed in competing departments. (See Fig. 12-12.)

Identification of workers by colored buttons helps to overcome difficulties in scoring. Since the members of different teams work together, they make sure that every case involving a competitor is charged against his group record.

## Intraplant or intradepartmental contests

By setting standards of performance, an intraplant or intradepartmental safety contest puts

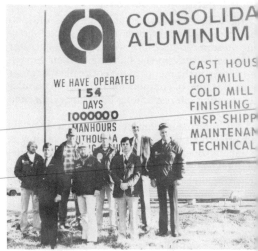

FIG. 12-13.—Plant safety team includes plant manager, industrial relations manager, production manager, and the safety supervisor; union is represented by the president of the local and two safety committee members.

*Courtesy Consolidated Aluminum Corporation, Hannibal, Mo., plant.*

**344**

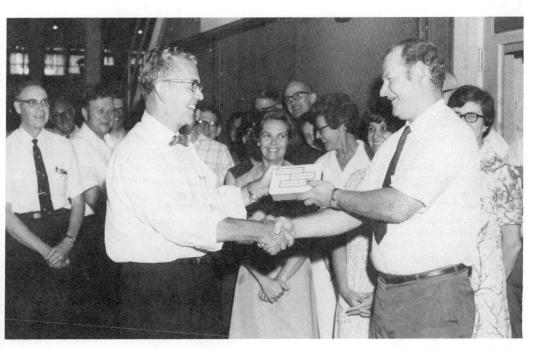

FIG. 12–14.—Everyone received a first aid kit when plant went two million workhours without a lost-time accident.

*Courtesy Mead Central Research Laboratory, Chillicothe, Ohio.*

conscious workers. Employees who are involved in disabling accidents (or drivers who have had a "preventable accident") during the period become ineligible for drawings.

Various sweepstakes plans have proved popular and effective in maintaining interest in a good record from month to month. One such plan was operated successfully by a branch plant of a well-known paper company. Here's how it worked.

On the payday prior to the beginning of each month all hourly employees received cards with serial numbers at the pay office window. The workers wrote their names and departments on the cards, tore off the stubs and put them in a box, and retained their portions of the cards. Names of employees in departments having no disabling injuries during the month then were drawn for prizes ranging from $5 to $25. The company contributed a total of $75 per month.

Since eligibility for the drawing depended on a perfect departmental record, each worker had to be careful about his actions. Workers frequently corrected others for unsafe practices that might spoil chances for prizes.

If no accidents occurred during a three-month period, supervisors participated in a drawing for prizes ranging from $5 to $15. This feature proved helpful in enlisting their cooperation.

Some companies give awards like first aid kits or trading stamps to those in every department that has worked a given period without accident. (See Fig. 12–14.) This approach is effective only if going a month, for instance, without an accident is unusual.

### Overcoming difficulties

A few difficulties in operating contests are rather easily overcome. One is that some departments are inherently more hazardous than others.

In some contests handicaps have been established, based on annual rates of insurance companies or on average accident frequency for the different kinds of work. This has been discussed previously.

Another method is to base standings on improvement over past records. Thus, a department with a past average frequency of 20 and a current frequency of 15 would be rated as having

**345**

made 25 percent improvement and would win over a department with a past frequency of 15 and a current frequency of 12—a 20 percent improvement.

Usually, in both methods an average of rates over three to five years is used as the base.

Another problem is that a department may have so many accidents at the beginning of the contest period that it is out of the running and loses interest. Having shorter contest periods helps to overcome this difficulty. Another remedy is to have different awards for different achievements. An award for the department having the longest run of injury-free workhours is an example.

Division of responsibility for the cause of an accident may become a problem; in other words, an unsafe act of one supervisor's worker (or an unsafe condition in this supervisor's department) may affect another supervisor's record. These situations must be anticipated and the contest planned to deal with them fairly, thus creating a favorable interest.

### Noninjury rate contests

Noninjury rate contests, such as safety slogan, poster, housekeeping, and community contests, can be just as effective in maintaining interest as contests based on injury rates. The objective in any case is to get the maximum number of people talking, thinking, and participating in safety. They are especially effective in promoting off-the-job safety.

Descriptions of various kinds of contests frequently can be found in the Council's monthly magazine *National Safety News*. On occasion, staff members or officers of the Council help judge such contests or assist in other ways.

**Slogan, limerick, and poster contests.** Safety slogan contests may be of various kinds. One can be for the best safety slogan submitted by an employee. Another may be run in which employees or their spouses are rewarded if they can repeat the "slogan of the week" or the message on a certain safety poster.

Company magazines may conduct contests to "finish the limerick" or "write a rhyme" or write "twenty-five words on the best way to be safe." Often these are open to both employees and family members.

The value of homemade posters is in their special application to a particular industry or company. If the posters are the result of an employee contest, their interest-creating value will be increased, possibly exceeding that of the tailor-made variety of posters. An important ingredient of such a contest is to get employees and their families participating in the planning and judging stages too.

Frequently, employee poster ideas—aside from the quality of the art work—are so good, that companies even submit the winning contest entries to the National Safety Council for possible conversion into printed safety posters.

**A housekeeping contest** often is conducted among departments. This type of competition is fundamental because it is aimed at accident *causes* and usually tries to eliminate unsafe practices and conditions.

Housekeeping contest plans differ from one company to another. The following plan is used successfully by a metals firm.

Once a week a committee of three representatives of management inspects each department and reports unsafe conditions to the superintendent. A copy is furnished to the works manager, and another is kept for the use of later inspection committees. A demerit for each unsatisfactory condition is charged to the department. If the condition is not rectified within one week, an additional demerit is chalked up.

At the end of the month the demerits for each department are totaled, and departments are rated on the basis of the proportion of demerits to the total number of employees in the department. If Department A employed 175 people and had 25 demerits, its rating would be 85.7. This figure is obtained by dividing 25 (number of demerits) by 175 (number of employees), multiplying by 100, and subtracting the product from 100. Standings are posted monthly on the bulletin boards in each department.

Awards are made at a mass meeting held after the lunch period. Names of employees in winning departments are placed in a box from which is drawn the name of the winner for the month. The winner's picture is posted on a special bulletin board, and a short talk on safety by a representative of management is broadcast throughout the plant. (A general rule prohibits an employee from winning more than one award during the contest.)

The name of the winning department is inscribed on a plaque each month. The head of the winning department receives the plaque from the

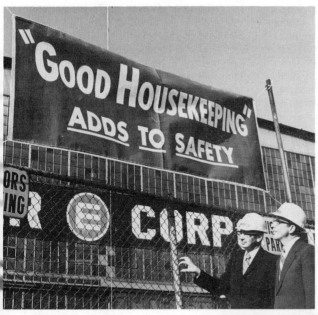

FIG. 12–15a.—Contest reminders should be placed about the plant in order to motivate employees. This banner is located near main plant entrance.

*Courtesy Edgewater Corp., Oakmont, Pa.*

FIG. 12–15b.—Company's program title is painted on the back of a huge fixed crane. In addition to signs, program uses booklets, contests, meetings, and visuals to encourage employees to develop a positive and continuing concern for safety both on and off the job.

*Courtesy Newport News Shipbuilding and Dry Dock Company.*

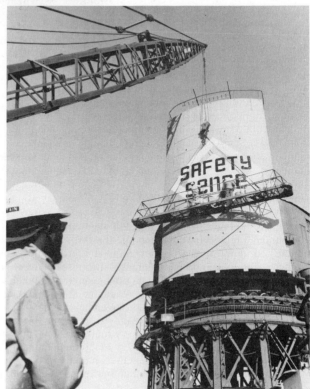

previous month's winner at the mass meeting, and at the end of the year the department that has won the plaque the greatest number of times receives it permanently.

**Community and family contests.** Many companies have stimulated interest by sponsoring safety essay or poster contests for children of employees, local school children, or young art students. The publicity before and after such contests plus the interest generated by the posters themselves and the judging not only stimulates the interest of employees but also promotes the company's community and public relations.

More than one company has launched a safety poster or essay contest for the children of employees with the full knowledge that the employees would give their children considerable help and that there would be much favorable discussion about the contest in locker rooms, lunchrooms, and car pools.

**Miscellaneous contests.** There is an endless number of different types of contest possibilities. Often they can be combined with injury reduction contests. Contests can be held for attending safety meetings, for wearing safety shoes, for reporting unsafe conditions or unsafe acts, or for off-the-job or public safety activities or individuals, departments, or branch plants.

Although contests are popular with both management and employees, the safety director always should attempt to determine before starting them whether or not they will require time and effort that should be spent on providing safer equipment or better training for supervisors and employees.

## Contest and other publicity

All stages of a contest should be played up as dramatically as possible. Placards and news stories should prepare for it. Standings should be announced at frequent intervals. Special signs, banners, and posters can be used for this purpose (see Fig. 12–15). Handout bulletins can be sent to individual employees urging care in keeping the record perfect. The company magazine and even the local newspaper and radio station can make good copy of a contest. Trade journals and National Safety Council newsletters are other outlets for contest publicity. In a smaller community, outstanding safety performance by a well-known company deserves—and usually

gets—excellent publicity.

The publicity value of a successful contest is considerable, although difficult to estimate. It is a fact that large companies invest literally thousands of dollars and hundreds of hours of planning time to set up awards, judge, and make elaborate presentations.

Publicity should be commensurate with the real significance of the occasion. The presentation of a watch or other personal award to an employee who has gone 25 years without a disabling injury has human interest value to a company paper and perhaps to a local newspaper or trade journal.

Recognition of an exceptionally fine "no injury" record made by a corporation (one million injury-free workhours would probably be a minimum), or presentation of a National Safety Council award to a company deserves a different and more impressive type of publicity.

Publicity (including photographs) can appear in the local newspaper. The information can be sent to the media in the form of a press release, which indicates the nature of the contest or award. See Chapter 13, "Publicizing Safety," for details of preparing a news release.

Some companies pay for radio or television time to announce the results of a contest. Others arrange for photographs and stories to go in their company papers, on their bulletin boards, and perhaps in local or trade association papers. One company had large campaign-type buttons made, and photos of children wearing them appeared in the local press.

## Meaningful awards

An award serves several purposes. It is an inducement, a builder of good will, a continuing reminder, and a basis for publicity. To serve these purposes, however, an award must be meaningful.

The winning and display of a multiplicity of awards may detract from the true value of the program, particularly if the awards are given too freely by sales-minded donors. Employees sense when awards are given only for sales or publicity purposes and are based on little or no safety effort.

The value of awards lies in their appeal to basic interest factors, such as pride, need for recognition, urge to compete, and desire for financial gain. Monetary awards, however, should not appear to be bribes. In general, select awards which are worthy of good publicity, which will photograph well, and which provoke conversation. The distribution of U.S. Savings Bonds or trade stamps for safe records gets away from the appearance of "bribery."

The originality or cleverness of an award or of its method of presentation is an important factor. Refreshments awarded to all employees in a department after the completion of one million injury-free hours probably might create more favorable comment than would the presentation of a fancy plaque to the department supervisor. The drawing of a small cash prize or a grab bag prize would attract more interest than a routine presentation of the same award. An award to an employee's spouse for completing a home safety checklist, for identifying a safety slogan, or for contributing to the company paper would create more interest than the same award given on the job.

• One of the Council's members reported an award idea that received an unusual amount of publicity, both within the plant and locally. A local automobile agency loaned the company a new car that was driven for a week by an injury-free employee whose name was drawn from the hat. The employee and the company received excellent publicity in the local papers; the employee had a special "reserved for John Doe" parking space in the company lot. The only cost to the employer was a few dollars to cover special insurance. Even a special parking space alone can be effective. (See Fig. 12–16.)

• Another way to gain interest is to let the employees participate in selecting the award, planning its presentation, and helping with publicity. Frequently, the employees will suggest a humorous or novel award or publicity approach that may attract more interest than one planned by management. In any case, the employees' participation is a wise investment in safety promotion.

• Payment of bonuses as a type of award for good safety records evokes considerable difference of opinion. Some managements and safety people feel that this approach is unwarranted; and some plans using it have proved unsuccessful or have been abandoned.

• Sums of money are divided into various amounts, or government savings bonds are purchased and raffled, particularly for outstanding achievements by departments and small plants. Some companies raffle household or sports mer-

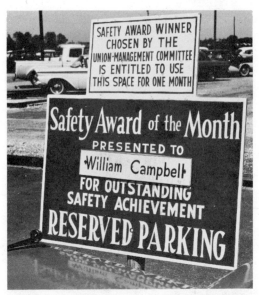

FIG. 12–16.—A "reserved parking" privilege at a choice location is an inexpensive but very effective award for contest winners and for employees who achieve outstanding safety records.

*Courtesy Kaiser Aluminum and Chemical Corp., Chalmette, La.*

chandise. Many employees value attractive pins or engraved cards commending them for years of employment without an accident. One company places a safety record sticker on the employee's hard hat. Others provide special badges, pins or shoulder patches to recognize safety achievement or service on a safety committee.

• Interest in safety among supervisors and workers often is developed by personal awards like wallets, knives, or key cases, often suitably inscribed.

In addition to contest awards, recognition should be given to those who have saved lives, served on safety committees, submitted valuable suggestions to the management, or made other significant contributions to accident prevention.

### Award presentations

Make an award presentation something special, and recognize it by well-planned publicity. One company rents an auditorium and invites civic and labor leaders, "main office" executives, other dignitaries, and employees' families to a large

**349**

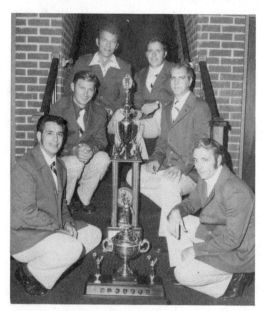

FIG. 12–17.—Winners of a National Mine Rescue and First Aid Contest pose with their trophy. Staircase affords a natural background that contributes to good photographic composition.

*Courtesy of Winding Gulf Division of the Westmoreland Coal Co., Tams, W. Va.*

celebration party. The presentation of even a modest award to an individual worker or supervisor would call for the participation of company officials and perhaps family members or other workers.

The president of the company himself, or some other high official, can present the awards at a general meeting, a picnic, or a dinner (or breakfast) that may even include entertainment. The reason for inviting VIP's is not only to add prestige to the presentation, but also to promote their interest and commitment to safety.

The presentation requires planning, and must be in keeping with the importance of the occasion. The place of the event should be appropriate and comfortable, not noisy or crowded. An award to an individual might be made in an executive office; a group award might be made in a conference room, private dining room, or in a company lounge or cafeteria (during a nonrush period).

Brief the participants on the agenda. Familiar-

ize those who make the presentation with the significance of the award, the achievement it recognizes and the background of the individual(s) who earned it. Arrange for reporting and photographing the event in order to get maximum publicity. Photographs can be specially posed after the actual presentation to take advantage of desirable backgrounds, such as the plant or company name, some prominent trademark, or other interest-catching effect. The award itself should be featured prominently in the picture. (Fig. 12–17.) (See the next chapter and the Council Data Sheet 619, *Photography for the Safety Professional,* for other ideas.)

For a group award—such as a company, a plant, or a department's completing an injury-free year—free refreshments, such as coffee and cold drinks, can be offered for a specified time—ranging from one coffee break (per shift) to a full 24-hour period (see Fig. 12–18).

Another, more elaborate award was given by the president of a company employing about 300. At the end of a year in which there had been no disabling injuries, he took the group to a major league baseball game. The following year, after his company maintained its no-injury record, he invited the group, plus their families, to an all-day picnic and cruise.

Such activities help build better employee and public relations, as well as promote more interest in safety.

## Posters and Displays

Posters and displays are meant to reach large numbers of people on the move with brief, simple messages, designed to accomplish one or more missions—to convey information, to change attitudes, and/or to change behavior. They are designed to communicate with people going about their normal activities and consequently the audience must be seized, the message conveyed, and the contact finished in a very brief span of time. (See Fig. 12–19.)

Safety posters are one of the most visible evidences of accident prevention work. Because of this, perhaps, some companies have mistakenly assumed that posters alone would do the safety job and have neglected such essentials as real management support, guarding, and job instruction. In fact, hit-and-miss use of posters in a plant where no other safety work is done is likely to have a negative influence, making employees feel that the company is not sincere. (See National

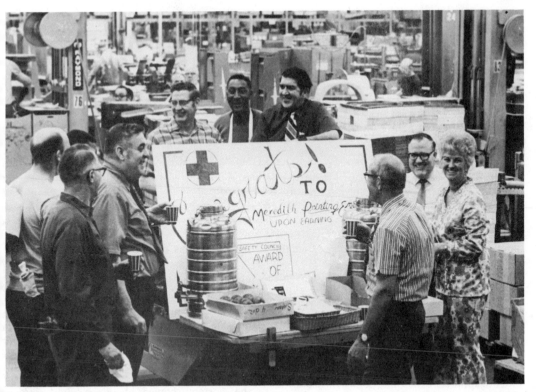

FIG. 12–18.—Coffee and doughnuts were served to all when this "mobile celebration" toured the plant in recognition of the company's receiving the National Safety Council's Award of Merit.

*Courtesy Meredith Printing Division, Des Moines, Iowa.*

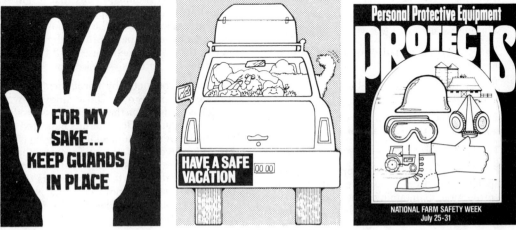

FIG. 12–19.—Poster messages should be brief and simple. They can be slanted to on-job, off-the-job, and special-interest activities.

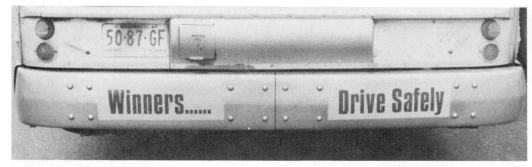

FIG. 12–20.—"Winners ... Drive Safely" reflector-type bumper stickers, used on B.C. Hydro Transit's Greater Vancouver fleet, are part of a safety campaign aimed at reducing traffic accidents. "Winners" refers to the awards that company has already earned for successful campaigns.

Safety Council Data Sheet 616, *Posters, Bulletin Boards, and Safety Displays.*)

## Purposes of posters

Posters properly used have great value in a safety program through their influence on attitudes and behavior. One has only to see the efforts that commercial advertisers make to acquire space in business areas or near factory gates in order to appreciate the value of posters *inside* the work place.

When posters are selected, it is well to have in mind their specific purposes:

1. To remind employees of common human traits that cause accidents

2. To impress people with the good sense of working safely

3. To suggest behavior patterns that help prevent accidents

4. To inspire a friendly interest in the company's safety efforts

5. To foster the attitude that accidents are mistakes and safety is a mark of skill

6. To remind employees of specific hazards

Posters are useful also in supporting special campaigns, for instance, using guards, wearing eye protection, maintaining good housekeeping, offering safety suggestions, or driving carefully (Fig. 12–20).

Posters promote traffic, home, and even pedestrian safety by encouraging safe work habits.

## Effectiveness of posters

A number of studies have been made on the effectiveness of posters for training and motivating.

• One study was conducted by the British Iron and Steel Research Association. Three posters that reminded workers to hook cable slings were displayed in six plants over a period of six weeks. A seventh plant was used as a control. Tallies made in the six plants before and after display of the posters showed about an eight percent increase in compliance with the rule. The seventh plant, in which the posters were not used, showed a very slight decrease in compliance.

Although use of the posters merely supplemented previous training, plants that originally had the lowest rates of compliance showed some of the best gains. Use of the test posters separately, on a biweekly basis, proved slightly more effective than simultaneous use of all three posters during the entire six-week test.

• In a survey conducted by a prominent casualty insurance company, over 200 employees were interviewed in depth on the effectiveness of safety posters, films, and leaflets. Results indicated that all the media were instrumental in bringing workers to a high level of safety awareness and that all were effective in sustaining that awareness. Employees were found to prefer posters to leaflets, although they acknowledged the value of leaflets for more detailed coverage of, for example, off-the-job safety.

• A survey of Council members indicated that about three-fourths of the nearly 800 respondents

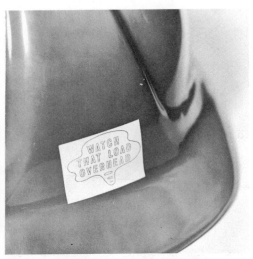

FIG. 12–21.—"Walking safety poster." Construction superintendent lets workers select own safety message, place it on their own safety hat.

*Courtesy Stone & Webster Engineering Corp.*

use a variety of poster subjects with one-third preferring cartoons and all-industry posters. Horror or shocker posters were least preferred.

Fifty-four percent of the respondents use posters to influence general attitudes; 27 percent to cover special operations; 18 percent, to meet special or seasonal problems; and 14 percent, to promote off-the-job safety.

Sixty-nine percent of the respondents in the Council's poster survey preferred posters of 8½ by 11½ in. and 17 by 23 in. size (21.5 × 28 cm and 43 × 58½ cm). Of these two sizes, the smaller was preferred six-to-one over the larger.

While there can be no question about the interest stimulated by a "sexy" photo, there may be some question as to the effectiveness of the safety message, particularly if the photo is unrelated to the message. Frequently, an unusually striking photo or overly elaborate (and expensive) artwork actually detracts from the safety message. This is not to say that "eye-popping" illustrations should never be used; occasional use may serve to attract attention to the more conservative, serious messages on other posters.

## Types of posters

Industrial posters available from the National Safety Council, insurance companies, associa-

tions, and other sources fall into three broad categories: general and special industry and special hazard.

• The general posters are concerned with such subjects as chance-taking, disregarding safety rules, forgetting to replace guards, and other human failures.

• Special industry posters, as the term indicates, have application only in specific industries, such as mining or logging.

• Special hazard posters, for example on lifting, ladders, the storage or handling of flammable liquids, are useful in every industry where the particular hazards are encountered. In some cases, a hazard is so serious that a special poster is

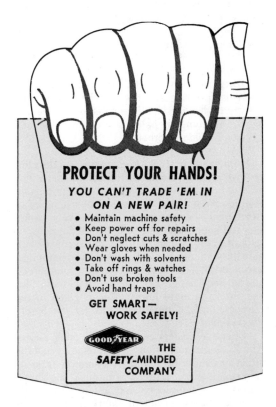

FIG. 12–22.—This die-cut pocket card has "fingers" that seemingly reach out of the pocket, tempt viewer to inquire about the message (which is revealed as card is pulled out).

*Courtesy Goodyear Tire & Rubber Co., Inc.*

developed because of the severity and not the frequency of exposure.

The National Safety Council carries more than 1000 different safety posters in stock at any one time. These range from pocket-size pressure-sensitive stickers to billboard-size jumbo posters. About 15 new posters are added each month.

Subject matter is roughly in proportion to the occurrence of certain types of accidents. For example, more posters are concerned with material handling than with chemicals and gases. (For illustrations of the many posters available from the National Safety Council, see the latest *Poster Directory.*)

**Other locations.** Posters and stickers can be mounted on delivery trucks, buses (Fig. 20–20), industrial trucks, mail trucks and carts, in elevators, and even on doors. Pocket cards or plastic pocket protectors, such as those available from the National Safety Council, might be called "walking safety posters." (See Figs. 12–21 and –22.)

**Other materials.** Safety messages need not be limited to printing and artwork. They can be very effective when used in illuminated or changeable signs. One company paints a safety message on a plywood welding screen.

**Homemade posters.** A company can develop its own posters to deal with special hazards not covered by posters available from outside sources. Even the smallest company can make an occasional special poster inexpensively, using colored paper, crayons, or felt marking pens, to call attention to a special hazard, to commemorate the winning of a safety award, or to point up a problem not likely to be covered by a commercial poster. See Chapter 14, "Audiovisual Media," for details. Even more information is given in the Council book, *Communications for the Safety Professional.*

Effective posters can be made using photographs of local conditions or accidents, even if the situations must be posed. A common type of homemade poster is the "testimonial" showing a photo of an employee and a close-up of his damaged safety glasses or safety shoes, with a brief statement explaining how this equipment protected him. (See Fig. 12–23.)

Homemade posters on new processes, new guards, or new rules personalize the safety pro-

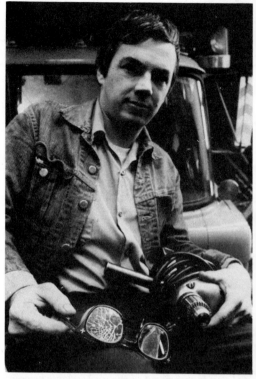

FIG. 12–23.—Photograph plus a brief statement makes an effective, personalized safety item that can be used as a poster or placed on a bulletin board. Glasses that stopped a fragment of metal thrown from a drill saved this person's eyesight. Quote that ran with the photograph when it was posted was, " 'That's one thing I wouldn't want to be without—my sight,' says Dave Lindorff, Central Shop."

*Courtesy* Public Employees Section Newsletter.

gram and augment even the best selection of commercial posters.

## Changing and mounting posters

No specific rule can be given for the frequency of changing posters because of varying definitions of the term "poster."

Some types of posters may well be mounted permanently. For example, a poster on artificial respiration can be kept in the first aid room, or one on the use of a certain kind of fire extinguisher can be posted near it.

Most companies change general interest posters at definite intervals, usually weekly, perhaps

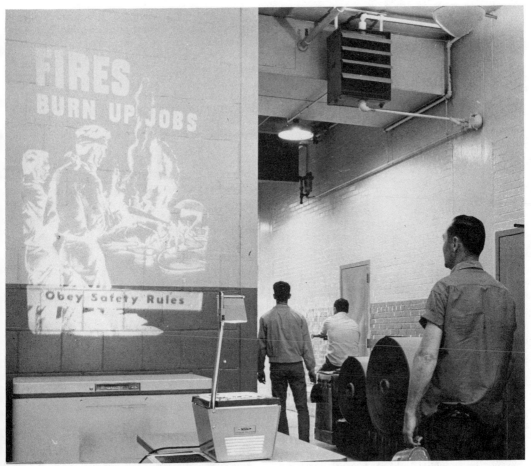

Fig. 12–24.—A novel method of displaying safety posters is shown here. A transparency made from a poster was placed on an overhead projector in this heavy-traffic area; projector threw the image onto a blank wall.

*Courtesy 3M Company.*

rotating them from one area to another or filing them and then reusing them after a year or so.

The type of posters displayed should be varied. Consecutive posting of several infection posters, for instance, or of machinery posters is not desirable unless a special campaign is being conducted. To secure proper balance, it is better to use an eye poster, than a machinery poster, next an infection poster, and so on.

For maximum effectiveness, posters not only must be selected carefully and changed on a definite schedule, but also displayed attractively in well-lighted locations where they will be seen by the greatest number of people. They should be placed on safety bulletin boards, near time clocks, in cafeterias, and at points of special hazard, such as paint storage rooms, rubbish cans, hazardous machinery, or dangerous intersections.

A novel idea for displaying posters is shown in Fig. 12–24.

### Bulletin boards

Bulletin boards should permit convenient change of posters and should be placed where employees can see them when they are momentarily at leisure, such as near drinking fountains

**355**

# 12—Maintaining Interest in Safety

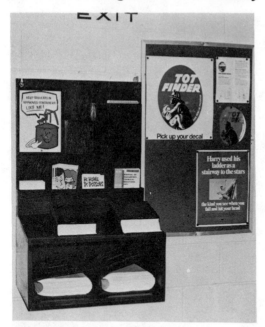

FIG. 12–25.—In addition to inspirational and educational safety bulletins, this "information station" carries pertinent chemical safety data as well as Council booklets for employee use.

*Courtesy Borg-Warner Corporation, Washington, W. Va.*

range from large, enclosed, illuminated boards with special sections for posters, safety bulletins, and other messages to a number of small frames or other inexpensive poster mounts installed at strategic points.

The National Safety Council has available black enameled poster frames to which clip-on literature racks can be added. This permits convenient distribution of leaflets and other pickup literature which support the safety message. (See Fig. 12–25.)

## Displays and exhibits

Personal protective devices, tools, and pieces of firefighting equipment can be used to make up displays or exhibits, with or without corresponding posters. (See Fig. 12–26.)

Another good interest-catcher is a combination of a Council poster, a seasonal topic, and a safety display.

Displays can also be used to promote off-the-job safety as well. For example, many companies try to motivate their employees to understand that a happy vacation must also be a safe vacation. (See Fig. 12–27.)

Signs with changeable letters, electric tape

(Fig. 18–2). They should be centered at eye level, about 63 in. (1.6 m) from the floor. They should be in a well-lighted place; if more light is needed, they can be specially lighted. A good size for a bulletin board is about 22 in. wide by 30 in. long (56 × 76 cm).

Boards should be attractively painted and glass-covered. One board at a location in the work place is usually desirable, but in lunchrooms or locker rooms several panels may be used effectively. Flashing lights, sometimes desirable in nonproduction areas, are likely to be objectionable in workplaces.

A bulletin board should be used for only one display at a time, but need not carry safety posters exclusively. Any program of mutual interest to company and employees may legitimately use the bulletin boards. In fact, safety posters may have a stronger appeal if they appear on a board on which employees occasionally see displays on other subjects.

Bulletin boards in the same company may

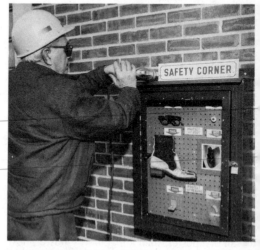

FIG. 12–26.—Here is one of 45 "Safety Corners" throughout a company's facilities. Displays are concerned with both on-job and off-the-job safety.

*Courtesy Newport News Shipbuilding and Dry Dock Company.*

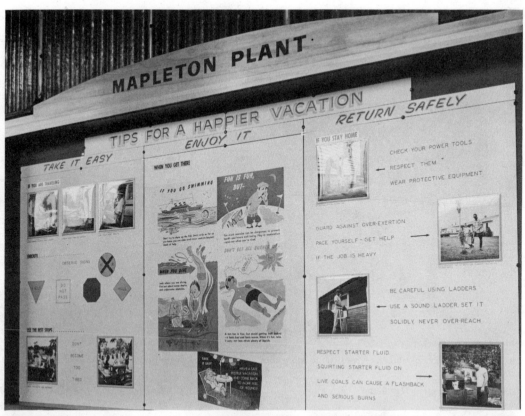

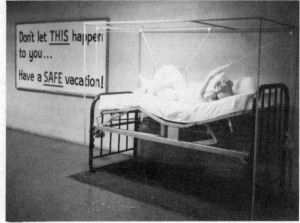

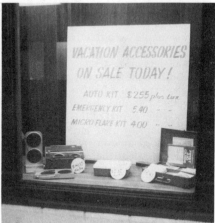

FIG. 12–27.—To implant the idea that "A happy vacation is a safe vacation," one company put up the display pictured at top. Its theme was three-fold: "Take it easy if you are traveling; Enjoy it when you get there; and Return safely." In addition to drawings, photographs showed actual plant employees. Realism was injected into the exhibit (photo at left) by a dummy undergoing traction; bed was borrowed from a local hospital. At right, first aid kits were sold to employees at cost.

*Courtesy* Metals Section Newsletter.

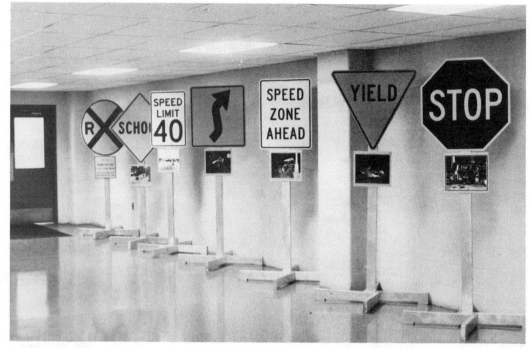

Fig. 12–28.—A display of traffic control signs, accompanied by photographs of traffic accidents, was placed near plant entrance.

*Courtesy* Metals Section Newsletter.

messages, or eye-catching lighting can be used for safety displays. (See Figs. 12–12 and –13.)

Many simple and attractive displays have been devised for presenting statistical data to workers. One is a safety clock, the face of which is marked off to indicate the frequency of disabling injuries. Twin clocks or dials often are used, one recording the present rate and the other the rate for the corresponding period of the past month or year.

One company used large thermometer-like boards, placed at every gate and clock-house. Arrows indicated the present and previous month's records. The comparative standings of departments were shown below.

An auto race was the theme of another display; each car represented a department. The cars moved daily to denote progress being made. Airplanes can be used similarly. Another exhibit featured race horses participating in a "Safety Derby" and named after items of personal protective equipment.

A display of highway signs with photographs

of accidents below them was placed near the plant entrance (Fig. 12–28) of another company.

## Other Promotional Methods

Other methods that can be used effectively to arouse and maintain interest in safety are campaigns, safety stunts, courses and demonstrations, publications, public address systems, and suggestion systems.

### Campaigns

Campaigns serve to focus the attention of the entire plant personnel on one specific accident problem. They are, of course, additions to and not substitutes for persistent accident prevention effort the year round.

Campaigns may be undertaken to promote the use of safety shoes, home safety, vacation safety, or fire safety. A "Clean-Up Week" may be held, or a "Stop Accidents" campaign may be run to promote safe attitudes both on and off the job.

The National Safety Council's nationwide campaigns "Win with Safety" and "Profit from Safety," (and others) included posters, films, booklets, and specialty items to promote and maintain the interest of employees. In addition, special campaign materials have been developed in collaboration with trade associations and for special problem areas such as "Stop Shock," and "Fight Falls." Information on current campaign material is given in Council catalogs and other publications and is available from the Council headquarters.

Moreover, large corporations have conducted extensive campaigns to promote safety on and off the job. Much of this safety awareness material is aimed at families of employees, local citizens, and even groups outside the U.S. One company's "Safety is Caring" program is shown in Fig. 12–29.

Suitable publicity should be planned for the campaign from kickoff to conclusion, similar to that discussed for safety contests earlier in this chapter. Signs, flags, desktop symbols, and other items can be used to dramatize the campaign. To wind it up, a special event can be scheduled, such as giving each employee an inexpensive novelty item, free coffee, or a free breakfast or dinner.

Many of the same promotion stunts or ideas that help maintain interest in contests also can be effective in special campaigns. For example, a first aid drill or a demonstration of artificial respiration may be given. Some companies use safety parades, exhibits of unsafe and safe tools and equipment, pledge cards, and other such features.

Timeliness may be an important factor in the way employees respond to a campaign. Successful safety campaigns have been linked to elections, World Series, the football season, Thanksgiving, and other special events.

See Council Data Sheet 616, *Posters, Bulletin Boards, and Safety Displays*, for more ideas.

## Off-beat safety ideas

Off-beat safety ideas or "stunts" capitalize on all the effective aspects of showmanship and thrive on an endless variety of ideas. They can be developed as separate devices for maintaining interest or can be used to supplement contests and campaigns. *National Safety News* and other publications regularly give details on various stunts.

Stunts that criticize or ridicule seem to belong to the past. However, if handled with a light touch

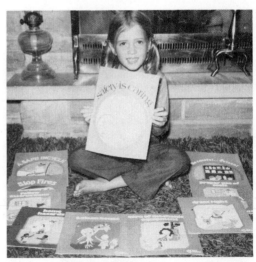

FIG. 12–29.—"Safety is caring" program provides materials for off-the-job safety program involving children. Four coloring books and six story books are geared to interest children. Programs are provided for each location where company has a facility; extra copies of the booklets are provided local libraries, schools, churches, and youth organizations.

*Courtesy Allied Chemical Corporation.*

and in a group that accepts them good-naturedly, stunts with a negative approach may have their uses. Typical of such stunts is the giving of an old broom to the department with the most demerits for poor housekeeping. It would be better, however, to give a new broom to the cleanest department.

Most companies agree that constructive stunts help inspire employees to high standards while stunts that ridicule may do more harm than good, particularly if the employees resent that they have been treated unfairly. More important, employees and supervisors who are the objects of ridicule may have just cause to blame management for not setting up safe procedures or providing safe facilities and equipment.

Safety stunts can involve an entire company, a department, a small group, or just the individual. A stunt may be humorous, novel, or dramatic, and occasionally even shocking.

A simple stunt is often most effective. A pivoted hammer, mounted over a pair of safety glasses in a display case, can be operated by a string to demonstrate the impact resistance of the

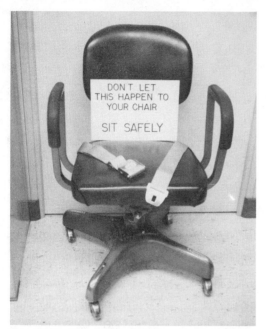

FIG. 12–30.—Four kinds of accidents involving office chairs were described in a bulletin distributed to all employees; the bulletin has this photo of an office chair equipped with safety belts—a tongue-in-cheek warning that employees be more careful with their seating habits if they want to avoid an accident or getting their chair equipped with a safety belt. When the chair itself was put on display at the various offices, the local press picked up the idea for a story.

*Courtesy Contra Costa County Civil Service Commission, Martinez, Calif.*

glasses. To dramatize the importance of eye protection, the "let's pretend" test can be used. Several volunteers are blindfolded and then asked to light a cigarette, eat, write, and move around. Another stunt is described in Fig. 12–30.

Stunts developed for the company safety program often can be used at company open houses or safety picnics and in community safety projects as well. Such stunts, when supported by visual aids, signs, and printed material, demonstrate the company's interest in accident prevention and give the employees a chance to participate in programs that help create safer attitudes on the job, too.

Off-beat "posters" are interest-getting. Fig. 12–22 shows a hand that reaches out of a pocket.

Fig. 12–31 shows a litter bag that is given to an employee on his last workday before vacation; this gives his supervisor a good opportunity to wish the vacation-bound employee an enjoyable and safe vacation.

A card, shown in Fig. 12–32, is used to alert a co-worker that he has exposed himself to an accident.

## Courses and demonstrations

Most safety professionals agree that courses in first aid, lifesaving, water safety, civil defense, and disaster control have bonus values that help prevent work injuries, too.

The worker who has gone through a course in first aid and has learned to give artificial respiration will be more mindful of the hazards of electric shock and more likely to help maintain electrical equipment in safe condition. Likewise, the employee who learns how to stop arterial

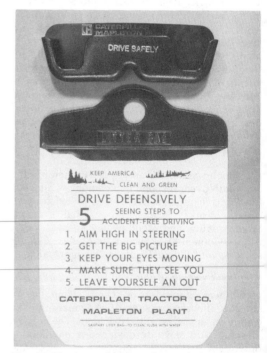

FIG. 12–31.—A reusable litter bag with five defensive driving steps is given to each employee by his supervisor on the last day before the employee takes his vacation.

*Courtesy Caterpillar Tractor Co., Mapleton Plant.*

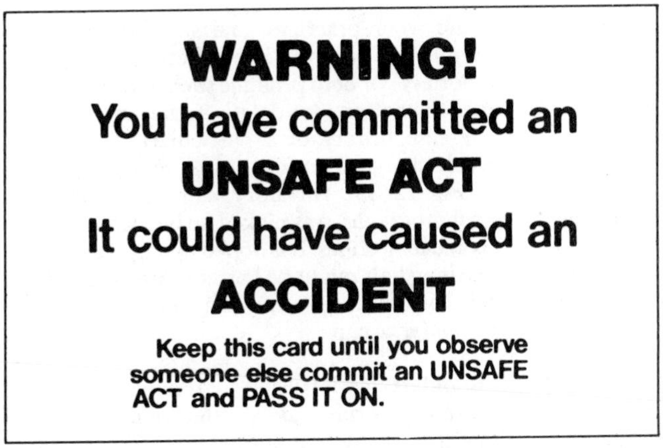

FIG. 12–32.—This plastic card, shown in its actual size, is handed to someone who has been observed committing an unsafe act.

*Courtesy Goodyear Danville Plant's Joint Safety Committee.*

bleeding better appreciates the consequences of using a saw or a power press without the guard.

Home study and extension courses, although designed primarily for training purposes, also serve to stimulate and maintain interest. They give the employee a better understanding of the job and do a great deal to dispel unsafe attitudes. Most safety training courses, in fact, are designed specifically to improve the attitudes of both supervisors and employees. The use of good visual aids will enhance the effectiveness of the courses; the use of video tape for a technical discussion demonstrates the progressive nature of the company as well. (See Chapter 14, "Audiovisual Media.")

The participation of the public in courses taught or attended by employees promotes community good will. Many industrial safety people are doing an excellent job of promoting safety and fire prevention through arranging courses on these subjects for the Boy Scouts and Explorer Scouts, the Girl Scouts, Camp Fire groups, Junior Achievement companies, and other youth or school groups.

The National Safety Council's "Defensive Driving Course" provides an excellent way to promote good employee and public relations. It stimulates safer attitudes both on the job as well as off.

Demonstrations of fire equipment have a practical value beyond that of teaching employees how to react in an emergency. The mere fact that the equipment is provided for their use reminds them of management's concern about their welfare. Moreover, the demonstrations make employees more aware of the dangers of fire and point up the need for obeying fire prevention rules.

Demonstrations of fire equipment by local fire departments or distributors of fire equipment are easily arranged. Many companies conduct their own demonstrations, using extinguishers that require recharging, or "not-in-service" extinguishers kept specifically for this purpose.

## Publications

**Reports.** The safety professional should make reports on safety program progress interesting to his superiors and to supervisors. Visuals can be effective. (See Chapter 14, "Audiovisual Media.")

Once a procedure for such reporting is set up, it may be administered routinely by an insurance department or an accounting department or even may be made a part of production cost figures.

The cost of accidents and, perhaps, the cost of prevention should be given in terms that are significant to management, such as medical and compensation costs, production losses, sales losses, increased maintenance costs, and the less tangible but perhaps more important hidden costs involved in administrative problems and in impaired public, customer, or employee relations. Reports need not be dull. Photographs, for example, can pin-point a company's major sources of disabling work accidents.

In one company a statement of accident losses and safety achievements may be included in the annual report, whereas in another a special annual or monthly safety report may be issued to top executives and supervisors. If departmental accident losses, like incidence rates, can be charged on an equitable basis, such as "per hundred thousand dollars of sales" or "per one thousand employee-days of production," the comparative standings of departments and improvement in departments or units are easy to evaluate. (See the discussion in Chapter 6, "Accident Records and Incidence Rates.")

The fact that such information is recorded and publicized is in itself an incentive to supervisors. It reminds everyone concerned that accident costs are just as much an integral part of profit and loss as production, sales, maintenance, distribution, and advertising.

Special charts, graphs, and statistical reports can be used to give the facts about accidents. One chart can show the number of disabling injuries, others the number of days lost, injury causes, accident causes, or body location of injuries. It cannot be too strongly emphasized that unless such charts are kept up to date they can do more harm than good.

**Annual reports.** In recent years, a great many companies have gone to considerable lengths to make their annual reports to stockholders interesting and clearly understandable. In many cases, annual reports are also distributed to employees so that they can become better acquainted with the company's purposes and problems. A section on aims and accomplishments in accident prevention attracts employee interest and further serves to emphasize the interest of management in the safety of its employees.

Publicity regarding a good safety record may be arranged in local newspapers or in trade journals. Such publicity is particularly valuable in a smaller community where the company is well known or where the quality of a product, so far as the public is concerned, is reflected somewhat in its safety record. (This discussion is continued in depth in the next chapter, "Publicizing Safety.")

**Newsletters.** Monthly or weekly newsletters are especially important as a means of maintaining interest. They keep employees and supervisors informed, particularly in decentralized or field operations where bulletin boards are not feasible. Such newsletters can give detailed information on standings in a safety contest and publicize unusual accidents or serious hazards. They can help explain safety rules, remind employees

of safe work practices, and support the safety program in general. If workers can serve as "reporters" or help produce such a newsletter, so much the better. (See details in the next chapter.)

A case history of a particularly unusual or spectacular accident can sometimes be featured (see Fig. 12–33). This story, with the accompanying photographs, was picked up by many newsletters and magazines. It is hoped that operators who have long hair might be better motivated to keep their hair in an upswept arrangement or, better yet, under a cap.

**Booklets, leaflets,** and personalized messages take many forms: safety rule booklets, special "one-shot" leaflets, monthly publications such as the National Safety Council's *Industrial Supervisor* magazine and its *Safe Worker* and *Safe Driver* for employees, and letters from management.

The content of an employee rule booklet, except for material involving company policy, may be developed with the help of safety committees or selected workers as a means of stimulating interest and helping ensure compliance with the rules.

Larger companies may have their own editors and artists, even their own printing facilities, and produce publications of professional caliber. Smaller companies, however, also can issue attractive booklets, leaflets, and personalized messages, and at negligible expense.

The National Safety Council, trade associations, and professional organizations publish a wide variety of booklets and leaflets that are authoritative, attractive, and relatively inexpensive. They cover a large range of subjects—material handling, first aid, housekeeping, fire prevention, vacation safety, safe driving, and the like. Such materials, carefully selected and regularly distributed, effectively supplement company-prepared publications.

Letters commending meritorious service, signed by the manager and addressed to individuals, make an excellent impression upon workers.

Safety calendars, published by the National Safety Council, together with Christmas letters from the manager have a direct appeal that reaches the workers' homes. Such mailings should include each employee. *Family Safety*, a quarterly publication of the National Safety Council, is sent to more than two million homes by managements who are interested in the welfare of both employees and their families.

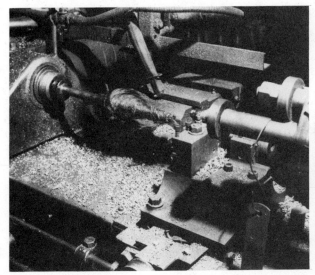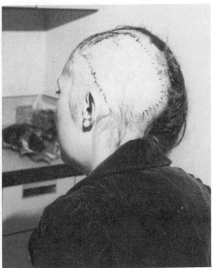

FIG. 12–33.—This particularly hideous accident was described in a Council Metals Section *Newsletter* and brought a lot of attention to the importance of operating rotating machinery safely. Here's the story. As this operator was bending over to clean the air ports on a lathe she was running, her hair (which was hanging down instead of being held up by a cap) became entangled in a rotating part (left photograph). Her hair and a large portion of her scalp was pulled out and she was pulled against the machine with such force that she was knocked unconscious. Fortunately, she was immediately taken to the hospital where she recovered; unfortunately, however, she will have to wear a wig for the remainder of her life.

**Buttons, blotters,** book matches, pencils, and other small novelties, all conveying a safety message, also may be used. For example, booklets of silicone tissues for cleaning glasses, imprinted with brief messages or safety rules, serve to remind employees of the rules and to encourage proper use of safety equipment.

### Public address systems

Public address systems often are used to broadcast announcements and page employees. Many companies have taken advantage of these installations to broadcast safety information.

Such messages should be planned carefully. Employees might readily lose interest in long speeches or too-frequent safety reminders. When the public address system is used for broadcasting music, safety announcements can be made between numbers.

### Suggestion systems

Because accident prevention is closely associated with efficient operation, many suggestions help not only to prevent accidents but also to lower production cost; not only to improve manufacturing conditions and methods, but also to better the health and change the outlook of workers.

Effective suggestion systems, like many other things in life, cost money. Many companies pay considerable sums for employee suggestions—one firm awards more than $10 million annually, but feels the money is well spent because of the value of the suggestions themselves.

Improved employee interest and personal involvement are additional benefits. Many companies prefer the positive, more enduring motivation of recognition and awards, to the "negative admonitions" of some safety publicity. Safety suggestions are also regarded as a highly desirable way to avoid safety grievances.

If a company does not have a general suggestion system, it is probably better not to establish one for safety suggestions alone. Setting safety apart from ordinary operating procedures may de-emphasize its importance.

Getting good suggestions is important and must be encouraged by all ranks of management.

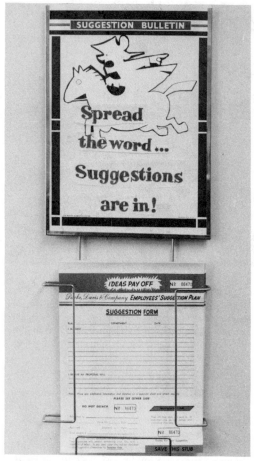

FIG. 12-34.—Posters and suggestion form racks can be placed in employee lounges, food service facilities, and other high-traffic areas. Companies usually distribute an information booklet that explains how the system works.

*Courtesy Parke, Davis & Company.*

Posters, contests, campaigns, merchandise incentives, direct mail, printed handouts, personal appeal, supervisory training, safety clubs, and press releases are employed to motivate employees to submit safety suggestions.

To merit an award, a safety suggestion, like a production suggestion, should be substantial, be practical, and be a real solution. Changing a method or material, guarding a hazard, inventing a safety tool or device are examples of suggestions worthy of awards. Erecting a sign, cautioning workers, or publishing slogans are examples of ideas usually not considered eligible for an award.

**Suggestion awards.** It is easy to measure the monetary value of suggestions that result in greater efficiency, lower material cost, decreased labor cost, or reduced waste. Usually awards for suggestions in these categories are in proportion to the savings derived by the company. Although some safety suggestions also have a monetary value, they are hard to evaluate; hence, payments for suggestions that contribute to the welfare of the employees, but result in no direct savings to the company, are most often estimates or composite judgments. Some firms have developed guidelines which consider such factors as the degree of hazard, originality, extent of application, etc. One company has also developed an award guide based upon disability cost experience.

Distinguishing between "safety awards" and others is a mistake that can result only in a feeling that safety is regarded by the company as a sideline of no great importance. Payment for a safety suggestion must be on the same basis as that for other suggestions—it should be based upon its real worth if it can be determined. If a suggested safety device enables an operation to be run at a speed that would be dangerous without the device, a saving may be measured. If a number of accidents have occurred on an operation and a suggested device will eliminate them, the cost of those accidents can be projected and a saving calculated.

Awards should reflect the merit of the suggestions. Most companies award cash and/or bonds. Some award merchandise, all-expenses-paid trips, company stock, certificates of merit, medals, gifts for the suggester's spouse and family, or recognition luncheons.

Some companies exclude superintendents, supervisors, designers, methods and systems personnel, and other supervisory or technical personnel from receiving awards, so that the other workers will have someone to whom they can go for assistance. Some companies feel supervisory personnel should not be excluded and several firms have separate plans and award schedules for salaried, supervisory, technical, and management personnel.

**Suggestion committee.** If necessary, a special subcommittee can be set up to determine the monetary value of safety suggestions so that employees will be rewarded for them exactly as they would be for other money-saving suggestions. However, some firms believe such special treatment sets safety ideas apart from other ideas.

Many old, established suggestion systems now in operation are producing excellent results in savings. No company should start a suggestion plan or decide not to start one without first studying carefully the plans now in existence. Further information can be obtained by contacting the Executive Director, National Association of Suggestion Systems. (See References.)

**Boxes and forms.** Suggestion boxes should be attractive and well placed, and stocked with special blank submission forms. (See Fig. 12–34.) It is essential that management acknowledge and resolve all suggestions promptly, to increase the interest of the employees and establish a spirit of cooperation and importance.

Commercial suggestion forms also are available.

## References

Alliance of American Insurers, 20 N. Wacker Dr., Chicago, Ill. 60606. "Tested Activities for Fire Prevention Departments," (latest edition).

Hannaford, Earle S. *Supervisors Guide to Human Relations,* 2nd ed. Chicago, Ill., National Safety Council, 1976.

Konikow, Robert B., and McElroy, Frank E. *Communications for the Safety Professional.* Chicago, Ill., National Safety Council, 1975.

National Association of Suggestion Systems, 435 N. Michigan Ave., Chicago, Ill. 60611.

National Safety Council, 444 N. Michigan Ave., Chicago, Ill. 60611.
    *Accident Facts* (annual).
    Catalog and Poster Directories.
    *Family Safety* Magazine.
    Industrial Data Sheets
        *Motion Pictures for Safety,* 556.
        *Nonprojected Visual Aids,* 564.
        *Photography for the Safety Professional,* 619.
        *Posters, Bulletin Boards, and Safety Displays,* 616.
        *Projected Still Pictures,* 574.
        *Writing and Publishing Employee Safety Regulations,* 664.
    *Industrial "Newsletter."*
    *Industrial Supervisor* Magazine.
    *National Safety News* Magazine.
    *101 Ideas that Worked.*
    *Safe Driver* Magazine.
    *Safe Worker* Magazine.
    *You Are the Safety and Health Committee.*

# Publicizing Safety

# Chapter
## 13

367

# 13—Publicizing Safety

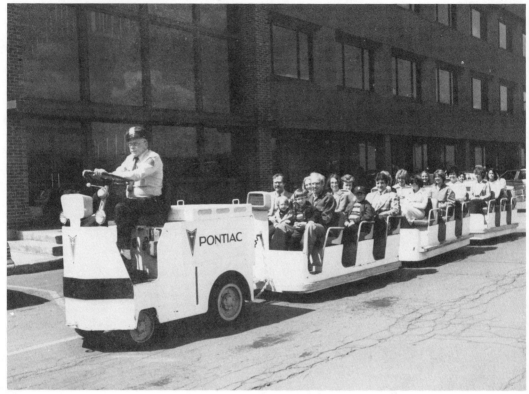

FIG. 13–1.—A plant tour—often an important part of a public relations program—can demonstrate a company's concern for the safety and well-being of visitors as well as employees. Providing in-plant transportation for visitors is one way of showing such conern.

*Courtesy Pontiac Division, General Motors Corporation*

The preceding chapter covered "internal" publicity. This chapter discusses how to influence the way a company looks to people on the outside, and how to keep people on the "inside" informed of what is going on. Favorable publicity is an unmistakable bonus to a good safety program. Why it is so often left uncashed is difficult to understand.

Any company likes to have some-one—especially a prospective customer—say, "I like what I hear about this company. I understand that it really takes care of its employees. So I figure it must treat its customers right; therefore, I'll be treated right."

One good way for a company to get a reputation for taking care of its employees is to be known as a really safe place to work.

Yet an amazing number of companies do little

or nothing to let their public—customers, stock-holders, the community—know that the safety and welfare of their employees are important to them.

That is what this chapter is all about. It is an effort to present a simple and sensible formula for letting people know that "at my company, the welfare and safety of the workers are important."

Most companies have a professional public relations department which handles the commu-nication program. In smaller companies, the safety director may have to generate his own publicity. In both cases, the information in the following pages should prove useful. The safety professional should be aware of overall company policies and programs and know when to turn over routine portions of his safety publicity to specialists, and when to ask for creative help.

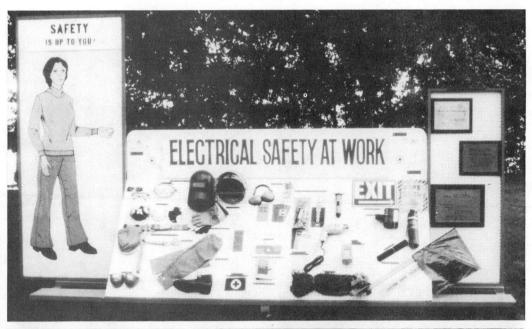

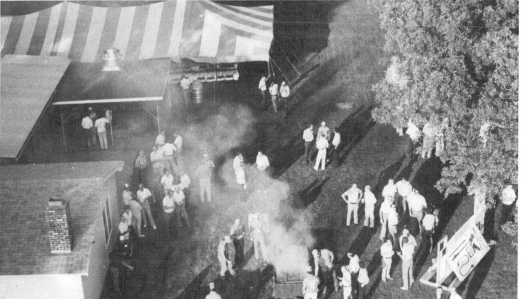

FIG. 13-2.—Joint labor-management sponsored family outing recognized new Alcoa plant safety record of more than 4.7 million safe work hours. Display (top photo) showed safety equipment, including electrical home safety items along with appropriate handouts. The picnic meal included roast pork prepared by local county pork producers (bottom photograph). Use of a bucket truck, normally used to transport electricians to elevated locations, was demonstrated by providing rides for guests. Theme for the ride was "Get high on safety!"

*Courtesy I.B.E.W. Local 1379, Alcoa, Davenport, Iowa, Works.*

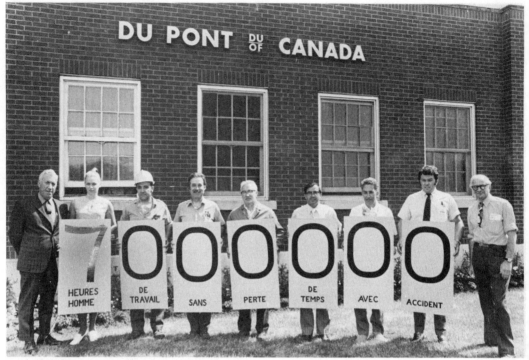

FIG. 13-3.—A seven million worker-hour record was publicized by featuring the record itself. *Courtesy du Pont of Canada, Ltd., Shawinigan Works.*

### Public Relations and Publicity

There is a difference between public relations and publicity—a big difference.

Public relations is the "management function which evaluates public attitudes, identifies the policies and procedures of an individual or an organization with the public interest, and plans and executes a program of action to earn public understanding and acceptance," according to the magazine *Public Relations News*. Every employee, every activity, every facility of a company contributes in many ways to the overall feeling that persons outside the company have about that company. This is true public relations.

Anyone concerned with accident prevention in any way—safety professional, supervisor, member of the plant safety committee, or officer of the school or community safety council—should realize that any time he communicates with someone outside his committee, department, or company, he is involved in public relations (Fig. 13-1). Even

a family picnic can strengthen public relations (Fig. 13-2).

Publicity is a specialized tool of public relations. It is the technique used to acquaint the public with something an organization or an individual is doing via editorial time or space in the mass or trade media. As such, it merely brings to light what is already happening. Although important to good public relations, publicity cannot do it alone.

Any public relations program has to be backed up by a sound organization. Public relations reflects the quality of an organization—but it cannot create that quality. Successful safety achievement merits and can result in good publicity, but canned publicity or publicity based upon inflated facts or specious statistics will be recognized for what it is—and can do more harm than good.

Publicity, to "click", need not always be red-hot news, but it must have an element of spot news, or human interest, or self-help. Then it will have feature value.

Activity—real, honest, legitimate activity—makes news. Of course, urgent need or dramatic circumstances help make news, too. Until they turn up, however, genuine effort will go a long way toward giving a program news and publicity value.

## Basis for success

The basis of a successful public relations program is a successful management—management that makes sure that staff and employees produce good products safely and efficiently, that they cooperate with each other and with the customers, and that all give the best and friendliest service humanly possible—and give it at all times.

The plain fact is that poor public relations is costing individuals and organizations in this country millions of dollars each year.

The remedy is simple: a better understanding and use of fundamental public relations on the part of everyone—and a sincere effort to put it into practical use.

For lack of good public relations, many a worthy cause has failed to get the support it deserves, and many an organization has failed.

A good public relations program need not cost a great deal of money. But it is worth time, effort, and a reasonable budget.

## The Voice of Safety

In any genuine, effective public relations (PR) program, emphasizing safety can be a real help. In fact, it is hard to imagine a PR program where sincere and effective concern for the protection of employees from accidents is not a top priority.

If a company does not have a safety program, it misses vital opportunities for good public relations and dramatically increases the chance for adverse public attitudes.

The safety professional should not only welcome publicity for his safety efforts, but should energetically seek it.

### Working within the company

First, it is essential to talk a little about the basic facts of public relations and publicity. There are two questions to be answered:

1. Does the company have a public relations department?

2. Is there an employee publication in the company?

If both answers are "yes," the safety professional should get in touch with both these units before doing anything about publicizing the safety program.

This step is important. It not only assures professional skill and consistency of efforts to publicize safety activities, but it will save confusion, avoid duplication, and possibly prevent misunderstanding.

Why does such an obvious procedure have to be mentioned? The reason too often is that there is little, if any, communication between a safety professional and the publicity department and publications editor.

Communication between the safety engineer and the publicity staff and editor is indispensable, for these three must work together, or safety is not going to get the attention it deserves and needs.

The safety professional should tell the publicity staff and editor, if he has not done so before, that he is more determined than ever to cut accidents in the company and that he realizes their help and advice are needed to reach this goal.

He should point out to them that he is fully aware of the necessity of employee and public acceptance of the safety program and that they are the people who can help get it.

There is a wealth of real news in safety, and there is a strong possibility that everyone in the safety business has been too quick in assuming that safety must by its very nature be on the dull side. In recent times, there has been more and more recognition by more and more writers and others that safety can be made interesting. It just takes the combined efforts of safety professionals, publicity people, and editors to turn the trick.

### Sixteen ways to make safety news

It might be useful to list some of the things that can make safety news in an organization and that editors and publicity staff ought to know.

1. No-accident records for the entire company or for any one unit—in terms of either days or worker-hours (Fig. 13–3).

2. Improved safety records for the company or any one unit, even if no prolonged no-accident period is involved.

3. An interplant safety contest, or an intercom-

pany contest—especially if anyone has dreamed up an unusual angle (like an out-of-the-ordinary prize).

4. Any unusual safety record for safety performance by an officer or employee of the company—either in length of time or character of the job done.

5. Innovations in safety programs of the company that will prevent accidents. An invention, too, has special news value if the company has been plagued with accidents the new gadget may prevent.

6. An unusual or highly valuable safety suggestion by an employee.

7. Safety conventions or meetings, either those held by the company or those held elsewhere, to which company representatives will go. A digest of such meetings should be publicized.

8. Other special safety events besides conventions—a safety banquet, a safety training course, fire and first aid demonstration, a special meeting, or an award ceremony.

9. Some unusual stunt intended to get the employees to take their safety training home to their families, or something the company is doing directly with the families of workers in an effort to promote around-the-clock safety. Open-house tours, local water safety shows or public showings of safety films are examples.

10. Some pronouncement or statement by the president or other high official of the company on some unusual or new safety device or company safety service, such as free inspection of employees' cars.

11. A speech by the head of the company or the safety professional at a local, regional, state, or national safety convention or conference. The editors or publicity staff should have advance copies of it. The person making the speech should be sure to say something worthy of public attention.

12. The company's annual report is the foundation for corporate communications. Stockholders *do* read these reports. A good paragraph or two on the safety record for the past year will go a long way in achieving sound publicity within the corporate family, as well as inform the analysts, who recommend stocks, what the company is doing

beyond its financial performance.

13. Any act of heroism by someone in the company. This is a sure-fire story for local papers as well as company publications. Maybe this type of news is not pure safety, but newspapers regard it as part of safety, and it can always be tied in with an indirect safety message. (See Fig. 13–4.)

14. A survey or study of some phase of accident prevention in the company. If the investigators discover that married people who own their own homes are safer than their single counterparts, they have provided a ready-made story.

15. Election or appointment of a company official or safety professional to an important post as a volunteer officer of the National Safety Council, American Society of Safety Engineers, Board of Certified Safety Professionals, local safety organization, or governmental agency.

16. A company or employee winning an award in a National Safety Council contest. Winners, not losers, are publicized.

A good rule of thumb is to stress the positive, rather than the negative side of an event. For example, instead of a story that says "single people are less safe," it could say that "a company study shows a need for special safety efforts by singles."

## Some Basics of Publicity

If a company does not have a publicity department, this fact need not prevent its chances of getting publicity into local papers or on the air.

It hurts, of course, because publicity people are more experienced in getting publicity and naturally know their way around in media circles better than the safety professional does. However, even in the absence of a company publicity department, the safety professional can get publicity for safety activities by going directly to the newspapers, magazines, and radio and TV. He might solicit and secure advice and help from local safety organizations, or even business or trade associations with such service. He should certainly, however, keep his manager or vice president informed of what is going on.

The safety professional should not pretend to the editors and the program managers that he is a

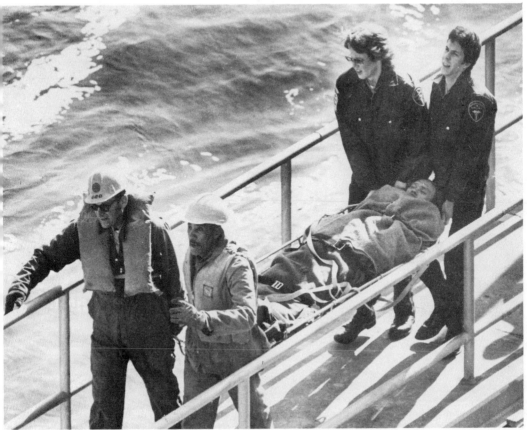

Fig. 13–4.—Rescuers carry a concrete worker whose small boat capsized, throwing him into chilly, turbulent water of the Mississippi River. He went over two spillways, one of them 30 feet long, before he was rescued. He was wearing a U.S. Coast Guard approved Type III work vest, which also had OSHA-required safety features and hypothermia protection.

*Courtesy the* Minneapolis Tribune.

publicity expert. On the contrary, he should take advantage of his innocence of the wiles professional publicists sometimes employ to get space or time.

Editors and program people are usually not difficult to approach—provided that the safety professional is courteous and friendly and admits that he lacks specialized knowledge of publicity techniques. Naturally, no editor or anyone else likes to have someone come charging in and pretend that he is doing a big favor by delivering the story the world has been waiting for.

Although the common sense and salesmanship needed for success in the safety field certainly are enough to enable the safety professional to present his case clearly and effectively to the paper or radio or TV station, he should, nonetheless, be willing to accept advice from publicity professionals on how to best tell his story.

## Select the publicity audience

"Who must be reached with safety publicity?" This seems like a fundamental question, but many companies never try to answer it.

Industrial or manufacturing companies, of course, would scarcely mind if the whole populace insisted on reading or hearing or looking at the company's publicity and taking it deeply to heart.

Because publicity cannot reach everyone, the

# 13—Publicizing Safety

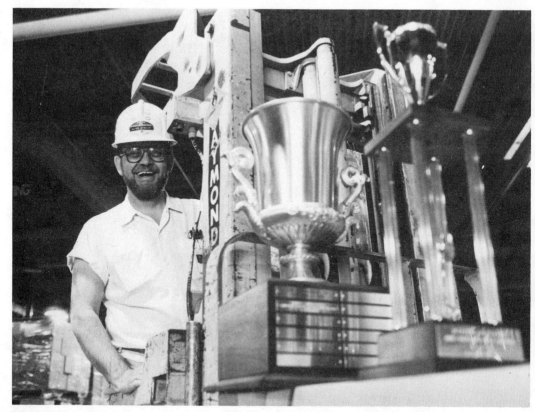

FIG. 13–5.—Awards can be displayed against meaningful backgrounds. Here, Clyde Nyquist, a senior warehouse specialist at Abbott Laboratories, North Chicago, Ill., poses with the trophies he won at the 10th annual International Materials Management Society Fork Lift Truck Rallye. News release that Abbott sent out stressed company's lift truck operator training programs, refresher courses, and good safety and production records.

*Courtesy Abbott Laboratories.*

audience must always be chosen carefully, especially if the budget is tight or time is limited. In that case, it is logical to assume that—in addition to the in-plant (company) audience—the company would prefer to reach people who might be in a position to buy the product, or help the company in some other direct and profitable manner.

## Use humor and human interest

It is worthwhile to try to brighten safety, to make it positive, rather than ponderous and dreary. It is even possible to evoke a chuckle now and then.

Editors are familiar with the solemn pro-

nouncement that "Safety is a serious subject, and must be taken seriously—safety is no laughing matter." No one can argue with that position. Of course, safety is a serious subject. Of course, an accident is no laughing matter. But does it follow, therefore, that no one can put into safety—the enemy of accidents—some of the same techniques, the same sales appeal, the same sparkle that are used so successfully to sell all the things people need to keep them shipshape? (See Fig. 13–5.)

If those techniques can sell shampoo or a personal care product or an automobile, is it unreasonable to expect they can also sell safety?

Or how about a cartoon treatment? This just

may brighten what might otherwise be a slightly dull and drab presentation.

The safety professional should not be too disturbed if someone points out that a cartoon has treated safety negatively. It may well have done just that. This is the very thing that gives a cartoon its punch. A "prat-fall" cartoon will draw attention to the slippery, icy sidewalk in a way that cannot be shown by a person walking and *not* falling. There is no need to dread being negative now and then. However, care should be taken to avoid ridiculing or negatively portraying ethnic or minority groups and victims of accidents.

It is even possible to get a cute child or baby into the act, or even a faithful, shaggy dog, in order to get that spark, that punch, that human touch that lifts safety activities out of an impersonal rut.

## Names, not statistics, are news

Remember that facts and figures about injuries and their frequency and severity are not really interesting in themselves. There must be a good-sized injection of human interest in safety news, and human interest means people.

The safety professional who wants publicity must talk more about people and safety, and less about things and safety. The quickest way in the world to drum up interest in a stuffy safety meeting, for example, is to develop a discussion or even an argument as to whether men or women can drive better or work better—"better" in this instance means safer.

## Friendly rivalry

Safety awards, safety records, safety contests, safety inventions, and "gimmicks"—these are only a few of the many things that make good safety news.

If the company is trying for a new injury-free record in its industry, it is headed for headlines. The editor and the publicity department must be kept informed all along the way. They will help arouse public interest in the performance, and also stimulate greater interest and greater effort among the employees themselves.

An award is worthless if kept a secret. It is worth only what is made out of it. Photos of award presentations are commonly used for publicity but they should be interesting and even unusual to attract special attention. (See again Figs. 13–4 and –5.)

In some instances, top safety awards have been accepted by some companies as if they were a "dime a dozen". On the other hand, other companies have made similar awards the occasion for some of the biggest, bell-ringing celebrations ever seen—and "safety stock" took a big rise as a result.

A public utility company in Michigan, for example, made so much of its intercity rivalry over the safety record of the various units throughout the state that an outsider might think the winning city had won the World Series.

At one banquet marking the celebration of such a victory, more than 1500 employees, from the top brass on down, jammed a big hall to "whoop it up."

During the closing months of this intercity contest, the excitement among employees was akin to pennant fever in the baseball leagues, and no one dared to violate a safety rule.

This victory got tremendous coverage in the papers and on the air throughout the entire state of Michigan. Here was publicity—and public relations—that any organization would welcome. Safety had made news; the publicity had made safety.

## Publicity techniques

These pointers are offered to the safety professional who wants to make the most of his public relations and publicity opportunities:

1. Be honest in what you say. Never exaggerate. Underplay instead of overplay, if you have to make a choice.

2. Deliver what you promise. If you say to the press that something is going to happen, make certain it happens—and as you said it would. This often calls for a "runthrough" in advance.

3. If for any reason there is a change in plans from what you have announced, notify the papers and radio and TV stations at once.

4. Be scrupulously accurate in your names, places, and other facts. There is no such thing as being too careful in this respect. If an editor misspells names, the only thing to do is to resubmit the names correctly spelled again and hope for the best.

5. Be reasonable in your requests for space and time. Complaining about your company PR department, or complaining that the local paper or station has treated your company shabbily will not only accomplish exactly

Office of the Commissioner
Department of Streets and Sanitation

Jane M. Byrne
Mayor

City Hall, Room 700
121 North LaSalle Street
Chicago, Illinois 60602
(312) 744-4611

John L. Donovan
Commissioner

April 25, 1980

For Immediate Release

SAFETY FIRST

The City of Chicago is presently undergoing organizational changes which will enable this City to provide the most effective services and the most comprehensive safety program of any city in the world. Some of these changes will be accomplished easily, others will be more difficult. None are impossible!

The Safety and Training Division of the Department of Streets and Sanitation in tune with this progessive restructuring is developing a series of new

FIG. 13–6.—News release should be double-spaced typewritten. Ordinary letterhead can be used.

nothing, but will make for a bad relationship.

6. Do not alert your PR department or publications editor (or put out anything yourself) unless you have real news or features to offer. You must not issue material just to be issuing it. Be reasonable with the amount of material you send out. You can wear out your welcome.

7. Tip off your local or industry association, safety councils, and your publicity department (or if you do not have one, the papers or radio and TV stations) to anything worthwhile you run across that might make an item or program for them, even though it has no relation to you or your company. They will appreciate it.

8. Above all, do things that make news. Almost every routine safety item can, with a little extra effort by the safety professional and the editor, become a more readable, more constructive piece. News will be published only if something is being done for safety that makes news. News can always be heightened by intelligent, imaginative treatment, but it must be there in the first place to be worth telling. Advertising space can even be purchased for special items.

9. Use good sense and an honest approach if the news is bad. Prove to press representatives and the public that you can roll with the punches. (Check with legal counsel and public relations officials on how far you need go, however.)

## Publicity by the safety office

If a safety professional must handle his own publicity with the local press, he should also know the following. These hints might seem unnecessary, but many stories have died because someone failed to observe them.

1. Timing is vital when calling on the editor or program director. It is considerate to call up first, suggest that the item might interest him, and ask him when it would be most convenient to drop in. One should never suggest he send someone out.

2. Generally, the person to contact is the city editor of the paper or the news director of the radio or TV station. Of course, if an item is specifically written for a certain columnist or commentator, it is better to contact him directly. If it applies only to a specialized area (finance or sports, for example), it should be brought to the attention of that editor.

3. Write not for your boss, but for your reader or listener. Answer objectively the questions: who, what, when, where, how and why. Do not load your releases with propaganda for the company. There is no surer way to kill your positive relations with the media.

4. Make your releases just as professional in style, appearance, and general quality as you possibly can. (Fig. 13–6 shows an example.) Often a lead time is required; one must ask a speaker, in advance, what he will say in order to write the release as though he has said it.

5. In writing a release, be brief and to the point. Newspaper space is limited, and costly. Try to "hold down" the piece to a page or a page and a half at most. Papers receive thousands of releases each month. These are skimmed, and only the best get into print.

6. If you are sending a picture with the release, the caption should be typed on a piece of plain white paper and pasted to the back or bottom of the photo. *Never* use paper clips, and *never* write with a pen or pencil on the back of the picture. Either of these will likely damage the photo and make it difficult to reproduce clearly.

## Safety on the air

Newspaper publicity is only half the battle. The safety professional who would mold opinion must get air-minded and see what can be done to get safety on radio and TV. (See Fig. 13–7.)

In the first place, it is amazing to find how much of a safety program lends itself to radio and TV. The publicity department can, of course, provide guidance, but the publicity people must know what they have to work with before they can offer it to the radio and television stations. A few possibilities are:

1. Why not a safety fashion show? If the station prefers to use its own models, the pros can model the safety clothing. TV viewers will then be able to see what the well-dressed worker wears on the job.

2. The publicity department can stage a wrong vs. right program on what the men and women working for the company should wear. This subject is a natural for company publications, and chances are, TV will nibble at it, too. Manage to "mug it up" enough so that the "wrong" examples are a little exaggerated.

3. If an employee has come up with an idea or a device for preventing accidents, and can demonstrate it visually, he is a possibility for a TV spot.

4. When one of the company's officials has been chosen for a state or national safety post, such as a director or officer of the National Safety Council, radio and TV may be happy to salute him as a local personality who has been tapped for a top job.

5. Any time the company can hang up a fine safety record, the local radio and TV stations should get a chance to interview some of the people responsible for it.

6. If an important person (in the safety field) comes to visit, the safety professional should see that advance word of his visit reaches the media.

7. Leave script writing to the script writers but check facts. If a radio or TV station requests material, send them the facts, figures, and whatever narrative is necessary. The people at the station will put it into the proper form.

## Hints for TV interviews

The safety professional must often be the spokesman for his company, not only for newspaper coverage, but also for radio and television. Although getting the facts correct and watching legal implications may be adequate for a newspaper interview, a television or radio interview reflects more of the company than merely what

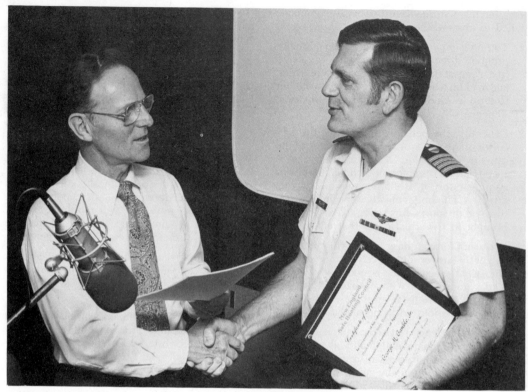

Fig. 13-7.—Known as "the voice of the New England Safe Boating Council," George M. Gamble, Jr. *(left)* records safe boating tips for use by more than 100 New England radio stations. Here he receives a commendation for his volunteer work from the U.S. Coast Guard.

*Courtesy Raytheon Company.*

the facts show. It projects a company image through the company spokesman. If you do not feel that you project a good image over the radio or television, pick someone who will, in your department, or in the public relations department.

Here are some tips that will help you give a better radio-TV appearance.

1. Remember that you are being interviewed for your knowledge, not for your personality, entertainment value, or good looks. Be yourself. Don't put on a special voice or worry how the lavaliere microphone looks with your clothes.

2. Don't worry about being nervous. Just don't

panic. Don't back out of the interview after the station crew has set up its equipment.

3. Go over with the interviewer in advance just what areas will be discussed. You can steer him away from areas you cannot discuss, and you can get help on questions that you might not be able to answer.

4. Using notes is OK. If you must read, read normally, but well. Do not rush or drag. Be sure to maintain eye contact with the interviewer or camera. Do not memorize a statement and rattle it off. You will waste everyone's time.

5. If you have a bad cold or sore throat, turn over the interview to a colleague.

## Handling an accident story

In any public relations or publicity program, it is just as important to know what not to do as to know what to do. In fact, it can be even more important.

The foremost warning is this: do not cover up bad news. Good press relations are of utmost importance. It is at such a time that a sound public relations program "pays off."

Every safety professional hopes the day will never come that an accident—a bad one—occurs and knocks the props out from under him and his safety record, but it has happened. In some instances, the repercussions of the way the accident was handled have been even more tragic than the accident itself—at least, to the company as a whole.

Here is an example of how not to handle a press representative: In a midwestern city some time ago, two workers were killed by a crane. This company enjoyed a first-rate relationship with the newspapers and radio and TV people in that city. It worked hard at safety and at public relations. It was good to its employees and had a fine reputation for playing its cards fairly and on the table.

On this particular occasion, however, someone in the company's higher echelons got "buck fever." So, when a young reporter came out to the plant to get what was to his paper a routine story of the accident, he ran into censorship at the plant.

The safety professional shoved him off to the personnel manager. This person switched him to the general manager, who gave him some "double talk" and tossed him to the company doctor. The doctor said the safety director was the person to talk to.

By this time the reporter's righteous wrath was rising. He knew he was getting the treatment, and what had started out to be just a routine assignment now had become a challenge to dig up something that, for some reason, appeared to be covered up by the company.

The reporter could not lose in a contest like this. Since the workers had been killed, the coroner would have all the facts. If they had been badly hurt, one of the hospitals would have the information. If the workers had not been killed or hurt badly, it was no story in the first place.

So the reporter got the facts from the coroner's office, and he wrote a story that was just as nasty toward the company as he could make it without committing libel.

The story was edited, headed, set in type, and lay in the composing room, awaiting its turn to get into the paper.

Now in this paper, as in every other paper, there is usually more news set in type than the paper can print. Each day dozens of items get left out—the "overset," as it is called in newspaper parlance.

The story of the accident might well have ended up as "overset" and, if printed, might not have been played up. These no longer were normal circumstances, unfortunately. The cover-up and run-around the reporter had received at the plant had changed all that.

This little story had been marked "must" when it was sent to the composing room. It thereupon became something very special—a story that was now given front-page prominence.

When there is bad news to report, the safety director will just have to swallow hard, grit his teeth, and back up his publicity department 100 percent in giving out the news as straight and fast and completely as if the tidings were all in the company's favor.

Along with the grief, a mention of the good things—that this is the first accident in months or years, that the company has a safety record far better than the national average for its type of operation, and that it has won a number of safety awards—will help take the curse off the story. Reporters are usually happy to include these facts, too.

It is not only fair and honorable, but downright smart to "lay it on the line" for press representatives whenever there is news, regardless of whether it is pleasant or unpleasant news. This principle is vital to a good public relations program.

It would be wise for a safety professional to anticipate that some day he may have to serve as a company spokesman at an accident or disaster scene. He should, therefore, seek legal counsel to make certain he knows how much he can say in a press interview.

News media can actually help during a big emergency. Families, friends, and neighbors will be clamoring for news and the media can get it to them fast. Details of any casualties must first be given to next-of-kin.

## Working with Company Publications

If the safety professional thinks that safety has been neglected in his company publication, it is time to correct the situation. He should ask the editor frankly how to get more news value and human interest into safety stories. He should tell the editor he wants the program to be just as newsworthy as it can possibly be and that he realizes he needs something besides cold facts and colder figures to make safety articles and pictures attractive to his readers.

The editor is just as eager as anyone to publish interesting news and features, and he will go more than halfway to think up ways to put news value and reader interest into safety doings.

Here is an example of how the safety professional and the editor can team up to make a routine safety happening more newsworthy.

Suppose one of the employees, Oscar B—, reaches his twenty-fifth anniversary of steady work without a day's lost time due to an injury. This achievement probably entitles Oscar to a button or a badge or a plaque or something.

The public relations-conscious safety professional asks, "Well, instead of just pinning this button on Oscar with a hearty handclasp and a few words of commendation, why not make a real thing out of it? Take the occasion to tell Oscar—and all the world—that at this plant there is nothing more important than recognizing the contribution to a safer, better way of work that Oscar has made through his personal example of safe practices over the years."

Spurred by the talk the safety professional and the editor have had recently about perking up safety news—or maybe just because he is an energetic sort, anyway—the editor does not merely publish a picture of Oscar and his award along with one flabby little item. The editor finds Oscar, sits down with him over a cup of coffee, and asks him a few questions about his career, about his opinions on safety "way back yonder" and now, and about any ideas he may have for making things even safer at the plant.

Now the foregoing is only one little example of what can happen when the safety man and the editor of the company publication get together to do a more imaginative and energetic job of publicizing the safety program.

A system can be used when one department of the company wins an interdepartmental safety contest. Instead of merely recording the results of the contest, the editor can dig into the program of the winning department, interview the people responsible for its sucess, and, perhaps, come up with a piece for his magazine that will give every

department some hints on how to improve its safety activities.

## Producing a publication

Materials, such as safety newsletters, instruction cards, bulletins, broadsides, booklets and manuals for communicating safety rules, information, and ideas in print, require careful planning and preparation. Among steps to be taken in planning both internal (to a company audience) and external (to the general public or other out-of-company groups) publications are:

1. Clearly define the objectives of the publication. Consider the type of audience to be reached by those objectives.

2. Determine how general or how restricted the message is to be.

3. Decide what form of publication will best convey the message.

4. Estimate cost of preparing and printing the publication in whatever forms, sizes, and quantities needed. An expenditure for a new publication must, of course, be provided for in the budget, whether or not the item is produced "in house."

If the objective is to place in the hands of the worker the specific rules he is to follow in doing his job safely and efficiently, an instruction card may be suitable. To stimulate general safety-consciousness, a broadside (single sheet printed on one side) may be effective. If a series of short reminders, for example, on fire prevention, is needed, posters may be the answer. To treat a topic of general interest, such as methods of materials handling, a leaflet may be used. Here, posters or leaflets from the National Safety Council, insurance company, or other organizations may be more effective, and more economical than "in house" produced material. For highly technical jobs or for more thorough coverage of a plant's safety policies and rules, manuals may be required. Even a company-wide (or plant-wide) public-address system would be appropriate.

When the form of the publication is being decided, it should be remembered that there is a direct relationship between the appearance of a printed piece and the degree of interest which it arouses. Most readers will react unfavorably to a bulletin, newsletter, or booklet with text in very small type, few or no illustrations, narrow margins, and long paragraphs.

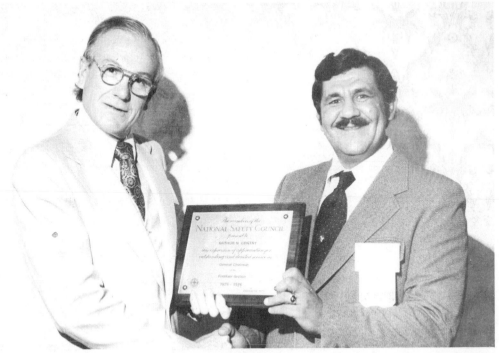

FIG. 13–8.—Award photographs are the "backbone" of safety publicity. Here, Art Gentry (left) is recognized for his work as chairman of the Council's Industrial Division Fertilizer Section.

*Courtesy Fertilizer Section* Newsletter.

Reasonably large type (10 point or 12 point), selected to fit the size of the page and, of course, to accommodate the volume of material, will help readability. For comparison, this column is set in 9-point type. Elite typewriter type is 10-point size. The *Safety Newsletters,* published by the various divisions of the National Safety Council, are set in 10-point type in 2¹/₈-inch wide columns. In addition, judicious use of white space and variety in size and placement of illustrations help make a publication both pleasing to the eye and easy to read. In safety, as in other fields, ideas conveyed in print are best received and best absorbed if they are well organized and attractively presented.

**Illustrations** serve to break up the text and help to get points across to the reader. Photographs which show action described in the copy add realism in instructional materials such as manuals. Human interest photos are desirable in newsletters. Line drawings and sketches are valuable to clarify technical points on instruction cards, in manuals, and in other training materials. Awards can also be publicized (Fig. 13–8).

If the printing process permits reproduction of photos and other illustrations, pictures of award winners, safety devices, and safe and unsafe practices can be used. To avoid embarrassing or ridiculing employees who have been injured or caught in an unsafe act, their features can be blocked out, or pictures specially posed (and so identified) by other employees can be taken of similar situations.

Since some states have laws that forbid publication of a person's photograph without his written permission, a signed release should be obtained from every person who appears in recognizable form in any picture. Often having a new employee sign a photo release is part of the employment routine. Asking for a photo release is just good manners. See Fig. 13–9 for a sample.

Details on illustrations are given in Chapter 14, "Audiovisual Media."

```
                                          RELEASE NO. _____


                                  Date _____

                                  Place _____

      For the consideration of _____ , the undersigned grants permission to
      _____and its assigns, to publish and reproduce the attached
      photographs of persons or objects shown therein.  It is understood that my name
      will not be used in connection with the aforementioned pictures.

      It is further declared that the undersigned has legal authority to sign this
      document.



                                  _____

                                  _____
      Description of photographs                              Witness
```

Fig. 13–9.—One form of model release. Some companies have each employee sign a release when he starts to work. It is suggested that legal counsel be sought before setting up any company procedure.

**Preparation of material.** Once the objectives, scope, and form of a publication are determined, the person preparing it should make an outline of the subject or subjects to be covered. For most types of material, the outline need not be elaborate, but it should be logical and complete, showing how each topic is a part of the overall plan.

Before gathering material, the writer might well spend some time studying the people for whom the message is intended so that he will know something of the knowledge and comprehension of the readers-to-be. In the interests of accuracy, completeness, and balance, material should be gathered from several sources—including articles, books, and especially supervisors, workers, and others in the company who have had experience in the matters to be treated. To ensure technical accuracy, it may be necessary to solicit help from specialists in specific areas.

No matter what the form of the publication, the writer should keep in mind certain basic rules of good writing. To get ideas across quickly and easily, short sentences, simple words, and brief paragraphs are recommended. Try to avoid being so simple that the copy reads like a second grade primer, however.

In a piece of some length, such as a booklet, a system of headings, kept as informal as possible, will both arouse the reader's interest and guide his thinking as he reads. In a piece designed to instruct, numbered lists of job steps, for instance, will prove helpful. In any case, the writer should follow closely the line of logical thought developed in his outline.

Copy should be written in a positive, constructive style. When the nature of the material and the form of publication permit, a friendly—but never condescending—tone can be used effectively. Personal references and names, as in a newsletter, will increase readership. Humor tied to the message and pitched to the employees' sense of what is funny can add a great deal to some types of publications. For instance, cartoon illustrations and a light touch in copy may be particularly

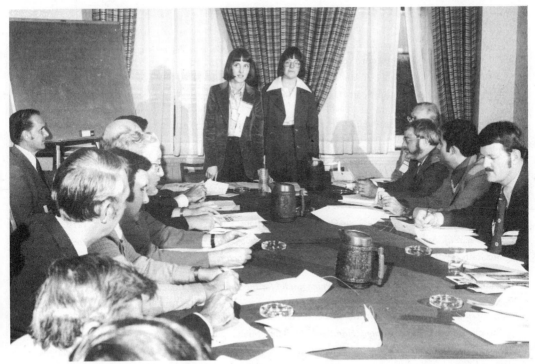

Fig. 13–10.—A training session for *Industrial Newsletter* volunteer editors is held at each National Safety Congress. Much of the information given is applicable to running a company publication.

effective in a rule booklet.

Readability of the proposed publication can be gaged by having a few of the people to whom it will be addressed test-read it for understanding.

**Production of publications.** For the technical details of printing, the advertising department or experts in the publishing field can be consulted. In layout and typography, readability should be the first consideration.

How the piece is to be used will determine its size, paper, binding, cover and similar details. For materials that are to be filed or for insertion of revised pages, loose-leaf binders may be used.

The in-company or outside editor or printer who will handle the job should be asked for technical advice.

**Getting ideas.** Everyone in the public relations and publicity business runs dry of ideas now and then. Anyone who is suffering from this affliction should not hesitate to call on others for help. Employee publications do not compete with one another; so ideas can be borrowed freely from them.

Some national agencies produce and supply safety material. See listings in Chapter 4.

The National Safety Council publishes in *National Safety News* a "Safety Clips" page, which contains stories and illustrations for editors of employee publications. Council Sectional Newsletters and other of its publications contain a wealth of interesting and informative material. The Council publication, "How to Run a Newsletter," single copies available on request, has additional ideas. Council poster miniatures and other Council materials usually are released for general use if the customary credit is given.

Volunteering to serve as an editor of a National Safety Council Industrial Division Newsletter is good practice. At each fall Safety Congress, a training session is held for incoming *Industrial Newsletter* editors (see Fig. 13–10).

**383**

# 13 — Publicizing Safety

## References

Ashley, Paul. P. *Say It Safely: Legal Limits in Publishing, Radio, and Television,* 5th ed. Seattle, Wash., University of Washington Press, 1976.

Black, Sam. *Practical Public Relations,* 4th ed. Brooklyn Heights, N.Y., Beekman Pubs, Inc., 1977.

Center, Allen H., and Cutlip, Scott H. *Effective Public Relations,* 5th ed. Englewood Cliffs, N.J., Prentice-Hall, Inc., 1978.

Farley, William E. *Practical Public Relations for the Businessman.* New York, N.Y., Frederick Fell Publishers, Inc.

Flesch, Rudolf, and Lass, A. H. *A New Guide to Better Writing.* New York, N.Y., Popular Library, 1977.

Forrestal, Dan. *Public Relations Handbook.* Chicago, Ill., The Dartnell Corp., 1979.

Harris, Morgan, and Karp, Patti. *How To Make News and Influence People.* Summit, Pa., TAB Books, 1976.

Lesly, Phillip, ed. *Public Relations Handbook,* 2nd ed. Englewood Cliffs, N.J., Prentice-Hall, Inc., 1978.

Lewis, H. G. *How To Handle Your Own Public Relations.* Chicago, Ill., Nelson-Hall, Inc., 1976.

Luedke, W. J. *Ayer Public Relations and Publicity Stylebook,* rev. ed. Bala Cynwyd, Pa., Ayer Press, 1979.

McGrath, Phyllis S., ed. *Business Credibility: The Critical Factors.* New York, N.Y., The Conference Board, Inc., 1976.

National Safety Council, Chicago, Ill. *Photography for the Safety Professional,* Industrial Data Sheet 619.

Nolte, Lawrence W., and Wilcox, Dennis L., eds. *Fundamentals of Public Relations: Professional Guidelines, Concepts and Integrations,* 2nd ed. Elmsford, N.Y., Pergamon Press, Inc., 1979.

Russell, Diane. *Public Relations Handbook.* Midland, Mich., Pendell Publishing Co., 1976.

Starr, Edward. *What You Should Know About Public Relations.* Dobbs Ferry, N.Y., Oceana Publications, 1968.

Turabian, Kate L. *A Manual for Writers,* 4th ed. Chicago, Ill., The University of Chicago Press, 1973.

*Understanding Public Relations.* New York, N.Y., Preston Publishing Co., Inc.

# Audiovisual Media

# Chapter
## 14

# 14—Audiovisual Media

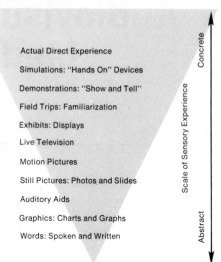

Actual Direct Experience

Simulations: "Hands On" Devices

Demonstrations: "Show and Tell"

Field Trips: Familiarization

Exhibits: Displays

Live Television

Motion Pictures

Still Pictures: Photos and Slides

Auditory Aids

Graphics: Charts and Graphs

Words: Spoken and Written

Concrete

Scale of Sensory Experience

Abstract

FIG. 14–1.—"Experience is the best teacher." In measuring the relative value of an audiovisual or other means of communication, remember that the more concrete the medium of communication is, the more effective it is.

Audiovisual (A/V) is a term used to describe instructional materials and equipment designed to facilitate teaching and learning by making use of both hearing and sight.

Commonly used audiovisuals include actual equipment and models; flip charts and posters; slides and other projected transparencies; recordings, filmstrips, videotapes, and motion picture films. Teaching facilities might include chalkboards, flannel boards, hook and loop boards, bulletin boards, and display cases. A/V equipment (hardware) includes simulators, projectors of all kinds, tape recorders for sound and video, cameras, monitors, and the full range of television studio equipment, and cable television hardware. Activities such as demonstrations and experiments are also usually considered part of audiovisual programs.

## Effectiveness of Audiovisual Media

Audiovisuals assist the communications/learning process by presenting information concisely and with impact. Visuals involve people more than do abstract words. Sometimes mere words and sentences, whether spoken or written, not only provide relatively little meaning, but may be misconstrued by learners.

Figure 14–1 rates various communications media on a relative scale of concrete to abstract experiences—the more concrete the communication, the more effective it will be. Designing a communication or training program to take advantage of more concrete resources, as they are needed, takes more ability than merely knowing the subject matter; it demands an ability to use audiovisuals effectively, and to know when each can be most productive with the intended audience. With properly defined objectives, their uses are endless. Only imagination—and budget—define the limits.

Safety professionals are using audiovisuals as tools in presenting information for:

New employee indoctrination

Training supervision in its role in accident prevention

Specific safety procedures, such as hot work permits, vessel entry, electrical and other power lockouts

Basic fire prevention techniques

Job safety analysis programs

Fire brigade training

Safety professionals should be aware of the range of audiovisual resources and their appropriateness both to transmitting the message content and to audience appeal.

Often more than one visual is necessary for the communications job. For this reason, many safety departments have numerous types of audiovisual products available.

Some of the most popular audiovisuals that are used in safety education today include slide presentations, demonstrations, flip charts, overhead projection, chalkboards, posters, films (8 or 16mm), videotape and closed circuit television. Accordingly, units that provide the capability of controlling more than one projector (multi-medium) are in demand.

## Use in training and motivating

Audiovisual materials are important conveyors of information. Photos of hazards or of unusually good conditions provide visual evidence useful in reports to supervisors and to top management. These, plus graphical presentation, can make routine reports and statistical analyses interesting and easy to understand. More than one safety professional has found a simple bar chart or colored graph to be more meaningful to his boss or to other supervisors than pages of detailed statistics.

A visual can emphasize the points of information in a safety talk; it can even provide a convenient "outline" for the speaker. Visual materials can be used to organize group thinking and to summarize safety committee action.

As a motivational tool, visuals that appeal to the emotions can help change attitudes, encourage safe work habits and compliance with safety rules, and remind employees of special rules or hazards.

Audiovisuals of all types are used widely to promote interest and obtain cooperation in special campaigns, safety contests, and similar activities.

### Selection of media

To be most effective, audiovisuals must be selected with care, after considering many factors. (See Table 14–A on next page.)

• What is the purpose of the communication—motivating, training, reporting, factfinding, entertaining? What result is wanted? Which medium (or combination) will serve this purpose best, within budget limits?

• Which medium will best convey the content of the message? For example, detailed technical figures can be communicated by a chart that can be held up, or projected in front of the audience, and held for some time while it is explained. A tape recorder or a movie projector would be of little help.

• What is the size and type of audience? What is their attitude toward you and toward your subject? How knowledgeable are they? How good are their communications abilities?

• How capable are the communicators? Do they need special training in either the subject matter or in the effective use of the audiovisual? Do they need other help?

• Where is the audiovisual to be used—in a training room, at a meeting, in the office or plant, in the field, or at home? Use of audiovisuals requires scheduling, preparation or purchase, dis-

tribution, and storage. Suitable facilities must be made available.

• How flexible (or how formal) must the audiovisual be? In some cases, a flexible type (which each speaker can adapt to his particular uses) may be desirable. In other cases, a formalized aid which offers careful planning, conformity of message with company policy, and uniformity of presentation may be preferable.

When a formalized visual is being considered, a number of questions, such as the following, should be asked: Will the entire message apply to many different audiences, even though they are located in different geographical areas or are confronted with different hazards? Will the material become dated, or can it be used almost indefinitely? Is it likely, for instance, that changes will be made in machines, processes, job layouts, or even personal protective equipment illustrated?

In some cases, a combination of flexible and formalized aids is desirable. For example, some speakers use a carrying case containing three-dimensional exhibits, charts, flannel boards, and other nonprojected material, as well as slides in a portable projector, to give road show presentations that can be changed to meet specific needs.

• How do the costs of the various audiovisual media compare? In the selection of audiovisual equipment, this point is especially important.

Whether or not the cost of an audiovisual is justified must be considered in the light of what it will buy. An investment of $50,000 or more in a well-planned sound movie might be justified for a long-range training program or public relations campaign. One of the advantages of such visual is that it can be used over a relatively long period of time as a means of communicating the same message to many people. The repeated showing of a $50,000 film to large audiences over several years might well bring the cost per viewer down to a few pennies.

In contrast, the apparently modest expenditure of $500 on a homemade movie developed without sufficient planning and applicable to only a handful of employees could be excessively high and perhaps ineffective. Moreover, the same amount of time, money, and effort devoted to a training program, individual job instruction, or perhaps production of an inexpensive safety rule booklet might get better results.

# 14—Audiovisual Media

Cost is only one of a number of factors to be weighed in the selection of a visual. An expensive visual is not necessarily the best one. For example, a simple paper pad or chalk board may be more effective than an elaborate printed brochure for presenting a safety report to a group of executives or for training employees in safe practices.

• How is the message to be supported? Not only must there usually be followup, but other people must often know what was communicated to whom, in order that they can reinforce the message, or at least not contradict it "accidentally."

## Commercial vs. homemade visuals

To determine whether it is more economical and practical to make audiovisual aids than it is to buy them, the same factors that affect selection of aids must be considered: the purpose for which the aid is to be used, the type and size of audience, and the degree of flexibility desired.

For an informal supervisors' meeting, for a report to a safety committee, or for a presentation to company officials, a homemade aid, such as a chalk board or hand-lettered flip chart, would be appropriate. However, for more formal talks or for a number of meetings at decentralized locations, a commercially prepared aid—a videotape, a set of slides with a script to be read, a filmstrip with a record or a tape, or a set of commercially painted charts—might be a wise investment.

Other points to be examined when a choice is being made between a commercial aid and a homemade aid are the costs involved and the availability of facilities, talent, and time. See Fig. 14-2.

It is a good idea to contact manufacturers of audiovisual-making and projection equipment; many will provide instruction booklets and other materials on how to make and use audiovisuals. See References at the end of this chapter for leads.

Still another factor is that participation of individuals or of committees in the planning and development of a visual may be highly desirable as a means of arousing and maintaining interest in accident prevention. The net effect of employee participation, in fact, may compensate for lack of the professional touch, provided that the quality of the finished product is not seriously affected.

When a final decision is being made, the various factors must be considered in terms of one another. For example, slides may be selected as

## TABLE 14-A—MAJOR FEATURES AND LIMITATIONS OF VARIOUS AUDIOVISUALS

| Type and Popular Size | Audience Size | Shipping and Handling | Limitations | Strong Points | Comments |
|---|---|---|---|---|---|
| MOTION PICTURES 16mm sound | Medium to large | Film easy and cheap to ship; projectors heavy, expensive to ship. | Camera and projector expensive; require trained operator, except for self-threading models. Film not easily changed or updated. | Effective for training and motivating. Uniform professional message. Optical sound nonerasable. Sharper image than 8 mm for given projection size. Single-frame, stop-motion projectors are available. | Silent version less costly, but less effective. |
| MOTION PICTURES 8mm sound and "Super-8" | Small to large | Low shipping cost; projector is lighter. | Safety subjects not as widely available as 16 mm. Not too suitable for large audiences. | Lower cost, lighter weight equipment than 16mm. Homemade movies more feasible. Instant cartridge-loading types are easy to use. Sound is available on Super-8. | Useful in rear screen projection and automatic continuous showings. |
| SLIDES 2 × 2 in. (35 mm, 126, or 127) 2¼ × 2¼ in. (120 film) 3¼ × 4 in. (magic lantern) | Small to large | Slides easy to store, handle, and ship. Projectors light to heavy. | Slides may get out of sequence, reversed, etc. Cardboard mounts not durable. | Effective for training and motivating. Less of a "canned" show since slides may be rearranged. Slides can be made and processed quickly. Color inexpensive. | Taped message or reading script easily added or changed. Remote control and multiple projection possible. |

| | | | | | |
|---|---|---|---|---|---|
| **FILMSTRIPS** 35mm sound | Small to large | Strips and recordings easy to handle. Projectors light to medium. | Strips and records not easily changed or updated. "Canned" measaage may not be effective or paced suitably for user. | Effective for training and motivating. Message uniform. Sound easily added on tape or disc. | Silent strips with script less expensive, but still effective. |
| **OVERHEAD PROJECTORS** 10 X 10 in. 7 X 7 in. | Small to large | Shipping costs of transparencies higher. Projector light to heavy. | Transparencies positioned by hand. Projector close to screen; it or user may block view unless screen is raised or set at an angle. Ready-made material not widely available. | Effective for training. User can write on transparency while facing audience. No need to darken room. Transparencies easily made and filed. Presentation informal and flexible. | Color transparencies or overlays easily made. |
| **OPAQUE PROJECTORS** 10 X 10 in. max. | Small to medium | Projectors heavy and bulky | Projectors require manual operation. Material in books may be difficult to store or ship. Room must be darkened. Copy may be too small. | Effective for training. No transparencies required; small objects, printed material, drawings, and photographs used "as is." | Copies or originals can be hinged or put on rolls to maintain sequence. |
| **CLOSED-CIRCUIT TELEVISION AND VIDEOTAPE** | Small to medium | Camera, recorder, and monitor require dolly or handtruck if they are to be moved about, except for light-weight models. | Initial investment expensive. Requires adequate lighting. In color or black and white. Copies must be made one at a time unless duped by lab. | Instant replay. Excellent for training situation where trainee must "see himself in action." Has relatively low operating cost. Can be shown in lighter room. | Small number of people can view screen. TV is a culturally natural transmission medium. |
| **FLANNEL, HOOK AND LOOP, MAGNETIC** 12 X 36 in. to 48 X 72 in. | Small to medium | Larger boards are bulky | Presentation requires advance preparation. Few ready-made presentations available. Flannel board material may fall off if not applied correctly or if board too nearly vertical. | Effective for training. Message easily changed, yet can be filed and reused. Permits informal presentation with desirable audience contact. Dramatic, "slap-on" effect builds interest. | Boards suitable for heavier displays; cost slightly higher than cards or pads. |
| **FLIP CHARTS AND CARDS** 36 X 48 in. 18 X 24 in. | Small to medium | Easels or charts may be bulky and heavy, but usually portable. | Limited to small groups. Limited as to amount of copy. Good lighting necessary. | Effective for training and informing. Prepared material can be arranged in sequence. Good audience contact. Material easily prepared; can be added during talk and can be saved. | Ready-made letters, color, sketches, cut-outs easily added. Colored paper effective. |
| **PAPER SHEETS AND PADS** 28 X 36 in. | Small | Pads usually disposable. | Speaker must print legibly. Good lighting necessary. Ink from felt markers may bleed onto adjacent sheets. | Effective for training or discussion; informal. Permits reference to other sheets during the discussion and for later writing of minutes. Low-cost pads easily obtainable. | Used in place of chalk boards, no erasing. |
| **CHALK BOARDS** (*portable and wall mounted*) 36 X 48 in., larger for wall mounted | Small | Portable boards bulky and heavy. | Board must be erased before reuse and recall not possible. Good lighting necessary. Ordinary chalk marks hard to see. Dust from chalk and erasers annoying. | Effective for training or for discussing a limited number of points. Presentation informal. Portable chalk boards also useful for holding charts or displays. | Colored or fluorescent chalk adds life to talk. Magnetic boards available. |
| **POSTERS AND BANNERS** 8½ X 11½ in., 17 X 23 in., and larger | Small or large | Easily filed, handled, and mailed. | Only one or two ideas can be presented at a time; considerable time needed for changing. | Effective for motivating; support training. Specific messages can be posted at points of hazard or to meet timely situations. Ample posters available. | Homemade posters supplement general posters. |
| **WORKING MODELS, EXHIBITS, AND DEMONSTRATIONS** | Small or large | May be hard to handle, store, and ship. | May require special training to use. Live action is subject to errors. | Action can closely simulate actual conditions. Permit group participation. | |

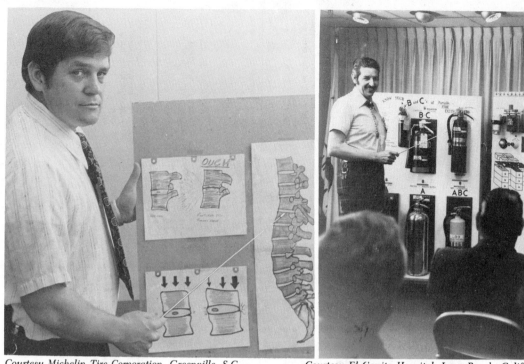

*Courtesy Michelin Tire Corporation, Greenville, S.C.*     *Courtesy El Cerrito Hospital, Long Beach, Calif.*

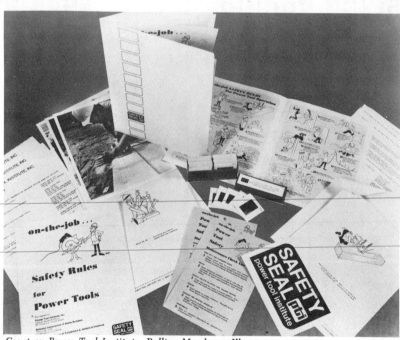

*Courtesy Power Tool Institute, Rolling Meadows, Ill.*

Fig. 14–2.—Here are three visuals that range from a completely home-made chart (upper left), through a display of actual firefighting and fire alarm items, to a complete educational program that can be purchased (above).

he type of visual to be produced. The speaker may have a suitable camera and lights, plus the ability and the time to do the job himself. However, the number of showings, the size of the audience, or the importance of the message may warrant the expense of professional input.

The same comparison can be made between professional and homemade charts, signs, and other visuals.

Even if a safety department alone could not justify a professional visual media staff, the needs of the department, when added to those in sales, training, and other communications areas, might justify such in-company, or in-plant, facilities and staff. The combined benefits and savings would make this worthwhile, not to mention the more effective visuals that would be available.

## Preparation of Audiovisual Media

Once an audiovisual medium that is suitable both for the job and within the limits of budget and time has been selected, the details of production must be worked out. The general procedure is to make an outline, develop script and picture descriptions, have pictures taken or art work made, and check content for accuracy. Often the length of the presentation must fit an instructional time frame. Deadlines must be set.

Many types of audiovisuals include written or spoken words; coordination between the illustrations and the message is essential. Both should complement each other for maximum effectiveness. Also, art work used for visuals might also be effective in printed brochures or magazine articles, as well as pass out instructional materials.

## Preparing a script

A videotape, a film, a set of slides, or other type of presentation requires good organization and a script suitable to the audience and the action desired from it. Here are some guidelines:

1. Identify target audience. Decide what needs to be taught (task analysis), the knowledge level of the audience, the detail needed, and the level and method of presentation. Write down the objective of the visual; perhaps discuss it with colleagues or with a committee assigned to help with the project.

2. Develop a simple outline of the subjects to be covered, indicating the approach (humorous or serious, for example) to be used, and the props, types of illustrations, and shooting locations needed. Check to see if these are available or must be obtained or made.

3. Conduct a formal planning session. Using a script or script outline, review in detail all information to be presented; concentrate on logical sequence, technical accuracy, and possible problems. Avoid the temptation to crowd too many ideas into the outline. Concentrate on the chief objective.

4. Determine how to open and close the story. In a training script, main points should be repeated and summarized.

5. Following the outline, write a rough draft of the script and of the picture descriptions, and then a final draft. Technical and/or management approval is usually required.

6. Develop a shooting list. Based on script or script outline, identify shots by location and approximate length of time. Identify supplementary materials needed, such as titles, cartoons, drawings, diagrams of equipment parts, and sound effects.

For a script to have maximum effectiveness, short words and simple sentences are usually recommended. The script should be kept brief and to the point. If a lengthy description for one shot is necessary, variations or different views of the scene or subject could be developed, thus obviating the need to hold one scene too long.

Story board technique. In preparing a script for a set of slides or for a motion picture or videotape, the story board (planning board) technique is recommended.

Usually, the copy is typed double space, down the right side of the page or illustration board, frame by frame (or scene by scene), with the corresponding illustrations or picture descriptions placed opposite.

Or each frame can be represented by a 4 × 6 in. (10 by 15 cm) card with the illustration on the left side and the script and production instructions on the other side. The cards can be mounted on a large piece of cardboard, laid out on a desk top, or placed in a planning board rack. This technique makes it easy to rearrange the sequence and to visualize the entire finished product. See Fig. 14–3.

When a set of charts or even a chalk-talk is

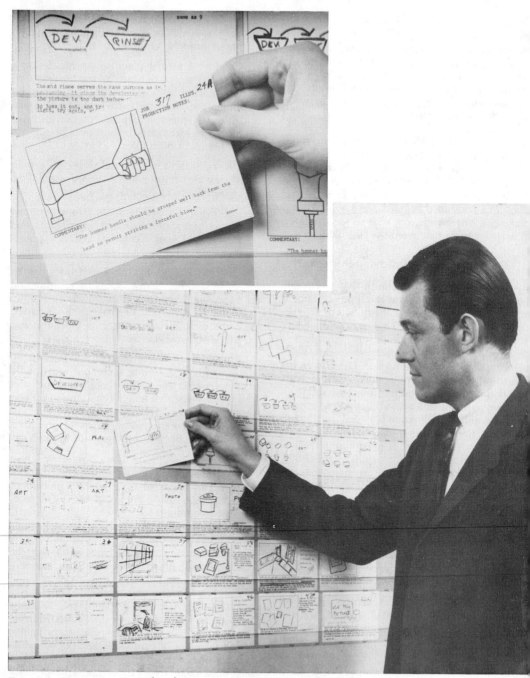

FIG. 14–3.—Planning board card (inset) gives the commentary and a rough sketch of the artwork or photograph needed. Cards can be sorted easily to make a logical sequence (larger picture).

*Courtesy Eastman Kodak Company.*

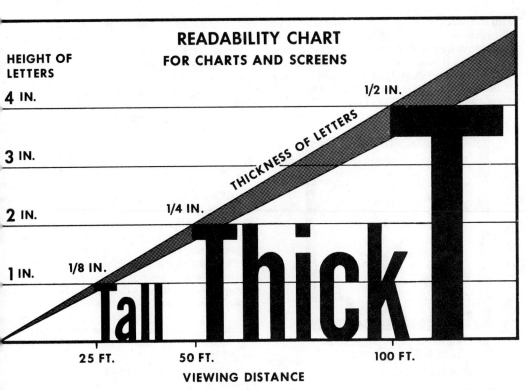

**FIG. 14-4.**—Readability chart for determining size and thickness of letters for nonprojected visuals. Size of lettering on projected visuals should be such that lettering is of adequate size when projected on screen. Make sure that thickness is proportional to height, that spacing between lines is about letter height, and that color aids readability, not fights it.

being prepared, rough sketches or notes can be made on a paper pad and scaled to size. Even in miniature, a rough sketch will give a good idea of the amount and size of lettering that can be used, the effect of color, and other aspects.

If the script is to be reviewed by safety committee members, company officials, or other persons, it can be typed and duplicated. Cards can be grouped and duplicated on pages. Deadlines for reviews must be set and followed. Of course, important points should be approved by key executives or other authorities.

## Lettering

The most common complaint regarding both nonprojected and projected visuals is that lettering is difficult to read—too small, too thin, too crowded—or even illegible. The best rule-of-thumb is to design lettering so that it can be read from the back row of the audience. Simplicity is the keynote.

Block letters show up better than handwritten copy. To be easily read at a distance of 50 ft (15 m) letters should be 2 in. (5 cm) high and 1/4 in. (8 mm) thick, as they are projected on the screen or show on a visual. (See Fig. 14-4.)

For use with overhead or opaque projectors, material typed with characters at least 1/4 in. high, with spacing of 1/4 in. between lines, will give a letter height of 2 in. on a screen 6 ft (1.8 m) wide and will be clearly visible at a distance of six to eight times the screen width.

The space between rows of letters should be at least one-half the height of the letters, preferably the same as the full height. For example, there should be at least 1/2 in. (and preferably 1 in.) spacing between letters 1 in. (2.5 cm) high.

Printed or typed material on 8½ by 11 in. (20 × 25 cm) sheets, such as record forms, will require larger lettering or typing on a machine with oversize (1/4 in.) characters. Material typed all-caps in an area 3 in. high by 4½ in. (7.5 × 11.5 cm) wide will be legible when converted to a 2-in. square slide. If possible, all illustrations and titles (art and lettering) should fit the horizontal format of the screen. That is, the width should be 1½ times the height. See (Fig. 14–5.)

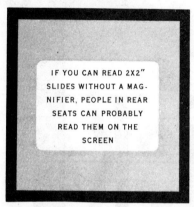

IF YOU CAN READ 2X2" SLIDES WITHOUT A MAG- NIFIER, PEOPLE IN REAR SEATS CAN PROBABLY READ THEM ON THE SCREEN

FIG. 14–5.—Rough rule-of-thumb for lettering to be shown on a 2 by 2 in. slide.

*Courtesy Eastman Kodak Co.*

Material on a visual should not be crowded, should be well organized, and kept simple. A simple rule for the amount of copy is: no more than 6 or 7 lines with 3 to six words of typed or lettered material per line. Typewriters which permit half-spacing (technically, "one-and-a-half spacing") are of special value here; use of a gothic typeface improves legibility.

A growing variety of ready-made lettering material is available in camera and art supply stores. Examples are plastic stick-on letters, rub-on transfer letters, gummed letters, and ceramic, cork, cardboard, or other letters which give a three-dimensional effect when lighting is from one side.

Most suppliers and many shipping rooms have stenciling equipment—either templates that are painted through or letters that are painted around—that can be used with either an ordinary stenciling brush or an inexpensive spray paint. Also, lettering guides are available for use with special lettering pens and felt-tipped marking pens. Often many styles of lettering can be made with one lettering set.

For a visual to be shown to a small group, large black or colored crayon may be used. For visual intended for larger groups, instructor chalk, broad-tip felt marking pens, stencils, cut out letters, or brush-painted letters are prefera ble. Background colors can be varied also. To much of any one color can be tiring. Try white o black or black on yellow.

**Use of color**

Color enhances both nonprojected and pro jected visuals. Contrasting colors always shoul be used. For example, black lettering shows u well on a white, yellow, or light-orange back ground, and worst on a dark blue.

With projected visuals, color adds realism provides contrast values that can bring out impo tant points, and gives a professional look to th completed visual. Full-color motion pictures ar expensive and are not always necessary. Whe emphasis is focused on the action, black and whit may even be more effective.

With color film or special titling film, fo instance, title frames can be made attractive an closeups can be shot against black or colore backgrounds for good contrast. Textured back grounds and colored lighting effects lend a profes sional touch.

For posters, dramatic effects can be obtaine with the high-visibility fluorescent paints, chalks and papers, particularly if "black" light is used

Color can be added with large blocks o instructor's colored chalk or with colored felt tipped pens that make a broad, heavy line Colored designs easily can be made by sprayin through stencils or simple cutouts. Spray cans ca be used also to give overall color, and powdere colored chalk can be daubed lightly over lettere material to give a tint.

Colored tape and ready-made arrows, circles and other stock designs can be used to make chart and graphs, and also to mark important parts i equipment photographs.

**Drawings and graphs**

Because of the size of type and the amount o copy, a graph, chart, or other line drawing ma become illegible when reproduced on film o viewed from a distance. Therefore reduce th details to those fundamentals required to illus trate the point.

The same rules that apply to lettering apply t drawings: the line work should be broad an

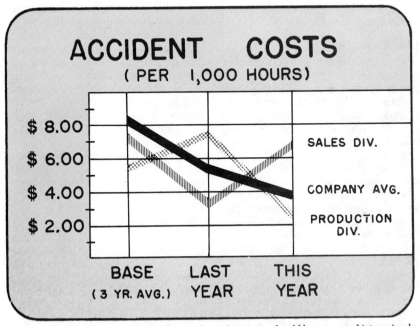

| ANNUAL SAFETY REPORT | | | |
|---|---|---|---|
| Accident Cost Factors by Departments | | | |
| (Incurred losses per 1,000 hours) | | | |
| Group | Base Period 3 Years | Last Year | This Year |
| Production Division | $5.40 | $7.10 | $2.50 |
| Sales Division | 7.20 | 3.25 | 6.70 |
| Company Average | 8.50 | 5.10 | 3.60 |

**ACCIDENT COSTS**
( PER 1,000 HOURS)

SALES DIV.

COMPANY AVG.

PRODUCTION DIV.

$ 8.00
$ 6.00
$ 4.00
$ 2.00

BASE (3 YR. AVG.)  LAST YEAR  THIS YEAR

FIG. 14–6.—For use as an audiovisual, complicated statistics should be converted into a simple graph for greater clarity. Typed slide (top) also shows poor spacing: top part is crammed while bottom portion is left blank. Other slide is better balanced, facts are easier to grasp.

opaque. Frequently a complex item can be constructed from areas cut out of colored paper. Colored paper is also effective for bars of a bar chart or areas under a curve. Graphs may be simply constructed from colored tapes ($\frac{1}{8}$ to 1 in. wide). Remember in presentations, graphs are frequently used to show a trend rather than specific points; hence the grid background should be omitted or should consist of only a few fine lines. Where accuracy is important, the actual numbers should be used.

Another inexpensive do-it-yourself technique is to draw a cartoon or chart. Varicolored chalk on a contrasting background lends an interesting fillip that is often lacking in conventional black-and-white material.

Try to show only one point at a time in building your overall story.

Depending upon the size of type and the amount of copy, a page of printed material may become illegible when reproduced on film. If such material must be used, it should be converted to a form more suitable for the purpose. The information given on a page of statistics, for instance, might be expressed in a few simple charts or graphs. Reduce the details to those fundamentals required to illustrate the point. Then do it effectively. See Fig. 14–6.

**Photographic illustrations**

The value of a visual depends to a considerable extent upon selecting the right illustrations and the quality of the illustrations. So far as photographs are concerned, the general principles of good photography are the same regardless of the type of camera or film used. Here are a few suggestions for taking good pictures.°

• The important part of the picture should be highlighted by means of a closeup, a supplementary sketch, a contrasting background, or by an arrow or sign placed by the item. For example, if a guard or a piece of safety equipment is being photographed, it can be painted (spray cans are handy) or shot against a colored background that provides effective contrast.

• It may sometimes be important to include an object of known size such as a pencil, automobile, or person to give an indication of the relative size of the object being photographed. Be sure to use a late model car so that the picture does not look dated.

• Both with motion and with still pictures, use o long shots, then medium shots, followed by close ups help establish the scene or situation.

• If material far in the background must b shown in detail, extra lighting must be used. A single flashbulb will not suffice. If background detail is not important, it can be kept out of th original picture, cropped out of the negative o the finished photo, or touched out of the print Off-to-one-side lighting will give a pleasant three dimensional effect and will keep light off th background, thus playing it down in the photo

• If there is doubt as to the possible result, it is good idea to take two or three different exposure at the time of the original shooting. Probably there then will be no need to come back later t get a better picture. Use of a Polaroid photo t determine exposure for black-and-white or colo film in difficult situations is often a help.

• Use of an exposure meter will help ensure goo results with both natural or existing light and wit floodlights or spotlights. A special exposur meter can be used for electronic flash. If a mete isn't used, exposures can be calculated on the basi of guide numbers provided by the manufacture of the camera flash unit or that are found in th instructions for the film. Numbers are for averag rooms. Large industrial areas require lower num bers (more light). Where possible, photos shoul be made outdoors, to take advantage of natura lighting, or in a studio under controlled light. I actual job situations are wanted, then shooting o location is called for.

• By using a "macro" (close up) lens, artwork ca be copied and made into a slide. If floodlight are used (as shown here), be sure to use "tungsten" (Type B) color film. (See Fig. 14–7.)

**Adding sound**

With either a set of slides or a filmstrip, soun can be added by means of a tape recorder o which a prepared sound track, with or withou commentary, is played. The slide or filmstri projector operator can follow a marked readin

---

°For a detailed discussion, see National Safety Counci *Photography for the Safety Professional*, Data Sheet 619

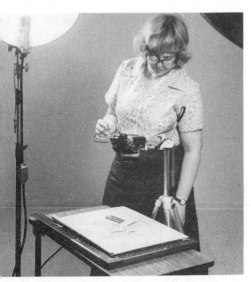

Fig. 14-7.—A 35mm single lens reflex (SLR) camera is used to copy artwork in order to make a 2 × 2 in. slide. When 3200 K lights are used (as here), the camera must be loaded with Type B color film. Be sure lights are equidistant from the copy and that no glare or bright reflections off the artwork spoil the slide.

cript, or a bell sound, "beep," or other audible signal can be used to tell him when to move the next picture into position. Using special equipment, inaudible signals can be inserted on the record or the tape to advance the slides or the strip automatically. Frequently, records are made with the audible signal on one side and the inaudible signal on the other.

If the slides are updated or rearranged or the filmstrip is revised, the tape easily can be remade.

A motion picture film can be made with either optical sound or magnetic sound. The magnetic sound requires a projector that plays it, but it is more easily applied and is finding increased use, especially on 8mm where optical sound is not available. Unless original super-8mm film is to be shot and projected, however, it is best to film on 16mm and reduce to 8mm optically for the print. The sound would be duplicated separately.

Videotape records sound as well as motion.

## Safety considerations

Photographers, whether professional or amateur, should observe certain precautions when taking pictures on location.

**Safe background.** Nothing can ruin the effect of a safety presentation more than unsafe, extraneous material in the background. For example, if the workers demonstrating a guarded grinding wheel are not wearing safety glasses, the photograph or movie sequence is likely to do more harm than good. Or, if the background shows poor housekeeping, fire hazards, or other employees not wearing the required personal protective equipment, it detracts from the safety message in the foreground.

**Safety equipment.** All photographers and their helpers should use the safety equipment required in the area. This means they should have safety glasses, safety shoes, and safety hats where required, not only for their own protection but to demonstrate a safe attitude.

**Observe safe practices.** These include not smoking and avoiding the use of flash equipment or the wrong type of electrical equipment in hazardous areas. Clearance should be obtained for work in hazardous areas.

**Electrical equipment.** Wiring should be in good condition and of the three-wire, automatic-grounded type with lock-type connections. Where possible, it should be strung over aisles or otherwise kept out of the way of truck and pedestrian traffic. If there could be any danger from operating machines, they should be locked out or have main switches pulled to prevent accidental starting. The services of a qualified maintenance worker or electrician to assist the photographer may at times provide an extra safeguard. Any electrical equipment that the photographer uses, other than a flash unit, should be UL-listed.

**Ladders.** Ladders or work stands should be available so that camera operators and helpers do not have to use makeshifts or climb on machines, tables, or other equipment unsuited for the purpose to get unusual angles. If they must work from heights, they should use safety belts and lifelines.

## Legal aspects

There are certain legal considerations in photographic production. It is customary to use model releases, discussed in the previous chapter, which permit employees (and others) to give written permission for the company to use photographs of them. Check with a legal counsel, industrial relations department, and local photographers for practical advice on using employees or the public in a film.

Consideration should also be given to copyrighting a slide show or film. This can be handled through a company's legal department. (For details, contact U.S. Copyright Office, Library of Congress, Washington, D.C. 20559; ask for form PA, "Application for Copyright Registration for a Work of the Performing Arts.")

## Presentation of Audiovisual Media

Even the best planned audiovisual will miss its mark unless the necessary facilities are at hand and unless the speaker checks them and rehearses with them.

If a company is planning on building a training room, it is best that the safety professional work with the designers at the earliest stages to make sure that the room incorporates all the features deemed necessary for effective use of audiovisuals.

### Room lighting

Nonprojected visuals require good general lighting. If a room has only indirect illumination, a portable floodlight or spotlight can be used on charts, exhibits, chalk boards, and other visuals. Such a light can be clamped to a chair or to a portable stand immediately in front of the visual, but placed so it will not interfere with the view of the audience.

A spotlight can be used also to put some light on the speaker so that he can maintain "eye contact" with the audience of the visual. But slides or a film, for instance, requires that the room be darkened.

Colored spotlights can heighten the dramatic effect of a visual. Revolving colored lights, like those used for Christmas displays, are suitable for more permanent exhibits, signs, or displays. "Black" or ultra-violet lighting used with fluorescent paint, paper, chalk, or ink gives a vivid effect.

If lighting must be dimmed for the showing of a projected visual, preparations must be made for darkening the room at the proper time, but "killing house lights" should not cut off power to the projector and reading lights. The location of the light switches must be noted, and someone should be asked to darken the room at a given signal. A shielded, reading light will be needed

when the house lights are turned off for the presentation. A small flashlight may come in handy if the reading light is not operative.

Window blinds or drapes should permit shutting out daylight.

Well in advance of the meeting, electric outlets should be located and electric equipment checked for safe working condition. Having spare bulbs and extra extension cords on hand may save embarrassment or prevent delay. Extension cords should be marked with high-visibility tape or placed so that they do not create tripping hazards.

### Use of pointers

A pointer is a necessary item when a speaker is using a chalk board or charts and may be helpful with other types of aids as well. A pencil or a finger is a poor substitute for a pointer.

Use of a pointer enables the speaker to face the audience and at the same time easily relate his words to the visual material. The speaker should not play with the pointer—this distracts from the presentation. He should not touch the visual or the projection screen with the pointer—it may move the visual or screen, or even mar it.

If visibility is a problem, a pointer with a fluorescent painted tip will be helpful. In a darkened or semidarkened room, a battery-operated or 110-volt flashlight-type pointer can be used to project a spot of light or a bright arrow onto a screen from a considerable distance.

A high visibility electric pointer is useful even in a fully lighted room when the speaker must stand at some distance from his chart or screen.

A telescoping, pocket-size pointer is useful for speakers who must carry a pointer with them.

### Amplifying and recording systems

If the acoustics in the room are bad or if outside noise makes hearing difficult, an amplifying system will be needed for successful presentation of an audiovisual. This is particularly important if there are a number of speakers and some may not be heard in far corners of the room.

If the speaker must move around, a lavaliere (chest-type), wireless, or lapel microphone is necessary. (Be sure the lavaliere microphone does not rub against a tie clip as this makes a lot of noise.) If the speaker can remain in one place, a pedestal or lectern microphone is satisfactory.

If audience participation is desired from a large group, floor microphones placed in the aisles or roving microphones carried by assistants vill enable members of the audience to be heard throughout the room. Otherwise, the speaker nust repeat questions and comments from the loor, using his microphone, so that the entire udience will know what has been said.

Before each use, an amplifying system should be checked for good operating condition and to be ure that reception is satisfactory throughout the oom. At all times while the system is being used, t should be supervised by an individual familiar vith electronic equipment to assure control of rolume and of annoying acoustic feedback.

Also see the discussion of public address systems at the end of this chapter.

## TelePrompters

TelePrompters may be rented for dramatic or ormal presentations in which actors, technicians, or executives are required to follow a prepared script.

Of course, technical help is needed to set up the TelePrompter, and those using it must be amiliar with the technique so that their presentation will have the desired natural effect.

## Screens

There are several basic types of screens used for projection:°

*Glass-beaded screens.* Usually portable, but often of the large pull-down variety, these screens have a high reflectance value but within a narrow angle of projection. (45 deg).

*Matte finish screens* do not give quite as bright an image as beaded screens. However, since they have a wider viewing angle (60 deg), they are more suitable for larger audiences, and for any room where some of the audience must sit at a considerable angle to the screen.

*Lenticular-surfaced screens* have embossed surfaces that reflect a high percentage of projected light on a viewing angle wider than that of beaded screens (70 deg), and reject stray incident light.

*Permanently mounted aluminum foil screens* are the brightest obtainable. Solid backed and slightly curved, they cannot be rolled up. The viewing angle is only 30 deg. maximum. The screen is designed for use with room light on; it is too bright for use in a darkened room, unless projector illumination is reduced.

*Rear projection screens* can be used in partially lighted rooms and have a wide viewing angle. However, any stray light behind the rear screen must be held to an absolute minimum.

The image on the screen should be neither dazzlingly bright nor dim. Generally, a 500-watt projector bulb is satisfactory for small and medium groups in either a darkened or partially darkened room, provided that the film, slides, or transparencies have good color and well defined material. A 1000-watt bulb in a 16mm movie projector is better for medium and larger groups. Special longer-burning bulbs are available.

Where possible, screens should be set slightly above the heads of the audience for maximum visibility. With some projectors, principally the overhead type that is set close to the screen, a keystone effect may be created, whereby the top of the image is noticeably wider than the bottom. This distortion can be reduced by slanting the screen slightly so that its plane is more nearly perpendicular to the projected light. Some screens now are equipped with a clip or bar which permits this adjustment. Such bars can also be purchased separately and attached to portable or wall screens.

Be sure that the area of the projected image fills the screen, if possible, but does not extend over on the background.

Although modern projectors equipped with powerful bulbs do not require complete room darkening, room lights should be dimmed (or some lights switched off) and windows shaded as needed. This leaves sufficient light for note-taking or script reading, if necessary. There is no need to completely darken a room for showing noncontinuous-tone images (such as graphs, diagrams, or lettering). A reverse-projection unit or a shadow box permits showing filmstrips, slides, or movies to a small group without dimming lights.

Slide projectors that must be located in or behind the audience should have a remote-control device, or be operated by someone other than the speaker (if the presentation does not have a recorded narration). There should be a subtle signal agreed upon for changing slides. When the speaker must say "Next slide please," or snap a cricket, he distracts the audience. Some offhand,

---

°Detailed information can be supplied by screen or projector manufacturers.

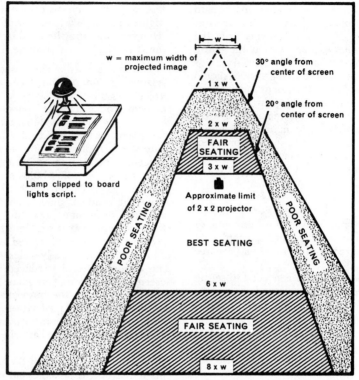

FIG. 14–8.—Shading indicates both good and poor seating areas when ordinary (beaded) projection screens are used. A lenticular screen would widen the angle, which is measured from centerline. Shaded reading light permits reading script without distracting audience.

but clear, gesture with the pointer or flashlight should suffice.

## Seating

A room in which an audiovisual is to be presented should be checked for safety features and for seating arrangement. Aisle space should be adequate, exits ready for emergency use, and ash trays provided if smoking is permitted.

The seating arrangement should be planned so that every member of the audience will have an unobstructed view of the visual. For meeting room or auditorium seating, allow 21 to 24 in. (53 to 61 cm) width for each chair and 36 in. (91 cm) for each row of chairs, or about 5 to 6 sq ft (0.46 to 0.56 m²) per viewer. In classrooms or conference rooms, allow twice as much space.

For viewing a projected visual, the most desir-able seating area is within a 30-degree angle from the projection axis with a matte screen and within a 20-degree angle from the axis with a beaded screen. See Fig. 14–8.

The recommended minimum viewing distance is at least twice the screen width, and the maximum no more than eight times the screen width, although a distance no more than six times the screen width is desirable. A 6-foot-wide (1.8m) image, therefore, could be viewed at a maximum distance of about 50 ft (15 m) by approximately 100 persons.

For extremely wide rooms, and if the seats cannot be arranged so the audience sits within the recommended viewing angle, it is possible to project images from slide projectors or over-head projectors simultaneously on two or three screens, separated by at least 25 ft (7 m).

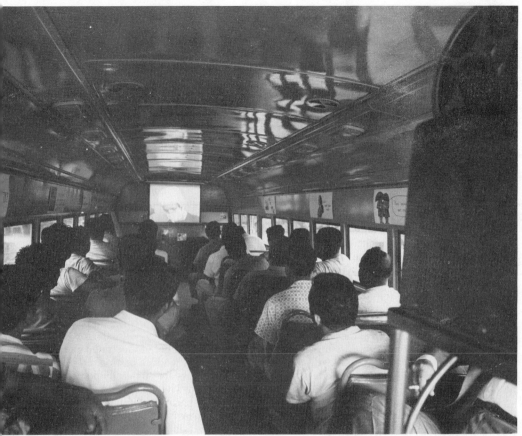

Fig. 14–9.—This 44-passenger bus has been converted into a mobile training room for up to 32 people. Courtesy Dillingham Corporation, Honolulu.

## Mobile presentations

Where good projection facilities are lacking, such as in the field or at branch terminals or plants, mobile presentations should be considered. Flip charts, flannel boards, and demonstrations can be used outdoors or in quarters not well suited to projected visuals.

Trucks, trailers, converted buses, (Fig. 14–9), and other large vehicles may be used as mobile classrooms. Rear screen projectors, mounted in station wagons or van wagons, facilitate the use of projected visuals in the field. For such small quarters, air conditioning should be used.

## Rehearsal

With even the simplest visuals, practice before use is imperative. It will help prevent the speaker from running overtime and will help assure smoothness of presentation.

Unrehearsed use of a visual may reduce its effectiveness considerably. A set of charts, for instance, may be well prepared, easy to understand, and attractive, but if they are shown in random fashion or must be fumbled with by the speaker, much of their impact will be lost.

Moreover, if the speaker wanders from the subject, the set of charts or transparencies, instead of serving as an "aid," may even prove distracting. If other material than that illustrated must be discussed, the speaker would be wise to cover the charts (or turn off the projector) until he is ready to return to them.

When items such as chalk, an eraser, and a pointer are needed, the speaker should make sure

**401**

in advance that they are at hand. A person who needs a marking pen should carry two pens in case one runs dry. Some training rooms have white chalkboards; if using a felt-tipped pen, be sure the ink can be removed by a damp cloth.

Training and rehearsal is particularly important with more complicated equipment such as a movie projector. Well in advance of the showing, a trained operator should make sure that the film is not broken and that the equipment is "ready to roll," and that extra bulbs are on hand. The projector should be threaded or slides inserted in correct projection position, the motion picture header run off, the sound adjusted, picture focused, and the screen set up at the proper distance. When a tape or a record is to be used with a film, a set of slides, or a filmstrip, the sound and picture should be synchronized. Arrangements for turning lights on and off should always be checked.

A film, a set of slides, or a filmstrip should be previewed and checked for good condition, and, in the case of slides, for proper sequence and right side up. When slides are in proper sequence, draw a diagonal line across the top of the pack—an out-of-place or mis-turned slide shows up at once.

The need for introductory remarks, discussion questions, and recall or followup materials should be considered.

If a script is to be read, the speaker should not indulge in lengthy ad-libs. He should stick to his plan of presentation, giving each chart, slide, or frame the time and attention it deserves, but no more. It is a good idea to preview all visuals that are required and have them on hand before the meeting starts.

The speaker should face the audience as much of the time as possible, particularly if he is using charts or a chalkboard. He should not talk when he is moving about or not facing his audience. Not only would the distraction be bad, but the audience would have difficulty hearing him.

If the speaker wishes to face the audience the entire time, he can arrange for an assistant to write on the chalkboard or turn the flip charts. Be sure that this doesn't become more distracting than useful. If the speaker is using a projected visual, he can operate the projector with a remote control cord or have another person run it for him.

It is more effective if the speaker has the full information of the slide in front of him so that he does not have to turn continually toward the screen and away from the audience.

## Nonprojected Visuals

Nonprojected visuals° include graphics, three dimensional exhibits and models, and live pre sentations. Among the various types of graphic are chalkboards (formerly called blackboards, paper pads, flip charts, display cards, flanne boards, magnetic boards, and hook and loo boards.

### Chalkboards and paper pads

Chalkboards are a well-known, basic visua. They come in several colors and charcoal, bu light green is considered standard. A dustles chalk should be used, preferably a yellow or othe bright color for maximum visibility since whit chalk does not show up well on a dusty chal board.

Large blocks of instructors' chalk or the side c stick chalk gives a heavier and wider line fo greater visibility. Different colors of chalk, par ticularly the fluorescent chalks with black ligh are very effective.

Paper pads (usually 2 by 3 ft [0.5 × 0.76 m provide inexpensive visuals for small group Pads, or a number of sheets of paper, clamped o light-weight wooden or aluminum folding easel (as flip charts are) are easily portable and alway ready to go. The speaker can keep training mate rial on the pad so that he can refer to it, or throw away, as he wishes. Some commercially availabl pads have faint cross-hatching to facilitate letter ing and layout of artwork on the paper.

Pads are of real value to those who must lea discussions or run "brainstorming"sessions. A each chart is filled, it can be tacked to a corkboar or clipped to a wire running along one side c the conference room. This (a) provides the grou with a continuous record of what has been dis cussed, (b) lets latecomers catch up to the discus sion, without having to stop the discussion an have a review, and (c) helps in writing a goo report of the meeting—the notes are right on th pad sheets.

Inexpensive rolls of white paper can be use for homemade charts. Even brown wrappin

---

° Posters, the most commonly used type of visual, ar discussed fully in Chapter 12, "Maintaining Interest i Safety," and in National Safety Council Industrial Dat Sheet No. 616 "Posters, Bulletin Boards, and Safet Displays."

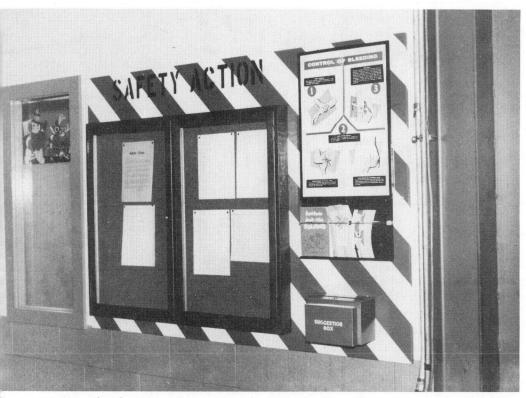

FIG. 14–10.—A poster (right) informs employees of the proper method to control bleeding. Bulletins and a suggestion box round out the display.

Courtesy Merideth Printing Co., Des Moines, Ia.

paper will do if material such as lettering is added in a contrasting color which will stand out. Material can be written so that it can be read as the chart is unrolled like a scroll.

## Flip charts and posters

**Flip Charts.** Flip charts are a refinement of paper pads. Usually charts are on heavier paper, prepared in advance, and used in more formal meetings; frequently, blank pages are also provided for "on-the-spot" additions. Flip charts might combine specially made material mounted on large sheets or hinged in briefcase-size easel-binders that are used for desk-top or bench-top discussion. Portable units are easy to make and are easy to take to different locations.

To help in making the presentation, brief notes can be written in lightly in blue pencil on the face of the card or flip chart. Notes are written small

enough so that the instructor can read them, but yet they are "invisible" to anyone in the audience, if he is more than 6 or 7 ft (1.8 or 2 m) away.

**Posters** are desirable to a successful safety program. They serve as reminders, warnings, and motivators (See Fig. 14–10). They deal with many accident problems, both occupational and nonoccupational, and they employ many types of art styles and formats. They are not used like a flip chart, but rather they are displayed at various locations throughout an establishment or plant.

Selected carefully and used discriminately, posters can help employees avoid hazards and unsafe acts and can help the company or plant have a more effective safety program. For more details, see the discussion of Posters and Displays in Chapter 12, "Maintaining Interest in Safety," and in Industrial Data Sheet No. 616.

**403**

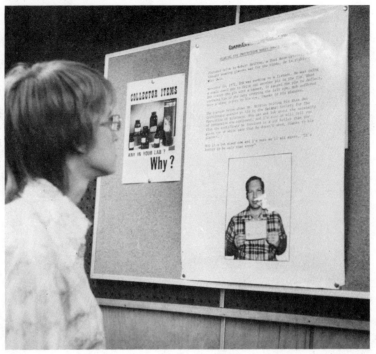

Fig. 14-11.—Two photographically produced posters grace this company's bulletin board. Photo at right presents a "silent sermon"— the case history of an employee whose eyesight was saved by his wearing safety glasses.

### Flannel boards

A flannel board is a plywood board, commonly 3 by 4 ft (0.9 × 1.2m) covered with dark flannel. A number of frames can be fastened together or placed close together to form multiples of the original size.

Roll flannel can be tacked, tied, or otherwise stretched over any large, flat, slightly inclined surface, including a chalk board. Art work or lettering can be made directly on a special velour-backed paper or on light-weight cardboard or heavy-weight paper to which flocking paper with felt adhesive or strips is affixed. In an emergency, sand paper can be used instead of the special flocking paper. The flocking or sandpaper grips the long-napped flannel with sufficient strength to hold light-weight cards.

These individual cardboards, with words, designs, or messages on them, can be "slapped on" or built up to create a dramatic effect not possible with other visuals.

### Hook and loop boards

A hook and loop board is a heavy-duty "slap board." The material covering the board contains countless nylon loops. These loops are caught by almost invisible nylon hooks that are on the small pieces of tape mounted on the back of signs or other objects used for the display. A tiny patch of the hook material fastened to a heavy or large object will hold it securely on the board.

Hook and loop boards are available commercially in sizes ranging from 18 by 24 in. (45 × 60 cm) to 48 by 72 in. (1.2 × 1.8 m).

### Magnetic boards

A magnetic board can be made of either a spray-painted sheet metal plate or a steelbacked chalk board. Small objects or cutouts mounted on small magnets or on magnetic tape can be placed on the board and then moved at will.

This type of visual often is used for training operators of vehicles such as forklift trucks. The mobility of the objects–toy vehicles or cutouts of trucks, together with the cutouts of aisles and loads–enables the instructor to give a realistic demonstration of safe practices.

## Photographs

Photographs need not be projected to be useful. Candid shots of safe and unsafe practices or conditions, photos of award presentations, meetings, new equipment, and the like, have excellent news value on bulletin boards, (see Fig. 14–11), in company (or plant) papers (house organs or safety magazines), and are even welcomed by national trade and professional magazines.

The "instant" photograph can be another excellent tool. It provides a record of hazards and is useful in accident investigation. See Council Data Sheet No. 619.

## Exhibits and demonstrations

Exhibits and models make very effective three-dimensional displays for use in instruction. Such exhibits can be made for the purpose of demonstrating the safe working of a machine or process. Examples of first aid equipment, protective clothing, rescue equipment, respiratory protective equipment and fire protection applicances can also be featured.

A small wooden dummy made with articulated joints and spine is often used for showing the correct and safe method of lifting and carrying heavy loads. See Fig. 14–12 for lifting instructions.

Demonstrations of firefighting can sometimes be organized with the assistance of the local fire service. (See Fig. 14–13.)

Demonstrations of good and bad lighting can be easily arranged in a lecture room. The effect of an impact on safety hats, safety shoes, and eye protection devices can be shown. The teaching of splinting by demonstration plays an important part in firstaid training.

## Projected Visuals

Projected visuals include slides, filmstrips, transparencies for overhead projectors, objects used in opaque projectors, motion pictures, television and videotapes.

This chapter will not go into great detail regarding slides, filmstrips, and movies, because excellent information is available from the manufacturers of film and projectors, camera stores,

libraries, schools, and publications. The *National Safety News*, for instance, frequently carries detailed articles on producing slide shows, using slides, and related topics. The National Safety Council also publishes a series of Data Sheets on the subject (see References).

## Slides

Slide presentations have become increasingly popular with the addition of sound. Programs can be recorded and sound synchronized to slides on a cassette recorder, which can automatically advance the slides with the narration.

Learner response is encouraged when cassette recorders are equipped with a "stop" button on the visual synchronizing mechanisms. The slide presentation can pose questions, be stopped for class response (oral or written), and then started again for correct answers and the explanations or discussions. To add a touch of professionalism, background music can be played.

One international organization has designed basic safety presentations available in half a dozen languages. For each presentation, locals receive a package consisting of the tape cassette, slides, and a printed copy of the narration for whoever will conduct the safety training session.

● Specific advantages include:

Slides can be easily updated

They are inexpensive

Almost anyone can make a slide

They can be geared to the needs of the audience by substituting specific slides

Audio tape for automatic advance is available

Can be coupled with other projectors both slide and film

Are easily stopped for discussion

● Potential disadvantages include:

Slides can easily get out of order

They can stick in the holding tray

Slides can easily be projected upside down or backwards

Poorly made slides are distracting

The simplicity of producing slides can give a sense of "false security" and result in poorly organized presentations

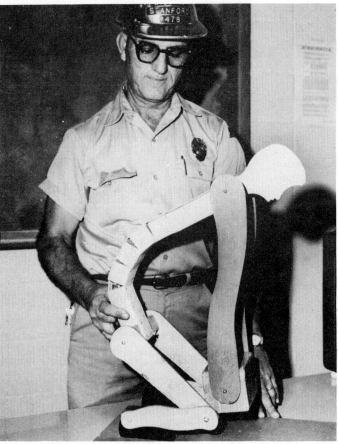

Photo courtesy Mississippi Chemical Corp., Yazoo City, Miss.

## Here Is How To Use It

There is a proper and an improper way to pick up a heavy object. The proper way is to keep the back straight, the knees bent and spread, and the load close to the body. The improper way is to reach way over and lift. (Twisting the back complicates the bad effect.)

To demonstrate this effectively, a special model can be used. If used with its block "spine" "locked," the model (dubbed "Junior") simulates lifting with strong leg muscles; the ribbon on the "spine" remains limp, indicating very little tension of the back muscles. It demonstrates that the back cannot be kept straight without bending the knees.

To demonstrate improper lifting, "Junior" is used as is shown in the photograph. The legs are bent only slightly (or held straight). One hand lifts the handle just ahead of the fulcrum at the "hips" in order to lift the weight in "Junior's" "hands." The back arches under the strain and visibly pulls each block apart.

Model can be made to show proper foot placement (see drawing at right).

---

Slide projectors range from inexpensive single slide viewers that can be held in the hand and looked at, to remote control or automatic-change projectors that have trays or magazines holding up to 140 slides. A small rear projection portable machine in a self-contained case, designed for table top use, is suitable for very small groups. With a taped or recorded message, this type is well suited to training one or two employees.

### Filmstrips

The term "filmstrip" is preferred to the term "slide film" because the latter may be mistakenly understood to mean the separate slides. A filmstrip is merely a strip of standard 35mm film on which has been photographed a series of single frame pictures whose area is about one-half that of a standard 35mm slide.

Filmstrips require even more careful planning than slides because it is impossible to rearrange the frames or to add new material to suit specific situations or changing times.

Because of this inflexibility and specialized equipment needed for their production and presentation, filmstrips are being used less and less; the ubiquitous 2 by 2 slide is now used for most slide shows.

## Construction Specifications

The spine is made with 9 blocks, each 2-in. square and 1⅝-in. high. Each is drilled at the center to accommodate a standard screen door spring. The T-shaped head and shoulder piece is about 8-in. long, 2-in. thick, and supports the arms on shoulders about 5-in. apart. The hip block is 2-in. square, with sloping sides so legs will spread open in front. Add a ⅜-in. spacer between the hip block and each leg.

Assemble the body by using wood screws to attach ends of spring to the head and hip pieces. Tack a piece of 2-in. wide belting to the *front* of the spine blocks to hold them in alignment.

The arms and legs can be shaped from ¼-in. plywood.

A block, approximately 5-in. square and 3½-in. high, represents the lifting weight. Elastic tape or multiple rubber bands are stretched from the shoulder to the hip, along the *back* of the spine blocks to represent the spine muscles.

A metal handle can be secured to the lower end of the hip block, as shown in the drawing.

"Junior" can be mounted on a 1×12-in. board, 18 to 24-in. long.

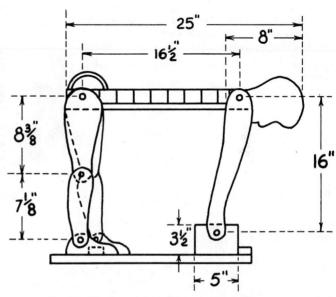

Fig. 14–12.—A model is used to demonstrate correct lifting.

## Overhead projection

Of the many ways to put visuals in front of people, overhead projection offers special advantages:

The speaker can present to any size group in a fully lighted room

He faces his audience at all times.

The material can be revealed point by point.

The audience is not distracted by the machine.

Overhead projection equipment is easy to operate and is readily available.

Overhead transparencies can be made quickly and inexpensively.

Lettering is a key to the effectiveness of a visual for overheads. Careless lettering can detract from even the best illustration while neat, wellplanned lettering can be effective by itself. Letters should be at least 1/4 in. high (if the original can be read from a distance of 10 ft (3 m), the transparency should project well). The letters can be applied to transparencies by hand, stencils, tracing, transfer letters and symbols, and lettering tape which is made from an imprinting machine.

It may be helpful to use color for clarity and

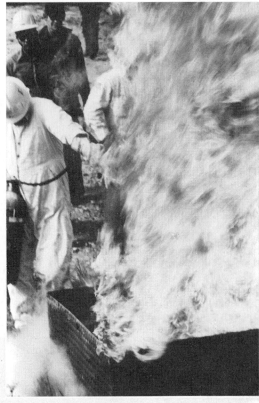

FIG. 14-13.—Training class for workers on the inland waterways not only teaches how to use an extinguisher properly, but gets them close enough to the fire's heat to overcome trainees' fears and establish their confidence in themselves and their equipment when and if the real situation should arise.

*Courtesy Inland Waterways Safety and Health Association.*

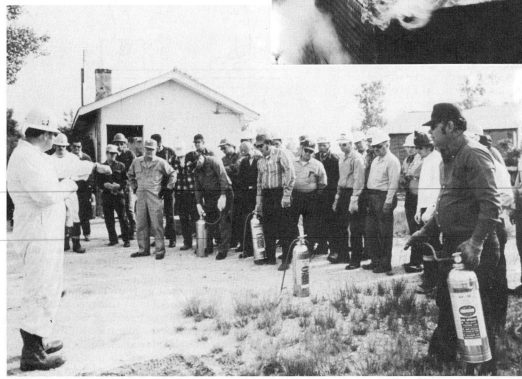

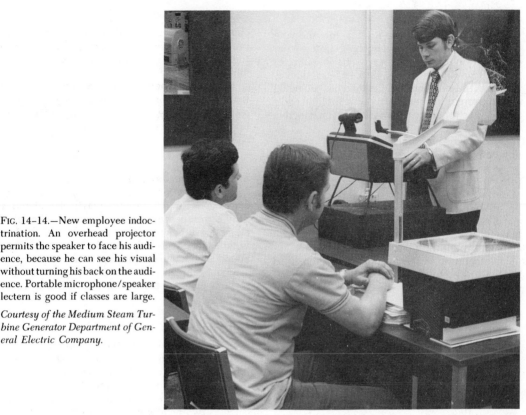

FIG. 14–14.—New employee indoctrination. An overhead projector permits the speaker to face his audience, because he can see his visual without turning his back on the audience. Portable microphone/speaker lectern is good if classes are large.

*Courtesy of the Medium Steam Turbine Generator Department of General Electric Company.*

emphasis of certain points. Color attracts attention, is eye-pleasing and provides variety.

Where possible, limit each original to one point or comparison. Break paragraphs into sentences, and sentences into phrases and key words. Use a maximum of six lines, and six or seven words per line.

Reproduction equipment is available for making transparencies from almost any original.

To add impact to projected transparencies, overlays can be used. This method helps simplify difficult concepts and also lets the presentor build the visual's story in a meaningful way. It involves two or more imaged transparencies used in sequence over each other. Using no more than two overlays and different colors for each makes this a very effective way to present step-by-step information. Overlay visuals are "hinged" to the frame on one side with tape to allow the base visual to be presented first, then the overlay flapped over it to complete the message.

On overhead projection the visual can be projected unframed, but there are good reasons for using frames: The frame blocks light around the edge of the visual, adds rigidity for handling and storage; and provides a convenient border for writing notes.

If a blank transparent sheet or roll of clear plastic film is used on the overhead, the speaker can use it as a pad to gather ideas or lead a discussion. Not only are ideas written down for all to see on the screen, but the sheets can be saved and used to keep a record of the meeting.

This visual technique has a number of important advantages. The speaker needs no assistant; he can face the audience, and the room can be either partially or fully lighted. He can use any opaque material as a cover sheet, which can be withdrawn to reveal data point by point, and he can point to items on the transparency—and therefore on the screen—with a pencil or other object. See Fig. 14–14.

**409**

## Opaque projectors

Opaque projectors are useful for showing printed material and even three-dimensional objects. Printed material up to 10 in. (25 cm) square or an object up to 2 1/2 in. (6.5 cm) thick is placed in the machine, and the image is projected onto the screen by means of a powerful light and a mirror. The room must be darkened for effective viewing.

With an opaque projector, material that cannot conveniently be transferred for overhead projectors or photographed for 2 in. slide projectors can be quickly shown. An example of such material would be a safety catalog or a safety poster in full color. Of course, to be suitable for use in an opaque projector, printed material must have type large enough to be legible to the entire audience when the material is projected.

Another use of the opaque projector is to project a picture, map, or other shape on to a pad or chalkboard so that it can be traced. The size of the projection can be varied to the exact size required. This results in a neat, professional-looking drawing that now can also be used as a flipchart.

## Motion pictures

Movies are rated excellent for training and motivating. Because of their higher cost compared with that of other visuals, they should be planned with special care. Usually, movies are important enough to justify commercial production or at least professional advice before and during production. Some homemade movies, however, have proved to be effective. See previous section on Making Motion Pictures.

The three principal sizes of motion picture film commonly in use are 35mm, 16mm, and 8mm, both standard-8 and super-8 sizes. The 35mm film is found almost exclusively in theaters. The 16mm size is widely used by industrial organizations, and the 8mm size is gaining attention because of its lower cost.

The development of magnetic and optical sound, improved color stock, rear-projection screen, self-threading cartridge, single-frame viewing, and super-8 equipment has resulted in greater use of motion pictures for in-plant training.

The super-8 (and standard-8) projectors and cameras are smaller and lighter than the 16mm equipment—an advantage where portability or size is a factor. These projectors can be used for continuous showing of safety films in such locations as cafeterias and lounges, with either a regular screen or small rear-screen self-contained unit.

A wide selection and variety of 16mm safety films are available from insurance companies, local safety organizations, commercial film libraries, industrial producers, and the National Safety Council.

**Polavision** . This Polaroid product consists of a camera, rear-screen playback unit, and other accessories. After the picture is made, the film cartridge is inserted into the playback unit and is fully developed in about 90 seconds. Then it is ready for projection. The cartridge runs 2-1/2 minutes in length and is available only in color. Sound is not available. Equipment is easily operated, but the projection area is limited because the screen's diagonal measurement is less than 12 in. (30 cm).

## Multi-Image.

Multi-image refers to the capability of using more than one projector simultaneously. Actually it is an expansion of the basic sound slide program format that has gained tremendous popularity. The presentation can be of the same medium (such as two or more slide projectors), or mixed media (slide/motion picture).

A programmer allows you to automatically turn slide and/or movie projectors on and off, advance slides, and change slide projector lamp currents from off to full on, at nearly any rate of change. These functions may be performed in any sequence you desire.

- Advantages include:

  Visual information can be presented both linearly and spatially, enabling the viewer to see not only the order but also the relationship of information.

  These programs compress the time needed to create an impression.

  They tend to develop greater viewer involvement and even excitement.

- Potential disadvantages are:

  Operator training is necessary

  They can require sizeable budgets

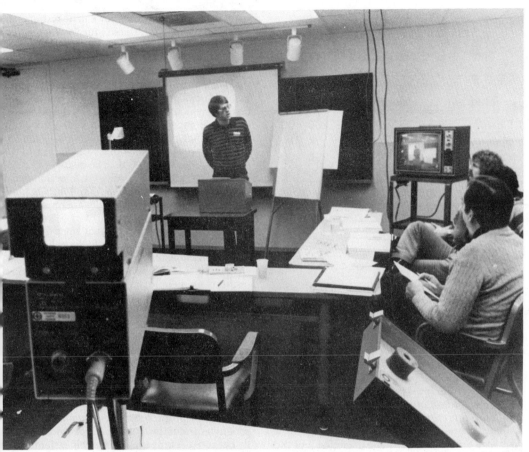

FIG. 14–15.—While this student of National Safety Council's Safety Training Institute makes a presentation, the talk is taped on closed circuit TV. Later, the presentation will be critiqued by both the class and the student.

They take time to develop

In summary, it should be remembered that each audiovisual system has properties peculiar to itself that represent a possible advantage or disadvantage when compared with another type of audiovisual system. The audiovisual decision-maker must weigh needs and objectives against all the other factors, including budget and audiovisual capabilities.

### Videotape and Closed Circuit Television (CCTV)

The word *video* may be used to describe any type of television equipment, such as video cam-eras, tape recorders, tape players, recording tape, monitors, and a full range of television studio equipment and cable television hardware.

As a greater effort is being made today to remove communication barriers and to assure that available information is properly learned and used, videotape is being recognized as one of the most effective communications and training methods available, both as a production medium and as a transmission medium. It can also be used as a means of self-analysis (Fig. 14–15). The following discussion is taken from "Using Video-tape to Conduct Safety Training," by Gerald H. Katz. See References.

## TABLE 14-B

### AVERAGE COSTS OF PROGRAM MATERIAL AND EQUIPMENT

| Medium | Cost per Minute* | Projection Equipment |
|---|---|---|
| Film | $3000 | $ 200-400 |
| Slides/Audio cassettes | $ 640 | $ 200-400 |
| Videotape | $ 600 | $1000-1500 |

*From "Federal A/V Report Reveals Some Amazing Facts," Video Systems, P.O. Box 12901, Overland Park, Kan. 66212. Vol. 5, No. 8, August 1979. pp. 34-36.

### Videotape advantages

The advantages of videotape lie in two areas: lower cost of production and a culturally natural transmission medium.

With reference to lower cost, Table 14–B presents data on the three most commonly used audiovisual media. The survey data indicate average costs of program material produced by out-of-house production companies.

The lower cost of video compared to motion pictures is due to two factors. First, video has the ability to play back instantly the field-recorded sequence to assure the technical accuracy of the visual material, and to verify that the proper focus, lighting, viewing angle, and composition have been achieved. If there is any problem, the activities can be immediately repeated, taped, and reviewed until the proper content has been recorded.

If motion picture or slide film is used, the image content is not known until the film is developed and reviewed, which may be days later. Any problems may require a return to the field shooting location several times, thus greatly increasing costs. In addition, much more footage may be shot than will actually be used to provide "insurance" in case some shots are unusable.

The second reason for the lower cost of video is the structuring and editing of the program material. (See Fig. 14-16). The video program is structured with all video footage taken for specific uses, and reviewed in the field prior to studio assembly. No time is spent choosing from alternate scenes later because they can be reshot right away if the first effort doesn't turn out as desired. Sometimes the audio can be rewritten to match the action, although the picture should be selected to meet script demands, especially if the script has already been approved by technical and management people. Compared to motion picture film which must be edited from the processed film, videotape is quickly edited electronically and does not require splicing.

Adding sound to slide programs increases the cost also. (See Table 14–B.) The quality of a slide is not known until it is developed; selection of the best slide from the many that are taken is time-consuming because 5 to 15 slides are required per minute of program time.

Another consideration is that since 1950, the television set has become the focus of household communication, bringing in the nightly news, entertainment, and cultural programming. As a result, many people have moved from a reading-oriented culture to a verbally and visually stimulated culture; people passively interact with the video screen (see McLuhan in References). For the majority of people, viewing a television set to obtain information is more natural than listening to a live presentation, watching a motion picture, or viewing a slide presentation.

### Videotape players

Although professional producers of television programs prefer the reel-to-reel recorder, primarily because the tape in this format is easier to edit, there is widespread distribution of already-produced subjects for the popular cassette tape player.

The two words, "cassette" and "cartridge," are often used interchangeably, referring to any container holding tape that can be used in a player without having to be threaded. Technically, a distinction is recognized. A cassette holds both the original reel and the take-up reel in the same case; a cartridge has only one reel on which the tape is wound. Its take-up reel is incorporated into the player, with the threading being done automatically.

But in operation, they are much alike. The plastic case with the tape is put into position, a switch or two is flipped, and the player goes to work. It picks up the signal and feeds it to the television set. They are not alike, however, in physical format. Be sure to use the cartridge or the cassette that is designed for the equipment on hand. There is a limited interchangeability.

The most commonly used systems are based on magnetic tape, but several types of presentations start out with film.

## In-house and out-of-house production

In deciding whether to create such programs within company or plant facilities or by using an outside firm specializing in such work, the *quality* of the presentation must be considered.

Because of familiarity with the household television set, the student using television as a learning tool is conscious of the quality of production. In order to hold the student's attention, the quality must be comparable to what the student has been watching, as opposed to "home movies" or merely "a talking head" appearing on the screen. Home movies are basically amateur productions that will not convey proper images either of the company or its safety practices. The talking head may as well be a live lecture, because the real advantage of the video medium—its ability to bring the job site directly into the classroom—is not being utilized.

To achieve the quality desired, two factors must be available: People to produce the programs, and equipment to record the program materials.

As a rule of thumb, if less than one video program is prepared each month, it may be advisable to consider an out-of-house training organization to produce the videotapes, *under the direction and control of an in-house coordinator.*

The "one program monthly" rule is the production load that can be used to justify three full-time people: a training program developer, a video director, and an equipment operator. If these positions are filled by part-time personnel, schedules will not be met, costs will increase, and production will probably fall into the "home movie" classification.

The necessary video equipment for production includes a video camera, video recorder, and an editing system. It can cost from $5,000 to hundreds of thousands of dollars (exclusive of physical facilities to house a video studio). The current minimum equipment investment for quality productions is $50,000 to $100,000. If the equipment is going to be stored in a closet and used only occasionally, consider the out-of-house training or production company.

A caution is in order here. A training company is different from a video production house. The

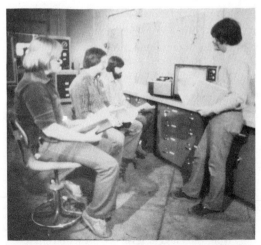

Fig. 14-16.—Employees view a training program on maintenance. Instructor explains the procedures step by step and refers to the training manual. The presentation is stopped periodically so students can ask questions.

*Courtesy Duke Power Company, Charlotte, N.C.*

training company will perform all the steps listed next. The video production house performs only steps 3, 5, and 7, and then only under close direction.

In addition to the six steps listed early in this chapter under Preparing a script, the following steps must be followed.

1. Develop program's scope. Identify the information to be covered, its sequence, and what is to be shown to take advantage of the dynamics of the medium; identify shooting locations, equipment, and personnel requirements. Get approval of budget.

2. Rehearse activities in the field. This permits identifying video camera locations and performer knowledge, and assures proper equipment operation and its availability.

3. Shoot field footage. Also, review technical accuracy and visual content of each piece of field video.

4. Write narrative script. This must be timed to the field video, and the script must then be submitted for review.

5. Studio assembly and editing. This will be performed by recording the audio track from

**413**

an approved script, and integrating it with the field video and the additional visual aids.

6. Review completed program. This is done with all persons who attended the formal planning session (step three under Preparing a script, earlier in this Chapter). Identify corrections of either the visual or audio portion of the program. If all prior steps were properly performed, these should be minimal.

7. Make corrections. This will be followed by the development of written materials for students and the instructor.

8. Train the instructor to use the program properly.

9. Run the program in the field and get feedback from the class in terms of presentation level, meeting objectives, and training effectiveness. If the target audience was correctly pinpointed and the program scope correctly defined, little modification should be needed. If modifications are needed, make them after pilot programs are complete.

10. Continue to monitor training effectiveness and document employee performance and program benefits.

## Audio Aids

Purely audio aids include tape recorders, radios, commercial recordings, and public address systems.

### Tape recorders

A tape recorder can be used many ways:

• One safety professional, using a battery-operated recorder, dictates a running commentary while photographing safe or unsafe operating conditions, new processes or equipment that require subsequent study. This method proves easier than writing notes. After being edited, the tape is used with the slides to make up a training tool.

• A tape recorder can record minutes in safety meetings, valuable discussion in training sessions, and on-the-job interviews which may prove useful later for bulletins, newsletters, and future meetings.

• Tape recorders and dictating machines are frequently used to record speeches and conferences. Pedestal or table microphones generally pick up extraneous sounds, as well as the desired ones; also it is sometimes difficult to identify a speaker. Those planning such discussion recordings should arrange for one-at-a-time discussion or for placement of recorders at different parts of the discussion table. It is a good idea to mention names frequently as one addresses a conferee, and to rephrase discussion points that may be unclear, either to meaning or to clarity (someone else talking at the same time, for example).

• A safe, efficient job procedure can be taped. Sufficient time is allowed for performing each task. The trainee, with the tape player nearby, follows the instructions as he performs the work.

A tape recording can be used with slides or other visual training material and used individually to train new employees at a remote location—for example, one restaurant of a chain of restaurants.

Foreign languages can be recorded on a tape for instruction of non-English-speaking employees. If audiovisuals are to accompany presentations that are given in two or more languages, it is best that they be strictly pictorial, having no languages written or printed on them.

• A polished speaker can even use a tape recorder to "argue" with himself" at meetings. This requires close timing.

### Radio

Radio can serve as a medium to promote accident prevention through scheduled programs on various aspects of home, traffic, and community safety. Spot announcements concerned with traffic safety, for instance, commonly are broadcast at frequent intervals by local stations during long holiday periods such as the Labor Day weekend.

### Commercial recordings

Music, special sound effects, and even dramatic episodes on commercial recordings can be added to safety talks, slide scripts, and the like, to give a professional touch.

### Public address systems

A public address system is a useful tool for making safety announcements, directing emergency evacuations, and perhaps even publicizing unusual safety achievements.

There is some question as to whether public address systems should be used to broadcast safety messages on the job. Some administrators feel that music or messages might prove dangerously distracting to workers at moving machinery or on other work which requires full attention. This technique may not be effective and may even draw complaints if used excessively.

Portable public address systems have been used by supervisors and safety professionals as an aid in on-the-job meetings, either to help overcome extraneous noise (Fig. 14–14), or to create a dramatic effect.

## References

Bowman, William J. *Graphic Communication.* New York, N.Y., John Wiley & Sons, Inc., 1967.

Byrness, S.J. "Corporate AV: Ups and Downs." *Audio-Visual Communications,* June 1977, p. 38

General Services Administration, National Archives and Record Service, National Audiovisual Center, Washington, D.C. 20409. "List of Audiovisual Materials Produced by the United States Government for Industrial Safety," 1980.

Horn, George F. *Visual Communication: Bulletin Boards, Exhibits, Visual Aids.* Worcester, Mass. 01608, Davis Publications, Inc., 1973.

Junghans, F.G. "Safety Training with Audiovisuals." *National Safety News,* January 1975, p. 62.

Kaiz, Gerald H. "Using Videotape To Conduct Safety Training." *National Safety News,* January 1980, pp. 45–50.

Konikow, R.B., and McElroy, F.E. *Communications for the Safety Professional.* Chicago, Ill., National Safety Council, 1975.

Mambert, W.A. *Presenting Technical Ideas.* New York, N.Y. John Wiley and Sons, 1968.

McLuhan, Marshall. *Understanding Media: The Extensions of Man.* New York, N.Y., McGraw-Hill Book Co., 1964.

"Multiply Your Images: How and Why To Get Started in Multi-Image." Rochester, N.Y., Eastman Kodak Company, 1979.

National Audio-Visual Association, Inc. 3150 Spring St., Fairfax, Va. 22030. *Audio-Visual Equipment Directory.*

National Education Association, Dept. of Audio-Visual Instruction, 1201 16th St. N.W., Washington, D.C. 20036.

National Safety Council, 444 N. Michigan Ave., Chicago, Ill. 60611.
*Communications for the Safety Professional.*
"Guide for Audiovisual Aid Development."
Industrial Data Sheets
*Motion Pictures for Safety, 556.*
*Nonprojected Visual Aids, 564.*
*Photography for the Safety Professional, 619.*
*Posters, Bulletin Boards, and Safety Displays, 616.*
*Projected Still Pictures, 574.*
"National Directory of Safety Films."
*Poster Directory.*

Shefter, Harry. *How to Prepare Talks and Oral Reports,* Pocket Books, Inc., 1 West 39th St. New York, N.Y. 10018.

U.S. Office of Education, Bureau of Adult and Vocational Education, 400 Maryland Ave. SW., Washington, D.C. 20202.

(Other data books and pamphlets are available from distributors and manufacturers of cameras, films, and other visual media equipment. Trade journals in the fields of photography, education, sales management, advertising, and training also contain excellent information.)

# Office
# Safety

# Chapter
# 15

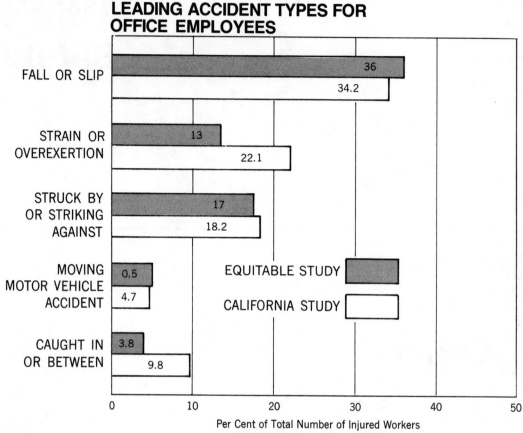

## LEADING ACCIDENT TYPES FOR OFFICE EMPLOYEES

FALL OR SLIP — 36 / 34.2

STRAIN OR OVEREXERTION — 13 / 22.1

STRUCK BY OR STRIKING AGAINST — 17 / 18.2

MOVING MOTOR VEHICLE ACCIDENT — 0.5 / 4.7

CAUGHT IN OR BETWEEN — 3.8 / 9.8

EQUITABLE STUDY

CALIFORNIA STUDY

Per Cent of Total Number of Injured Workers

FIG. 15–1.—A comparison of two studies of accidents occurring in the office worker population.

Office safety programs are necessary for several reasons:

• Many large organizations today consist almost entirely of office workers (insurance companies and banks are good examples). Accidental injuries are just as painful, severe, and expensive to office workers as to production workers. Unless an organization has an effective office safety program, however, accidental injuries are far more likely to occur.

• An injury to an office worker can break the safety record of a manufacturing plant just as effectively as can an injury to a production worker. In the aerospace industry, for example, the injury frequency rate for office workers sometimes has been greater than for production workers.

• A company safety program cannot be fully effective if it covers only a portion of a company's employees. A safety program that is not vigorously pursued in company offices probably will not be vigorously pursued in the factory, shop, or plant. If office workers are exempt, then production workers often feel that following rules to avoid hazards is an unnecessary burden, and, perhaps, an unfair exercise of authority by management. Exempt office workers seldom understand the importance of safety and may scoff at or criticize production-oriented safety activities, especially in front of production employees.

• To emphasize what was written in Chapters 3

## TABLE 15–A

### DISABLING ACCIDENTS FROM FALLS IN OFFICE WORK

| Equitable Life—8,000 employees (a eight-year study) | Disabling Accidents | Days Lost |
|---|---|---|
| *In hallways and work areas, caused by running, slipping, tripping over wires, desk drawers, file cabinet drawers, etc.* | 53 | 553 |
| *From chairs* | 21 | 120 |
| *Stairs* | 16 | 117 |
| *Escalators or elevators* | 8 | 55 |
| **Total** | 98 | 845 |

| California Survey—1,000,000 employees (a one-year study) | Disabling Accidents By Category | Totals |
|---|---|---|
| *FALLS* | | 4,360 |
| *FALLS OR SLIPS ON STAIRS OR STEPS* | 752 | |
| *FALLS FROM OTHER ELEVATIONS* | 370 | |
| *FALLS ON THE SAME LEVEL* | 3,238 | |

and 5, the safety professional who expects to "sell safety" to management must get management involved in a total safety program—get them involved in preventing office accidents as well as production accidents. Any management that preaches safety must also practice it.

### Seriousness of Office Injuries

One reason that office safety programs are not more widespread is that many people believe office injuries are inconsequential.

This is not true. One aerospace firm, for example, paid out $102,000 over eight years at one facility just for injuries incurred by people falling out of chairs. Approximately 25,000 people worked at the plant, and more than half were office workers. Of the 14 chair accidents that occurred, the two worst totaled $97,000. Not only are medical and wage replacement benefits costly for long-time accidents, but there are also hidden costs such as the loss of productivity. (See Chapter 7, "Accident Investigation, Analysis, and Costs.")

Studies made by the State of California Department of Industrial Relations, and the Equi-table Life Assurance Society of the U.S. (see "References"), show that this is not an isolated incident. (Fig. 15–1).

The California State Department of Industrial Relations in 1978 analyzed reports filed by more than 3000 California employers (together employing more than one million office workers) on disabling injuries to employees. When extrapolated to nationwide scale, on-the-job office accidents would annually amount to about 40,000 disabling injuries at a *direct cost* (indemnity benefits and medical expenses) of about $100 million. (This figure does not include any indirect costs for employers, workers, or the nation.)

Of the many accidental workdeaths occurring to office workers, approximately, half are work-connected automobile accidents. However, this amount can be significantly reduced by using a defensive driving program, (DDC), such as that developed by the National Safety Council.

"Office worker" is defined in the California study as "a person primarily engaged in performing clerical, administrative, or professional tasks indoors in an office at the employer's place of business." This definition does *not* cover salespersons, claims adjusters, social workers, medical

## TABLE 15–B

## PERCENTAGE OF DISABLING WORK INJURIES*
## AND ILLNESSES TO OFFICE WORKERS BY
## OCCUPATION AND LENGTH OF SERVICE

| Occupation | Total Disabling Work Injuries | Length of Service | | | | | |
|---|---|---|---|---|---|---|---|
| | | 1 mo. | 2 mo. | 4-6 mo. | 3-5 yrs. | 6-10 yrs. | 11-20 yrs. |
| Professional Technical & Kindred | 1,418 | 1.5 | 2.5 | 7.5 | 17.7 | 15.7 | 12.1 |
| Managers & Administrators | 2,000 | 1.4 | 2.4 | 3.4 | 18.1 | 16.0 | 18.9 |
| Clerical & Kindred | 12,858 | 2.1 | 4.3 | 4.0 | 17.1 | 15.7 | 9.2 |
| Totals | 16,276 | 2.0 | 3.9 | 8.2 | 17.2 | 15.7 | 11.0 |

*These figures are true only for the 1978 California Study.

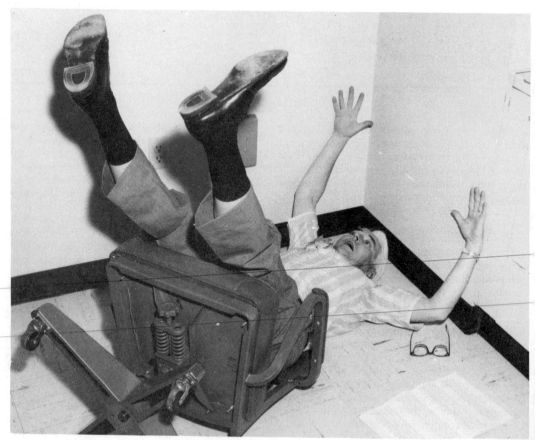

FIG. 15–2—Falling from a chair is extremely dangerous because a person is totally unprepared. It can be bad because in falling backward, the head is  exposed to serious injury.

and teaching personnel (other than clerical or administrative), and certain stock, order, and inventory clerks. The California study did not cover employees of the federal government, maritime workers, and railroad workers in interstate commerce. The Equitable Life Assurance Society study, on the other hand, *did* include salespeople, claims adjusters, medical personnel, and supply and warehouse personnel. The insurance company study covered approximately 8000 employees of one company working in one building, about 5 percent of whom were maintenance personnel. During the eight year study period, the injury frequency rate was 2.3, and severity rate was 15 for the office workers, using ANSI Z16.1 method of calculation; see Chapter 6, "Accident Records and Incidence Rates." The average days charged per disabling injury was 5.9.

See Tables 15–A and –B for details of the studies.

## Complacency—prime cause of injury

Office injuries may seem to be inconsequential because they lack dramatic impact.

The person who is injuried falling backward from a chair (Fig. 15–2) seems to merit little sympathy or attention. The image of an office worker slipping and crashing to the floor on his back seems amusing to some people.

Industrial accidents are commonly considered to occur more frequently and with greater severity—amputations, lost eyes, and broken bones—than office accidents. But who is likely to be absent from work the longer? The office worker who sustains a severe compression fracture of one or more lumbar vertebrae from a bad fall, or the production worker whose hand is amputated?

Complacency—the attitude that office accidents do not amount to much—is one of the prime causes of office accidents. The average office worker gives little thought to safety because office work is not perceived as being hazardous.

On the other hand, the well-instructed worker in a plant manufacturing flammable, toxic chemicals knows that it is a risky business—and understands why safe procedures must be used and safety equipment worn. The worker's safety attitude and training is his best defense. As a result, the production department may have less accidents than the plant office.

The office worker, therefore, has to be informed of the hazards to be guarded against, and of safe work procedures that must be used. The employee must also be shown that management provides a safe environment and safe equipment to encourage a proper safety attitude. The worker must be willing to adopt safe procedures, and be encouraged to do so. Even more important, office supervisors must understand the nature of office hazards and unsafe practices and take necessary preventive measures.

## Who gets injured?

The California and the Equitable Life studies pointed to whom most injuries occurred, and how they occurred.

**New surroundings.** These studies showed the importance of teaching office workers to look for new hazards and to correct them. It was also found that there was a substantial increase in the number of injuries in the first year a company moved into a new office building. The change upset established routines and presented unknown hazards. Even going to and from work became more hazardous as employees had to explore new routes.

**New and young employees.** A recent California study (1978) has found that the new and younger employee does not have a higher accident rate than the longer-employed and older worker—at least in California (see Table 15–B). In California, office employees who had been on the job for 1 and 2 months had an injury percentage rate of 2.0 and 3.9, respectively. At the same time, those that had been employed for 3 to 5 years had the highest accident percentage rate (17.2 percent). As for age, the study showed that only 3 percent of the injuries occurred in the 18 to 19 years bracket.

**Sex of employee.** In the 1978 California study, 70 percent of the disabling injuries occurred to women, who comprised 68 percent of the office labor force. Compare this percentage with that of California industry—women accounted for 22.6 percent of the job injuries, even though they represented about 41 percent of the work force.

The 1978 study shows that for office occupations, the estimated disabling work injury rate for women was very close to the injury rate for men. The rate was approximately 7.8 disabling injuries per 1000 women employed in office work compared with 7.1 for the same number of men. This

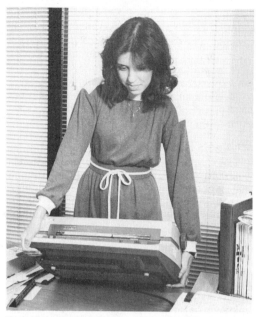

FIG. 15–3.—Moving office equipment should be left to the properly designated personnel. Even a typewriter can slip, fall, and cause serious injury. A strained back can also result.

slips and falls. The 1978 California survey showed that 39 percent of all disabling injuries to women were caused by falls and slips; men sustained only 22 percent of their injuries from this source.

• Most chair falls came when a person was sitting down, rising, or moving about on a chair. A few were caused by people leaning back and tilting their chairs in the office or cafeteria, or putting their feet up on the desk. Although stairs seem more hazardous than chairs, people seem to recognize the hazard and are more cautious. Furthermore, people are not as often exposed to the stair hazard as they are to a chair.

• A final category was falls from elevations, caused by standing on chairs or other office furniture and by falls from ladders, loading docks, or other miscellaneous elevations. These falls (not including stairs) accounted for approximately two percent of the disabling injuries in the California study, whereas falls on stairs accounted for almost 5 percent.

**Over-exertion.** Almost three-fourths of the strain or exertion mishaps occurred while employees were trying to move objects—carrying or otherwise moving office machines (Fig. 15–3), supplies, file drawers and trays, office furniture,

differs greatly from the 1963 California study where the injury rate for women was twice the injury rate for men.

The injury statistics the California study were similar to the Equitable study, which was compiled from carefully made reports. The rate of injury accidents per thousand male employees was about the same as it was for female employees. However, the rate of total days lost from disabling injuries was 2½ to 3 times higher for the men than for the women.

## Types of disabling-injury accidents

**Falls** are the most common office accident, and account for the most disabling injuries, as shown in both surveys, Fig. 15–1. They cause from 2 to 2½ times as high a disabling injury rate among office as among nonoffice employees. Falls were the most severe office accident and were responsible for 55 percent of the total days lost because of injuries.

The most common accidents resulting in injury occurring to women office workers were

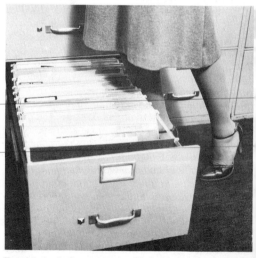

FIG. 15–4.—It does not seem likely that someone would trip over something as obvious as a drawer left open, but it can happen easily enough if a person is distracted.

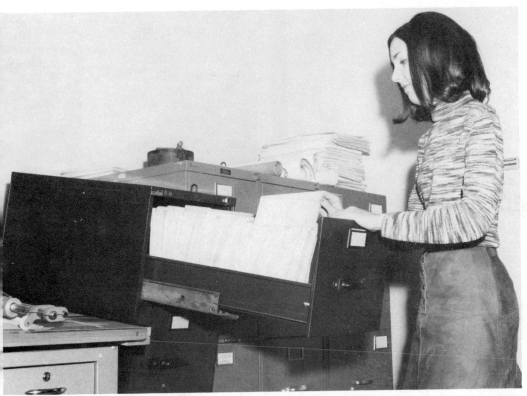

FIG. 15–5.—Pulling a file drawer out, even the top one can be hazardous, particularly if the lower drawers are empty causing a top-heavy condition.

heavy books, or other loads. Often, the employees were making unauthorized moves without the knowledge or consent of their supervisors.

A significant number resulted from the sudden or awkward movement of the employee himself, and did not involve any specific agency. Reaching, stretching, twisting, bending down, and straightening-up were often associated with these injuries.

Striking against objects caused approximately seven percent of the office injuries in both studies discussed here. Two out of three of these injuries were the result of bumping into doors, desks, file cabinets, open drawers, and even other people (Fig. 15–4) while walking. Hitting open desk drawers or the desk itself, while seated at a desk, or striking open file drawers while bending down or straightening-up caused most of the rest of these injuries.

Other incidents of striking against objects included bumping against sharp objects such as office machines, spindle files, staples, and pins. Also, cuts a worker would receive in handling paper, file drawers, and supplies often became infected.

Objects striking workers accounted for about 11 percent of injuries to office workers in both studies. Most of these injuries were sustained when the employee was struck by a falling object—file cabinets that became overbalanced when two or more drawers were open at the same time, file drawers that fell when pulled out too far, (Figs. 15–5 and -6), office machines and other objects that employees dropped on their feet when attempting a move, or typewriters that fell from a folding pedestal or rolling stand.

In addition, a number of employees were struck by doors being opened from the other side.

**423**

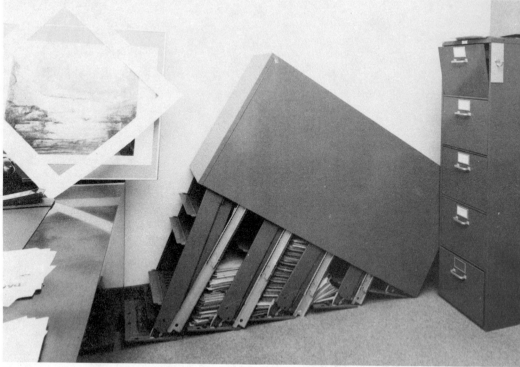

Fig. 15-6.—An excellent view of what can happen when file drawers fall.

Office supplies or other material and equipment sliding from shelves or cabinet tops caused a few injuries in this classification.

**Caught in or between.** The final major classification was accidents where the worker was caught in or between machinery or equipment. Mostly, this was getting caught in a drawer, door, or window. However, a number of employees got caught in duplicating machines, copying machines, addressing machines, and fans. Several got their fingers under the knife edge of a cutter.

**Miscellaneous office accidents** included foreign substances in the eye, spilled hot coffee or other hot liquid, burns from fire, insect bites, and electric shocks.

## Controls for Office Hazards

To control office accidents, the first necessary steps are to eliminate hazards or reduce exposure to them. The best times to take these steps is when the office is laid out, when equipment is purchased, or when office procedures are set up.

### Layout and ambience

Offices should be laid out for efficiency, convenience, and safety. The principles of work flow apply to offices as well as to factories.

An office machine should not be placed on the edge of a table or desk. Machines that tend to creep during operation should be secured either directly to the desk or table or placed on a nonslip pad. And, particularly, typewrites on folding pedestals should be fastened to the pedestal.

Heavy equipment and files should be placed against walls or columns; files can also be placed against railings. File cabinets should be bolted together or fastened to the floor or wall so that they cannot be tipped over (see Figs. 15-5 and -6). If they are moved, they can be temporarily fastened together by stout adhesive tape and then rebolted as soon as possible.

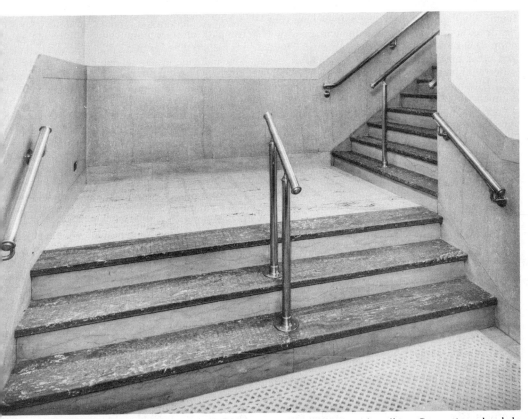

FIG. 15–7.—Heavy duty, slip-resistant stair treads and sturdy handrails facilitate safe walking. Contrasting colors help delineate each step.

*Courtesy The R. C. Musson Rubber Co.*

Floors in office are one of the major causes of office accidents. They should be as durable and maintenance free as possible. Floor finishes should be selected for anti-slip qualities. Well-maintained carpet provides good protection against slips and falls. Defective tiles or boards or carpet should be repaired immediately. Worn or warped mats under office chairs and rubber or plastic floor mats with curled edges or tears should be replaced or repaired as these conditions can create tripping hazards.

Slipperiness is characteristic of highly polished and extremely hard but unwaxed surfaces such as marble, terrazzo, and steel plates. Slip-resistant floor wax can give these materials a higher coefficient of friction than they already have and can reduce their slipping hazard. However, wax must not be applied so thickly that a smeary coating results. Also, an oil mop should not be used on a wax floor because a soft and smeary coating will result. Chapter 21.

Special anti-slip protection should be used on stairways (Fig. 15–7) and at elevator entrances, and these specially hazardous areas should always be maintained in the best possible condition. Floor mats and runners often provide a better, more slip-resistant walking surface. Their use is discussed in the National Safety Council's Industrial Data Sheet 595, *Floor Mats and Runners.*

Refer to Chapter 21, "Nonemployee Accident Prevention."

**Aisles and stairs.** A suggested minimum width for aisles is four feet. Passages through the work area should be unobstructed. Waste baskets should be kept where people do not trip over

**425**

them. Telephone and electrical outlets should not be placed so that when in use, the wire creates a tripping hazard in passages that people use. These and other obstructions, such as low tables and office equipment should be placed against walls or partitions, under desks or in corners. Stepoffs from one level to another in an office should be avoided. If one exists it should be well marked and guarded with a railing.

File drawers should not open into aisles, particularly narrow ones, unless extra space is provided. Pencil sharpeners and typewriter carriages must not jut out into aisles.

Stairways and exits (including access and discharge) should comply with NFPA 101, *Life Safety Code;* floor and wall openings should comply with ANSI *Safety Requirements for Floor and Wall Openings, Railings, and Toe Boards,* A12.1. Handrails, not less than 30 in. or more than 34 in. (7.5 and 9 m) above the upper surface of the tread, are specified for one side of stairs up to 44 in. (1.1 m) wide, and both sides for stairs wider than 44 in. For stairs wider than 88 in. (2.2 m) add an intermediate (center) rail. (See Fig. 15–7.)

Exits should be frequently checked to be sure that stairways are unobstructed and well illuminated. Exit doors, if locked, shall not require the use of a key for operation from inside the building.

**Doors** are another frequent source of accidents in offices. Glass doors should have some conspicuous design, either painted or decal, about 4½ ft above the floor and centered on the door so that people will not walk into it. (See Chapter 21 for details.)

Safety glass complying with American National Standard Z97.1 should be installed particularly in doors, rather than plate glass. Sometimes local codes specify the type that must be installed.

Solid doors also present a hazard, because they can be approached from both sides at the same time, and one person can be struck when the door opens. Frosted glass in doors gives a view through for accident prevention, but still preserves privacy. Employees should be warned of this hazard and instructed (a) to approach a solid door in the proper manner, that is, out away from the path of an opening door; (b) to reach for the door knob; then, if the door is suddenly opened from the other side, it is the hand that receives the brunt of the impact rather than the face.

Another hazard is the door that opens directly

onto a passageway. If the door opens directly into the path of on-coming traffic, somebody might bump into the edge of the door. If doors that open onto hallways cannot be recessed, they should be protected with short-angled, deflector rails or U shaped guardrails which protrude about 18 in. (46 cm) into the passage way, or the area the swing over can be marked as suggested in the paragraph preceding. Another procedure is to place storage lockers or benches along the wall near the door, which (in effect) recesses the door.

Some offices that have a tile floor rather than some type of carpeting paint white or yellow stripes or apply commercially available tape to floors to separate traffic or to guide people away from a rapidly opening door. The floor in front of a swinging door can also be marked or painted as a warning. A sign could also be posted as warning. As a final precaution, it is good practice to have the door hinges on the upstream side of the traffic that is, on the right hand side as one faces the door from the hallway.

Doors are covered in the *Life Safety Code* NFPA 101.

**Adequate light,** ventilation, washrooms, and other employee services have an important influence on employee morale. Growth of a business sometimes results in installing more desks and other equipment than original plans called for. Overcrowding is bad from the standpoints of both appearance and physiological effect on employees, especially if it overtaxes ventilation facilities. Smaller offices can be made to appear larger and less crowded, if walls, woodwork and furniture placed against the walls are the same color.

Illumination levels recommended by the Illuminating Engineering Society for an office are listed in Table 15–C. Also see especially Chapter 1, "Industrial Buildings and Plant Layout," of the *Engineering and Technology* volume of this Manual.

Employees should not face windows, unshielded lamps, or other sources of glare. Indirect, shielded fluorescent lamps are particularly desirable to produce high levels of illumination without glare.

Walls and other surfaces should conserve light, while avoiding annoying reflections.

If offices depend largely on daylight, employees engaged in the visual tasks should be located near windows. North light is preferred by draftsmen and artists. Ceiling walls and floor act as

## TABLE 15-C  LEVELS OF ILLUMINATION FOR OFFICES

| | Recommended Illumination* (Footcandles) |
|---|---|
| Cartography, designing, detailed drafting . . . . . . . . . . . . . . . . . . . . . | 200 |
| Accounting, auditing, tabulating, bookkeeping, business machine operation, reading poor reproductions, rough layout drafting . . . . . . . . . . . . . . . . . . | 150 |
| Regular office work, reading good reproductions, reading or transcribing handwriting in hard pencil or on poor paper, active filing, index references, mail sorting . . . . . . . . . | 100 |
| Reading or transcribing handwriting in ink or medium pencil on good quality paper, intermittent filing . . . . . . . . . . . . . . . . . . . . . . . . . . . . . . . . . . . . . . . | 70 |
| Reading high-contrast or well-printed material, tasks and areas not involving critical or prolonged seeing such as conferring, interviewing, inactive files, and washrooms . . . . | 30 |
| Corridors, elevators, escalators, stairways . . . . . . . . . . . . . . . . . . . . . . | 20 (or not less than 1/5 level in adjacent areas) |

*Minimum on task at any time.

*From Illuminating Engineering Society.*

secondary large area light sources and if finished with the recommended reflectances, will increase the utilization of light and reduce shadows.

Some accidents may be attributed to poor illumination. However, many less-tangible factors associated with poor illumination are contributing causes of office accidents. Some of these are: direct glare, reflected glare from the work and harsh shadows, all of which hamper seeing.

Excessive visual fatigue itself may be an element leading toward accidents. Accidents may also be prompted by the delayed eye adaptation a person experiences when moving from bright surroundings into dark ones and vice versa. Some accidents which are attributed to an individual's "carelessness" can be traced to difficulty in seeing, from one or more of these mentioned causes.

**Illumination evaluation.** As a uniform means of evaluation, a standard procedure, entitled "How to Make a Lighting Survey" has been developed in cooperation with the U.S. Public Health Service. (This publication is not part of the ANSI standard, *Practice for Office Lighting,* A132.1, but is presented as background material for the use of the standard.) Table 15-C shows the illumination levels recommended by the Illuminating Engineering Society and approved by the American National Standard *Practice for Office Lighting.*

**Ventilation.** Window ventilation is often unsatisfactory compared with comfort (or air) conditioning. Persons near windows may feel cold; those farther away may be warm. This is particularly true in the modern "all-glass" office building. Where there are large interior spaces, forced ventilation usually is needed, if the space is to be used for office purposes.

All mechanical ventilation and comfort conditioning systems require careful planning and installation by experts. Private offices installed around the outer walls of a large office space should not cut off light and ventilation from the other employees.

If fans are used in an office, they should be secure and placed where they cannot fall.

**Electrical.** There should be protection against the electrical equipment hazards in an office. In some cases, the hazard can be avoided completely, such as not using electric-key switches. People have been known to try to pick the locked switch with hair pins or paper clips. Dictating machines, electric typewriters, desk lamps, and other equipment require outlets and extension

**427**

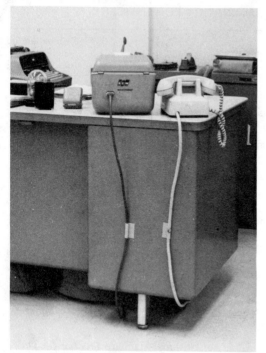

FIG. 15–8.—Clipping or taping electric cords keeps them from being a tripping hazard.

*Courtesy* Trades and Services Newsletter.

cords arranged to avoid tripping hazards.

A sufficient number of outlets (receptacles) should be installed to eliminate the need for extension cords. Cords that are necessary should be clipped to backs of desks or taped down (Fig. 15–8). If cords *must* cross the floor, cover them with rubber channels designed for this purpose.

Outlets should accommodate 3-wire grounding plugs to help prevent electric shock to operators. Floor outlets should be located, if possible, so that they are not tripping hazards, and also should be placed where they will not be accidentally kicked or used as a foot rest. A floor outlet that protrudes above the level of the floor is frequently shielded by a desk or some other piece of furniture. However, when the desk is moved, the outlet becomes an immediate tripping hazard unless it is appropriately covered (see Fig. 15–9). Such floor design is not common any longer; underfloor or cellular floor raceways are usually used in new construction.

Electric equipment in photographic laboratories, particularly, should be grounded because the lab worker is close to both water and electricity in the darkroom.

The use of poorly maintained or unsafe, poor quality non-U.L.-listed coffee makers, radios, lamps, etc., provided by or used by employees particularly in out-of-the-way locations, should be prohibited. Such appliances can create fire and shock hazards.

Cords for electrically operated office machines, fans, lamps, and other equipment should be properly installed and inspected frequently to see whether there are any defects which may cause shocks or burns. Switches should be provided, either in the equipment or in the cords, so that it is not necessary to pull the plugs to shut off the power. Extension cords should be used sparingly but when used they should be free from splices and they should be disconnected by grasping the plug, not by pulling on the cord. The fact that office equipment is operated on 110-volt circuits is no assurance that serious injury will not occur. Fatalities can be caused by current as low as 100 milliamperes if it passes through the vital organs. (See Chapter 15, "Electrical Hazards," in the *Engineering and Technology* Volume.)

Keyed metal light sockets may be especially dangerous when located near plumbing or other grounded equipment. Such sockets should be grounded or replaced by a non-conducting type, such as porcelain, plastic, or rubber. Wall receptacles should be so designed and installed that no current-carrying parts will be exposed, and outlet plates should be kept tight to eliminate possibility of shock or collision injury. Cords should not rest on steam pipes or other hot or sharp metallic surfaces.

In the installation or repair of any electrical equipment, the work should be done by qualified workers using only approved materials. Because defective wiring may constitute both shock and fire hazards, all recommendations of the *National Electrical Code*, NFPA 70, should be observed.

**Materials stored** in offices sometimes cause problems. In general, materials should be stored in areas specifically set aside for the purpose. Whenever the storage area is located, it should be where the traffic patterns are not crossed to reach; also, nothing should be allowed on the floor in a passageway where it could become a tripping hazard.

Materials should be stacked or piled neatly in stable piles that will not fall over. The heaviest and largest pieces should be on the bottom of the pile. Where materials are stored on shelves, the heavy objects should be on the lower shelves. Objects should not be stacked on window sills if there is a danger of breaking the window or falling out.

No smoking should be allowed in mailing, shipping, or receiving rooms, and in other areas where there may be large quantities of loose paper and other combustible material, and in areas where flammable fluids are used, such as duplicating rooms or artists' supply areas.

Flammable and combustible fluids and similar materials should be stored in safety cans, preferably in locked and identified cabinets. Only minor quantities should be left in the office and bulk storage should be in properly constructed fireproof vaults. (See Chapter 16, "Flammable and Combustible Liquids" in the *Engineering and Technology* volume of this Manual.)

### Safe office equipment

A good quality of office furniture not only contributes to the safety of the office but also to its appearance. This, in turn, improves the attitudes of both employees and visitors.

**Chairs,** especially, should be comfortable and sturdily built with a wide enough base to prevent easy tipping. The casters on swivel chairs should be on at least a 20-in. (0.5 m) diameter base, but a 22-in. base is preferred. The casters should be securely fixed to the base of the chair and well constructed because loose or broken casters are a frequent cause of chair falls (Fig. 15–2). About 20 percent of the chair falls in the 1978 California study were due to chair defects.

Adjustment features on chairs should be well designed and well made so that they will work properly. Chairs with poor adjustments should be replaced or fixed so that they are safe.

**Desks and files.** Spring-loaded typing desks should be selected carefully. If some models are opened without due care, the typewriter table will snap out and cause a bruise or a cut.

Also, even if good quality desk and file cabinets are purchased, it is still possible that occasionally one will have a sharp burr or corner on it. Office furniture should be inspected when

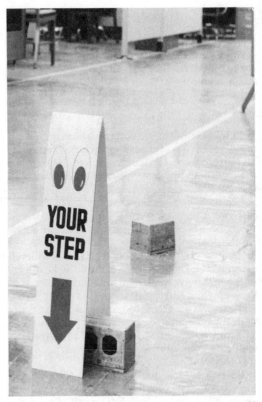

FIG. 15–9.—Although newer offices do not have outlets such that shown here, many older offices still have to contend with hazards such as these.

received and such burrs or corners should be removed immediately.

Drawers on desks and file cabinets should have safety stops.

Purchase office machines, such as rotary files, copying machines, paper cutters, and paper shredders, with well-designed guards.

Glass tops on desks and tables can crack and cause safety hazards. Durable synthetic surfaces are free from this trouble.

A sufficient number of noncombustible waste baskets should be furnished for litter. Also enough safety-type ash trays should be available and they should be large enough and stable enough to safely contain smoking materials.

**Office fans** should have substantial bases and convenient attachments for moving and carrying. If located less than 7 ft (2.1m) from the floor, they

**429**

should be well guarded, front and back, with mesh to prevent the fingers from getting inside the guard.

Many cut fingers have resulted when people try to move fans by grasping the guard, or try to catch falling fans. Fans should not be handled until the power is turned off and the blades stop turning.

**Computers.** If a computer is to be installed in a building that has overhead sprinklers, keep sprinkler protection in service throughout the area, but get advice on necessary protection against both fire and water damage. Actually, water damage is not to be feared as much as previously thought. For one thing, most new computers are less susceptible because of their solid state circuitry. In addition, tests have shown that water does not harm magnetic tape. Most of the damage suffered by computers in a fire results from the heat. One of the best ways to prevent a damaging fire is to keep combustible materials such as paper, tapes, and cards at an absolute minimum in the room with the computer. When safeguarding such an investment, call in a fire protection adviser, as well as a computer installation expert.

**Rolling ladders** and stands used for reaching high storage should have brakes that operate automatically when weight is applied to them. Small step ladders should have nonskid feet.

**Chemical products.** If possible, substitute nontoxic and nonflammable solvents for those used in printing and duplicating or other operations. (Details are given in *Fundamentals of Industrial Hygiene*, part of this Occupational Health Series.) If chlorinated bleaches are purchased for cleaning purposes, make sure that they will not be mixed with strongly acidic or easily oxidized materials. Purchase a good grade of slip-resistant floor wax.

**Purchasing equipment.** As discussed in Chapter 3, p. 78, and Chapter 5, pp. 151-155, the company safety professional should work with the purchasing agent in buying office furniture and equipment. Both should be aware that sometimes office equipment is advertised in such a way that safety features are stressed, but the machines may be delivered without them. Mechanical hazards of heavy office equipment can be ascertained by careful, expert inspection before purchase. These hazards can almost always be eliminated or minimized, although sometimes at substantial expense.

The purchasing department must also be made aware of precautions to be taken in connection with chemicals, dyes, inks, and other supply items. Particular attention should be paid to toxic, irritant or flammable properties. Where hazards are unavoidable, labels and specific instructions for careful handling should be supplied or issued when the material is received.

The purchasing department should gather all pertinent information from the manufacturer on equipment design, and should try to determine the composition of proprietary compounds. This they can forward to the safety professional (or safety department) for an opinion concerning inherent safety hazards before purchasing new equipment or supplies.

**Office machines.** All machines that have external moving parts that could be hazardous should have enforced safety procedures; constant training and retraining of operators is necessary.

Employees should be told that if any office machine gives a shock, appears defective, or if it sparks or smokes—turn it off, pull the plug, and tell the supervisor.

## Printing services

**Larger offset presses.** Check the operation of offset presses. Is the operator putting his fingers on the blanket while the press is in motion? One offset press department had seven finger injury accidents in the first two weeks of operation, all caused by press operators who put their fingers in the running press to remove dirt or other particles from the plate.

Presses should meet all guarding regulations imposed by local, state or provincial, and federal agencies.

The area around the presses should be free from clutter and be well lighted, the flooring should be resilient or rubber mats should be provided to minimize operator fatigue and to prevent slipping.

Only qualified operators should operate presses. Loose clothing and long hair are hazardous around these machines. Low flashpoint flammable liquids or toxic solvents should not be used to clean the presses; office supervisors and press operators should understand the fire and health hazards involved and follow all instructions for

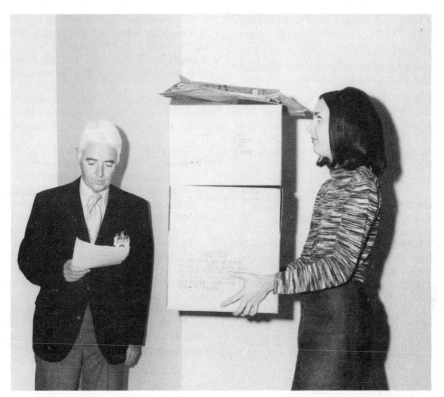

FIG. 15–10.—A person should never carry more than is convenient (*a*) even if light, a stack might hinder vision, and (*b*) a heavy load can cause muscular injury if not handled properly as well as making it difficult to move easily.

*Figs. 15–2, –5, –6, –10, and –11 were taken from "Play It Safe in the Office," Lewis News, Lewis Research Center, NASA, Cleveland, Ohio. (Used with permission.)*

afe use, storage, and disposal of such flammable nd/or toxic substances.

**Gathering and stitching machines.** Guards hould be installed on open sprockets and collec- or chain drives of gathering and wire stitching (or tapling) machines to protect employees from and and body injury. The operating arm on the nd of the gathering machine should be guarded.

Hinged drop-guards should be installed to ·over any exposed operating mechanism which ·reates nipping hazards under the machine and .long the working area where operators fill the ·ockets. The floors and work platform at this area hould be covered with nonskid material.

Operators should be trained to open signatures n the middle and place them on the saddle or rod

between the hooks on the moving chain. If the hook is not put on the rod or chain correctly, *no attempt should be made to straighten it out until the machine has been shut off.* The machine should also be shut down when threading stitcher heads, making any adjustments or removing jams.

**Folding machines.** Here are specific points to be stressed for safe operation of folding machines:

1. Before jammed paper is pulled from the machine, shut the motor off to avoid getting hands in the feed rollers.

2. Finger clearance at the folding knife should be checked before pulling out paper, putting tape on rollers, or adjusting plates and roller pressure.

**431**

3. Workers should walk down the steps of folder feeder platforms facing forward, never backward.

4. On large-size folders, all steps and platforms should be protected by railings.

Defective staples protruding from reports or booklets should be removed to avoid cuts from them while books are being jogged, trimmed, or wrapped. Workers should be trained to cup their hands over the work when removing defective wire staples.

Employees engaged in this operation should wear eye or face protection, and passers-by should be protected against flying staples by screens or by isolation of this work.

## Enforced safety procedures

Because the major category of office accidents is slips and falls, running in offices, for whatever reason, should be prohibited.

A number of office accidents can be prevented if everybody walking in passageways would keep to the right. As discussed under Doors earlier in this chapter, collisions at doors also can be prevented if people do not stand directly in front of the door, but away from the path of its swing when they go to open it. (Details were discussed earlier in this chapter.)

People carrying material must be sure they can see over and around it when walking through the office (Fig. 15–10). They should not carry stacks of materials on stairs; they should use the elevator, if available, if not, make two trips. People should not have both arms loaded when using stairs; one hand should be free to use the handrail.

When using stairs, outside at night or in a dimly lit area, workers should be instructed to go single file, to keep to the right, and to always hold the handrail. People should not crowd or push on stairways; they should pay attention to where they are going. Commonly, falls on stairs occur when the person is talking, laughing, and turning to friends while going downstairs.

Other safety rules for stairs include: do not congregate on stairs or landings, and do not stand near doors at the head or foot of stairways.

Good housekeeping is essential to prevent falls. Littering should not be allowed. Spilled liquids must be wiped up immediately, and pieces of paper, paper clips, rubber bands, pencils, and other loose objects must be picked up as soon as they are spotted.

Broken glass should be swept up immediately. It should not be placed loose in a waste container, but it should be wrapped in heavy paper and marked BROKEN GLASS. Glass which shatters into fine pieces can be picked up with damp paper towels.

Tripping hazards, such as defective floors, rugs, floor mats, should be reported to the maintenance department and fixed immediately.

**Chair falls.** Habits that lead to chair falls (Fig. 15–2) must be discouraged. Scooting across the floor while sitting on a chair should be forbidden. Leaning sideways from the chair to pick up objects on the floor is dangerous and should be discouraged. Leaning back in the chair and placing the feet on the desk should be discouraged.

People should seat themselves properly in their chairs. They should form the habit of placing a hand behind them to make sure the chair is in place. Sitting down on the edge of the seat rather than in the center, or backing too far without looking, or kicking the chair out from under can result in a sudden fall to the floor. Standing on a chair to reach an overhead object is particularly dangerous and must be forbidden.

**Filing cabinets,** as discussed earlier in this chapter, are a major cause of injuries including bumped heads from getting up too quickly under open drawers, mashed fingers from closing drawers improperly, and hand injuries and strains from moving the cabinets around.

Some precautions are necessary against these accidents.

• First, people should never close file drawers with their feet or any other part of their body. They should use the drawer handle to close the cabinet, making sure their fingers are not curled over the edge when the drawer closes. All file drawers should be closed immediately after use.

• Second, only one file drawer in the cabinet should be opened at one time in order to prevent the cabinet from toppling over. As previously indicated, where possible, file cabinets should be bolted together or otherwise secured to safeguard against this chance of human failure.

• Third, when one person has a file drawer open, he should warn other persons working in the area so that they do not turn around or straighten up quickly and bump or trip over an open drawer (see Fig. 15–4).

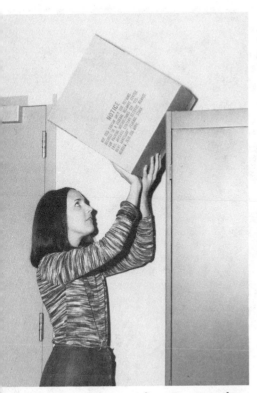

FIG. 15–11.—Store boxes, records, equipment, and any other item that needs storage in their proper designated place. Do not put them on top of lockers.

• Fourth, climbing on open file drawers must be forbidden.

• Fifth, small tools used in filing areas are tripping hazards when left in passageways. Any person who sees one out of place should put it where it cannot cause a fall.

• Sixth, filing personnel should wear rubber finger guards to eliminate cut fingers from metal fasteners or paper edges.

Desks or files should never be moved by office personnel; they should be moved by maintenance workers preferably using special dollies or trucks made for such moving. In general, furniture should not be rearranged without authorization or checking with office management. When desks or cabinets are moved, thought should be given to floor obstructions and necessary aisle space before making the move. When a telephone terminal box on the floor or electrical outlet box is exposed after moving furniture, the box should be marked with a tripping hazard sign until it is removed (Fig. 15–9). The outlet must be removed and, if it is needed, relocate it; it is far cheaper to do this than to pay for a fall.

Electric cords are for temporary use only. If laid under rugs, they sometimes come out because of traffic movement and form tripping hazards. New outlets should be installed to eliminate the necessity for extension cords.

**Materials storage.** There are a number of precautions to be taken when storing materials. Neat storage makes it easier to find and recover materials without dropping or knocking over other materials. Supervisors must keep employees from stacking boxes, papers, and other heavy objects on file cabinets, desks, and window ledges, or from placing these materials carelessly on shelves so that they could spill off like in an avalanche (Fig. 15–11). If heavy objects spill toward a window, the glass might even break and cause a serious accident.

Card index files, dictionaries, or other heavy objects should be kept off the top of file cabinets and other high furniture. Movable objects such as flower pots, vases, and bottles should not be allowed on window sills or ledges.

Razor blades, thumb tacks, and other sharp objects should not be thrown loosely into drawers. They should be carefully boxed. Blades and points should be kept stuck in foamed-polystyrene blocks.

**Other hazards.** Some additional hazards are as follows: (a) never allow a spindle (spike) file in the office, (b) never store pencils in a glass on the desk with points outward, (c) never leave a knife or scissors on a desk with the point toward the user, and never hand sharp-pointed objects to anyone, point first, (d) paper cutters should be equipped with a guard that affords maximum protection (bar guards or single-rod barriers found in some cutters are not considered full protection), and (e) do not leave glass objects on the edge of desks or tables where they can easily be pushed off.

Office machinery should be operated only by authorized persons. This was discussed in an earlier section.

Some offices have an employee lounge or eating area that has a hot plate for brewing coffee and/or a microwave oven for warming lunches.

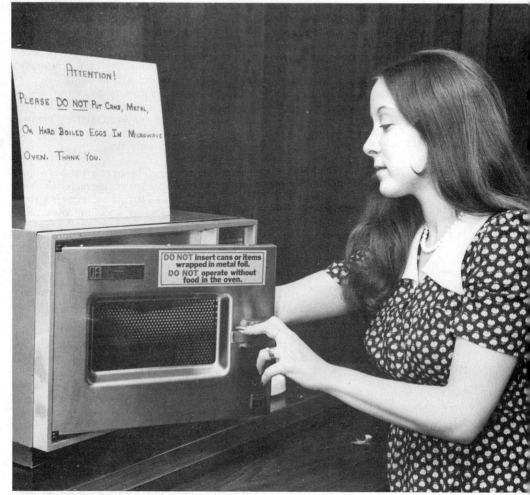

FIG. 15–12.—Some offices have hot plates and/or microwave ovens to allow the employees to warm up a hot beverage o lunch. Signs should be posted to use only opened containers, and not to put metal objects or food wrapped in metal foil in microwave oven.

Spilled beverages can be a burning and a tripping hazard. Microwave ovens must be properly used (Fig. 15–12). (See the discussion in Chapter 18 under Food Service.)

**Office supervisors** should make sure that all materials are kept in their proper places. All litter must be placed in waste baskets, and all drawers not being used must be kept closed.

Supervisors are just as responsible for training their people in the safe procedure as they are in

training them for efficiency.

Supervisors should encourage employees t report all broken chairs, or missing casters, stuc drawers, cracked glass, and other hazards fo correction. A policy of immediate correction o these defects should be followed.

### Fire protection

**Fire hazards.** Solvent-soaked or oily rags use for cleaning duplicating equipment should b kept in a metal safety container. Smoking shoul

**434**

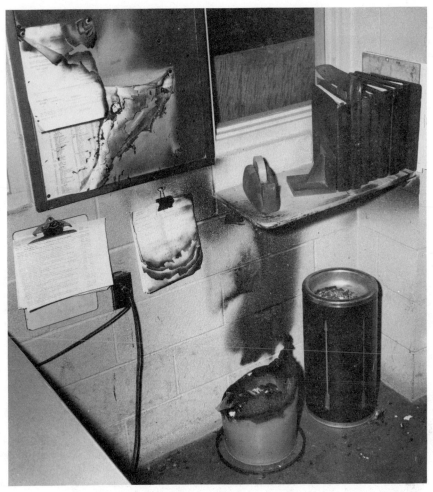

Fig. 15–13.—Still-warm ashes from smoking materials were dumped into an office wastebasket that contained paper—with these results.

*Courtesy* Printing and Publishing Newsletter.

be prohibited within 10 ft (3 m) of where flammable solvents are used in duplicating or any other office operation. Solvents should not be handled carelessly because there is danger of splashing them in the eyes.

Never allow smoking on elevators.

Do not throw matches or cigarettes into waste baskets; the contents are usually very combustible (Fig. 15–13).

Procedures should be established in order that cleaning and maintenance personnel avoid collecting possible smoldering combustible material from ash trays in other combustible containers, such as cardboard boxes or cloth bags.

Some waste containers made from plastic or other flame-resistant material may actually be combustible if subjected to fire or intense heat. If such combustion occurs, dangerous toxic gases and dense smoke may be generated that can easily endanger a whole office. In order to avert this hazard, metal or fire-safe tested materials, designed to contain the fire should be used.

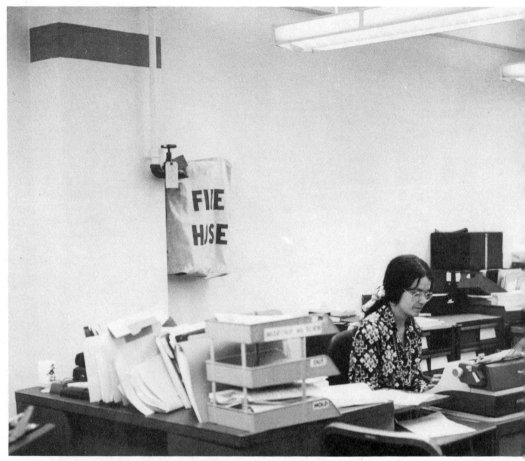

FIG. 15–14.—Fire hose in office areas is identified by bright red stripe over the location, whether protected by a cabinet or canvas cover. Because this type of hose rots easily, water should never be turned on except in a fire emergency.

**Fire extinguishers.** Portable fire extinguishers in a fully charged operable condition should be kept in their designated places at all times when they are not used. (See Chapter 17, "Fire Protection," in the *Engineering and Technology* volume of this Manual, for correct type of extinguishers for specific office hazard areas.)

Employees, in general, should know what to do in case of fire.

It is important that certain employees be trained to operate extinguishers and fire hoses if provided (Fig. 15–14), and know how to react in case of fire or other emergency. (Panic and confusion can be as dangerous as flame and smoke.)

When a fire is discovered, an employee should do three things: (*a*) turn in the alarm (no matter how small the fire is), (*b*) alert fellow workers, and (*c*) if trained to do so, use the proper firefighting equipment.

**Emergency plan.** Every office should have a written emergency plan. Monitors should be appointed in every area to guide people safely out of the building. Every department should be assigned a specific route—and also an alternate in case the exit is blocked. A surprise fire drill may save lives in an emergency situation in the future.

When the alarm sounds, fire monitors should

direct the show, but every employee must play his part. The group should move calmly along in a businesslike manner, without hurrying or pushing, and wait on a different floor or outside the building for the signal to return. In a real emergency, the officials in charge would authorize return to the building. (See Chapter 16, "Planning for Emergencies").

## Safety Organization in the Office

The supervisor is, of course, the key person in the office safety program. However, even the hardest-working supervisor will have difficulty maintaining full-time interest in safety all alone. The office safety committee can serve as a work horse in maintaining interest in the accident prevention program, but it cannot substitute for good management.

**Safety committee** In planning an office safety program, representation on the safety committee should be on the same basis as that of any other company department or division. The office should be on the inspection itinerary of the company's safety person. The office supervisor should accompany the safety inspector on every inspection, along with an office safety committee member. (See Chapter 4 for inspection procedures.)

The committee assists all supervisors in maintaining safety, reporting directly to the safety director or whoever is in charge of the program. Along with the department head, it can make periodic inspections of the office to look for accident or fire hazards. It makes recommendations, many of them based on suggestions from supervisors and other employees. It also can help prepare and revise company safety rules.

Often the committee is in charge of office-wide communication and incentive programs designed to maintain peak interest in safety, using such means as posters, bulletins, and contests.

The organization of the office safety committee can be the same as that of the company and joint safety committees discussed in Chapter 3, p. 87.

**Accident records** are absolutely necessary if a safety program is to succeed. Not only do accident investigations and analysis of records spotlight problems that must be corrected, but the records show whether or not progress is being made in accident prevention.

Office employees, like plant workers, should report every accident, no matter how minor the injury. The reports should be detailed, and made as quickly as possible following the accident or near accident. Unsafe conditions or procedures that are indicated in the reports should be corrected as quickly as possible, because near-miss accidents are warnings of worse accidents to come.

Records are the concrete foundation of the safety structure. They tell the "who, what, when, why, and how" of accidents in your office—and help you to prevent repeat performances. Accurate records also provide guidelines on which company insurance rates are based.

The average office will not have enough major injuries to warrant extensive investigation and analysis. However, it's urgent that records be kept to pinpoint problems and prevent future accidents.

If, for instance, a large number of falls are injuring workers, supervisors can double-check possible hazards and devote special attention to the problem in meetings and other communications.

Standard report forms are available. They were discussed in Chapter 6, "Accident Records and Incidence Rates." Accident investigation was discussed in Chapters 4 and 7.

**Instruction.** In order to develop proper safety attitudes, safety instructions should be properly given to new office employees, regardless of age. The personnel or industrial relations department can provide an accident prevention brochure or a set of printed rules. They should also arrange for all explanations of procedures as quickly as possible during the employee's early work days. Motivation and training were covered in Chapters 10 and 11 and 9, respectively.

Unfamiliar surroundings, new equipment, or altered work tasks increase the likelihood of accidents, even among veteran employees. Therefore, these people too should be instructed upon entering a new job. There should be specific instructions for each piece of equipment. No one should ever be permitted to use a machine unless he has been fully instructed in its operation, and also he should know the location and use of fire equipment as well as how to summon medical aid.

Instruction for supervisors in safe office operation is necessary because they are likely to have the same lack of recognition of accident potentials as the employees. However, prevention of accidents requires the dedicated vigilance of the supervisor throughout every working day. If he fails to carry out this function, accidents due to unsafe acts by his employees will continue, undiminished.

In developing a good attitude toward safe behavior, it is important to promote off-the-job safety also. Safe attitudes and behavior are not merely "put on" when an employee enters the office, and "taken off" when he walks out the front door. (See Chapter 11 for details.)

**Good example.** All office employees who must enter production areas where safety hats, eye protection, and hearing protection are necessary should be provided with these items and should be required to wear them. Every employee who visits the plant should have a card of the general safety rules that apply to the plant, and should be familiar with them. The same requirement should be enforced for all visitors. Safety rules should apply to everyone if the program is to be successful.

**Full management backing.** Finally, to repeat what has been said in previous chapters, a company safety program cannot succeed unless it has the wholehearted backing of its top management. The supervisor must know that his accident prevention performance is watched and that good performance is appreciated. The Council's *Supervisors Safety Manual* has some good information that can be used.

## References

American National Standards Institute, 1430 Broadway, New York, N.Y. 10018.
   *Performance Specifications and Methods of Test for Safety Glazing Material Used in Buildings*, Z97.1.
   *Practice for Office Lighting*, A132.1.
   *Safety Requirements for Floor and Wall Openings, Railings, and Toe Boards*, A12.1.

Baldwin, Doris. "Caution: Office Zone." *Job Safety and Health*, Vol. 4, No. 2 (Feb. 1976).

"How Safe Is Your Office," *National Safety News*, Vol. 112, No. 4 (Oct. 1975).

Kiefer, Norvin C. "Office Safety," *Journal of Occupational Medicine*, Vol. 9, No. 11 (Nov. 1967).

"Industry's Orphan—Office Safety," *Environmental Control Management* (Dec. 1969).

National Fire Protection Assn., 470 Atlantic Ave., Boston, Mass. 02210.
   *Life Safety Code*, NFPA 101 (ANSI A9.1).
   *National Electrical Code* NFPA 70.

National Safety Council, 444 N. Michigan Ave., Chicago, Ill. 60611.
   Industrial Data Sheets
         *Electric Cords and Fittings*, 385.
         *Escalators*, 516.
         *Evacuation System for High-Rise Buildings*, 656.
         *Falls on Floors*, 495.
         *Flammable Liquids in Small Containers*, 532.
         *Floor Mats and Runners*, 595.
         *Off-the-Job Safety*, 601.
         *Power Lawn Mowers*, 464.
   *Motor-Fleet Safety Manual.*
   "A Safety Handbook for Office Supervisors,"
   *Safety Manual for the Graphic Arts Industry.*
   *Supervisors Safety Manual.*

State of California, Dept. of Industrial Relations, Div. of Labor Statistics and Research, 455 Golden Gate Drive, San Francisco.
   "Disabling Work Injuries to Office Employees," 1963 and 1978 editions.
   "Work Injuries and Illness in California, Quarterly."

*Statistical Abstract of the United States*, U.S. Department of Commerce, 1979.

Terry, George R. *Office Management and Control.* Homewood, Ill., Dow Jones-Irwin, Inc. 1975.

# Planning for Emergencies

# Chapter
## 16

# 16—Planning for Emergencies

No industrial, commercial or mercantile organization is immune from disaster. Emergencies can arise at any time and from many causes, but the potential loss is the same—people and property. Advance planning for emergencies is the only way to minimize this potential loss.

Planning in advance is necessary—it is not a luxury, rather it is good insurance. Where professionally trained emergency help and assistance may not be available, the need for emergency planning is intensified. A comprehensive management plan is intended to take care of all expected emergency situations. This includes both the spectacular (such as a tornado) and the common accident situation. Quite often emergency planning is assigned to the safety professional. This is fine, but there is a real need for the corporate management to be fully involved in the many decisions that must be made.

The safety of employees, visitors, and customers must be the first concern in planning for an emergency. Care for the injured must be available immediately. In some disasters, evacuation may be necessary.

Next, consideration should be given to protecting the property and the operation. In a new plant, consideration should be given to arranging and locating certain facilities and operations to provide greater inherent safety to the entire operation. In general, all emergency plans will include cleanup details necessary for the situation.

Finally, planning may be concerned with restoring business to normal. In emergencies likely to damage or wipe out a unit or plant, the question of resuming operations under conditions of temporary wiring, lack of heating, or repair and construction work should be considered.

Regardless of the size or type of organization, management is responsible for developing and operating a program, which is designed to meet these eventualities. An effective plan requires the same good organization and administration as any business undertaking. There is no one emergency plan that will do all things for all organizations. Each company must therefore decide on a plan that fits its needs and can be afforded.

Emergency plans involve organizing and training of small groups of people to perform specialized services, such as firefighting or first aid. Small, well-trained groups can serve as a nucleus to be expanded to any size needed to meet any kind of emergency. Even with outside help available, a self-help plan is the best assurance that losses will be kept to a minimum.

An organization will need to develop several plans to control different types of emergencies. Although certain basic elements would be common to all plans, the same complete plan could not, for example, be used for both a tornado and a nuclear attack.

Before an organization initiates an emergency plan, it is necessary to evaluate the potential disasters that might occur. The next section, Types of Emergencies, discusses these in detail.

The next step is to assess the potential harm to people and property. Again some adjustments, perhaps a range in the extremes of most likely and most unlikely, could be compiled. The time of day and the event itself are other factors that should be considered in assessing the potential damage. Planning should encompass all shifts and catastrophes that might occur during weekends or holidays when no one or only a skeleton staff may be on hand.

In trying to estimate potential damage to property one would follow the same general procedure. A building may be strong enough to resist a tornado, but a sudden 7-in. (17 cm) rain storm might cause dangerous flooding. On the other hand, an exploding boiler located in an adjacent building would probably not harm the main plant.

Next, probable warning time should be considered. For example, a flood may build up over a period of several days while a "bomb scare" affords only a few minutes warning from a telephone call. This warning time should permit some chance to alert personnel and mobilize the plan. It may be desirable to have two different plans, depending upon the actual time available.

The amount of change that must be made in the operations is another factor. For example, in anticipation of a heavy snow storm, it may be necessary to send employees home early. And some equipment may be left turned on or idling, instead of being shut down completely.

There needs to be consideration to power supplies and utilities that may be involved, particularly those controlling fire protection, lighting, ventilation, and communications.

A basic emergency preparedness plan will usually include—a chain of command, an alarm system, medical treatment plans, a communications system, and shutdown and evacuation procedures.

This chapter points out the various elements involved in developing emergency and personnel-protective plans. Not every element discussed will apply to every organization. Also several of the functions may well be combined and handled by one person, particularly in a smaller company. Generally the text is directed to the more elaborate and expanded type of organization and planning.

## Types of Emergencies

Before a company begins an extensive planning, organizing, and training, it is necessary to determine just what disasters are most likely to occur. In some areas, floods are no problem; in other regions, hurricanes or earthquakes are of little concern. However, work accidents, fire or explosion, sudden shutdowns, or acts of aggression might occur anywhere.

There are many sources of information to help determine the possibility that such an event might occur in your locality—weather records, accident and fire statistics, and industry or local authorities. After listing the potential disasters, some reasonable assessment must be made of the likelihood of occurrence. Some adjustments should be made to allow for the seasonal nature of certain events.

### Fire and explosion

Except where fires result from large-scale explosions, warfare, or civil strife, the fire emergency usually allows a short time for marshaling of firefighters and organizing an evacuation if necessary. Many conflagrations originate as small fires; therefore, prompt action by a small, trained group can usually handle the situation. However, plans should include the marshaling of extensive fire fighting forces upon the first indication of any fire growing beyond the "small fire" stage (that is, fires that could positively be controlled by inhouse personnel).

The main point is this: *small fires must be checked as soon as they start.* The first five minutes are considered the most important. Good housekeeping, prompt action by trained people, proper equipment and common-sense precautions will prevent a small fire from becoming a disaster.

Specific information on fire extinguishment and control is in Chapter 17, "Fire Protection," of the *Engineering and Technology* volume.

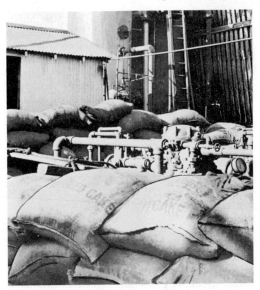

FIG. 16-1.—Installations subject to high water can be protected by a barrier made of piled sandbags.

## Floods

When a company or plant is located in an area that can flood, it should have the protection of dikes of earth, concrete, or brick construction. The probable high-water mark can be obtained from the U.S. Weather Bureau or the U.S. Army Corps of Engineers. The latter group also provides valuable assistance in planning flood water control.

Floods—except "flash" floods caused by torrential cloudbursts, or bursting of a storage tank, dam, or water main—do not strike suddenly. Ordinarily, there is enough time to take protective measures when a flood seems imminent. (See Fig. 16-1.)

## Hurricanes and tornados

Areas most frequently exposed to winds of destructive hurricane force are the Atlantic and Gulf coasts. However, inland locations are not immune to this type of disaster.

The U.S. Weather Bureau and other agencies have developed improved methods of detecting and tracking hurricanes; thus ample warning can be given for maximum protection of property and evacuation of personnel from threatened areas.

Companies regularly exposed to this hazard

have developed a system of tracking the hurricanes on a map. At predetermined locations, a specified alert condition becomes effective and each supervisor completes a checklist for that alert. As the hurricane progresses through the 100-mile (160 km) circle, 50-mile (80 km) circle, etc., the plant is shut down in an orderly manner.

Buildings constructed in areas where hurricanes occur should be built strong enough to withstand these destructive winds and tides.

Basic preventive measures include equipping with storm shutters or battens which can be promptly applied, at least on the side from which the storm is expected to approach. If this is not done, failure of windows may lead to lifting of the roof and destruction of the building. Where the roof is lost or damaged, building contents are drenched by the heavy rain that accompanies the storm and by water from broken sprinkler pipes. To prevent this, roofs should be securely anchored and tall structures (such as chimneys, water towers, and flag poles) designed to withstand high wind velocities.

Although the central Mississippi Valley is considered the tornado area of the country, almost every state has experienced them. The damage is inflicted quickly and is usually restricted to a small area, but the destruction can be massive.

Although the U.S. Weather Bureau has effectively increased its forecasting of tornado conditions and determining possible areas of danger, it is not possible for them to give as much advance warning or to pinpoint the strike area as accurately as they can with hurricanes. Therefore, a company must be prepared to protect its personnel on short notice and to take corrective action to protect and restore undamaged equipment and materials.

U.S. National Weather Service radio bands can be monitored during likely days. In one Midwest city, several large companies have set up a cooperative warning network. A lookout is stationed atop the city's tallest building. Through a central network, not only the member companies, but also the city's radio stations and civil defense, are alerted in the event of an approaching tornado.

Tornado and hurricane experience indicates that emergency plans should include:

1. Procedure for getting personnel to a safe place. If the building is not constructed to withstand

the forces, emergency shelters should be located close to the work area. All personnel should be instructed in the procedure to follow, with and without advance warning.

2. Assignment of trained personnel to take care of power lines—dangling wires are a serious hazard.

3. Assignment of trained people to remove wreckage to prevent injury to salvage and repair workers.

4. Schedule regular meals and rest for the repair crews.

## Earthquakes

Most seismic areas in the United States are around the Pacific Coast. Earthquakes generally occur without warning and affect the entire community or large areas thereby making community services unavailable for assistance.

"Earthquake-resistant" construction consists of building a structure so that it "floats" above the bedrock, ballasting it as a ship is ballasted, by making lower stories heavy and upper stories light. Utility lines and water mains should be flexible and laid in trenches that are free of the building, rising in open shafts and connected to fixtures by flexible joints.

The principal dangers from earthquakes are the collapse of buildings, fire originating from broken gas mains, and lack of water to fight any fire. Water reservoirs or emergency water sources should be provided for fighting fire if the municipal supply mains are broken or water pressure is likely to be disrupted.

## Civil strife and sabotage

Riot or civil strife is a recent addition to the list of reasons why a company should plan in advance for an emergency.

**Civil strife.** While the same considerations for organizing against and combating natural forces are involved, particularly fire, there is one additional element which makes this type of emergency different. The difference is that people are involved. This raises the questions of the right to protect property and the individual's legal right to assemble. A company should obtain from an elected legal authority in the community (district attorney) a statement explaining the company's rights in protecting its property and the company's legal responsibility for the safety of employees and other people— such as customers, supplier salesmen, and visitors—who may be on the company property. A company's legal department can be helpful in determining such a position, but its opinion does not have the force of law.

Some of the problems involved are: business disrupted when an office or plant area is invaded by outsiders; protection against a mob intent on destroying company property; neighboring companies request for assistance of your personnel during a riot; rights and responsibilities of armed company guards.

This type of emergency can be just as disastrous as any other type and should receive advance planning by manufacturing, mercantile, or commercial establishments.

**Sabotage.** Protection against sabotage is also an important consideration. The saboteur may be a highly trained professional or an amateur. He may be anyone—usually one of the least-suspected members of the organization. Because physical sabotage is frequently an inside job or requires the assistance—knowingly or unknowingly—of someone inside the plant, the principal measures of defense must be against entry of persons bent on sabotage. Evidence of sabotage should be reported to the FBI and if defense work is involved, to the Department of Defense.

## Work accidents and rumors

The "chain reaction" from a so-called "routine" work accident can result in an emergency situation. (Examples would be a break in a chemical line or toxic vapors from outside the plant entering the ventilating system.) Panic caused by a rumor or lack of knowledge can also create an emergency.

Some of the points to be considered are: auxiliary areas in the building to be used for medical treatment, method of notifying employees of the actual situation, method of quickly taking a head count, and sources of oxygen supplies available on short notice.

## Shutdowns

Although a shutdown is not an emergency per se, it can result from an unscheduled action, such as a disaster or strike; hence a fast shutdown procedure should be covered under an emergency plan. This plan should be based on a priority checklist. That is, all of the tasks to be assigned and functions to be performed should be arranged in order of importance so that if time is short, at least the most vital precautions are completed. This "crash" procedure is usually an adaptation of the routine procedure used for scheduled shutdowns, such as for vacation or renovation. Naturally the amount of warning time controls the speed of shutdown. Whenever a plant or other unit or building must be shut down, safeguards against fire take on added importance. Few employees, if any, will be present to discover and deal with a fire which might start. The extent of these measures will vary with the size and purpose of the plant. It is important to organize a formal program for instructing personnel. Examples of items which need attention include removal of lint, dirt, and rubbish; draining and cleaning of dip and mixing tanks and other equipment where flammables have been used; cleaning spray booths, ducts, and flammable liquid storage; closing of gas and fuel line valves; opening switches on power circuits which will be out of service; checking for serviceable condition of sprinkler systems, fire extinguishers, hydrants, alarms, and other protective apparatus; and anchoring cranes.

Prior to the closing, employees are alerted by special instructions to keep their work stations clean and fire-safe.

During the shutdown, continuous inspection of any maintenance or special operations, such as remodeling, must be maintained. Gas cutting and welding should be carefully supervised. Employees who remain on duty—the plant protection force, watchmen, maintenance workers, supervisors, or executives—should be briefed in effective countermeasures in case a fire breaks out.

If there has not been sufficient notice to effect a normal shutdown, it may become necessary to allow personnel into the area to perform necessary functions.

Company management should designate someone to authorize the admittance of personnel necessary to handle emergencies arising within the area. The chief of protection or the fire chief should arrange with local police and fire department officials for assistance if an emergency gets beyond local control. It is especially important that arrangements be completed for expediting the admittance of firefighters and their equipment.

Some companies use plant protection service agencies to prevent loss from theft, fire, and accident hazards during shutdowns. Similar plans

**443**

should be worked out with these people so that police and fire assistance is expedited when it is needed.

## Industrial civil defense

One of the main differences between planning for peace-time emergencies and planning for emergencies resulting from warfare conditions is that war may cripple an entire community. This difference makes it more important that emergency plans take into account self-sufficiency because the outside sources of help—fire and police departments, hospitals and doctors, regular sources of supply for material and equipment—would not be so readily available.

Industrial civil defense consists of the plans and preparations engaged in by managements of business and industry to achieve a state of readiness. This would enable their plants and facilities, and their employees, to cope with the effects of nuclear attack.

Even if a particular area is not attacked, plants in an area that has been spared may be requested to furnish transportation to evacuate the injured from damaged areas and to house and feed the evacuees. Plant emergency squads may also be required to go to the assistance of stricken plants. In a major catastrophe, there would probably not be enough hospital space available, making it necessary to keep the injured in temporary shelter for a considerable time. In such cases, employees with the proper training might be required to administer sedatives and plasma and to treat minor and major injuries.

Under general plans of the Office of Preparedness, Government Service Administration, authorities in that group would handle the investigation of areas dangerously contaminated with radioactivity, if this were the cause of the trouble. However, it is advisable that plant personnel with responsibility for health and decontamination have some knowledge of this work. Company personnel can be trained in this subject, as well as many others, by the National Staff College, Defense Civil Preparedness Agency, Battle Creek, Mich. 49016.

This chapter cannot give detailed survival plans for a nuclear attack or for protection against chemical or biological warfare. However, it is suggested that the disaster program director consult with the Office of Civil Defense (state, or city offices), which has material and trained personnel to assist a company in formulating its own program. The main point, as far as this Manual is concerned, is that top management must initiate and actively support the program. (Additional program details are given in the next section, Radioactive materials. Specific hazards of ionizing radiation are discussed in the National Safety Council's book, *Fundamentals of Industrial Hygiene.*)

It is incumbent upon industry to engage in preparations to protect itself and its employees in event of nuclear attack so as to ensure continued economic production or early resumption of that production.

## Hazardous materials

Because there are many chemical substances being used today, there must be concern with the potential usage and handling problems. There are many rules and procedures to be observed, but again ask the question, what if a safeguard fails? What if the container cracks and substances leak out?

In addition to normal hazards, are there potential chemical reactions with other substances that cause still further dangers to people and property?

Chemical hazards are discussed in the Council's *Fundamentals of Industrial Hygiene.*

## Radioactive materials

Fires and other emergencies involving radioactive materials are becoming more common as the peaceful use of isotopes becomes more widespread.

**Radioactive elements and fire.** Giraud (1973, see References) makes the following observations.

Radioactivity cannot by itself cause fires, but neither can it be destroyed or modified by fire. A fire may, however, change the state of a radioactive substance and render it more dangerous by causing it to spread in the form of a gas, aerosol, smoke, or ash.

Furthermore, fires can cause structural disruptions in stocks of fissile materials and in the special equipment for their treatment or use. Such disruptions may, at worse, result in a nuclear chain reaction and a criticality accident may then occur.

Radioactive elements are found in various forms, depending on their uses. The human eye can detect no difference between an inactive

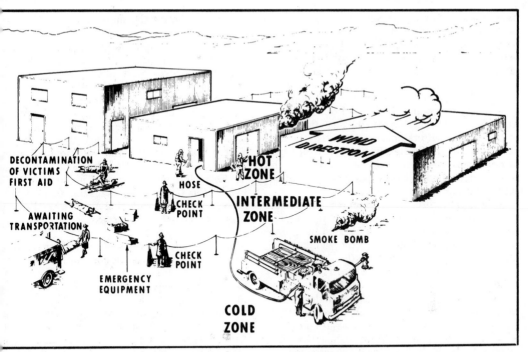

FIG. 16–2.—This diagram of an emergency situation involving a radioactive hazard shows some of the necessary precautions. Note the barricades and check points separating the "hot" and "intermediate" zones from the "cold" zone, and the air masks and extra protective clothing on the firefighters operating in the hot zone. The smoke grenade is a far more sensitive indicator of wind direction than is a windsock, and wind is extremely important. It will blow dangerous particles toward emergency personnel or away from them, depending upon how well organized is the operation.

Courtesy National Fire Protection Association (Kerr, 1977). Used with permission.

element and the same element when rendered radioactive. Both appear equally harmless. A fundamental distinction must, however, be made between so-called "sealed" and "unsealed" sources.

In the case of sealed sources, the radioactive substance is *not* accessible. The container has sufficient mechanical strength to prevent the substance from spreading during normal conditions of use. The capsule is made of stainless steel. The sources are of small dimension—approximately one centimeter.

In unsealed sources, however, the radioactive substance *is* accessible. In normal conditions of use, there is no means of preventing it from spreading. Solid substances are kept in aluminum tubes, and liquids are kept in flasks, and gases in glass ampules.

The fact that a substance is radioactive does not affect its general physical properties nor its behavior when heated to an abnormally high temperature—as, for instance, during a fire. The substance will, on contact with fire, undergo the normal transformations, depending on its initial form—*i.e.* solid, liquid, or gas. The melting, boiling, and sublimation—with the formation of combustion products corresponding to the chemical properties of the substance, in the form of slag, ash, powder, dust, mists, aerosols, fumes, or gases—can be expected.

These combustion products are generally finer and less dense than the original substance, so they disperse more easily. Although the change in the physical state of the substance will not have affected its radioactivity, the radiation hazard will be more difficult to control.

The protective containers currently in use

**445**

have a widely varying resistance to fire. The protection afforded to the contents will, therefore, depend on the type of container used. In general, sealed sources have a good fire-resistance, and radioactive elements thus contained are well-protected.

Unsealed sources, however, and solutions or gases in fragile containers easily fall victim to fire. The urgency of the action to be taken in the event of an accident with radioactive materials can be determined by the firefighting staff once the type of container is known, and the nature of such action will depend on the properties of the radioactive substance concerned.

When, as the direct or indirect result of a fire, the protective container has been broken, the radiation hazards for rescue workers at the point of the fire, or for personnel in the vicinity, are likely to be more serious than the danger connected with the spreading of the fire to parts of the building presenting conventional fire risks.

Accordingly, the person in charge of the rescue work will sometimes be obliged to over-ride the normal firefighting procedures to assure the protection and confinement of the radioactive elements threatened. If they are already affected by the fire, further hazards may arise.

The release of radioactive elements may result in contamination of surface areas. This may be caused by the spilling or splashing of radioactive substances or by the spreading of solid radioactive substances in paste, powder, or dust form. All possible precautions must be taken to prevent any further spread of the contamination. The means to be used, however, will differ with each case. In the first (spilling or splashing) absorbent materials should be used—such as powder, earth, sand, etc. In the case of spreading, the substances should be slightly dampened with a spray of water—unless it is otherwise specified on the container.

Liquids can be prevented from spreading by the methods normally used by the firefighting brigade. The contaminated area will be clearly marked and roped off to prevent the entry of unauthorized personnel. (See Fig. 16-2.)

Contamination of the atmosphere is caused by radioactive elements in the form of dust, aerosols, fumes, and gases. The spreading of such contamination is determined mainly by the prevailing weather conditions, and it is difficult to control. Such atmospheric contamination may lead to other toxic or corrosive hazards associated with the particular chemical. The most serious danger is that of inhaling the substance when it is suspended in the air. Firefighters, accordingly, should wear self-contained breathing apparatus.

The danger of internal irradiation is always present whenever there is contamination by a source of penetrating radiation. It may also occur by accidental release of an alpha or beta emitter from its protective container, or by the destruction (even partial) of the protective container.

The following material was adapted from "Preplanning for a Nuclear Incident," by James W. Kerr, FPE, which appeared in the April 1977 issue of *Fire Command!*® magazine. Copyright© by National Fire Protection Association, Boston, Mass. Reprinted with permission.

**Hazards.** How serious is the radiation problem? Although everyone is constantly exposed to radioactivity from cosmic rays and natural sources, the levels are very low. Only exposures that go much higher are of concern. The effects of radiation on living organisms — specifically people — seem to be most noteworthy when a large dose is received in a short time. If the same dose is spread over a longer time, as with workers in a factory using radioactive materials, the physical problems may be similar, but the effects show up differently.

Basically, overdoses of nuclear radiation start by causing simple symptoms that could be due to anything — even seasickness or the flu. By the time enough radiation has hit a person to cause such obvious problems as nausea and vomiting or diarrhea, some less visible changes in blood or nerve tissue also have happened. The tables in the book, *Nuclear Hazard Management for the Fire Service* (see References), make it obvious that it is vital to keep the radiation doses of those involved as low as possible.

On the fireground, do not expect immediate incapacitation of any firefighters from the radiation. The physiological effects do not appear for some time. Even lethal exposures do not cause nausea until after a few hours.

**Planning.** Regardless of the size of the nuclear event, the basic rules are always the same:

Notify the proper authorities,

Identify the hazards,

Find the limits of the area involved,

Reduce risk of exposure to people.

**446**

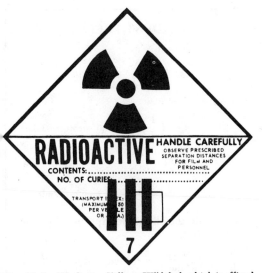

FIG. 16–3.—"Radiation Yellow–III" label, which is affixed to each package of highly radioactive material. Different labels are required for different intensities and quantities of radioactive material. See Title 49—Transportation, *Code of Federal Regulations*, Part 172, Hazardous Materials Table and Hazardous Materials Communications Regulations, for details.

These steps are always required, whether for a small spill at a laboratory, a train wreck, a reactor explosion, or fallout from a nuclear testing or war. Only the degree differs, and perhaps the "proper authority" to be notified. A major help for preparing preplans relating to medical matters is NFPA 3M, *Health Care Emergency Preparedness* (see References).

The experts in radiation usually are found in the Department of Defense, the Energy Research and Development Admistration, or the Nuclear Regulatory Commission. ERDA provides regional maps showing the proper telephone number for emergencies. The Chemical Emergency Center (CHEMTREC) can provide response/action information through a nationwide telephone number — 800/424-9300. (See the discription on p. 470 and in Chapter 24, "Sources of Help.") For the wartime case, Civil Defense is the obvious contact.

Plan to keep people — including your own forces — away from the immediate area. Except for essential suppression and rescue work, 500 yards (460 m) is a good safety distance for planning purposes. Any sightseers should be kept even farther away.

Plan to hold for proper medical evaluation anyone who may have been exposed or contaminated. Reentry to the restricted area must be controlled. Be sure to keep masks on everyone involved. Firefighters must avoid smoke, dust, and vapors, insofar as possible. (See Fig. 16–2.)

The first warning of a radiation problem could be the radioactive placard shown in Fig. 16–3. It features a black or purple "propeller" on a yellow background. Always be alert for it. All areas in the plant or laboratories that use or store isotopes should be known to the safety professional and to firebrigade personnel.

Decontamination is like any other technical operation: get expert advice. Otherwise, the radioactive material may be washed somewhere where it will do more harm than if left in place. Finally, obtain some knowledge of radiation instruments. Check with the scientific or engineering people who are using these materials. The local civil preparedness office is a prime source for requesting instruments and for training in their use.

**Operations.** There is nothing magic about nuclear radiation, nor about the means to cope with it in an accident situation. The accompanying drawing shows some of the necessary precautions. Invisible in the background is a pattern of fallout extending downwind; it has the same cigar shape as projections of fallout from nuclear war. It is similar to the smoke and combustion byproducts that are generated by every fire. Use common sense and experience, and keep upwind.

A few factors demand special attention. First, rescue requires extra speed. Radiation hazards, even more than the typical fire or toxic threats, require fast approach and fast exit. Victims need respirators, or at least eight thicknesses of gauze, to filter their air. Radiation monitors, using standard Civil Defense Preparedness Agency instruments or the equivalent, must check every person and item exiting from hotter to cooler zones.

Risks must be assessed mathematically. For example, criticality (the likelihood of a nuclear explosion) depends upon the amount of fissionable material on hand. But, because laws forbid having this much on a single transport, most emergency services need not be concerned about performing the calculations for this situation. Yet hazard from radiation — as distinguished from a nuclear explosion — can be calculated quite easily

**447**

## SAMPLE CALCULATION FOR A NUCLEAR INCIDENT PREPLAN

Problem: A research laboratory within your response area houses Cobalt–60. The fire inspector determines that the maximum source strength that will be on the premises is 10,000 curies, and that the cobalt is located 24 ft (7.5 m) from the entrance to its compartment.

If a fire starts in the room, how long can a firefighter stay at the doorway fighting it?

(Use a maximum allowable dosage of 25 Roentgens per man for any one incident.)

Procedure:

1. Determine the dose rate using Table 16–A. The table indicates a dose rate of 1.47 roentgens per hour per curie at a distance of 3 feet.

2. Calculate the total dose rate at 3 feet: 1.47 Roentgen/hour/curie $\times$ 10,000 curies = 14,700 roentgens/hour.

3. Calculate the dose rate at the specified distance, using the inverse square formula:

$$\frac{\text{Radiation at distance 1}}{\text{Radiation at distance 2}} = \left(\frac{\text{Distance 2}}{\text{Distance 1}}\right)^2$$

Radiation at 24 ft =

$$\left(\frac{3 \text{ ft}}{24 \text{ ft}}\right)^2 \times \text{(radiation at 3 ft)}$$

Radiation at 24 ft =

$$\left(\frac{1}{8}\right)^2 (14{,}700 \text{ roentgens/hour})$$

$$= \frac{14{,}700}{64} = 230 \text{ roentgens/hour}$$

$$= \frac{230}{60} = 3.8 \text{ roentgens/minute}$$

4. Calculate the allowable exposure time for firefighters:

$$\frac{25 \text{ Roentgens/person}}{3.8 \text{ Roentgens/minute}} = 6.6 \text{ minutes/person}$$

Assume a maximum exposure time at the door of 6 minutes per person for safety. If firefighters enter the room, the allowable exposure time must be recalculated.

Fig. 16–4.

*From Kerr (1977), see References.*

if the source strength is known. In a building emergency, a preplan inspection usually would have recorded the source strength. For transportation incidents, the label, the bill of lading, or both will indicate the source strength. Of course, fire or other effects of the accident could eliminate these sources of information, or render them illegible or inaccessible.

Calculating the allowable exposure time for emergency personnel is simple, provided that the source strength is known. The example shown in Fig. 16–4 is conservative, in that it ignores shielding, as by walls, containers, etc. It also assumes a point source rather than a more diffuse source. Note that it follows a rule of thumb limiting each person to 25 roentgens exposure per accident. Volumes could be written on this limitation. [Check latest exposure level limit.]

**Training and prevention.** Medical aspects of the problems resulting from exposure to radiation are complex, but early symptoms are simple. The real solution is not cure, but prevention, although decontamination can help to reduce total exposures.

Two important factors are obvious:

• Preplans must identify hazardous places and define the potential problem.

• Emergency personnel must understand the threat, and the principles of survival time and distance.

Training in the use of radiation instruments is neither complex nor expensive, and local civil preparedness offices are ready to help with it. Most other technical aspects of dealing with radiation incidents are largely covered in standard emergency procedure drills. Rules for prevention of casualties to emergency personnel *after* the incident also are well defined. (See References.)

Prevention of the accident depends on human

TABLE 16–A

RADIATION CHARACTERISTICS OF
COMMON ISOTOPES

| Isotope | Half Life | Dose Rate* |
|---------|-----------|------------|
| Sodium–22 | 2.6 years | 1.34 |
| Sodium–24 | 15.0 hours | 2.15 |
| Manganese–52 | 5.7 days | 2.14 |
| Manganese–54 | 300.0 days | 0.54 |
| Iron–59 | 45.1 days | 0.71 |
| Cobalt–58 | 72.0 days | 0.62 |
| Cobalt–60 | 5.3 years | 1.47 |
| Copper–64 | 12.9 hours | 0.13 |
| Zinc–65 | 245.0 days | 0.31 |
| Iodine–130 | 12.5 hours | 1.37 |
| Iodine–131 | 8.1 days | 0.25 |
| Cesium–137 | 30.0 years | 0.36 |
| Iridium–192 | 74.5 days | 0.61 |
| Gold–198 | 2.7 days | 0.27 |
| Radium–226 | 1622.0 years | 1.005 |

*Roentgens per hour per curie of source strength, measured at a distance of 3 ft (0.9 m) from a point source.

behavior—adherence to rules and procedures, and possession of basic skills. It obviously helps if management enforces laws and codes.

To avoid contamination from radioactive materials, follow these recommendations.

Avoid direct beams of X-ray or other machines.

Keep masked, to prevent ingestion of radioactive dust.

Avoid extreme fields of nuclear radiation.

Rotate personnel on an accident scene to prevent overdoses of a single person or team.

Know extinguishment procedures for the problem materials.

Know where to locate guidance and help.

Allow the "decay" of radiation intensity over a period of time to work for you.

## Weather extremes

Throughout a year, there may be some unusually severe and unexpected weather events that may require some changes in normal operations. Some examples follow.

In North Dakota, the temperature may occasionally drop to 35 degrees below zero (-30 C), yet most activities and travel are not normally affected. But, if the wind increases in strength or the temperature drops suddenly, there may be a need to assist people in travel or other outside activity. (See Fig. 16–5 for a windchill chart.) A special alert might be made to employees prior to their leaving from work. They should also know when or how they are to be notified about the company opening in the morning.

On the other hand, in the event of extremely heavy snowfall, what changes might be made in operations? What should employees be told prior to leaving for home?

Or suppose an unusually heavy rain strands hundreds of customers in a store just a few minutes before closing. Are supervisors and clerks prepared to handle the situation? May they allow telephone calls in and out? How do they control the crowd?

Hail or wind may start breaking glass windows while customers are shopping. What is the immediate action?

Suppose that adverse weather caused a power failure or someone suddenly shut off all power and lights while crowds were shopping? The emergency lighting system may operate as intended but employees, particularly key supervisors, must understand emergency plans and be prepared to act responsibly.

## Plan-of-Action Considerations

Following the assessment of potential emergencies, the next step is to translate these needs into a plan of action. Management should be in charge of drafting a policy and getting the plan underway. It will usually be necessary that the union leaders (if any) be involved in the planning process. Generally, someone should be appointed emergency planning director or coordinator, perhaps with help from an advisory committee. Usually because of their experience and training, the safety, medical, fire, and security departments will be involved. Of course, because production and maintenance will be affected, they must be consulted. Also, the legal staff needs to be aware of the plan.

And finally, contacts with local law-enforcement agencies, fire, and civil defense are necessary.

The cost and effort involved in giving immediate attention to emergency planning can be justified by weighing the cost of preparedness against the possibility of contributing to the yearly losses

CHART 46-B   WINDCHILL FACTORS

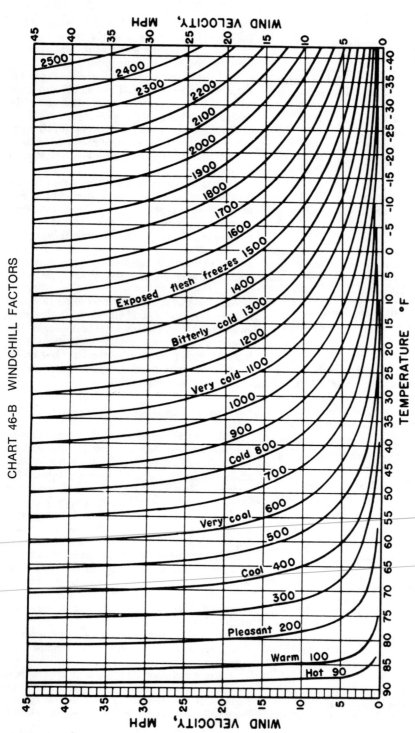

FIG. 16–5.—Windchill factors. The human body senses "cold" as a result of both temperature and wind velocity. The numerical factor that combines the effect of these two is called "the windchill factor," shown by the curves in the above nomogram of dry-shade atmosphere cooling. Take the line marked "very cold 1100," for example. This shows that a person can feel just as cold when the temperature is 35 F and the wind velocity is 45 mph as he can at −35 F and a wind velocity of only 1½ mph. When the windchill factor reaches 1400, flesh that is exposed to the wind will freeze in only a few seconds; out-of-door exposure is not recommended at all. Because of the extra clothing that people wear in cold weather, their physical size is greater than it is in warm weather. Be sure that equipment and controls are of adequate size and simplicity so that they can be run effectively and safely by persons wearing heavy clothing. See Table 10–B in Chapter 10 for approximate dimensions of heavy clothing.

*From Engineer and Development Laboratories, The Engineer Center at Fort Belvoir.*

from accidents, fires, floods and other catastrophes.

## Program considerations

The preliminary aspects of emergency planning have now been discussed—the need for advance planning and an evaluation of the type of emergencies and their potential harm to people and property. The next step, then, is to translate this need into a working plan within the organizational structure. In some cases, this requires working with other local agencies to most fully protect your operations.

Advance planning is the key. It is necessary to develop a written set of plans for action. The plans should be developed locally within the company (and corporate structure) and be in cooperation with other neighboring or similar organizations and with governmental agencies. It may not always be possible for them to fully cooperate or participate, but through planned action each organization should be aware of certain available assistances. And as a result, the company may need to plan to be largely dependent upon its own resources to provide the internal safety.

Often an emergency manual or handbook will be developed for the plant or organization. The following outline covers many of the items that might be included, but other items may be needed as dictated by the expected emergencies and the available resources.

1. Company policy, purposes, authority, principal control measures, and emergency organization chart showing positions and functions.

2. Some description of the expected disasters with a risk statement.

3. A map of the plant, office, or store showing equipment, medical and first aid, fire control apparatus, shelters, command center, and evacuation routes. (See Fig. 16–6.)

4. A list (which may also be posted) of cooperating agencies and how to reach them.

5. A plant warning system, type of signals.

6. A central communications center, including home contacts of employees.

7. A shutdown procedure, including security guard.

8. How to handle visitors and customers.

9. Locally related and necessary items.

Some of these items will be discussed in more detail on the following pages.

The plans should be rehearsed. Realistic conditions should be used so to further learn the effectiveness of the plan. For example, maybe the emergency lights failed when needed, or the telephone service failed; but such are also the conditions that might occur in a real disaster. Therefore planning should include all possible, as well as probable contingencies.

## Chain of command

Once the decision has been made to establish a disaster plan, a director or coordinator should be appointed and an advisory committee, representing various departments established.

The director should be a member of top management, whether it be a one-building or one-plant company or a national corporation, because he will have to be able to delegate authority, and speak for the company. The head of the disaster-control organization must be a cool, quick-thinking person and should be sufficiently robust to withstand the arduous duties that will fall upon him if an emergency arises. The emergency director's regular duties should be such that the greater part of his time will normally be spent at the unit he is responsible for. However, an alternate is always named in the plan—and the alternate should be a person who has the authority and qualifications similar to the director and he should be trained with the director.

The director (and his alternate) should be the first to be trained in his duties. Continuous liaison should be maintained with local Civil Defense authorities, if possible, to make sure that the company plans are coordinated with those of the community and to keep the company informed on new developments.

The director may be responsible for:

Communications
Firefighting
Rescue service
Guard service and warden service
First aid and medical service
Demolition and repair
Transportation
Investigation
Public relations.

All of these functions are likely to be essential although some may be combined. The person

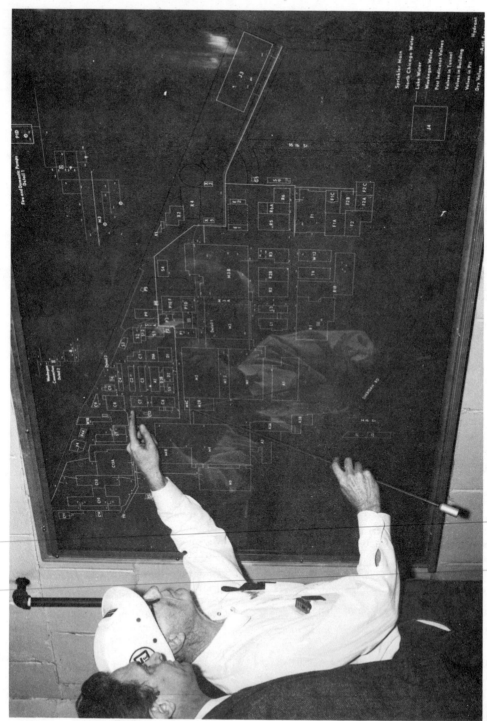

Fig. 16–6.—Safety specialist and fire chief check fire protection diagram in preparation for periodic training of fire brigade. Map shows sprinkler lines, pump houses, underground water supply systems, outdoor hose cabinets, fire hydrants, post indicator valves, and fire alarm and sprinkler systems.

*Courtesy Abbott Laboratories*

(and alternates) responsible for each function should be selected with great care and trained by the director. These chiefs should be familiar with all parts of the plan and should have experience in the fields in which they are to serve.

Assigned personnel must be trained to carry out their duties in accordance with the overall emergency plan. In small operations, where there may be no regular guards or firefighters, the operating personnel will be the people trained to take care of these duties. Of course, the number of members on each of the teams depends on the circumstances of each plant. Each team captain should select his own personnel from the available volunteers, supervise their training, and procure their equipment. Stronger people can be assigned to service in rescue squads because the work usually demands strenuous physical effort; those who are not so strong could be used in light salvage operations.

Because wholehearted cooperation of personnel is necessary to the successful operation of an emergency plan, shop stewards or other employee representatives should take part in the planning. They must be made to see that whatever measures are taken are for the protection of the lives and jobs of the workers as well as for protecting property.

Provisions should be made for emergency reporting centers so that employees will know where to report should the disaster occur while the employees are away from the plant. Reporting centers give employees a feeling of security and continuity, and aid the company in taking a "roll call." To facilitate these arrangements, each employee should carry an identification card which gives specific instructions on where to report, list of other reporting centers, basic employment record, and designation of the employee's next of kin in case they must be contacted or receive money due him. The reporting center will keep a duplicate record for each employee assigned to report there.

A one-plant company or a small company can consider using the home of a member of management, a supervisor, or an employee.

## Training

One of the most important functions of the director and his staff, on both the corporate and plant levels, is training. Training for each type of disaster is essential in developing a disaster-control plan and keeping it functioning. Employees must be taught to realize that an emergency plan is vital and real—it cannot exist usefully if it remains a remote idea. Training and rehearsals are time consuming, but they keep the program in good working order.

Training of key people will be of little value unless it reaches down to all employees. The better informed and prepared the work force is, the less chance of panic and confusion during the emergency.

Practice alerts should be conducted to make sure that the employees know where to report and what their duties are. Even the most carefully prepared plans can develop flaws when put into practice, and only rehearsals can show them up. The first one or two practices should be announced—lest there be a panic—but there should be no warning of succeeding ones. Officials should determine to their complete satisfaction that the disaster plan will work under emergency conditions. Once this has been determined, the plan should be maintained with periodic tests, staff discussions, and an occasional disaster problem. If this is not done, all the planning effort will have been wasted (see Figs. 16-6 and 16-7).

Management should assure employees that the company is doing everything possible to prevent injury to them, that every employee is an essential and necessary part of the team, and that the disaster-control organization is ready for any emergency. Such assurance will go a long way toward developing a state of mind that will not panic. Then when disaster strikes, emergency forces snap into action, workers file quietly into their shelters or other designated areas, firefighters are ready with hoses and equipment, and first aid squads stand by ready to aid the wounded.

Such planning is further evidence of management's concern for employees.

## Command headquarters

The average command headquarters will not withstand a direct nuclear attack, but it should still be planned for any of the other emergencies which may occur.

Coordination of the disaster control organization should come from a well equipped and well protected control room. The headquarters should be equipped with telephones, sound-powered phones, public address system, maps of the plant,

---

## IN CASE OF FIRE OR OTHER EMERGENCY

✔ **KEEP YOUR HEAD** — avoid panic and confusion.

✔ **KNOW THE LOCATION OF EXITS** — be sure you know the safest way out of the building no matter where you are.

✔ **KNOW THE LOCATION OF NEARBY FIRE EXTINGUISHERS** — learn the proper way to use all types of extinguishers.

✔ **KNOW HOW TO REPORT A FIRE OR OTHER EMERGENCY** — send in the alarm without delay; notify the **CHIEF OF EXIT DRILLS.**

✔ **FOLLOW EXIT INSTRUCTIONS** — stay at your work place until signaled or instructed to leave; complete all emergency duties assigned to you and be ready to march out rapidly according to plan.

✔ **WALK TO YOUR ASSIGNED EXIT** — maintain order and quiet; take each drill seriously — It may be "the real thing."

REMEMBER — IT IS PART OF YOUR
JOB TO PREVENT FIRES

---

FIG. 16–7a.—Sample emergency exit notice for general posting.

emergency lighting and electric power, sanitary facilities, a second exit, and two-way radios for communication both locally and with Civil Defense authorities. (See Fig. 16–8.)

Good communications are necessary for effective control and flexibility in a disaster situation. Communications include the telephone, radio, messengers, and the plant's alarm system (discussed separately later in this chapter). The disaster plan should provide for adequate telephones in emergency headquarters to handle both incoming and outgoing calls. Panic and disintegration of the organization will develop quickly if these calls are not handled with dispatch. An accurate log is kept of all incoming and outgoing messages (Fig. 16–9).

Some means of communication independent of normal telephone service must be available during an emergency, such as provided by a battery-operated radio. The disaster plan must anticipate the possibility of losing normal telephone communications and electric power.

### Emergency equipment

An emergency checklist should include equipment and material to be ordered as well as shutdown actions to be performed.

• For example, where it is not feasible to keep on hand the necessary emergency equipment and materials, a list should be maintained of sources from which these items can be obtained on short notice. These sources must be outside of the immediate area because of the rush for such material which would occur after receiving a flood alert. This equipment and material would consist of sandbags, battens for windows and doorways, boats, tarpaulins, fuel-driven generating equipment (such as gasoline-powered arc welding machines or motor-generator sets), standby pumping equipment, a supply of gasoline in safety containers to fuel this equipment, lubricating oil and grease, rope, life belts, portable battery-operated radio equipment, and audio speakers.

# EMERGENCY EXIT INSTRUCTIONS
## MACHINE SHOP – DAY SHIFT

### Read Carefully

The following persons will be in command in any emergency, and their instructions must be followed:

CHIEF OF EXIT DRILL—H. C. Gordon, General Sup't.
MACHINE SHOP EXIT DRILL CAPTAIN—R. L. Jones, Foreman
MACHINE SHOP MONITORS—Dave Thomas and A. L. Smith

### In event of FIRE in machine shop

✔ **NOTIFY THE GENERAL SUPERINTENDENT'S OFFICE**

✔ **PUT OUT THE FIRE, IF POSSIBLE**—If the fire cannot quickly be controlled, follow instructions given by Exit Drill Captain R. L. Jones or by the shop monitors. Leave by the exit door at the south end of the shop; if it is blocked by fire, use the door through the toolroom to the outside stairway.

### In event of FIRE or EMERGENCY in other sections of building

The general alarm gong will ring for two 10-second periods as an "alert" signal. Continue work, but be on the alert for the "evacuation" signal, which will be a series of three short rings. At the evacuation signal:

✔ SHUT OFF ALL POWER TO MACHINES AND FANS

✔ TURN OFF GAS UNDER HEAT TREATING OVENS

✔ CLOSE WINDOWS AND CLEAR THE AISLES

✔ FORM A DOUBLE LINE IN THE CENTER AISLE AND FOLLOW MONITORS AND EXIT DRILL CAPTAIN TO EXIT—Walk rapidly, but do not run or crowd; do not talk, push, or cause confusion!

After leaving the building, do not interfere with the work of the plant fire brigade or the city fire department. Await instructions from the General Superintendent or your foreman.

### Returning to the building

Return-to-work instructions will be given over the loudspeaker system or by telephone from the Superintendent's office.

FIG. 16–7b.—Sample individual instruction notice for general posting.

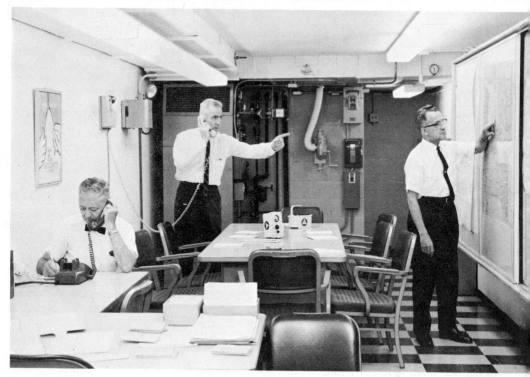

FIG. 16–8.—Underground emergency command headquarters has direct lines to company and municipal emergency service centers.

*Courtesy Western Electric Company.*

• Some of the items on the shutdown part of the checklist would be: closing of valves; protection of equipment that cannot be moved; doors, windows, ventilators closed and battened to keep out looters as well as water; vents and breather pipes plugged. Included with the checklist should be a list of telephone numbers of supervisors and key employees to be notified.

Provision should be made for moving tank cars to higher ground and anchoring them if there is any possibility that they still might not be out of the flood area. Portable containers should also be moved above the high-water mark, as should buoyant materials and chemicals that are soluble in water.

Storage tanks under the probable high-water mark (including underground tanks) should be specially anchored to prevent floating. Auxiliary dikes of sandbags or dirt should be built around key areas (see Fig. 16–1).

Other procedures that must be included: electric and gas utility services that should be shut off at the *main line* before any water reaches them. Hot equipment should be cooled before water reaches it. All machine surfaces should be coated liberally with heavy grease, especially around openings to bearings. (This step applies even to machines which may not be under water, because dampness affects equipment.) Open flames should be eliminated so that any flammable liquid floating on the flood waters will not be ignited.

• If at all possible, a salvage crew should remain at the site to continue preventive operations after the plant or facility has been shut down and take further necessary steps if the flood shows signs of exceeding the estimated high-water level.

### Personnel shelter areas

While there could be times during natural disasters when employees would be moved to shelter areas, shelters are more often associated

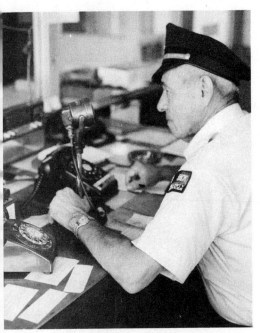

FIG. 16–9.—An important function of the communications setup is keeping an accurate log of in-coming and out-going messages, both radio and telephone, during the emergency.

*Courtesy A.B. Dick Company.*

with a bombing or nuclear attack.

The average company would find it impractical to build a shelter to provide protection against a direct hit or "near miss," but consideration should be given to shelters for protection against fallout or other disasters. A shelter designed and equipped to provide protection against radioactive fallout will also serve as a personnel refuge for other types of emergencies a company might face. Shelters are designated by the sign shown in Fig. 16–10.

Basements, tunnels (if they cannot be flooded), and inside areas of multistory buildings of concrete construction are examples of possible shelter areas in existing buildings. The denser the shield, the better it protects.

Many companies have not seriously considered constructing employee shelters because they do not think that the expense could be justified by the limited use. However, this is not necessarily the case; the shelter can have daily use as a locker room, training room, meeting room, cafeteria, or employee lounge. There might also be a psychological value in having employees use the shelter area on a daily basis; the familiarity tends to minimize any depressing effect which use of the shelter might have in an actual emergency. Although most industrial employee shelters are designed to give protection only from fallout, companies who have incorporated shelters in the construction of new buildings have found that they can also protect against blast effects.

Each employee shelter will have to have one person, with assistants, designated as the shelter manager. These managers will have to be carefully trained because they will be faced with all the psychological problems of life in close quarters, plus mass feeding, distribution of water, arranging sleeping accommodations, assigning duties, control of supplies, bolstering morale, and handling the personal problems that each individual will bring with him. The shelter manager may also be faced with emergency medical problems where training in first aid procedures is necessary.

### Alarm systems

In most industrial operations a definite fire alarm system is set up, using existing signaling

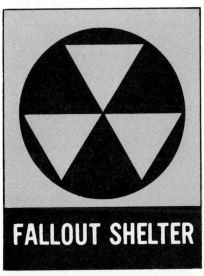

FIG. 16–10.—Civil Defense Fallout Shelter designation is used nationwide to mark shelters in both public and private buildings. Shelters are surveyed and approved by the Office of Civil Defense.

**457**

systems such as a plant whistle; however, to avoid confusion with the regularly used signals, some plants have special codes or other signaling devices. This type of signal also may indicate the location of the fire, or separate signaling devices may be used for the different building or working areas within the company property.

The alarm system that activates the emergency plan may or may not go through the communications center, but rather should be touched off in the emergency headquarters office. Alarm systems should be provided in all buildings.

In hospitals, or other locations where both employees and nonemployees can hear an audible page system, a code name can be used to announce a fire and its location, for example, "Doctor Red wanted in . . . ." Employees must be trained to be alert for this subtile signal.

Electric alarms are preferred to mechanical ones except in a shop having one large open area where there is only one alarm-summons station and one alarm-sending device, such as a manually operated gong. Manually operated alarms should supplement electric alarms (Fig. 16–11). Closed circuit systems of the type specified by National Fire Protection Association (NFPA) standards are recommended; see References at the end of this chapter.

Companies in areas where municipal fire departments are available usually have a municipal alarm box close to the firm's entrance or in one of the buildings. Others may have auxiliary alarm box areas, connected to the municipal fire alarm system, at various points on the premises. Another system often used is a direct connection to the nearest fire station which may register by a water alarm in the sprinkler system or be set off manually. If possible, the fire alarm system should be connected with the local firefighting alarm, and have an independent power supply.

In large cities private central station services are available and provide excellent protection. These central stations receive signals from plant fire alarm boxes, watchmen, sprinkler head operations, and other hazard control points in the plant. Being able to give undivided attention to matters of plant security, they can relay information to fire or police departments without delay. The signal received at the fire department or assistance agency should locate specifically the site of the fire, or at least the building or area, so the fire can be found quickly.

Automatic sending stations (thermostatic

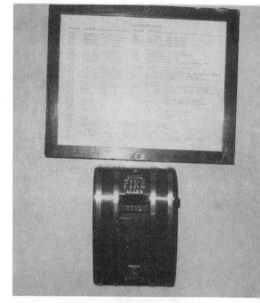

Fig. 16–11.—Manual alarm systems should supplement electric alarms. Employees should know how to activate a manual alarm. A code/location directory and fire plan is posted above the alarm.

*Courtesy Rush, Presbyterian, St. Lukes Hospital, Chicago.*

detectors) may be used, but should not interfere with the sending of the manual alarm.

Regular checks should be made on the alarm system. All stations should be inspected on a monthly basis by a responsible person, and the overall system should have a daily test to ensure it is in proper operating condition. These daily tests should be conducted at a prearranged time and under a variety of wind and weather conditions to determine whether the signal can be heard in all parts of the plant at all times.

### Fire and emergency brigades

Because a fire can start from so many causes, fire prevention and fire protection must receive major attention in any emergency program. Advance planning is important (Fig. 16–6).

The company fire chief must be able to command people as well as have special training in fire prevention and protection. A person who has had experience in city or volunteer fire department work, or a military service veteran with experience in firefighting is a good choice. In a

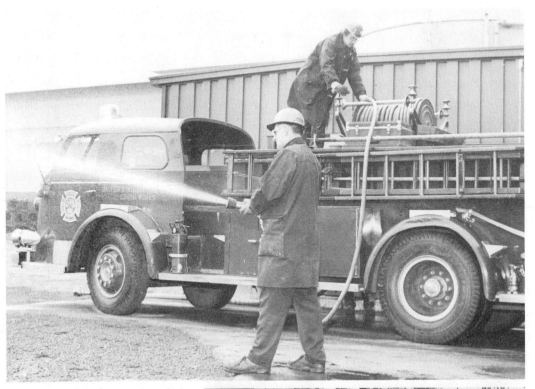

FIG. 16–12a.—Many companies have found they can add a combination rescue-truck to their emergency equipment without exhorbitant cost by obtaining a used truck from a local fire department that may have "outgrown" it. The company equips the truck to handle its particular anticipated problems.

*Courtesy U.S. Steel Corp., Central Steel Division.*

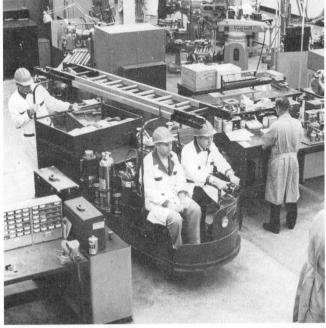

FIG. 16–12b.—A fire and rescue truck for in-plant use carries hose, fire extinguishers of various types, and miscellaneous emergency equipment. Unit can travel at 30 mph.

*Courtesy Taylor-Dunn Manufacturing Company.*

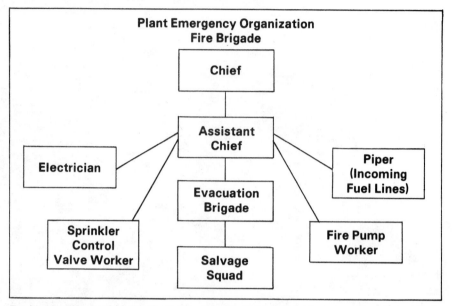

Fig. 16–13.—Because of the complexity of response needed to cope with an emergency, duties must be divided among plant emergency organization members to avoid confusion. Here is one plant's organizational chart.

*Courtesy* Textile Section Newsletter.

smaller company or plant, a master mechanic, maintenance department head, or other employee with mechanical experience can be a good part-time fire chief.

The fire chief should have one or more assistants who should have complete knowledge of the plant and equipment, command the respect and obedience of those under them, and are qualified to perform the duties to the chief officer if he is absent.

The size of the plant and the fire potential presented by the occupancy determine the kind of plant firefighting brigade. The majority of plants may required only first aid firefighters under the direction of departmental foremen or managers. In larger plants, the fire brigade organization, directed by a full-time fire chief, is composed of full-time and emergency members. The full-time members maintain fire brigade equipment and are responsible for the permanent fire protection of the plant. Emergency members report for fire duty when the alarm is sounded.

The fire brigade apparatus should be selected only after a study has been made of plant conditions, to thus make sure it will be adequate for any

emergency. Advice and assistance can be obtained from the local fire department, the NFPA, Office of Civil Defense, insurance companies, or perhaps a neighboring plant. Two fire and rescue trucks are shown in Fig. 16–12.

The large plant fire brigade is usually organized into squads, each with specific duties. One company's organization chart is shown in Fig. 16–13.

**The evacuation squad** evacuates all employees from the emergency area as quickly and orderly as possible, without injury. They search closed areas, such as washrooms, to determine that everyone has been evacuated.

**Utility control squad** members are usually maintenance personnel, who are familiar with plant piping systems and the control of process gases, flammable liquids, and electricity.

**Sprinkler control squad** members must understand the automatic sprinkler system—the direction of rotation of the valve they are to operate, the use of sprinkler stops, and the replacement of sprinkler heads, if this is not a maintenance

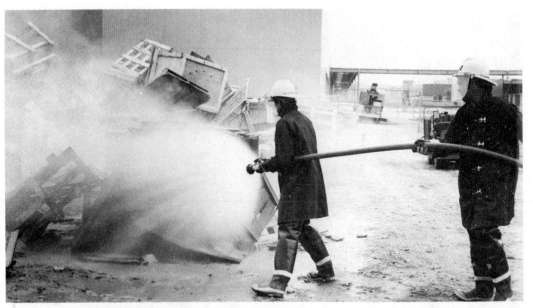

Fig. 16–14.—Fire brigade hose drill provides familiarity with equipment—makes the group more effective under actual emergency conditions. "Hands-on training" is the best teacher and should complement classroom study.

*Courtesy Michelin Tire Corp., Greenville, S.C.*

department function.

**Extinguisher squad.** Portable fire extinguishers are frequently operated by designated employees who work in the vicinity. However, as the size of the plant increases, it is advisable that special squads be selected for handling fire extinguishers.

**Hose squad** members are trained to operate fire hydrants and hoses. They should drill frequently with wet hose lines so they have the feel of a charged hose. After they become proficient in handling the hose, drills once or twice a year may be ample (Fig. 16–14).

**The salvage squad** is trained to protect as much stock and equipment as possible by controlling the directional flow of water and by covering stock with tarpaulins. Training should include proper methods of throwing tarpaulins and planned use of them in directing the flow of water. Members should also be familiar with the location of sawdust or other absorbent material and be aware of its value in controlling water on floors.

**The brigade-at-large or rescue team** consists of maintenance personnel or specially trained people.

The main functions of this unit are to extricate casualties and eliminate hazards to other workers involved in the control of the emergency. Members respond to all alarms with a utility truck containing such rescue equipment as: ropes, chains, block and tackle, ladders, cutting torches, saws, axes, and jacks. The amount of equipment, of course, will depend upon the size of the plant and the hazards involved, but every effort should be made to anticipate possible problems. Under the direction of the brigade officer, personnel in this unit also control utilities, ventilating fans, and blowers; they close fire doors, windows, and other openings in division walls; they open windows and doors leading to fire exits; and, where escapes are the swinging section type, they should be the first to operate the escapes and to secure the steps to the ground.

Depending upon the size and inherent hazards of the plant facility, it may be necessary to train squads in the handling and erection of ladders, use of foam lines, recharging of foam generators, and specialized rescue techniques.

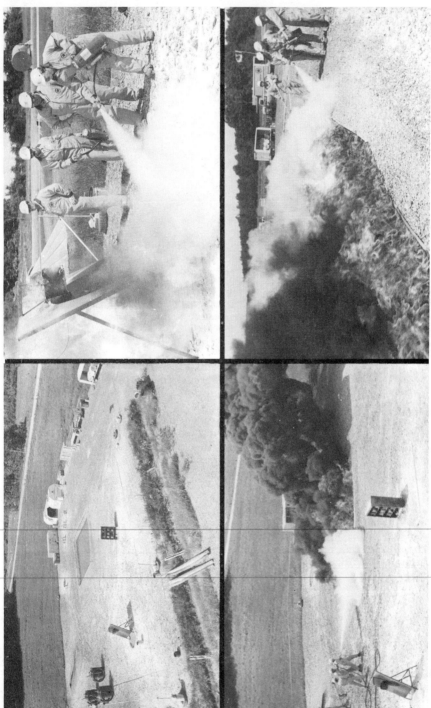

FIG. 16–15.—A special fire training site near Montreal International Airport is serving to train air transport industry personnel in emergency firefighting techniques. The site's characteristics, special props, and equipment enable 12-person classes to tackle simulated types of fires they are most likely to encounter. The gravel-base site (*upper left*) provides for ample drainage, isolation, storage of fuel and material, and a wind direction indicator. Types of fires simulated include (*upper right*), a running spill fire with fuel in a suspended bucket and on the ground; (*lower left*), a large pit fire in a 12-inch pit containing eight inches of water and 15 gallons of fuel; and (*lower right*) a trench fire, in an eight-inch trench with six inches of water and eight gallons of fuel. Spill fires on level ground and cabinet fires are also simulated. Three-man teams fight each type of simulated emergency.

*Courtesy of Eastern Region Air Canada and Montreal International Airport.*

**Manning of fire pumps.** There should be at least two competent persons for pump duty in the main pump room, and a person assigned to each pump located elsewhere.

**Training of firefighters.** The newly organized brigade should go through complete drills, preferably weekly. Later, less elaborate drills may be held at less frequent intervals. Drills should be held at unannounced times. They should be thorough in every respect, closely approximating fire conditions. (See Fig. 16–15.)

No matter how thoroughly the industrial fire brigade is trained, there still must be close cooperation between it and adjoining or nearby plants and the public fire department. As stated before, *it is recommended that the municipal fire department be called immediately upon alarm of every fire.*

Watchmen should be instructed in case of fire to open yard gates and be ready to direct fire apparatus. Where plants have railroad tracks, cars should not be permitted to block crossings that may be needed in an emergency.

The brigade chief will be in full charge at a fire until the officer in charge of the public fire department takes over. He then serves as an advisor on plant processes and special hazards.

**The fire station** itself should be centrally located, but not exposed to possible fires. It should be of fire-resistant material or located in a sprinklered part of the plant and protected with portable extinguishers. A larger plant may require mobile units, such as light hand-drawn trucks outfitted for the special hazards of the plant.

## Plant protection and security

Industrial security is management's responsibility. Government agencies can provide assistance and advice in establishing a policy. Since the basic problems of security are protection of property and control of persons, a company does not have to establish a new department to handle this function. A company's emergency security force could be built around the present security force.

Personnel need training in maintaining order, handling crowds, and coping with the threat of panic. They should also be prepared to prevent looting. They map emergency routes to shelters, both inside and outside the plant grounds.

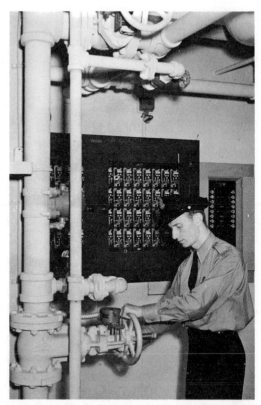

FIG. 16–16.—Watchmen and guards should be acquainted with sprinkler system controls. The control panel behind this guard indicates if there is tampering with any master sprinkler control valve in building.

A watchman of low mentality may be more of a liability than an asset. Fires have often been caused by watchmen smoking while on duty, or overlooking fire causes. Their failure to discover fires promptly, their shutting off of sprinklers without ascertaining whether the fires have been extinguished or their ignorance of the proper sprinkler valves to close after a fire is extinguished is often responsible for heavy water loss.

As a supplement to automatic alarm and signal systems, the employment of an intelligent and physically fit watchman can prevent or minimize fire loss. The watchman should be trained and made aware of his responsibilities. Because fires which start when the plant is idle produce more damage, the watchman becomes an important part of the fire prevention and detection organization (see Fig. 16–16).

**463**

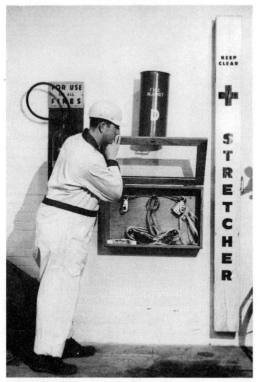

FIG. 16–17.—Standby rescue and first aid equipment should be neatly stored and available for immediate use in case of emergency.

*Courtesy Polymer Corp., Canada.*

The guard or watchman functions include protection against pilferage, burglary, vandalism, and espionage. The time of the inspection rounds should occur irregularly. The entire inspection should not create a detectable pattern.

The first round immediately after the plant closes is the most important. Most fires are likely to start just after employees have left, from machines or processes running unattended, or from careless smoking.

The guard or watchman should have enough time on his rounds to make a thorough inspection of the premises. His route should require no more than 40 minutes and should take him close to all hazardous occupancies. He should be provided with an approved flashlight or other illuminating device, and, where practicable, plant lights along his route should be left on.

The watchman can also look for violations of smoking rules, improper storage of flammable material, leaking oil, gasoline, gas, or other flammable materials, and he should report unsatisfactory conditions to the management. He should be physically capable of turning in a fire alarm, dealing immediately with small fires, and with such matters as shutting off gas and closing fire doors.

Failure of a guard to report on schedule at the end of his patrol calls for immediate investigation.

Additional protection and security measures call for closing off certain windows and other openings in plants which are not vital to operation and limiting the number of plant entrances and exits. (All measures must be consistent with good fire prevention practices.) Installation of protective wire mesh over windows along public thoroughfares is recommended. Floodlighting of critical parts of plants at night is necessary for good protection.

## First aid and medical

A helpful publication in establishing a disaster medical service is the *Guide to Developing an Industrial Disaster Medical Service* compiled by the American Medical Association's Council on Occupational Health. This guide can also assist a company in evaluating its readiness and will reveal weak areas. Examples of forms and casualty tags are included. Although the guide is designed to combat peacetime disasters, it provides a basis on which to expand the medical services to meet the devastation following a nuclear attack.

First aid and medical service should be headed by the company doctor, if available, as discussed in Chapter 19, "Occupational Health Services."

In the organization of the medical phase of the emergency plan, those responsible must select and train personnel; decide what measures, equipment, and supplies are needed; and establish first aid stations and a treatment center. (See Fig. 16–17.)

All employees should be encouraged to enroll in a first aid course. People assigned to first aid and medical units should pass standard and advanced first aid courses. Local chapters of the American National Red Cross provide excellent training in this regard.

If a major disaster occurs, there may not be enough trained doctors and nurses available. In such an eventuality, care beyond the first aid level will have to be provided by nonmedical people.

who have received additional training. Such a medical team can be developed by recruiting volunteer medical aides, preferably with some experience. In addition to first aid training, more advanced instruction by regular medical personnel or local hospitals should be provided.

A major consideration to keep in mind when establishing an emergency medical program, is that while most of the medical aid will be given in a central medical station, some of it may be given on the job site, possibly under hazardous conditions.

Plans should be made for representatives of the medical team to check all personnel at the disaster scene for trauma and to provide a written clearance for them to leave the plant when they are able to leave. In this duty, representatives of the investigation team may interview personnel before they leave to be sure that any needed eyewitness information is recorded.

Welfare and medical service includes the investigation of needs for prevention of epidemics, food inspection, and sanitation inspection. In the planning stages, company trucks, if any, should be designated as ambulances and the necessary equipment for them supplied. Two-way radio communication for such ambulance service is essential. Provision should be made for nonperishable food and water rations. There should be close coordination of plant first aid measures with the local civil defense, health, and medical services.

The chemical service responsibility of this unit requires that gas masks be provided in case tear gas is used as part of the sabotage effort and that trained personnel, equipment, and supplies for chemical defense and decontamination be on hand. There should be a plan for priority sequence in decontamination of the plant—that is, water supply, power plant, machinery areas, warehouse areas, etc. Medical team personnel will also be responsible for any radiological monitoring thought to be necessary after a nuclear attack. The mere knowledge that such monitoring equipment is available is a morale-builder.

After disaster, no one should be permitted to drink water until it has been examined.

## Warden service and evacuation

The warden service is responsible for maintaining employee control during emergencies, including (a) guiding employees to shelter, (b) directing employees away from hazardous areas, and (c)

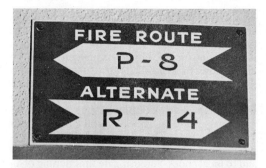
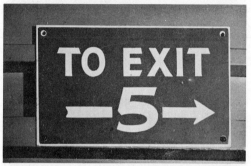
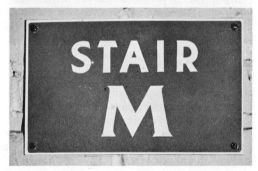

FIG. 16–18.—Exit routes and escape passages properly identified expedite rapid evacuation. Especially important is provision for an alternate exit path if the primary route is blocked by flame, hot gases, or debris.

*Courtesy Dunwoody Institute.*

averting panic. In smaller companies, the wardens could also have the responsibility of taking charge of shelters. In some cases, the warden service may be responsible for seeing that shutdown of processes and equipment is carried out smoothly.

This type of service was devised primarily for areas of high population densities, such as commercial structures and factories with a great many employees, and residential areas. Some plants have a high concentration of employees. For these, the use of warden teams is certainly a good idea. In some plants, however, the concentration is very low. In such plants or departments with low personnel concentration, warden service is not necessary. In these cases, the operators themselves will have to be trained in shutdown details.

Management, in checking and providing for safe exits and evacuation drills, should refer to the National Fire Protection Association's standards and to local codes. Smooth, safe functioning of an evacuation plan requires a thorough knowledge of all plant operations and types of employees, number and types of exits available, width of exits, proper location of exits, possible alternate exits, and location of hazards, as well as a knowledge of warning and evacuation facilities (see Fig. 16–18). The subject of building exits is coverd in Chapter 15, "Office Safety," in Chapter 1, "Industrial Buildings and Plant Layout," in the *Engineering and Technology* volume, and in the *Life Safety Code*, NFPA 101.

Most plants have a rigid rule that only especially appointed people on the fire brigade shall go to the vicinity of the fire, and that everyone else shall proceed on signal to a refuge location in accordance with the organized evacuation plan.

### Transportation

Disrupted transportation facilities or restrictive traffic regulations could make it impossible for many employees to get to work. The company may need to provide transportation with company trucks and cars. Advance planning for car pools and pick up stops will greatly facilitate such a step.

The transportation responsibility includes arrangements for ambulance service, preparation for transportation of employees to and from work, and movement of emergency service crews as needed.

The transportation unit should consist of a group of regularly assigned drivers. Station wagons, from which the seats can be removed, and company trucks can be used when it becomes necessary to handle stretcher cases in evacuating any injured. The unit will be the means of getting auxiliary firefighters, first aid teams, and salvage and rescue workers to the scene of the disaster at the earliest possible instant. The unit will also be used to deliver needed equipment and material from outside suppliers.

Planning for adequate transportation service and traffic control requires liaison with the public police department, civil defense authorities, and possibly the military.

A source of motor fuel will have to be anticipated. One company used oversized underground gasoline storage tanks for the company service pump. Its emergency electric generating equipment also used gasoline-run engines because, in this case, gasoline is more readily available than is diesel fuel.

### Security from Personal Attack

Protecting the employee from muggings, rapes, and robberies is a concern of the safety professional when they occur on company property. Even if these attacks occur elsewhere, the side effects are brought into the workplace.

### Coping with the crime problem

Safety personnel are not professional crime fighters. However, the on-the-job welfare of the work force is their responsibility, as is often the security of the physical property of a company building, or plant. If a woman is attacked while waiting in her car for her husband to clock-out on the late shift, or if a man is mugged in the company parking lot on payday, or if some part of the office or plant is burglarized, the safety of an employee can be jeopardized.

Employee attitudes and emotions can range from alarm and anger on the one hand to apathy on the other when such an incident occurs to someone who works along side them. Distraction or preoccupation of any kind, if only momentary, can result in a serious accident.

Because the modern industrial worker is an adult, he should not be coddled in an effort to avoid overt emotional displays. How then does the safety director cope with security and crime problems that chip away at the safe environment he has established within the confines of his plant or building? Further, how does a safety organization incorporate this area of concern with other phases of the profession? And, further still, how does he reconcile any ensuing economic expenditures?

There are no pat answers to these questions. Each must be answered in terms of a particular industry, location, and workforce. All should be answered, however, with an attitude of commonsense and practicality that addresses itself to the welfare of the employee.

## Study the building and premises

What does the building or plant look like at night? Is it swathed in a bath of floodlights? Does an armed guard open electronic gates to the plant yard? Or, is it a small building set back from the street in an open, landscaped industrial park? Whatever the physical setup, know it, and know it well. Is there unguarded access to the parking area from a busy street or highway? Is there a viaduct or catwalk that allows easy entrance to a restricted area?

In surveying the outside physical layout of an industrial concern, note that not all crimes of the mugging–burglary nature take place in dark secluded areas, but a large percentage are in those locations simply by the obvious reason that discovery is less likely. Thus a security survey of an industrial complex should probably center on secluded or remote areas. Tunnels between buildings, street underpasses, poorly lighted stairwells, dock areas, and freight elevators are all possible covert indoor hiding places for unauthorized persons.

Don't overlook washrooms and locker room facilities. Burglars have been known to hide in toilet stalls until after hours and then shop through the plant and offices for valuables.

## Implementing the survey

Once a list of security problems has been drawn up, priorities must be established and plans for implementing them must be made.

Installing lights and a fence around the parking lot may deter a car thief from the area or a sex offender from hiding in the back seat of an unlocked car. In addition, the fence and gate may slow up employees from leaving the area and make shift-change traffic more organized, and safer. Adequate lighting in a stairwell would reveal a lurking figure waiting to accost a female employee. Similarly, slipping and tripping would be less likely.

Often the plant or building survey reveals security gaps that can be closed by the maintenance department. For example, broken windows can be replaced; or if unused, boarded up. Trash barrels or anything that could be used by an intruder to stand on to squeeze through a window or trap door should be placed so as not be be an invitation. For small business or industrial operations that may be housed in one building, lights around the periphery of the structure are a relatively low cost method of deterrence. Decals prominently displayed in a window warning of an on-premise security alarm may be enough to dissuade the young or novice intruder. (Many establishments display such a decal whether or not an alarm system is actually installed for the psychological effect.)

## Professional assistance

The experience of local law enforcement agencies can be a major source of help in resolving a company's security needs. In addition they can advise of any local laws or codes that require compliance.

Some police departments, particularly in suburban or rural areas, patrol industrial areas throughout the evening hours. Find out what your local force does. At the same time they can give you an idea of the types of crime in your area and recommend special procedures suited to a particular setup.

For instance, maybe an adjacent race car track brings large crowds of people to the track across the street from your plant, which has a large fleet. Burglars may use the diversion of the sporting event to help themselves to tools and parts in your plant's garage complex.

Even the unpredictability of weather should be considered in a security program. Do heavy rains, snow, or fog render some security procedures inoperable? If so, the procedures may have to be changed. The police (and fire department) may advise of the special operations that they are required to take in the event of unusual weather conditions that would nullify some security procedures. Find out if bus routes or traffic must be rerouted behind your plant or building if the viaduct floods or the prairie catches fire.

Based on the discussion with the law enforcement agencies, it may be necessary to work with additional security professionals. This can include watch service companies, insurance firms, burglar alarm and detector manufacturers, and lighting companies. Naturally, any security equipment selected will be based on needs.

Just as multi-plant industrial complexes share core medical facilities, cooperative security plans are worth investigating. Expenses for additional lighting, fences, and watch patrols may be shared by several companies. However, this should be done only with the approval of the insurance carriers.

**467**

## Protecting personnel

Once the "bricks and mortar" of a plant are secure under the supervision of watchmen and guards or detector systems, much of the personal security of employees is also provided. Not all unauthorized persons questioned by a plant guard or detected on a surveillance system are there to steal. Some are on the premises (or in the area) to harm an employee, often just a person who is there by chance.

A well-organized employee identification system is basic to company and plant security. All too often it is assumed that the person sauntering through an area, be it restricted or not, has a legitimate reason for doing so. He may be thought of as being a repairman, delivery person, or from the superintendent's office. So goes the thinking of the average employee when he sees a stranger in his work area.

By challenging the stranger's presence in an area and asking him for a company identification card or, if cards are not used, asking for verification from another employee, this problem can be stopped. At first, employees may object to "police overtones" of "identify or else," but selling security to them on the basis of, "It's for your own protection," meets with little resistance. Supporting this approach with examples of little or no security measures usually quells even the strongest resisters.

Wearing photo-identification cards clipped to a shirt pocket or collar can be made a condition of employment. In addition, asking the employees themselves about improving security can often bring forth ideas that fit in well with a specific plant's set up. The "we want you on the job safely" approach is a more positive way of selling security to employees than the proverbial "No admittance beyond this point," or "Don't do this."

## Female employees

Rape is hideous to women. It can occur at any place, at any time. It is the one crime in which the victim must prove her innocence and relive every detail in court; often the victim is left with serious emotional scars and/or physical injuries.

Seen as a power crime by a male expressing his hatred for women, a rape case can trigger strong emotional reactions amongst coworkers. Currently there is much dialogue on the subject from all areas of society—law, sociology, psychology, security—all with a goal of improving the lot of the victim and understanding the rationale, or lack of rationale, of the accused.

Keeping in mind that the presence of other persons and the "light" of easy detection are obvious deterrents, security can be geared to these axioms. Women employees should know that rape victims are often the victims of chance, not necessarily because they know or recognize the assaulter.

Tell female employees about self-protection during a safety meeting set up just for the subject of security. Don't mince any words on the subject, but set the tone of the program with, again, "we want you on the job safely."

Encourage comments from the women, particularly with suggestions they may have on ways they will feel more secure. Don't let them leave the meeting empty-handed. Distribute National Safety Council's *Safety on the Streets* (see References) or similar literature that may be available from your local law enforcement agency, and perhaps a whistle. A number of cities have met with success after the establishment of whistle campaigns. While stopping rape is one of the reasons for using the whistle, it can be used by both men and women in an emergency situation.

The whistle is to be used when a person sees something suspicious happening, or when he is personally threatened, and when it is physically safe to sound the whistle.

Sometimes to guarantee further the safety of a workforce, additional security measures must be taken for the in-transit employee. Cabs and mini-bus rides from the plant gate to public transportation are standard procedures in many work situations. Guard escort from the plant gate to the employee's car is not unheard of in some high-crime areas. For the most part, these efforts have been set up to protect female employees who work evening shifts. Similar protection is afforded the female office worker by the frequent policy of "safety in numbers," or requiring the presence of a supervisor or several other people to be present during over-time hours.

However, in-transit security is just as sensible a procedure for preventing muggings and robberies of male employees as it is to deter an attack on a female employee.

## Mutual assistance

Cooperation with surrounding plants, local law enforcement authorities, and transportation systems can expedite in-transit security. The cost of operating a minibus service from several plants or establishments to the local bus or train can be shared by the participating companies. Or, a similar agreement can be made with a local taxi company. Some companies located in high-crime areas have borne the expense of taxi rides to the home of the employee in an effort to maintain a safe and qualified workforce.

This brings to mind a final reason for establishing an effective security program. Few people will work in an area that threatens their sense of security on a daily basis. Avoid the additional problems of rapid turnover and unqualified personnel because of the poor desirability of the company's location. In addition to reducing the occurence of crime in the area, it is simply good economics to attract a stable and competent workforce.

## Outside Help

A company's chance of survival and recovery is greater when knowledge, equipment, and personnel are pooled with its neighbors. Therefore, emergency plans should include a provision for exchanging aid with other plants in the industrial community.

### Mutual aid plans

A number of industrial communities are organized to assist their members in the event of emergency or disaster. These organizations include manufacturing plants, large offices, stores, hotels, utility companies, chemical plants, law enforcement organizations, hospitals, newspapers, radio stations, and television stations. They operate independently of or as supplements to any civil defense groups.

One thing that has been learned from past disasters is that it is impossible to have adequate supplies available for a really large disaster. The best defense is to have adequate supplies in other areas committed for standby use, with communication channels and a plan for their rapid transportation to the stricken area. Especially important are adequate medical supplies and firefighting equipment. A plan for rapid and accurate communication is a necessary, as was discussed earlier in this chapter.

Planning with neighboring companies and community agencies for mutual aid during a disaster should include establishment of an organizational structure, standardization of an identification system, a communication system, standardization of procedures and equipment (such as fire hose couplings), formulation of a list of available equipment, stockpiling medical supplies, sharing facilities in an emergency, and cooperative test exercises and training.

Frequently these "cooperatives" establish a task force composed of personnel from each member company. Training is supplemented by detailed written instructions. Bulldozers, floodlights, and tools are marked by each plant for emergency use of crews. Training on a community basis might include instruction by members of the public fire department to plant fire brigade members and also some actual training by members of a construction or wrecking company to show the salvage and rescue teams how to handle heavy weights and to work safely among debris.

### Contracting for disaster service

Some companies contract for disaster service. The service is paid for by a fixed annual retainer, plus additional pay for the actual hours worked. For example, a wrecking company can be engaged to supply the men and equipment necessary to clear debris created by a disaster. Contracting for such a service removes the burden of providing trained personnel and maintaining a great deal of idle emergency equipment that could easily be damaged in the very disaster it was designed for.

### Municipal fire and police departments

Firefighters from the station most likely to respond to an alarm should be fully acquainted with all fire hazards in the plant. Cooperation may be encouraged by inviting local fire officials to inspect the company area. As a result, they can become familiar with the location, construction, and arrangement of all buildings, as well as all special hazards, such as flammable gases, liquids, and materials. They can make sure that company equipment is compatible with the municipal equipment. Therefore, the local fire department can formulate an efficient plan of attack before a fire occurs. Such procedure is far better than waiting for fire to break out, and then running the risk of misunderstanding the situation and initiating improper firefighting methods.

Public fire department rescue equipment can supplement plant rescue units. Local fire and police departments can also help in training company forces, as discussed previously.

The public police force can aid in putting down large-scale disturbances and in assisting with evacuation from the plant premises in the event of a major disaster. Planning for this outside help should include arrangements for traffic control, particularly where a plant parking lot empties immediately onto a public highway.

### Industry and medical agencies

Details of the following services are given in Chapter 24, "Sources of Help," under Emergency and Specialized Information.

- In 1970, the Chemical Manufacturers Association created the Chemical Transportation Emergency Center (CHEMTREC). Under this program a national center located at 2501 M Street, NW., Washington, D.C. 20037 (CMA headquarters) can relay pertinent emergency information concerning specific chemicals upon request in particular information on the hazards, and information to take immediately to control the emergency. A phone is available for 24 hour service—800/424-9300. It is intended primarily for use by those who transport chemicals, but others may have need for the information.

- The Toxicology Information On-Line Network (TOXLINE) has been designed to provide current and prompt information requests on the toxicity of substances. It is intended to be used by health professionals and other scientists working with pollution, safety, drug, health, and other disciplines. The service is under the auspices of the National Library of Medicine, 8600 Rockville Pike, Bethesda, Md. 20014. The service is accessible via terminals on line through a national telephone-based network. A fee is required for use.

There are a number of other emergency and specialized information sources listed in Chapter 24, "Sources of Help."

### Governmental and community agencies

During a community-wide disaster, a large number of governmental and private agencies are available to assist industries; these include the Office of Civil Defense, the U.S. Army Corps of Engineers, the Salvation Army, the American Red Cross, the U.S. Public Health Service, and the U.S. Weather Bureau. To be effective in coping with an industrial community disaster, the efforts of all of these groups must be coordinated and directed toward a common end. Therefore each plant should have an up-to-date listing of all cooperating agencies; the administrator's name, address, and telephone number; and the task assignment of the agency. If possible, these people should meet periodically to discuss mutual problems and disaster control techniques.

The company's emergency planning director should become thoroughly familiar with the authority, organization, and emergency procedures that are established by law and which will become effective upon declaration of a civil defense emergency.

In wartime, the federal, state and local governments are responsible for relief measures to meet needs resulting from enemy attack. The Red Cross has offered to assist the government in providing food, clothing, and temporary shelter on a mass-care basis during the emergency period immediately following enemy attack. In many communities, local Civil Defense officials have requested Red Cross chapters to assume all or part of this responsibility, acting under Civil Defense authorities.

In natural disasters, the American Red Cross is responsible for assisting families and individuals to meet disaster-caused needs that cannot be met through their own resources. These relief operations are coordinated with the activities of the local, state, and federal governments. When a disaster occurs, the local chapter of the American Red Cross aids disaster sufferers. The resources of the national organization are available to supplement chapter assistance.

### References

American Insurance Association, Engineering and Safety Service, 85 John St., New York, N.Y. 10038. *Fire Hazards and Safeguards for Metalworking Industries*, Technical Survey No. 2. *Fire Safeguarding Warehouses*, Technical Survey No. 1.

American Medical Association, Council on Occupational Health, 535 North Dearborn St., Chicago, Ill. 60610. *Guide to Developing an Industrial Disaster Medical Service.*

The Conference Board, 845 Third Ave., New York, N.Y. 10022.
    *Studies in Business Policy*, No. 55, "Protecting Personnel in Wartime."

Factory Mutual System, 1151 Boston-Providence Turnpike, Norwood, Mass. 02062.
    *Handbook of Industrial Loss Prevention.*
    *Loss Prevention Data.*

Giraud, Raymond. "Radioactive Elements," *National Safety News*, June 1973. Adapted from author's article
    in *Revue Technique du Feu*, Enterprise moderne d'edition, 4 rue Cambon, 75 Paris 1, France.

Hatcher, Harry. *Fire Brigade Organization and Training*, North Chicago, Ill., Abbott Laboratories, 1974.

International Association of Fire Chiefs, 1329 18th Street NW., Washington, D.C. 20036. *Nuclear Hazard
    Management for the Fire Service*, 1975.

Kerr, James W. "Preplanning for a Nuclear Incident." *Fire Command!* April 1977.

National Fire Protection Association, 470 Atlantic Ave., Boston, Mass. 02210.
    *Auxiliary Protective Signaling Systems*, NFPA 72B.
    *Central Station Protective Signaling Systems*, NFPA 71.
    *Explosion Prevention Systems*, NFPA 69.
    *Facilities Handling Radioactive Materials*, NFPA 801
    *Fire Protection Handbook*, latest ed.
    *Guard Operations in Fire Loss Prevention*, NFPA 601A.
    *Guard Service in Fire Loss Prevention*, NFPA 601.
    *Health Care Emergency Procedures*, NFPA 3M.
    *Industrial Fire Brigades Training Manual*, 4th ed., SPP-13.
    *Life Safety Code*, NFPA 101.
    *Local Protective Signaling Systems*, NFPA 72A.
    *Management Control of Fire Emergencies*, NFPA 7.
    *Management Responsibility for Effects of Fire on Operations*, NFPA 8.
    *Private Fire Brigades*, NFPA 27.
    *Remote Station Protective Signaling Systems*, NFPA 72C.
    *Sprinkler System Installation*, NFPA 13.
    *Sprinkler System Care and Maintenance*, NFPA 13A.

National Petroleum Council, 1625 K. St. NW., Washington, D.C. 20006.
    *Disaster Planning for the Oil and Gas Industries.*
    *Security Principles for the Petroleum and Gas Industries.*

National Safety Council, 444 North Michigan Ave., Chicago, Ill. 60611.
    *Fire Protection Guide.*
    *Fundamentals of Industrial Hygiene*, 2nd ed.
    Industrial Data Sheets
        *Fire Brigades*, 588.
        *Fire Prevention and Control at Construction Sites*, 491.
        *Fire Prevention in Stores*, 549.
    "Safety on the Streets: A Manual of Safe Practices for Women."
    (See other appropriate topics treated in both volumes of this Manual, especially those pertaining to
        organization, training, medical and nursing services, fire extinguishment and control.)

National Staff College, Defense Preparedness Agency, Battle Creek, Mich. 49016.

"Security from Personal Attack," *National Safety News*, July 1973.

Underwriters Laboratories Inc., 333 Pfingston Rd., Northbrook, Ill. 60062.
    *Classification of Fire-Resistance Record-Protection Equipment.*
    *Gas Shutoff Valves—Earthquake.*

U.S. Defense Civil Preparedness Agency, Washington, D.C. (Available through Superintendent of Docu-
    ments, U.S. Government Printing Office, Washington, D.C. 20402.)
    *Attack Environment Manual*, DCPA CPG2-1A1 through CPG2-1A9, June 1973.
    *In Time of Emergency*, DCPA H-14, March 1968.

# Personal Protective Equipment

## Chapter
## 17

# 17—Personal Protective Equipment

The OSHAct makes it mandatory for each employer to furnish to each of his employees a place of employment that is free from recognized hazards that can cause (or are likely to cause) death or serious physical harm, and to comply with occupational safety and health standards promulgated under the Act.

This places a burden on management to take prompt steps to eliminate any hazardous situation. Extensive engineering revision of processing or manufacturing methods may be involved, or only a simple change in material handling methods may be necessary.

A machine so designed, for instance, that it effectively confines flying particles eliminates a cause of accidents. This is a more basic treatment of the problem than the use of goggles designed to prevent injury, because confinement stops particles at their source.

Reducing noise to acceptable levels by quieting down a machine or enclosing it is far superior than depending on personal hearing devices. (See Chapter 9 in the Council's text *Fundamentals of Industrial Hygiene.*)

Likewise, dangerous solvents, chemicals and other vapor or fume hazard substances should be confined to a pipe or closed tank, or their vapors or fumes should be exhausted mechanically, instead of depending on a respirator to protect an operator required to work in a hazardous environment. Protection by mechanical means is generally more reliable than protection dependent upon human behavior.

If it is impractical to eliminate a cause of accidents by engineering revision or by safeguarding, or to limit exposure time to hazardous dusts, mists, vapors, or excessive noise to acceptable levels by administrative procedures, use of personal protective equipment is mandatory.

## Equipment Selection and Use

Once it is decided that personal protective equipment is needed:

1. Select the proper type of equipment

2. Implement a thorough training program

3. Make certain the employee knows the correct use and maintenance of the equipment.

### Selection of proper type

After the need for personal protective equipment has been established, the next problem is that of selecting the proper type. Two criteria should be used: the degree of protection that a particular piece of equipment affords under varying conditions, and the ease with which it may be used.

Unfortunately, with the exception of respiratory protective devices (Fig. 17–1), few items of personal protective equipment available commercially are tested and approved by an impartial examiner according to published and generally accepted performance specifications. Satisfactory performance specifications exist for certain types of personal protective equipment, notably safety hats, devices to protect the eyes from impact and from harmful radiations, and rubber insulating gloves, but there are no approving laboratories to test equipment regularly according to these specifications.

A proposal has been made that private testing laboratories be accredited in accordance with criteria established by the National Institute for Safety and Health (NIOSH). Such equipment would bear an approval label.

In any event, unless the safety professional has ample testing facilities available to him, he must rely upon the equipment manufacturers' endorsement for devices that may fill his needs. Fortunately, the manufacturers have been aware of their responsibility in this respect, and have a remarkable record of reliability. Their representatives can usually be called in to demonstrate their products and discuss their conformance to safety standards.

The succeeding pages discuss seven major areas of personal protective equipment—head, eyes and face, ear, respiratory, hands, feet, and trunk. Each section will provide the latest information on the standards available or proposed, some details about the equipment available, suggestions for selecting equipment to meet the job hazard, and some case histories in the development and use of specific devices.

### Proper training and use of equipment

The next problem is that of getting the workers to wear the personal protective equipment (if necessary), once it has been chosen. It is no longer a matter of choice, it is now required by law. Several factors influence the solution of this problem, among them are: (a) the extent to which the personnel who must wear the equipment understand its necessity, (b) the ease and comfort with which it can be worn with a minimum of

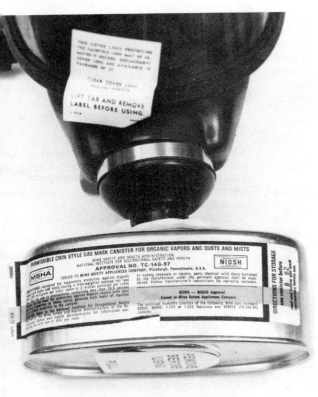

FIG. 17–1.—The National Institute for Occupational Safety and Health and the Mine Safety and Health Administration approve respiratory equipment. Approval label must appear on the device.

interference with normal work procedures, and (*c*) the available economic, social, and disciplinary sanctions which can be used to influence the attitudes of the workers.

In an organization where workers are accustomed to wearing personal protective equipment as a condition of employment, this problem is minor. People are simply issued equipment that meets the requirements of the job and is easy to wear, and are taught how and why it must be used. Thereafter, periodic checks are made until use of the issued equipment has become a matter of habit with the workers.

When a group of workers are issued personal protective equipment for the first time or when new devices are introduced, the problem may be more difficult. A clear and reasonable explanation as to why the equipment must be worn must be given. Traditional work procedures may have to be changed. If such changes are required, a good deal of resistance, justifiable or not, may be generated. Also, workers may be reluctant to use the equipment because of bravado or vanity.

It should be pointed out to them that the Occupational Safety and Health Act (OSHAct) requires "each employee to comply with occupational safety and health standards, and all rules, regulations, and orders issued pursuant to this Act which are applicable to his own actions and conduct."

The practice of having supervisors and foremen try out new protective equipment and devices prior to actual adoption, and getting their comments and discussing the advantages, has been successfully used in many operations.

A good deal of the resistance to change can be overcome if the persons who are going to use it are allowed to choose the particular style of equipment they will wear from a group of different styles which have been preselected to meet the job requirements. In some situations, it may be advisable to have a committee from the work

**475**

force help select suitable devices. Management's desire to standardize on one style of equipment may not be realized immediately, and several styles may need to be stocked. In the latter case, the cost, though higher than the cost of stocking only one style, will be small compared to the potential cost of accidents resulting from failure to use the equipment.

For the convenience of their employees, some companies maintain equipment stores on the plant premises.

## Who pays?

Policies differ with respect to who pays for personal protective equipment. The OSHAct states that the employer is responsible for the employees' use of the equipment, but the question of "who pays for it?" depends upon individual company's employer-employee arrangements.

The cost of eye protection equipment that has prescription-ground lenses, such as safety spectacles, is often shared by worker and employer. For instance, a National Safety Council survey showed that 27 percent of the companies supplying employees with prescription goggles gave them free, and 60 percent assumed part of the cost or made them available at below retail.

Most companies do not furnish safety-toe shoes free. Many industrial firms maintain shoe stores for the convenience of employees and make the shoes available at cost. In some instances, to encourage purchases, safety shoes are offered at below-cost prices.

In some areas, shoemobile service is available where a vendor comes into the plant with a trailer completely equipped and stocked to fit and sell safety shoes. These shoes are normally offered at an industrial price.

It is difficult to determine when management should pay the cost of personal protective equipment and when workers should. Factors are the probability and expected severity of injury, the willingness of workers to wear the equipment, its length of life, and the degree to which it may be depreciated by nonoccupational use, and provisions of collective bargaining agreements.

For example, the welder's helmet is almost universally supplied by management, for the job could not be performed at all without it. Work gloves sometimes must be purchased by the user. On the other hand, welder's or other special purpose gloves are usually considered as being a necessary part of the job work tools and are issued free.

## Responsibility

No matter what decision is made, it remains management's responsibility under the law to develop and enforce the program.

Here is one firm's policy on wearing of personal protective devices:

For safe use of any personal protective device it is essential the user be properly instructed in its selection, use, and maintenance. Both supervisor and workers shall be so instructed by competent persons.

Minimum training shall include the following:

1. Instruction in the nature of the hazard, whether acute, chronic, or both, and an honest appraisal of what may happen if the proper device is not used.

2. Explanation of why more positive control is not immediately feasible. This shall include recognition that every reasonable effort is being made to reduce or eliminate the need for personal protective equipment.

3. A discussion of why this is the proper type of personal protective device for the particular hazard.

4. A discussion of the device's capabilities and limitations.

5. Instruction and training in actual use and close and frequent supervision to assure that it continues to be properly used.

6. Classroom and field training to recognize and cope with emergency situations.

Training shall provide the workers an opportunity to handle the personal protective device, have it fitted properly, and test its wearability in normal air for a familiarity period, and, finally, in test atmospheres.

All equipment must be inspected periodically before use and after each use. A record should be kept of all inspections by date, with the results tabulated. The recommendations of the manufacturer for inspection should be closely followed, so too, should the recommendations of the manufacturer for the maintenance of the device, and the repair and replacement of parts supplied by the manufacturer of the product.

## Recognition 'clubs'

As an added incentive to wearing equipment, several organizations sponsor recognition awards for those who have been spared injury by wearing personal protective equipment. The oldest one of these is the Wise Owl Club, sponsored by the National Society to Prevent Blindness. The National Safety Council keeps an up-to-date list of U.S. and Canadian "clubs." It is available on request.

## Head Protection

Although every worker should be encouraged to use his head to absorb knowledge—he should not use it to absorb blows. Those who are exposed to head hazards must be provided with head protection (Fig. 17–2). Particularly hazardous operations are: tree trimming, construction work, shipbuilding, logging, mining, overhead line construction or maintenance, and basic metal (steel or aluminum) or chemical production.

Safety professionals should be aware of changes in operations that may create a need for head protection. For example, a firm undergoing a slack season might transfer some employees from relatively safe jobs to duties requiring safety hats or caps. In addition, construction, maintenance, and odd jobs requiring heat protection often occur in the normal operations of many companies.

### Safety helmets

Safety helmets (hats or caps) are rigid headgear of varying materials designed to protect the worker's head from impact, penetration, and electric shock or any combination of the three. They can help shield the hair from entanglement in machinery or exposure to irritating dusts. Bump caps (for less-hazardous exposures) are discussed later in this chapter.

Helmets (see Fig. 17–3) have been classified by ANSI into two types: (a) full brimmed, and (b) brimless with peak. The types have been further broken down into four classes: Class A, limited voltage resistance for general service, Class B, high voltage protection, Class C, no voltage protection, Class D, protection for firefighters helmet.

All helmets that meet American National Standards (ANSI) Z89.1 or Z89.2, shall be identified on the inside of the helmet shell with the manufacturer's name, American National Stan-

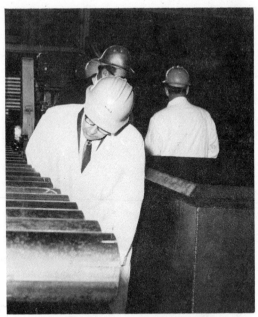

FIG. 17–2.—Head protection is needed where there is a possibility of falling objects, or bumping into suspended or traveling stock.

dard designation, and class (A, B, C, or D).

Materials used in the construction of Class A and B helmet shells should be water resistant and slow burning. Materials in Class D helmets shall be fire resistant (self-extinguishing when tested in accordance with ASTM Standard D-635), and nonconductors of electricity.

Class B (electrical worker) headgear do not have holes in the shell or any metal parts at all.

The helmets designed for use around electrical hazards are proof tested at 20,000 volts ac (rms), 60 Hz, for three minutes and leakage currents not exceeding nine mA. When tested to breakdown, the Class B helmet shall not fail below 30,000 volts.

The other classes have a less strict requirement: 2200 volts AC (rms), at 60 Hz for one minute with no more than 9 milliamperes leakage.

The thinnest section of Class A and B helmet shells will not burn at a rate greater than 3 in. per minute. After a 24-hr. immersion test, water absorption of the shell will be no more than 5.0 percent (by weight) for Classes A and D, and 0.5 percent for Class B.

**477**

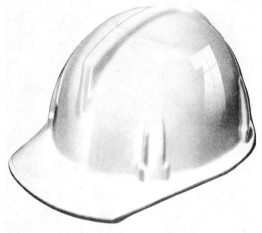

a. Protective cap molded of high dielectric plastic.

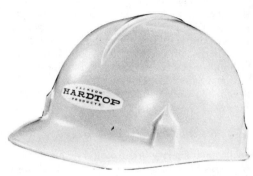

b. Protective cap molded of glass fiber and plastic.

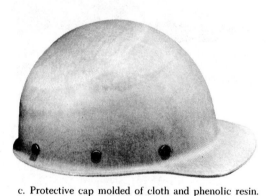

c. Protective cap molded of cloth and phenolic resin.

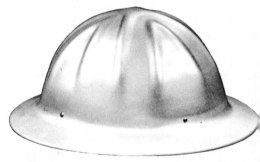

d. Protective hat constructed of aluminum alloy.

FIG. 17-3.—Various types of protective headgear.

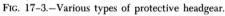

All helmets are designed to transmit a maximum average force of not more than 850 lb (385 kg) when tested for impact resistance. No individual helmet shall transmit a maximum average force of not more than 1000 lb (454 kg).

When properly selected and used, these helmets will greatly reduce injury from falling objects as well as exposure to electric burns.

Metal helmets should never be used where electrical hazards or substances corrosive to aluminum are present (see ANSI Z89.1.)

**Weight and shape of hat.** American National Standard Z89.1 specifies the weight for Class A and C helmets shall not exceed 15 oz (425 g), including suspension but excluding winter liner and chin strap. Class B helmets can weigh 15½ oz (439 g), as specified in ANSI Z89.2.

A brim all around the helmet (Fig. 17-3d) provides the most complete protection for head, face, and back of the neck. For use where a brim may be in the way, the cap type (Fig. 17-3a, -3b, and -3c) is frequently preferred. This type may also be equipped with lugs to support a welding mask (Fig. 17-4a and -4d), if a welder works on jobs which expose him to head injury.

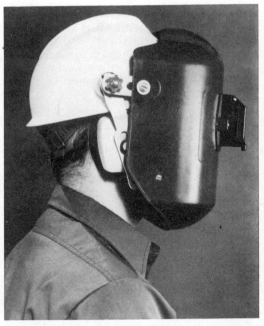

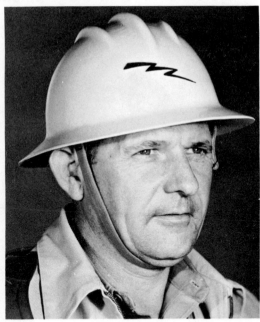

a. Protective cap with attached welding face mask and earmuffs.

b. Man wearing chinstrap to secure protective headgear in place.

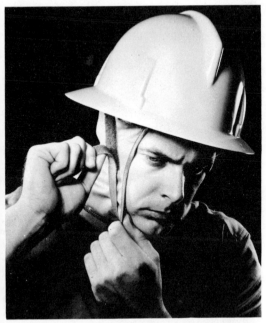

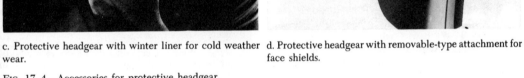

c. Protective headgear with winter liner for cold weather wear.

d. Protective headgear with removable-type attachment for face shields.

Fig. 17–4.—Accessories for protective headgear.

**479**

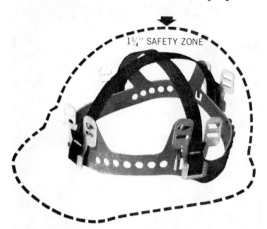

FIG. 17–5.—The crown straps of this safety hat are preset and unadjustable in order to guarantee clearance for impact protection. Underside of hat should be no less than 1¼ in. above head.

**Suspensions, liners, and chinstraps.** The suspension, working with the shell, absorbs the force of an impact. It is important that the suspension be adjusted to fit the wearer and keep the hat itself a minimum distance of 1¼ in. (3.2 cm) above the wearer's head (Fig. 17–5). Suspension bands should be nonirritating to the wearer.

Liners are available so that protective helmets may be worn in comfort in cold weather (Figs. 17–4c and 17–6).

Various types of leather, fabric, and elastic chinstraps are available. Often hats are bumped or blown off, or come off during a fall; a chinstrap affords full protection (Fig. 17–4b). A nape strap (provided with most helmets) helps keep the headgear from falling off during normal use.

Employees should not carry anything inside the helmet. A clearance must be maintained inside the helmet for the protection system to work. In the event of a blow to the head, that space is necessary to help absorb the shock of the blow.

## Bump caps

Another form of protective headgear is the bump cap, a thin-shelled, light-weight plastic affair (Fig. 17–7). It was originally conceived for use by aircraft workers, laboring in the close quarters of a fuselage—where a brim might get in the way.

Although some industries have adopted them, there are no specifications covering them. Authorities warn that, although they are fine for some applications, they are *not* a substitute for helmets. Use of such caps should be strictly limited.

## Hair protection

It is important that persons with long hair or beards who work around chains, belts, or other machines protect their hair from contact with moving parts (Fig. 12–33 p. 363). Besides the danger of direct contact with the machine, which may occur when they lean over, they are exposed to the hazard of having their hair lifted into moving belts or rolls that develop heavy charges of electricity. Since it is difficult to remove this hazard completely by mechanical means, people with long hair should be required to wear protective hair covering.

Hair nets, bandannas, and turbans are frequently unsatisfactory for hair protection because they do not cover the hair completely. Protective caps should completely cover the hair (Fig. 17–8). If the wearer is exposed to sparks and hot metals, as in spot welding, the cap should be made of flame-resistant material. Disposable flame-proof caps are provided in some chemical plants.

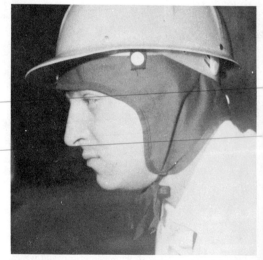

FIG. 17–6.—Winter liners rather than ordinary headgear are required for use with safety hats in inclement weather. Liners do not interfere with the inside clearance.

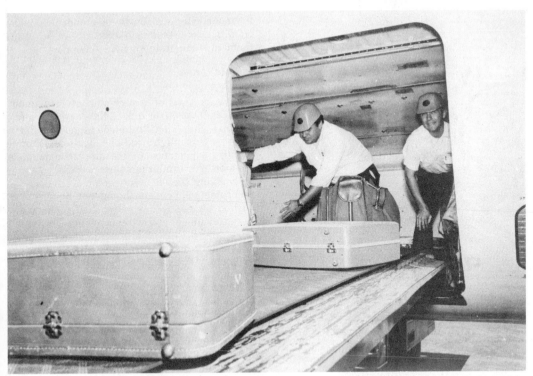

FIG. 17-7.—Bump caps offer limited protection for those who work in close quarters. They must not be substituted for a "safety" hard hat where the job requires such protection.

FIG. 17-8.—Cap protects hair of people in general factory work. The visor serves as a feeler guard to prevent injuries from contact with machines and objects. The netting construction on the top provides adequate comfort ventilation.

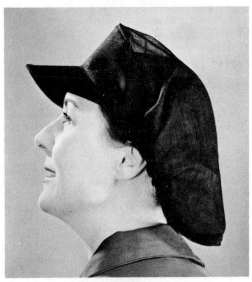

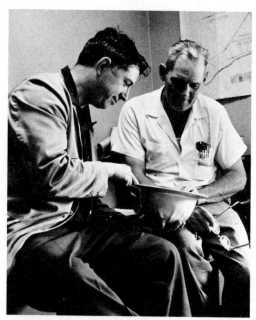

FIG. 17–9.—Periodic inspection of safety hats and suspensions is part of a maintenance program.

No standards have been accepted for protective caps, but they should be made of a durable fabric to withstand regular laundering and disinfecting. Design should be simple so that they can be pressed or ironed by machine, and they should be available in a variety of head sizes or should be adjustable to fit all wearers.

A cap should have a visor long enough and rigid enough to provide warning before the head itself comes into contact with a moving object, such as the spindle on a drill press.

In order to encourage its use, the cap should be as attractive as possible. It should be cool and lightweight. If dust protection is not required, the cap should be made of open-weave material for better ventilation.

After a suitable cap has been chosen, its use should be required and enforced. It is common practice among workers, for reasons of vanity, to wear the cap on the back of the head so that part of the hair over the forehead is exposed. Sometimes this practice can be discouraged by a realistic demonstration of what may happen when the hair comes in contact with a revolving spindle.

Convincing workers that caps preserve hair from the effects of dusts, oils, and other shop conditions has resulted in some success in getting them to wear protective hair covering.

## Maintenance

Before each use, helmets should be inspected for cracks, signs of impact or rough treatment, and wear that might reduce the degree of safety originally provided. Prolonged exposure to ultraviolet rays (sunlight) and chemicals can shorten the life expectancy of thermoplastic helmets. Helmets that exhibit less surface gloss, chalking, or cracking should be discarded.

Protective helmets should not be stored or carried on the rear window shelf of a vehicle because sunlight and extreme heat may adversely affect the degree of protection. Another good reason not to carry hats there is that in case of an emergency stop or accident, the helmet might become a hazardous missile.

Once damaged, a protective helmet should be discarded. Alterations of any sort impair the performance of the headgear.

At least every 30 days, safety hats (in particular, their sweatbands and cradles) should be washed in warm, soapy water or a suitable detergent solution recommended by the manufacturer and then rinsed thoroughly.

Before reissuing used helmets to other employees, they should be scrubbed and disinfected. Solutions and powders are available which combine both cleaning and disinfecting. Helmets should be thoroughly rinsed with clean water and then dried.

Keep the wash solution and rinse water temperature at approximately 140 F (60 C). Do not use steam, except on aluminum helmets.

Removal of tar, paint, oil, and other materials may require the use of a solvent. Because some solvents can damage the shell, the helmet manufacturer should be consulted as to what solvent should be used.

Pay particular attention to the condition of the suspension because of the important part it plays in absorbing the shock of a blow. Look for loose or torn cradle straps, broken sewing lines, loose rivets, defective lugs, and other defects (Fig. 17–9). Sweatbands are easily replaced. Disposable helmet liners made of plastic or paper are available for hats used by many people (such as visitors).

An adequate number of crowns, sweatbands, and cradles should be stocked as replacement

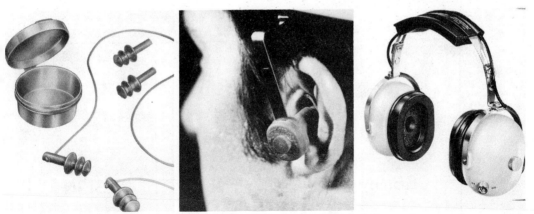

FIG. 17–10.—Three of the basic types of personal hearing protection. *Left*: One of three types of aural inserts. *Center*: Superaural. *Right*: Circumaural.

parts. Some companies replace the complete suspension at least once a year.

Many companies make use of colored safety hats to identify different working crews. Many colors are available; some colors are painted on and others have the color molded in. Before painting a hat, consult with its manufacturer so that a coating can be chosen which will not only last but which will not reduce the dielectric properties or attack and soften the shell material. Lighter colored hats are cooler to wear in the sun or under infrared energy sources. Safety people usually wear a white hat.

### Hearing Protection

Increasing attention is being paid to the problem of excessive noise in industry. See Chapter 9, "Industrial Noise" in *Fundamentals of Industrial Hygiene* in this Series.

Where it has been proven that engineering controls are not feasible as a permanent method of control, personal protective devices for noise control are acceptable. Their use, however, should be accompanied by an adequate hearing conservation program.

Some state regulations and portions of the OSHA legislation require audiometric testing of employees exposed to excessive noise. It is recommended that an audiometric testing program be initiated and maintained for employees who are exposed to noise levels in excess of 90 dBA. In fact, it is a good idea to test and maintain a record on all employees.

It is believed that a properly carried out audiometric testing program will determine whether the hearing protective devices worn by the employees are in fact protecting their hearing from noise damage.

### Types

Hearing protectors in general use fall into four types: enclosure, aural insert, superaural, and circumaural (see Fig. 17–10).

**Enclosure.** The enclosure type (Fig. 17–31) completely surrounds the head; the astronaut helmet is of this type. Attenuation of sound is achieved through the acoustical properties of the helmet. Additional attenuation can be achieved by wearing inserts with the enclosure type. Cost as well as bulk normally preclude use of this type for general use.

**Aural insert type.** The plug or insert type are generally classified in three broad types: (*a*) formable, (*b*) custom molded, and (*c*) molded type.

- *The formable type* fits all ears. Many of the formable types are designed for a one-time use only then thrown away. Material from which these disposable plugs are made include very fine glass fiber, wax-impregnated cotton, and expandable plastic.

- *Custom-molded* hearing protectors, as the

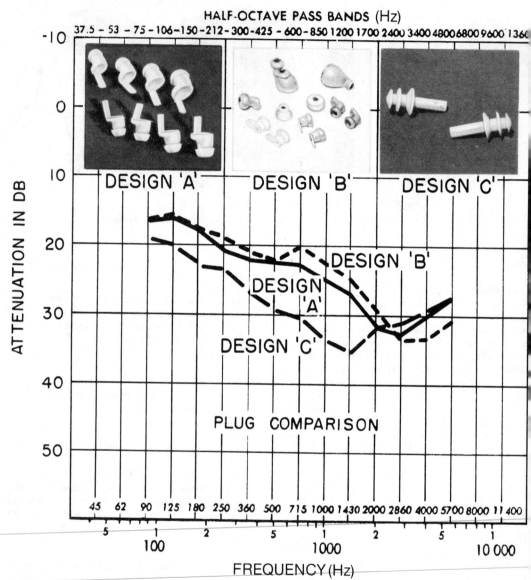

FIG. 17-11.—Attenuation (noise-reducing) characteristics of plug or insert type hearing protection. Curves are for plugs of design shown in photographs above.

name indicates, are made for a specific individual. A prepared mixture is carefully placed in the person's outer ear with a small portion of it in the ear canal; as the material sets, it takes the shape of the individual's ear and external ear canal. Only trained personnel should attempt the process of forming these hearing protectors.

• *Molded type* (or premolded) aural inserts are usually made from a soft silicone rubber or a plastic. The most important aspect of this type is to get a good fit. The hearing protector must fit

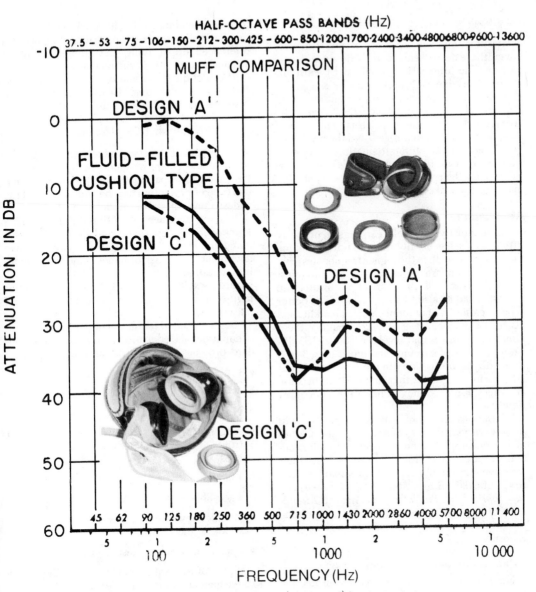

FIG. 17–12.—Attenuation characteristics of cup or muff type (circumaural) hearing protectors.

*Data from J. C. Webster and E. R. Rubin, U.S. Navy Electronics Laboratory.*

snugly in order to be effective. For some persons, this may cause some discomfort because of the irregular shape of the ear that some people possess. Also, these earplugs must be kept clean to avoid infection; also, by cleaning them—with a mild soap and water—their life is prolonged.

**Superaural** type of hearing protector depends on sealing the external edge of the ear canal in order to achieve sound reduction. A soft rubber-like material is used to make the caps, as they are sometimes called. They are held in place against the edges of the ear canal by a spring band or a head suspension.

**Circumaural type.** Cup (or earmuff) devices cover the external ear to provide an acoustic barrier. The attenuation provided by earmuffs varies widely due to differences in size, shape, seal material, shell mass, and type of suspension. Head size and shape also influence the attenuation characteristics of these protectors. The type of cushion used between the shell and the head has a great deal to do with attenuation efficiency. Liquid- or grease-filled cushions give better noise suppression than plastic or foam rubber types, but may present leakage problems.

### Attenuation

Commercially available earplugs if properly fitted and used, generally reduced noise reaching the ear by 25-30 dB in the higher frequencies (Fig. 17–11), which are conceded to be the most harmful. This will provide ample protection against sound levels of 115 to 120 dB. The better type of earmuffs may reduce noise an additional 10 to 15 decibels (Fig. 17–12), making them effective against sound levels of 130 to 135 dB. Combinations of earplugs and muffs give 3 to 5 more dB of protection. In no case will total attenuation be greater than about 50 dB because at this point, bone conduction becomes significant.

Variations from one model to another will provide varying degrees of noise reduction. Manufacturers supply attenuation data for their products so the safety professional can evaluate their effectiveness for use in a given situation. The ANSI Standard S3.19, *Method for the Measurement of Real-Ear Protectors and Physical Attenuation of Earmuffs*, gives methods for determining the efficiency of a specific device for a given noise exposure.

### Selection of hearing protectors

No matter how good a hearing protective device may be, its comfort has a great deal of influence on how well it will be accepted. Some people cannot wear earplugs for physical or psychological reasons. Others may not be able to wear the earmuff type of hearing protector. Consequently, many hearing conservation programs will include both types so the user may select the one most acceptable to him.

An aid in the selection of hearing protectors is the EPA requirement that calls for all protectors to have a label indicating its NRR (Noise Reduction Rating). As the NRR approaches a theoretical referenced upper limit, the amount of likely attenuation afforded will increase.

(For detailed information on this subject see *Industrial Noise and Hearing Conservation*, National Safety Council, Chicago, 1975.)

### Face and Eye Protection

Protection of the eyes and face from injury by physical and chemical agents or by radiation is vital in any occupational safety program. In fact, this type of protection has the widest use and the widest range of styles, models, and types.

The eye and face protection standard, Z87.1, *Practice for Occupational and Educational Eye and Face Protection*, is a fairly comprehensive document. It sets performance standards, including detailed tests, for a broad area of hazards—excluding only X rays, gamma rays, high-energy particulate radiations, lasers, and masers.

Besides general requirements, applying to "all occupations and educational processes," the standard provides requirements on the following:

- Rigid welding helmets
- Welding hand shields
- Nonrigid welding helmets
- Attachments and auxiliary equipment—lift fronts, chin rests, snoods, aprons, magnifiers, etc.
- Flammability
- Face Shields
- Goggles—eyecup (chipper's), dust and splash, welder's and cutter's
- Spectacles—metal, plastic, and combination.

Some of the requirements of the standard are stated generally. For example: "All shell material in helmets and shields shall be thermally insulating, and meet the requirements for slow burning, in accordance with paragraph 6.2.4 of ANSI Z87.1."

Other requirements are more precise. As regards flammability, for example, "The material shall not burn at a rate greater than 76 mm (3 in.) per minute."

**Changes in the standard.** However, the most

## Selection Chart for Eye and Face Protectors for Use in Industry, Schools, and Colleges

This Selection Chart offers general recommendations only. Final selection of eye and face protective devices is the responsibility of management and safety specialists. (For laser protection, refer to American National Standard for Safe Use of Lasers, ANSI Z136.1-1976.)

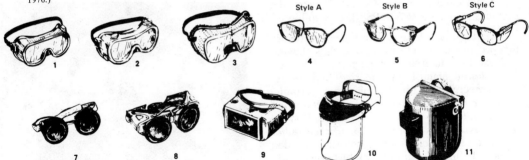

1. GOGGLES, Flexible Fitting, Regular Ventilation
2. GOGGLES, Flexible Fitting, Hooded Ventilation
3. GOGGLES, Cushioned Fitting, Rigid Body
*4. SPECTACLES, without Sideshields
5. SPECTACLES, Eyecup Type Sideshields
6. SPECTACLES, Semi-/Flat-Fold Sideshields
**7. WELDING GOGGLES, Eyecup Type, Tinted Lenses (Illustrated)

7A. CHIPPING GOGGLES, Eyecup Type, Clear Safety Lenses (Not Illustrated)
**8. WELDING GOGGLES, Coverspec Type, Tinted Lenses (Illustrated)
8A. CHIPPING GOGGLES, Coverspec Type, Clear Safety Lenses (Not Illustrated)
**9. WELDING GOGGLES, Coverspec Type, Tinted Plate Lens
10. FACE SHIELD, Plastic or Mesh Window (see caution note)
* 11. WELDING HELMET

*Non-sideshield spectacles are available for limited hazard use requiring only frontal protection.
**See Table A1, "Selection of Shade Numbers for Welding Filters," in Section A2 of the Appendix.

| APPLICATIONS | | |
|---|---|---|
| OPERATION | HAZARDS | PROTECTORS |
| ACETYLENE—BURNING ACETYLENE—CUTTING ACETYLENE—WELDING | SPARKS, HARMFUL RAYS, MOLTEN METAL, FLYING PARTICLES | 7, 8, 9 |
| CHEMICAL HANDLING | SPLASH, ACID BURNS, FUMES | 2 (For severe exposure add 10) |
| CHIPPING | FLYING PARTICLES | 1, 3, 4, 5, 6, 7A, 8A |
| ELECTRIC (ARC) WELDING | SPARKS, INTENSE RAYS, MOLTEN METAL | 11 (In combination with 4, 5, 6, in tinted lenses, advisable) |
| FURNACE OPERATIONS | GLARE, HEAT, MOLTEN METAL | 7, 8, 9 (For severe exposure add 10) |
| GRINDING—LIGHT | FLYING PARTICLES | 1, 3, 5, 6 (For severe exposure add 10) |
| GRINDING—HEAVY | FLYING PARTICLES | 1, 3, 7A, 8A (For severe exposure add 10) |
| LABORATORY | CHEMICAL SPLASH, GLASS BREAKAGE | 2 (10 when in combination with 5, 6) |
| MACHINING | FLYING PARTICLES | 1, 3, 5, 6 (For severe exposure add 10) |
| MOLTEN METALS | HEAT, GLARE, SPARKS, SPLASH | 7, 8 (10 in combination with 5, 6, in tinted lenses) |
| SPOT WELDING | FLYING PARTICLES, SPARKS | 1, 3, 4, 5, 6 (Tinted lenses advisable; for severe exposure add 10) |

CAUTION:
- Face shields alone do not provide adequate protection.
- Plastic lenses are advised for protection against molten metal splash.
- Contact lenses, of themselves, do not provide eye protection in the industrial sense and shall not be worn in a hazardous environment without appropriate covering safety eyewear.

Fig. 17-13.—Selection chart for eye and face protectors. See also Table 17-A.

*Courtesy American National Standards Institute.*

significant changes of the Z87.1-1979 from the previous standard, Z87.1-1968 are as follows:

*Special-purpose lenses.* This is a new category for specialized visual tasks, such as glass blowing and checking melt in metal or glass furnaces. Variable-tint plano (noncorrective) and corrective-protective (Rx) phototropic (photochromic) lenses *are not allowed for indoor application and are only allowable for outdoor tasks which do not involve hazardous ultraviolet or infrared radiation.* Phototropic lenses, which were not included in the old standard, must now all be permanently and distinctly marked with the symbol "V" as well as the manufacturer's monogram.

*Side shields.* The new standard lists three types of protective spectacles:

- Style A—without side shields. "The addition by users of accessory side shields which are not firmly secured does not upgrade or change the classification of Style A spectacles."

- Style B—with cup-type side shields. "The side shields shall not be easily detachable from the frame front and, in particular, accessory snap-on or clip-on types of side shields shall not be considered in compliance unless firmly secured."

- Style C—with semi- or flat-fold side shields. "Self-locking, slide-on side shields are acceptable. The side shields shall be firmly secured to protect against accidental removal."

*Tinted lenses.* A paragraph has been added recommending that "Tinted lenses should not be worn indoors unless called for by the nature of particular occupations, or when prescribed for individuals by ophthalmic specialists."

*Contact lenses.* Added to the old standard: "Contact lenses, of themselves, do not provide eye protection in the industrial sense and shall not be worn in a hazardous environment without appropriate covering safety eyewear."

*Product selection guide* (see Fig. 17–13). The three notes of caution have been added: (*a*) on face shields, (*b*) plastic lenses, and (*c*) contact lenses.

*Welding filter plates.* All welding filter plates must be hardened.

*Face shields.* The new standard emphasizes that face shields are not to be worn alone but are to be worn "over suitable basic eye protection."

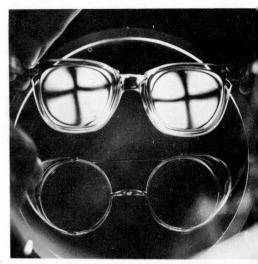

FIG. 17–14.—Photograph taken with light passing through two polarizing filters shows lack of heat treating in imported glass lenses (*below*). Safety glasses (*at top*) exhibit the proper crosspatterns.

*Product marketing.* Eye protection products must be marked with both the manufacturer's logo and a legible and permanent "Z87" logo.

*Protection limits.* A new qualifying statement has been added: "Nor should these requirements be interpreted to mean that protectors described herein are capable of affording greater protection than is specified in this standard."

*Glass breakage pattern.* Paragraph 6.3.4.2.3 of the old standard (Z87.1-1968) has been deleted. The paragraph had stated that hardened protective lens "shall break predominantly with radial cracks with a minor tendency toward concentric cracks." It is possible for a satisfactorily heat-treated lens to break in patterns other than as described in the old standard.

The Z87.1 standard also contains editorial clarification, an appendix that covers visible light transmission and a haze test for plastics, the selection of shade numbers for welding filters, and fitting details for goggles and spectacles.

### Background and supervision

Eye protective devices must be considered as optical instruments, and they should be carefully selected, fitted, and used.

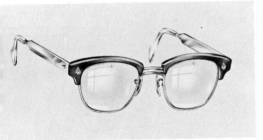

a. Plastic and metal frame safety spectacles, designed after regular streetwear glasses. The etched manufacturer's trademark on the lenses identify them as safety glass.

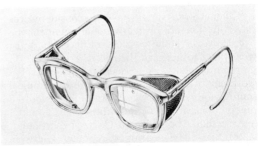

b. Plastic-frame safety spectacles with screened sideshields.

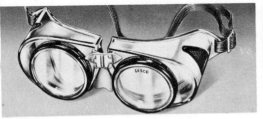

c. Rigid plastic chipper's goggles with standard round lenses.

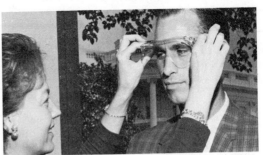

d. Light-weight, all-plastic visitor's spectacle.

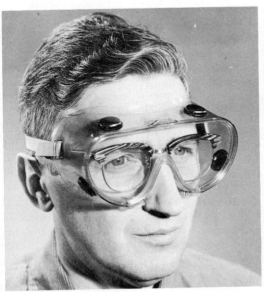

e. All-plastic, frame cover goggle with shielded vents.

FIG. 17–15.—Representative types of eye protection.

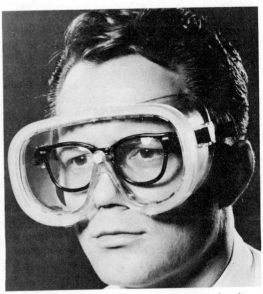

f. All-plastic frame chemical splash goggle with indirect and filtered ventilation for protection against heavy splash and driven mist.

Contact lenses should never be considered as a substitute for safe protective equipment for the eye. However, some workers, of necessity, must wear them to perform their jobs. Those that do must consequently exercise extra care. When the work environment entails exposure to chemical fumes, vapors, or splashes; intense heat, molten metals, or highly particulate atmosphere, contact lens use should be restricted. OSHA, in particular, states that the "wearing of contact lenses in contaminated environments with a respirator shall not be allowed." Workers have had their eyesight permanently impaired and have even been blinded by corrosive chemicals or small particles getting between the contact lens and the eye.

If corrective lenses are required, goggles, which cover ordinary spectacles, may be worn, but they require cups deep and wide enough to admit the whole spectacle. Goggles may also be worn over contact lenses.

The amount of money spent to acquire and fit eye protective devices is small when measured against the savings afforded by the protection given. For example, the purchase and fitting of a pair of impact-resistant spectacles may cost upward from 10 or 15 dollars; compensation costs for a lost eye may range from 5000 to 20,000 dollars.

If the eye protection program is supervised, directly or indirectly, by an industrial ophthalmologist, on either a full-time or consultation basis, there will be an additional return from proper utilization of the visual abilities of the work force.

Unfortunately, there is no impartial testing laboratory set up to approve eye protection devices according to generally known and accepted minimum performance specifications. Be sure that equipment is purchased from reputable manufacturers (Fig. 17–14).

## Impact protection

Three general types of equipment are used to protect eyes from flying particles encountered in such jobs as chipping, and grinding—spectacles with impact-resistant lenses, flexible or cushion-fitting goggles, and chipping goggles. (Refer to Fig. 17–15.)

**Spectacles** without sideshields are not recommended since they provide only frontal protection. Where side as well as frontal protection is

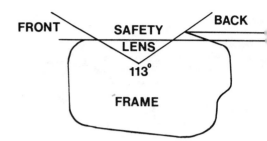

FIG. 17–16.—Cross section of safety lens in a safety frame.

required, the spectacles must have sideshields. Full-cup sideshields are designed to restrict the entry of flying particles from the side of the wearer. Semi-or flat-fold sideshields may be used where only lateral protection is required. Snap-on and clip-on sideshield types are not acceptable unless they are secured.

**Flexible fitting goggles** should have a wholly flexible frame forming the lens holder.

**Cushion-fitting goggles** should have a rigid plastic frame with a separate cushioned fitting surface on the facial contact area.

Both flexible and cushion goggles usually have a single plastic lens. These goggles are designed to give the eyes frontal and side protection from flying particles. Most models will fit over ordinary ophthalmic spectacles.

**Chipping goggles,** which have contour-shaped rigid plastic eyecups, come in two styles—one for individuals who do not wear spactacles, and one to fit over corrective spectacles. Chipping goggles should be used where maximum protection from flying particles is indicated.

## Selection of eyewear

Factors that should be considered in the selection of eyewear to protect from impact include the protection afforded, the comfort with which they can be worn, and the ease of keeping them in good repair. Styles now available (see Fig. 17–15a, –15b, and –15d) are similar to regular eyewear and are cosmetically pleasing. Flexible types are preferred by many because of their light weight and convenience. One drawback to the latter is they generally have a shorter wear-life than the more sturdier frame and glass lens type.

Proper eye protection devices should be selected, and their use should be impartially enforced so as to give maximum protection to the user for the degree of hazard involved. On certain jobs, 100 percent eye protection must be insisted upon.

Hardened glass ophthalmic lenses are no substitute for safety lenses. They generally are 2 mm thick instead of 3 mm for safety lenses. The lens bezel which fits the groove of the safety frame is ground to an 80 degree angle as contrasted to the 113 degree angle of a safety frame and safety lens. (See Fig. 17–16.)

Face shields are not recommended by ANSI Z87.1 as basic eye protection against impact. To get impact protection, face shields must be used in combination with basic eye protection. Face shields have their purpose, and are discussed later in this section.

## Plastic vs. glass lenses

When making a decision between plastic and glass lenses there are a number of things to consider:

● Both can pass impact tests when of certain formulation and thickness.

● Glass has a lower resistance than plastic to breakage from sharp objects.

● Tests show plastic lenses to have more favorable resistance to small objects moving at high rates of speed than glass.

● Abrasion resistance, while not good with plastic, is improved when the plastic is coated.

● Plastics are resistant to hot materials. Hot metal invariably shatters glass but not plastic. Hot metal also tends to adhere to glass.

● Plastics generally show surface reaction to some chemicals but satisfactorily stop splashes and protect the eyes.

● Whereas fogging occurs on both glass and plastic, it usually takes longer for plastic to fog.

Plastic goggles are available with a hydrophylic coating which tends to prevent fogging. There are also double-lens plastic goggles which operate on the Thermopane principle and suppress fogging to a large extent except under conditions of extreme humidity or cold. For extreme conditions of humidity, wire screen lenses of face shields may be suitable.

Spectacle frames should be rigid enough to hold the lenses in the proper position in front of the eyes. Plastic frames for safety glasses have the back of the groove slightly higher than the front to prevent the lenses from being pushed in; see Fig. 17–16. Frames should be constructed of corrosion-resistant material that will neither irritate nor color the skin. The simpler the design, the easier the spectacles are to clean.

Cup goggles should have cups large enough to protect the eye socket and to distribute the impact over a wide area of the facial bones. Cups should be flame-resistant, corrosion resistant, and nonirritating to the skin.

If lenses are to be exposed to pitting from grinding wheel sparks, a transparent and durable coating may be applied to them. Welding lenses should be protected by a cover lens of glass or plastic.

Lenses must not have appreciable distortion or prism effect. ANSI Z87.1 and Federal Specification GGG-G-50lb (*Federal Standard Stock Catalog*) limits the nonparallelism between the two faces to $1/16$ prism diopter (4 minutes of arc) and both the refraction in any meridian and the difference in refraction between any two meridians to $1/16$ diopter.

Both when supported in the eye cups of goggles and when supported on a rubber gasket on a wood tube, lenses are required to withstand the impact test described earlier in this section. (Additional information on eye protection can be found in the National Safety Council book, *Fundamentals of Industrial Hygiene*, 2nd ed.)

## Comfort and fit

To be comfortable, eye-protective equipment must be properly fitted. Corrective spectacles should be fitted only by members of the ophthalmic profession. An employee can be trained to fit, adjust, and maintain eye-protective equipment, however, and each employee can be taught the proper care of the device he uses.

To give the widest possible field of vision, goggles should be fitted as close to the eyes as possible, without bringing the eyelashes in contact with the lenses.

Various defogging materials are available. Before a selection is made, test to determine the most effective type for a specific application.

In areas where goggles or other types of eye protection are used extensively, goggle-cleaning

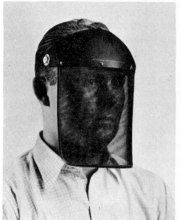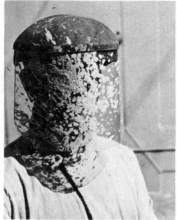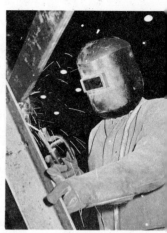

FIG. 17–17.—Three types of face shields. *Left*: Metal-screen face shield affords protection to furnacemen and others exposed to radiant heat. *Center*: Chemical-resistant full-face shield stopped a splash of boiling caustic. *Right*: Sturdy, nonflammable helmet with specified cover and filter plates protects welder from sparks, flying particles, and injurious rays.

stations can be conveniently located. Defogging materials and wiping tissues can be provided there along with a receptacle for discarding them.

Use of sweatbands helps prevent eye irritation, aids visibility, and eliminates work interruptions for face mopping.

Sweatbands are usually made of a soft, light, highly absorbent cellulose sponge. An elastic band holds the sweatband in place on the wearer's forehead so that it does not interfere with glasses or goggles. Evaporation from the exposed surface produces a cooling effect which adds to comfort.

## Face protection

Face shields are available in a wide variety of types to protect the face and neck from flying particles, sprays of hazardous liquids, splashes of molten metal, and from hot solutions (see Fig. 17–4a and –4d and 17–17). In addition, they may be used to provide antiglare protection where required. As a general rule, face shields should be worn over suitable basic eye protection.

Three basic styles of face shields include headgear without crown protectors, with crown protectors, and with crown and chin protectors. Each of the three is available with one of these replaceable window styles:

Clear transparent

Tinted transparent

Wire screen

Combination of plastic and screen

Fiber window with a filter plate mounting.

The materials used in face shields should combine mechanical strength, light weight, nonirritation to skin, and the capability of withstanding frequent disinfecting operations. Metals should be noncorrosive and plastics should be of the slow-burning type. Only optical grade (clear or tinted) plastic, which is free from flaws or distortions, should be used for the windows. And plastic windows should not be used in welding operations unless they conform to the standards of transmittance of absorptive lenses, filter lenses, and plates.

The metallic bindings on some plastic face shields help prevent the plastic from splitting and cracking. However, a slight bend in the binding will introduce an optical fault in the shield, making it unusable.

On some jobs, such as the pouring of low-melting metals, protection against radiation is not necessary, but it is desirable to protect the head and face against splashes of metal.

A face shield similar to an arc welder's face shield, but made of wire screen (which provides much better ventilation than a solid shield), can be used. *Federal Standard Stock Catalog* GGG-H-171 *Specifications* require a screen of 28-, 30-, or 36-mesh with wire 0.012 to 0.017 in. (0.30 mm to 0.43 mm) in diameter.

This shield is commonly used without a window because the plain wire will not fog under high termperature and high humidity. A metallized plastic shield that reflects a substantial percentage of heat has been developed for use where there is exposure to radiant heat.

## Acid hoods and chemical goggles

Head and face protection from splashes of acids, alkalis, or other hazardous liquids or chemicals may be provided in a variety of ways, depending upon the hazard. Good protection is given by a hood made of chemical-resistant material with a glass or plastic window (Fig. 17–18). In all cases, there should be a secure joint between the window and the hood materials.

Hoods are extremely hot to wear, but can be obtained with air lines for the wearer's comfort. When a hood is so supplied, the wearer should have a harness or belt like that on an air line respirator for support of the hose. A device based on a vortex principle has been developed to provide temperature-conditioned air.

If protection is necessary only from limited direct splashes, the wearer can don a face shield made of a material unaffected by the liquid or a flexible-fitting chemical goggle with baffled ventilation, if the eyes are not exposed to irritating vapor.

For severe exposures a face shield should be worn in connection with the flexible-fitting chemical goggles.

Face shields should be shaped to cover the whole face. They should be supported from a headband or harness, so they can be tipped back and clear the face easily. Any shield should be easily removed in case it becomes wet with corrosive liquid.

If goggles worn under the shield are of the nonventilated type for protection against vapor as well as against splashing, they should be of the nonfogging type (described earlier).

## Laser beam protection

No one type of glass or plastic offers protection from all laser wavelengths. Consequently, most laser-using firms don't depend on safety glasses to protect an employee's eyes from laser burns. Some point out that laser goggles or glasses might give a false sense of security, tempting the wearer to expose himself to unnecessary hazards.

Nevertheless, researchers and laser technicians do frequently need eye protection.

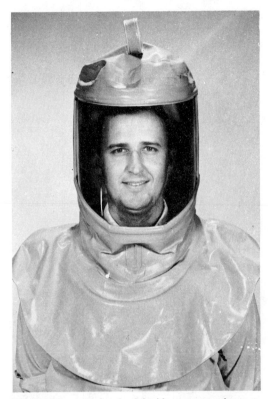

FIG. 17–18.—Acid hood of highly resistant plastic is designed for protection from acids and other corrosive chemical solutions. Rear-shielded ventilation ports can be used where ambient air is respirable. Where air is not, use air-fed models.

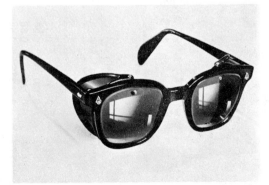

FIG. 17–19.—Laser protective spectacles. To designate specific wavelength protection, frames should be distinctively colored and optical density should be shown on the filter.

**493**

## TABLE 17-A
## TRANSMITTANCES AND TOLERANCES IN TRANSMITTANCE OF VARIOUS SHADES OF ABSORPTIVE LENSES, FILTER LENSES, AND PLATES

| Shade Number | Optical Density | | | Luminous Transmittance | | | Maximum Infrared Transmittance | Maximum Spectral Transmittance in the Ultraviolet and Violet | | | |
|---|---|---|---|---|---|---|---|---|---|---|---|
| | Maximum | Standard | Minimum | Maximum Percent | Standard Percent | Minimum Percent | Percent | 313 nm Percent | 334 nm Percent | 365 nm Percent | 405 nm Percent |
| 1.5 | 0.26 | 0.214 | 0.17 | 67 | 61.5 | 55 | 25 | 0.2 | 0.8 | 25 | 65 |
| 1.7 | 0.36 | 0.300 | 0.26 | 55 | 50.1 | 43 | 20 | 0.2 | 0.7 | 20 | 50 |
| 2.0 | 0.54 | 0.429 | 0.36 | 43 | 37.3 | 29 | 15 | 0.2 | 0.5 | 14 | 35 |
| 2.5 | 0.75 | 0.643 | 0.54 | 29 | 22.8 | 18.0 | 12 | 0.2 | 0.3 | 5 | 15 |
| 3.0 | 1.07 | 0.857 | 0.75 | 18.0 | 13.9 | 8.50 | 9.0 | 0.2 | 0.2 | 0.5 | 6 |
| 4.0 | 1.50 | 1.286 | 1.07 | 8.50 | 5.18 | 3.16 | 5.0 | 0.2 | 0.2 | 0.5 | 1.0 |
| 5.0 | 1.93 | 1.714 | 1.50 | 3.16 | 1.93 | 1.18 | 2.5 | 0.2 | 0.2 | 0.2 | 0.5 |
| 6.0 | 2.36 | 2.143 | 1.93 | 1.18 | 0.72 | 0.44 | 1.5 | 0.1 | 0.1 | 0.1 | 0.5 |
| 7.0 | 2.79 | 2.571 | 2.36 | 0.44 | 0.27 | 0.164 | 1.3 | 0.1 | 0.1 | 0.1 | 0.5 |
| 8.0 | 3.21 | 3.000 | 2.79 | 0.164 | 0.100 | 0.061 | 1.0 | 0.1 | 0.1 | 0.1 | 0.5 |
| 9.0 | 3.64 | 3.429 | 3.21 | 0.061 | 0.037 | 0.023 | 0.8 | 0.1 | 0.1 | 0.1 | 0.5 |
| 10.0 | 4.07 | 3.854 | 3.64 | 0.023 | 0.0139 | 0.0085 | 0.6 | 0.1 | 0.1 | 0.1 | 0.5 |
| 11.0 | 4.50 | 4.286 | 4.07 | 0.0085 | 0.0052 | 0.0032 | 0.5 | 0.05 | 0.05 | 0.05 | 0.1 |
| 12.0 | 4.93 | 4.714 | 4.50 | 0.0032 | 0.0019 | 0.0012 | 0.5 | 0.05 | 0.05 | 0.05 | 0.1 |
| 13.0 | 5.36 | 5.143 | 4.93 | 0.0012 | 0.00072 | 0.00044 | 0.4 | 0.05 | 0.05 | 0.05 | 0.1 |
| 14.0 | 5.79 | 5.571 | 5.36 | 0.00044 | 0.00027 | 0.00016 | 0.3 | 0.05 | 0.05 | 0.05 | 0.1 |

*Courtesy American National Standards Institute.*

Both spectacles and goggles are available—and glass or plastic for protection against nearly all the known lasers can be had on special order from eyewear manufacturers. Typically, the eyewear will have maximum attenuation at a specific laser wavelength—with protection falling off rather rapidly at other wavelengths.

Laser protective goggles or spectacles (Fig. 17–19) or an "anti-laser eyeshield" (Fig. 17–20) attenuate the He-Ne laser light (wavelength 6328 A or 632.8 ) by factors of 10 (O.D. = 1), 100 (O.D. = 2), 1000 (O.D. = 3), or more. An optical density (O.D.) of three or four still renders the beam visible in bright sunlight. The goggle-type of protective eyewear used in the laboratory is often unsuitable in the field because of fogging.

The American Conference of Governmental Industrial Hygienists cautions that laser safety glasses or goggles should be evaluated periodically to make sure that maintenance of adequate optical density is kept at the desired laser wavelength. There should be assurance that laser glasses or goggles designed for protection from specific laser wavelengths are not mistakenly used with different wavelengths of laser radiation. The optical density values and wavelengths should be shown on the eyewear. Eyewear storage shelves can also carry this notation.

Laser safety glasses or goggles exposed to very intense energy or power density levels may lose effectiveness and should be discarded.

Technical details, uses, hazards, and exposure criteria for lasers are given in *Fundamentals of Industrial Hygiene*, National Safety Council, Chicago, 1979. Also see ANSI Z136.1, *The Safe Use of Lasers*.

### Eye protection for welding

In addition to damage from physical and chemical agents, the eyes are subject to the effects of radiant energies. Ultraviolet, visible, and infrared bands of the spectrum are all able to produce harmful effects upon the eyes, and therefore require special attention.

Ultraviolet rays can produce cumulative destructive changes in the structure of the cornea and lens of the eye. Short exposures of intense ultraviolet radiation or prolonged exposures to ultraviolet radiations of low intensity will produce painful, but ordinarily self-repearing corneal damage.

Radiations in the visible light band, if too intense, can cause eyestrain and headache, and

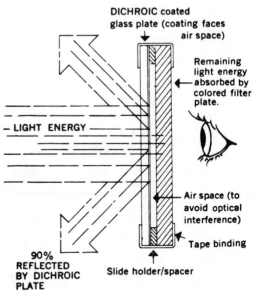

FIG. 17–20.—Diagram shows how "antilaser eyeshield" deflects laser beam.

can destroy the tissue of the retina.

Infrared radiations transmit large amounts of heat energy to the eye, causing discomfort. The damage produced is superficial.

The filtering properties of filter lenses have been established by the National Bureau of Standards. The percentage transmittance of radiant energies in the three bands—ultraviolet, visible, and infrared—is established for 16 different filter lens shades (Table 17–A). Also see Table 13-B in the *Accident Prevention Manual, Engineering and Technology* volume, for type of operation for which each lens shade is recommended.

Photochromic lenses (they darken in sunlight and fade indoors in low light levels) should not be used as a substitute for established filter lens shades. They have high transmission in the near-ultraviolet and infrared.

Welding processes (see Chapter 13, "Welding and Cutting" in the *Engineering and Technology* volume) emit radiations in three spectral bands. Depending upon the flux used and the size and temperature of the pool of melted metal, welding processes will emit more or less visible and infrared radiation—the proportion of the energy emitted in the visible range increases as the temperature rises. At least one manufacturer

**495**

produces an aluminized cover for the usual black welding helmet. Its purpose is to reduce infrared absorption and the resulting heat stress to the wearer.

All welding presents problems, mostly in the control of infrared and visible radiations. Heavy gas welding and cutting operations, and arc cutting and welding exceeding 30 amperes, present additional problems in control of ultraviolet. Welding helmets must be used to provide head and face protection (Fig. 17–17, far right).

Welders may choose the shade of lenses they prefer within one or two shade numbers. Following are shades commonly used:

SHADES NO. 1.5 TO No. 3.0 are intended for glare from snow, ice, and reflecting surfaces; and for stray flashes and reflected radiation from cutting and welding operations in the immediate vicinity (for goggles or spectacles with side shields worn under helmets in arc welding operations, particularly gas-shielded arc welding operations).

SHADE No. 4, the same uses as shades 1.5 to 3.0, but for greater radiation intensity.

For welding, cutting, brazing, or soldering operations, use the guide for the selection of proper shade numbers of filter lenses or windows in Chapter 13 of the *Engineering and Technology* volume. (Recommendations are also in ANSI Z87.1, *Eye and Face Protection*.)

To protect the filter lenses against pitting, they should be worn with a replaceable plastic or glass cover plate.

Eye protection having mild filter shade lenses or polarizing lenses, and having opaque side shields, are adequate for protection against glare only. For conditions where hot metal may spatter and where visible glare must be reduced, a plastic face shield worn over mild filter shade spectacles with opaque side shields should be specified.

It is permissible to combine the shade of the plate in a welder's helmet with that of the shade of the goggle worn underneath to produce the desired total shade. This procedure has the added advantage of protecting the eyes from other welding operations or from an accidental arc when the helmet is raised (Fig. 17–21).

To protect against ultraviolet and infrared radiation as well as against visible glare in inspection operations, protective lenses should be installed in a hand shield or welder's helmet. The

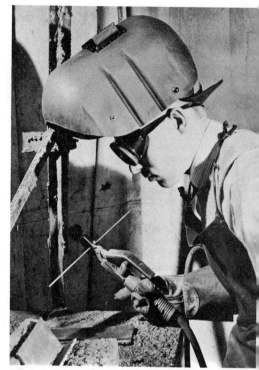

FIG. 17–21.—Double eye protection in electric welding. Flash goggles have No. 4 shade lens; they protect welder's eyes from the arc of other welders when he lifts his helmet to inspect work.

shield should be made of a nonflammable material, which is opaque to dangerous radiation and a poor conductor of heat. A metal shield is not desirable, because it heats under infrared radiation.

Some tinted lenses used in special work afford no protection from infrared and ultraviolet radiations. For instance, most melters' blue glass used in open-hearth furnaces and the lenses used at Bessemer converters afford no protection against either type of harmful radiation. Probably no harm will come from continued use of these lenses if the exposures are of short duration. However, new personnel learning these flame reading skills should be provided with lenses that protect in these two portions of the spectrum.

The chemical composition of the lens rather than its color provides the filtering effect; this factor must be considered when selecting a filtering lens.

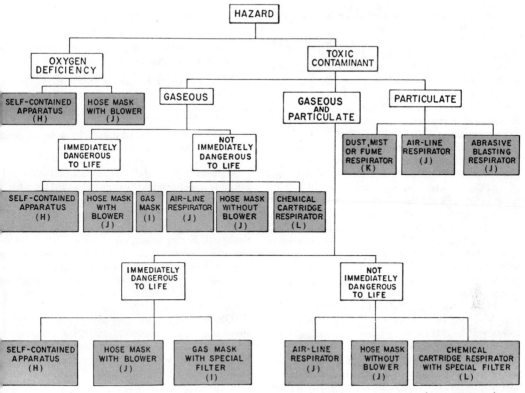

Fig. 17-22.—Suggested outline for selecting respiratory protective devices. Letters in parentheses (in shaded boxes) refer to Subparts of Title 30, CFR, Chapter I, Part 11, which discuss the items.

## Respiratory Equipment

The National Institute for Occupational Safety and Health (NIOSH) of the U.S. Department of Human Resources and the Mine Safety and Health Administration (MSHA) of the U.S. Department of the Interior have established minimum performance requirements for many respiratory protective devices. Following the enactment of OSHAct in 1970, Title 30, *Code of Federal Regulations*, Part 11 was jointly promulgated by NIOSH and MSHA's predesessor. This regulation prescribes approval procedures, establishes fees, and extends the requirements for obtaining joint approval of respirators.

NIOSH is now the testing and certifying agency for respirators, as well as a variety of other personal safety devices. This action removed primary responsibility for respirator testing and approval from USBM.

Use of the terms "approved" and "certified" reflects the applicable departmental regulations. Those regulations issued under the authority of the Coal Mine Health and Safety Act of 1969 refer to "approval" of respiratory protective devices. NIOSH regulations issued under the authority of *OSHAct* refer to "certification."

Part 11 of Title 30 CFR also placed an end-date of June 30, 1975, on the manufacture of USBM-approved respirators. However, users having such devices at the cut-off date are permitted to continue using them under a "grandfather" clause.

Most manufacturers will continue to furnish parts for the devices used under the grandfather clause.

NIOSH maintains a testing laboratory and issues approval certificates to manufacturers for particular respiratory devices in their entirety. Individual components, such as face pieces, hoses, or canisters, are not approved separately. An approval number appears on each component of the certified assembly, where feasible. A label appears on the device; Figs. 17–1 and –23.

The requirements for approval are contained in the Department of Interior's "Respiratory Protective Apparatus; Tests for Permissibility; Fees," contained in the Title 30, *Code of Federal Regulations*, Chapter 1, "Mine Safety and Health Administration," Subchapter B, Part 11. In some respects, these requirements are more stringent than the former Bureau of Mines requirements. The subparts of Part 11 that discuss various types of devices are shown in Fig. 17–22. NIOSH/MSHA are the official agencies for testing respiratory protective equipment—they test and certify mechanical filter respirators under Subpart K of Title 30 CFR, Part 11. This schedule discusses respirators for one or any combination of particulate hazard-nuisance, fibrosis-producing, or toxic dusts, mists, fumes, and radionuclides.

Although the NIOSH-MSHA certification system does not extend to every type of hazard, whenever there is a choice between certified and uncertified devices, the certified devices should be selected. Additional information on respirators can be found in Chapter 23, "Respiratory Protective Equipment," *Fundamentals of Industrial Hygiene*, 2nd ed.

## Respirator selection

Proper respiratory selection shall be made when engineering controls are not feasible, or if they are feasible, while they are being instituted, as noted in the OSHA regulations—see § 1910.134(a)(1) and (c). ANSI Standard Z88.2 can be of great value for this purpose because much of the OSHA respiratory protection standard was taken from it. In addition, the manufacturer of the respiratory devices should be consulted.

Among the many factors to be considered in the selection of the proper respiratory protective device for any given situation involving air contamination are the following. (The general principles for selecting respiratory protective devices are outlined in Fig. 17–22.)

1. The nature of the hazardous operation or process

2. The type of air contaminant, including its physical properties, chemical properties,

physiological effects on the body, and its concentration

3. The period of time for which respiratory protection must be provided

4. The location of the hazard area with respect to a source of uncontaminated respirable air

5. The state of health of personnel involved

6. The functional and physical characteristics of respiratory protective devices.

**Misuse.** The safety professional should become familiar with the type of hazard for which a given type of respiratory equipment is approved, and should not permit its use for protection against hazards for which it is not designed. *For instance, particulate filter respirators are of no value as protection against solvent vapors, injurious gases, or lack of oxygen. Their use under these conditions is one of the most common and most dangerous abuses of respirators.*

Other common misuses of respiratory equipment are to use chemical cartridge respirators where gas masks are required or to use chemical filtering types where atmosphere-supporting or self-contained units are necessary.

**Double hazards.** Some substances require protection against (a) damage to the respiratory system and also (b) systemic injury through the skin. All substances should be investigated to learn whether this double hazard is involved. Some common substances which are hazardous through both the respiratory system and the skin are:

Ammonia
Aniline
Carbon disulfide
Cresol (cresylic acid)
Dichloroethylene-1,1
Decalin (decahydronaphthalene)
Diethylene oxide (dioxane-1,4)
Diethylphthalate
Dimethylaniline
Dinitrobenzene
Dinitrochlorobenzene
Hydrogen cyanide (hydrocyanic acid)
Iodoform
Lead tetraethyl
Mercury and its compounds
Nicotine

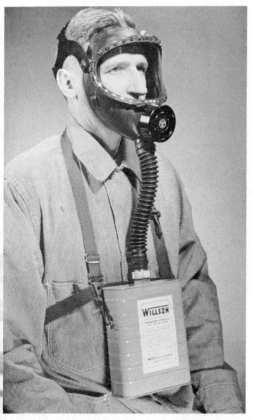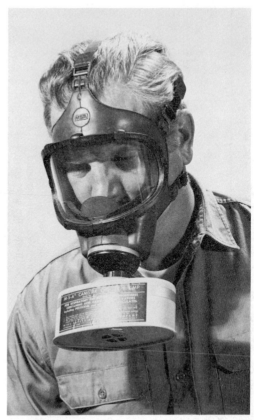

FIG. 17–23.—Two different designs of canister-type gas masks. Note the speaking diaphragms and the face pieces which allow wide, panoramic vision. *Left*: Mask makes use of a rigid, adjustable head harness. *Right*: Mask has conventional strap-type head harness.

Nitrobenzene
Nitroglycerine
Organic phosphate insecticides
Phenyl hydrazine
Tetralin (tetrahydronaphthalene)

Protective clothing should also be worn when appreciable amounts of hazardous substances, such as those listed above, are present. See the Council's book, *Fundamentals of Industrial Hygiene*, 2nd ed.

**Health.** Some workers consider respiratory equipment a nuisance, not realizing that failure to wear it may endanger their lives. Usually, the attitude of such people can be changed if someone in authority will clearly explain why the equipment is necessary, show them how to fit it in

position, and explain its operation. If such educational efforts fail, the alternative is discipline, for the risk of injury is serious.

Excellent health and thorough training in the operation and maintenance of equipment are essential for persons who are to use respiratory protective devices. Anyone in questionable physical condition should be prevented from entering environments presenting respiratory hazards, and thus avoid having to wear any emergency breathing apparatus for protection.

**Air and oxygen.** From the standpoint of fire hazard, neither pure oxygen nor air containing more than 21 percent oxygen is to be preferred to ordinary air for use in atmosphere (air) supplied respirators or open-circuit (demand) type self-

**499**

TABLE 17-B. CHARACTERISTICS OF GAS MASKS AND THEIR CANISTERS

| Mask | Type | Max. Con. of gas (% by vol.)° | Color of Canister (OSHA-NIOSH)† | Materials in Canister | Remarks |
|------|------|-------------------------------|----------------------------------|-----------------------|---------|
| ACID GAS (for protection against gases such as hydrogen sulfide, sulfur dioxide, chlorine, hydrocyanic acid) | A | 2% | White | Soda lime or soda lime and activated charcoal | The time of protection decreases rapidly as the concentration of gas increases. (See Notes 1, 2, 3, 5) |
| ORGANIC VAPOR (for protection against vapors such as aniline, benzene, ether, gasoline, carbon tetrachloride, chloropicrin) | B | 2% | Black | Activated charcoal | (See Notes 1, 2, 3, 5) |
| AMMONIA GAS | C | 3% | Green | Silica gel or porous granules impregnated with metallic salts such as those of copper or cobalt | (See Note 4) |
| CARBON MONOXIDE | D | 2% | Blue | Hopcalite | The air becomes noticeably warmer as the percentage of carbon monoxide increases (See Notes 1, 2, 3.) |
| DUST FUMES, MISTS, FOGS AND SMOKES in combination with any of the above gases or vapors | AE, etc. | 2% | Any of above, plus top grey stripe | Any of above plus mechanical filter | (See Note 6) |
| COMBINATION ACID GAS AND ORGANIC VAPOR | AB | 2% acid gases 2% organic vapors | Yellow | Activated charcoal and soda lime | (See Notes 1, 2, 3, 4) |
| COMBINATION ACID GAS, ORGANIC VAPOR AND AMMONIA GAS | ABC | 2% acid gas 2% organic vapor 2% ammonia | Brown | Soda lime, activated charcoal and silica gel or impregnated porous granules | As the number of gases increases, the service time of the canister decreases (See Notes 1, 2, 3.) |
| COMBINATION ACID GAS, AMMONIA GAS | AC | 2% acid gases 3% ammonia | Green with white stripe at bottom | Soda lime, silica gel or porous granules impregnated with metal salts such as those of | |

contained breathing apparatus, for ventilating, or for other purposes. A flammable substance in the presence of oxygen requires only a small fraction of the energy to ignite it as does the same substance in the presence of air, and an ensuing fire or explosion is much more violent.

Air or oxygen provided by or supplied to any respiratory equipment must be free from contaminants; quality as well as quantity is important. Respirable air should comply with the Compressed Gas Association *Commodity Specification for Air*, G-7.1-1966 (ANSI Z86.1), Grade D. This specifies that the maximum impurities be as follows: condensed hydrocarbons, 5 mg/m³ of gas at NTP; carbon monoxide, 10 mg/m³; and carbon dioxide, 1000 mg/m³. The presence of a pronounced odor renders the air unsatisfactory for breathing. The standard gives methods of verification and other details.

Oxygen should meet the requirements of the *United States Pharmacopoeia*. (See References.)

**Classification.** Respiratory protective devices can be classified as follows.

1. Air purifying devices

2. Atmosphere (air) supplied respirators, and

3. Self-contained breathing devices.

In turn, these are divided into a number of subclasses.

### 1. Air Purifying Devices

The air purifying device cleanses the contaminated atmosphere. Chemicals can be used to remove specific gases and vapors and mechanical filters can remove particulate matter. This type of device is limited in its use to those environments where there is sufficient oxygen to sustain life and the air contaminant level is within the specified concentration limitation of the device. The useful life of an air purifying device is limited by the concentration of the air contaminants, the breathing demand of the wearer, and the removal capacity of the air purifying medium.

#### Gas masks

The gas mask type of air purifying respirator consists of a facepiece connected by a flexible tube to a canister (Fig. 17–23). Contaminated air is purified by chemicals in the canister.

Because no one chemical has been found that will remove all gaseous contaminants, the canister must be carefully chosen to fit the specific need. A canister designed for a specific gas or vapor (or a single class of gases or vapors) will give longer protection than a same-sized canister designed for protection against a multitude of gases and vapors.

NIOSH-MSHA tests and certifies gas masks for a number of gases and vapors and combinations of these hazards. Gas masks that protect against airborne particulates, in addition to gases and vapors, are available. Table 17–B lists the general characteristics of gas masks and their canisters.

To meet the needs for protection from contaminants, industrial-type canisters are available to take care of acid gases, organic vapors, and combinations of the two general classes. They are identified as chin-style, industrial, and super-size. In addition, canisters have been developed for specific gases—such as chlorine, ammonia, and hydrocyanic acid.

Mechanical filters also are used when it becomes necessary to protect against dust and smoke, as well as toxic gases. (Combination respirators are discussed later in this section.)

It is usually more practical and economical to use an industrial-type of chin-style mask where protection is required from only one type of gas. All-around protection—for emergency repairs where almost anything can be encountered, and where it would not be practical to change the canister—is provided by a mask designated as Type N. It is distinguishable from other industrial masks by two features—an indicator for service life against carbon monoxide, and its red color. Table 17–B lists the approved color code for cartridges and gas mask canisters, as listed in American National Standard K13.1, *Identification of Air Purifying Respirator Canisters and Cartridges.*

The Type N mask protects against a broad spectrum of smokes, gases, and fumes, including ammonia and carbon monoxide, where known measured concentrations do not exceed the limits for canister masks, and where there is sufficient oxygen present to support life.

The more recently developed models of Type N masks feature a very efficient mechanical filter capable of removing fine particulate matter and chemical dusts. Their canisters have several layers of chemicals so that successive types or classes of gases and vapors are removed as the air progresses through them and emerges in a breathable state.

Canister gas masks with full facepiece are for emergency protection in atmospheres immediately dangerous to life. They do *not* provide protection against oxyygen deficiency; their effectiveness is limited to use in atmospheres containing at least 19.5 percent (by volume) oxygen, and not more than 2 percent of those toxic gases for which they are designed (except for ammonia, for which the limit is 3 percent, and phosphine, for which the limit is 0.5 percent).

Gas masks should not be used for firefighting in accordance with the NFPA Standard 19B, *Respiratory Protective Equipment for Firefighters,* because of the possibility of oxygen deficiency. Self-contained breathing apparatus should be used; see the sections that follow on hose masks and self-contained breathing devices.

The period of protection that a gas mask provides depends upon (a) the type of canister, (b) the concentration of the gas or vapor, and (c) the activity of the user.

Each person who must use a gas mask should first undergo a physical examination, especially of his heart and lungs.

**Train carefully.** Because the gas mask is ordinarily used in emergencies, where there is strain and excitement, those who use it should be carefully trained.

One of the first lessons should be how to make sure the mask will fit. To do this, the wearer should:

1. Remove the seal from the bottom of the canister and put on the head piece.

2. Adjust the head straps until the mask fits closely and comfortably.

3. See that there are no kinks in the tubes or the hose.

4. Breath naturally and observe the amount of resistance to inhalation.

5. Grasp the hose tightly and close off the air intake. Breathe deeply until the facepiece collapses. If correctly adjusted, the facepiece will remain collapsed until the intake is opened.

In training practice, the user should wear the mask long enough to become accustomed to the

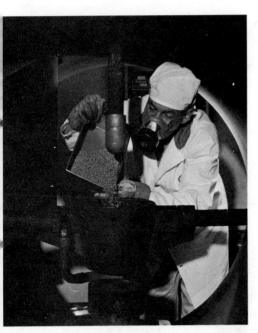

FIG. 17-24.—Single cartridge chemical respirator. Twin-cartridge units are also available and give longer life and less breathing resistance.

breathing resistance.

As a further check on the fit of the mask and the effectiveness of the canister, the user of a gas mask should enter the contaminated area cautiously. If the mask leaks or the canister is exhausted, the user will usually know by odor, taste, or irritation of eye, nose, or throat, and should immediately return to fresh air.

If the canister is used up, it should not be left attached, but removed, and a new one should be selected and fastened in place. When a respirator is worn in a gas or vapor that has little or no warning properties, like carbon monoxide, it is recommended that a fresh canister be used each time a person enters the toxic atmosphere.

Gas masks that offer respiratory protection against carbon monoxide must have an indicator that shows when the canister should be changed for protection against that gas. This is needed because water vapor renders useless the chemical (used for carbon monoxide removal), whether or not carbon monoxide is present. Nonwindow-type canisters should not be used; tests on nonwindow-type canisters that had been unsealed

for some time showed they had lost their ability to remove carbon monoxide, even though the inhalation resistance of most canisters was the same as for fresh canisters.

Canisters are usually supplied with seals to prevent air from entering them until they are to be used. These seals should be removed when the canister is installed in the mask.

**Storage.** If a universal Type N canister having an indicating window is used for protection against carbon monoxide, it should be discarded as soon as the color change in the window indicates that the canister will no longer convert carbon monoxide to carbon dioxide.

A card should be set up for each mask to indicate the date of the latest inspection and replacement of the canister, and the amount of use which the canister has had. If the mask is for emergencies only, it is wise to replace the canister after each use.

Gas masks should be kept easily available for emergencies. For instance, in an ice plant that could have an ammonia leak, the mask should be placed just inside or outside one of the exit doors so that it can be reached quickly without disabling exposure to the gas. It should not be kept too near the ice machine or ammonia piping.

Masks should be stored away from moisture, heat, and direct sunlight, and should be regularly inspected.

### Chemical cartridge respirators

Chemical cartridge respirators consist of a half-mask facepiece connected directly to one or two small containers of chemicals (Fig. 17-24). Chemicals used are similar to those found in gas masks, but cartridge respirators are for use only in nonemergency situations; that is, for atmospheres which are harmful only after prolonged or repeated exposures.

Previously, Bureau of Mines approval has been given *only* for Type B (organic vapor) and Type BE (dusts, fumes, and mists in combination with organic vapors). These types are approved for concentrations not in excess of 1000 parts of organic vapor per one million parts of air. Now, Subpart K (23c) of Title 30—Mineral Resources, *Code of Federal Regulations*, Part 11, permits certification of respirators providing respiratory protection against certain other gases.

Four important "don'ts" apply to chemical cartridge respirators:

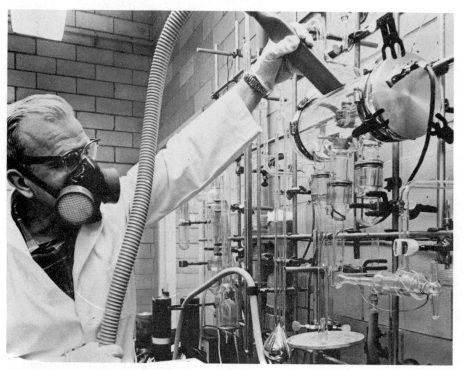

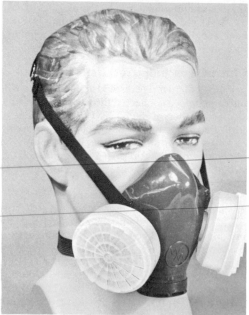

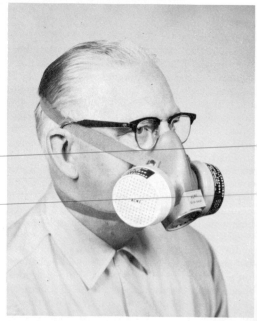

FIG. 17–25.—*Top*: Dust respirator and safety glasses protect employee during laboratory cleaning operation. *Lower Left*: Twin-cartridge dust respirator. *Lower right*: Twin-cartridge organic vapor respirator.

1. Don't use them for protection against gaseous materials that are extremely toxic in very small concentrations.

2. Don't use them for exposures to harmful gaseous matter that cannot be detected clearly by odor, or by nose or throat irritation.

3. Don't use them against any gaseous material in concentrations that are highly irritating to the eyes.

4. Don't use them for protection against gaseous material that is not effectively halted by chemical cartridges utilized, regardless of concentration.

### Particulate filter respirators

A particulate (mechanical) filter respirator can be designed to give satisfactory protection against any kind of particle (Fig. 17-25). The major items to be considered are the resistance to breathing offered by the filtering element, the adaptation of the facepiece to faces of various sizes and shapes, and the fineness of the particles to be filtered out.

Low breathing resistance requires a fairly large area of filtering medium. Fineness of the filter is fixed by the permissible leakage for various dusts. It is important that breathing resistance be low even after the respirator has had considerable use under dusty conditions. Excessive breathing resistance wastes energy and may be the source of lung injury if long continued.

Filters of high porosity may give low breathing resistance with small filter area, but they will not stop fine dust. All such filters do is to improve comfort by catching the larger particles, which are usually caught in the nose and throat.

Breathing out against resistance does not engender the psychological effect that resistance to inhalation does. However, it can be detrimental in that it is physically tiring.

Filters should be replaced whenever breathing becomes difficult due to plugging of filters by retained particulates.

### Combination respirators

Combination chemical and mechanical filter respirators utilize dust, mist, or fume filters with a chemical cartridge for dual or multiple exposure. Normally, the dust filter plugs up before the chemical cartridge is exhausted. It is therefore preferable to use respirators with independently replaceable filters. Carefully attach the filter to the chemical cartridge.

The combination respirator is well suited for spray painting and welding.

## 2. Atmosphere (Air) Supplied Respirators

### Hose masks

Hose masks are available with blower (power driven or hand operated, Fig. 17-26), without a blower, or connected to a source of respirable air under pressure. None of the respirators is approved in an *immediately dangerous to life or health (IDLH)* atmosphere.

The danger is considered immediate if, in the event of failure of the equipment, escape from the dangerous (toxic, flammable, and/or oxygen deficient°) atmosphere would be impossible or could not be made without serious injury.

In case of failure of the air supply on a hose mask with blower, it is still possible to breathe through the hose while making an escape.

Hose masks with blowers can be certified with a maximum of 300 ft (91 m) of hose for each person. For hose masks without blowers, the certification is for a maximum of 75 ft (22.9 m) of hose.

Most blowers for hose masks have two outlets so that two workers, each with a maximum of 300 ft of hose, can be supplied.

A hose line is not intended for use as a life line, but as a breathing tube. When a hose mask is used, a helper should be assigned with no duties other than to observe the man in the hazardous atmosphere, tend the life line, and rescue the first man if necessary. The helper, too, should be equipped with a harness and life line, in addition to a self-contained breathing apparatus. When hose masks with blower are used, a blower operator also must be provided. Be sure the blower intake is located outside the contaminated area.

The body harness needed to pull the hose lines requires inspection prior to each use. The minimum requirement for certification is that the component parts of the harness shall withstand a pull of at least 250 pounds (1110 newtons). Parts

---

° Almost every flammable gas and vapor is toxic; however many toxic gases and vapors are nonflammable. See Appendix C, "Chemical Hazards," in *Fundamentals of Industrial Hygiene*, 2nd ed., for several examples.

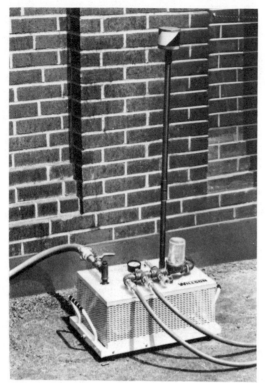

FIG. 17-26.—An air line respirator blower unit requires a fresh air source.

which are to be used subsequently should not be tested by being pulled, but only should be examined for signs of wear or deterioration. If a condition is found which appreciably reduces strength, the harness should be replaced.

NIOSH-MSHA certification requires that 50 liters/min (106 cu ft/hr) be delivered to each facepiece through the maximum length of hose at not more than 50 rpm of the blower crank. Under most working conditions, this amount would furnish enough air to the wearers.

To eliminate dust and fumes that may have accumulated within a mask, air line and breathing tubes should be blown out with air before a mask is put on. The couplings in the hose lines should be tested for tightness.

The hose mask should bear the certification number printed upon the container, and marked upon the facepiece and other parts of the equipment. (See Fig. 17-1). This number establishes that the equipment was properly designed to do

its job and will be safe to use if well maintained.

Where hose masks are supplied as emergency and rescue equipment, frequent and thorough training in their use should be given to all individuals who may use them.

The hose mask (Fig. 17-27) should be used by anyone entering tanks or pits where there may be dangerous concentrations of dust, mist, vapor, or gas, or insufficient oxygen. Inadequate oxygen should be suspected in any confined space, particularly in an iron or steel tank, unless a test shows that the supply with support life. Rusting of the walls of an otherwise clean tank may have depleted the oxygen supply.

No one should enter or remain in a tank or similar space that tests show has less than 16

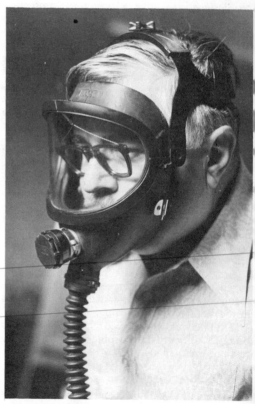

FIG. 17-27.—Spectacle mount permits the use of full facepiece air line respirator by those who wear prescription glasses. Special spectacle frame is spring-mounted to provide optically correct vision and eliminate the possibility of leaks from glasses' temples.

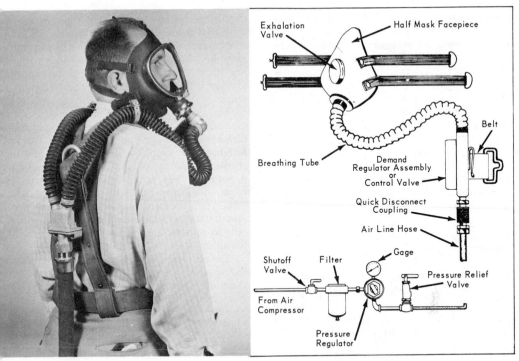

Fig. 17–28.—Air line respirator. Photograph at left shows full-face mask. Diagram (*right*) shows parts and connections.

percent oxygen in its atmosphere at any time unless he wears approved respiratory protective equipment, such as a air line respirator with egress cylinder or self-contained breathing apparatus.

Insufficient oxygen and dangerous gases should also be suspected in a tank which has held organic materials such as grain or grain products, oil, or food material.

These materials, as well as a variety of others, may eventually react with the air to reduce its oxygen content and produce dangerous oxidization products.

Before a worker enters an enclosed space having an atmosphere that may contain toxic or flammable contaminants or that may be deficient in oxygen, the atmosphere should be tested with appropirate instruments. Instruments for determining the percentage of combustible gases are tested and approved by the U.S. Bureau of Mines. If the amount of any contaminant in the enclosure is more than its maximum acceptable concentration, or if the amount is within or close to the explosive limits, or if oxygen is deficient, the tank

or enclosure should first be ventilated. This ventilation should never be done with oxygen because it could make an extremely hazardous atmosphere if flammable materials or gases were present.

After being purged of flammable or toxic concentrations and then reventilated, the tank or similar enclosure should be retested for contaminants in its atmosphere at intervals throughout the period that men are required to work in the space.

The hose mask with blower should be worn until the tank or similar enclosure has been thoroughly cleaned of scale and sludge and the flammable gas or vapor concentration has been reduced to 0.1 percent or less. Where there is a toxic gas or vapor and duration of stay in the enclosure is extended, the hose mask must be worn until the atmosphere is at or below the maximum acceptable concentration of the gas or vapor. It would be safer to use the device at all times in the confined space because the concentration of the hazardous gas or vapor can change suddenly.

**507**

The fit of the mask should be carefully checked before the worker enters the enclosure. Corrective glasses may cause a problem unless a spectacle mount is provided. (See Fig. 17-27.)

## Air line respirators

The air line respirator type of atmosphere (air) supplied respirator (Fig. 17-28) has a hand-operated, quickly detachable coupling on the belt or body harness with which the operator can connect to a compressed air hose; it also contains a device to limit air flow.

There are three basic classes of air line respirators—constant flow, demand flow, and pressure demand flow.

• Constant or continuous flow units have a regulated amount of air fed to the facepiece, and normally are used where there is ample air supply, such as provided by an air compressor. Constant flow air line respirators with facepieces only are used where respiratory protection only is needed. A hood can be added to the facepiece for protection against standblasting or a helmet with a hood or cape affixed to it may be added.

• Demand-type flow air respirators with half-masks or full facepiece deliver airflow only during inhalation. Such units are usually used where the air supply is restricted to high-pressure compressed air cylinders. A pressure regulator is required to reduce the air flow to proper pressure for breathing.

• Pressure demand flow respirators are designed for conditions where possible inward leakage is not permissible, and where there can be relatively high air consumption by the constant-flow units. Pressure demand air line respirators provide a positive pressure during inhalation as well as exhalation.

NIOSH/MSHA has certified air line respirators under Title 30 CFR, Part 11, Subpart J, which spells out such important factors as maximum hose length for which approval is given, and the maximum permissible inlet pressure.

The approved pressure range is noted for each certified device on the test certification or on the instructions supplied with each device. The ranges vary according to the type of equipment worn—respirator only, or with helmet or hood.

The air line respirator furnishes complete protection against any atmosphere not immediately dangerous to life or health, and for such conditions is the most desirable protection for industrial operations requiring continuous use of a respirator. Although other types of respirator may give adequate protection, they offer breathing resistance not present in the supplied air type and are consequently more fatiguing to wear.

The air line respirator's limitations should be understood. Respirable air (grade D, Compressed Gas Association Air Specification, G-7.1 or better) must be supplied to the user. A pressure regulator with an attached gage is required if the pressure in the compressor line exceeds the required delivered pressure. In addition, there should be a pressure relief valve set at a predetermined value, which will operate if the regulator fails to prevent high-pressure air from reaching the user.

The air supply must be free of carbon monoxide or other gaseous contaminations. To obtain clean air, the compressor intake must be kept away from all sources of contamination, including internal combustion engine exhaust. (See Fig. 17-26.)

Low-pressure blowers which do not use internal lubricants are preferable to conventional high-pressure compressors as a source of respirable air. If an internally lubricated compressor is used, it should be well maintained and must not run hot; dangerous amounts of carbon monoxide can be produced by decomposition of the lubricating oil in a hot compressor.

To safeguard against the hazard of carbon monoxide in compressed air, there should be a temperature-actuated alarm on the compressor or a carbon monoxide alarm in the air line.

The air delivered to the mask should be of comfortable temperature and humidity. Compression and re-expansion often produce a temperature and a relative humidity widely different from that of the air entering the compressor. To lower its temperature, air can be passed through a cooler. Some states require both interstage and aftercoolers together with a high-temperature alarm.

On a job which requires an employee to move from place to place, he will be hampered by dragging an air hose. This is usually a nuisance rather than a hazard, but it will have an effect upon efficiency which should be recognized in advance. Care must be exercised to prevent damage to the hose. For instance, it should not be permitted to lie in oil.

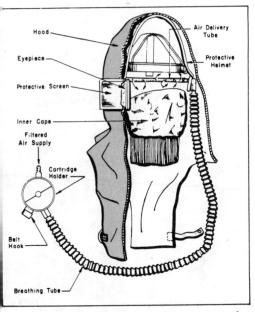

FIG. 17–29.—Diagram shows parts and connections for lightweight hood designed for use by persons doing abrasive blasting.

Labels in figure:
Hood
Eyepiece
Protective Screen
Inner Cape
Filtered Air Supply
Cartridge Holder
Belt Hook
Breathing Tube
Air Delivery Tube
Protective Helmet

## Abrasive blasting respirators

Abrasive blasting respirators are used to protect personnel engaged in shot, sand, or other abrasive blasting operations, which involve air contaminated with high concentrations of rapidly moving abrasive particles.

The requirements for abrasive blasting respirators are the same as those for an air line respirator of the continuous flow type, with the addition that mechanical protection from the abrasive particles is needed for the head and neck (Fig.17–29). NIOSH-MSHA tests and certifies such equipment.

There are two forms of abrasive blasting respirators that cover the head and neck, and even the shoulder and chest.

These units use a rigid helmet to encase the user's head. The eyepiece is of impact-resistant safety glass or of plastic covered by a metal screen. An adjustable knitted fabric collar, covered with rubber- or plastic-coated fabric, fits over the metal helmet and down over the user's neck, shoulders, and chest in order to give additional protection. A flexible tube brings air to the helmet. Air, exhausted from the helmet, flows between the collar and the user's neck.

In both units, the eyepiece (window) and the protective screen should be easily replaceable, preferably without the use of tools.

## Air supplied hoods

For some long-term operations where a completely enclosed suit is not necessary, an air supplied hood may be used. These are particularly useful in hot, dusty situations, Fig. 17–30.

Respirable air under suitable pressure should be delivered to a hood at a volume of at least 6 cfm (0.0028 m³/s).

## Air supplied suits

The most extreme condition requiring respiratory equipment is that in which rescue or emergency repair work must be done in atmospheres extremely corrosive to the skin and mucous membranes, in addition to being acutely poisonous and immediately hazardous to life, such as atmospheres containing ammonia, or hydrofluoric or hydrochloric acid vapors.

For these conditions, a complete suit of impervious clothing, with a respirable air supply, is available (Fig. 17–31). Complete units with self-

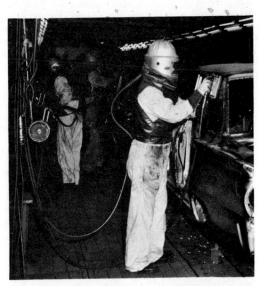

FIG. 17–30.—Solder grinders wear hoods to prevent foreign matter from entering their eyes, ears, noses, or mouths. Filtered air is supplied to the hoods at 12 to 15 psig and is exhausted around the bottoms.

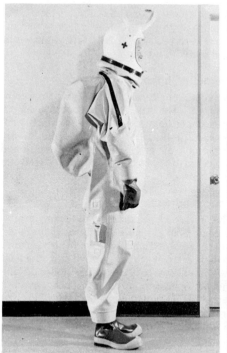
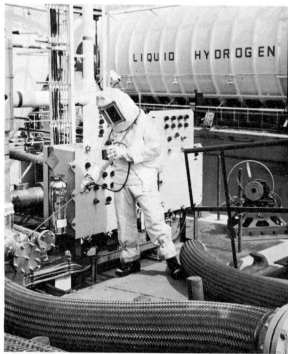

FIG. 17–31.—Environmental rocket fuel and corrosive chemical suits where complete protection from hazardous gases, mists, corrosive chemicals, or dusts is required. These suits include self-contained breathing apparatus. Suit at left has liquid air system which provides a certain amount of pressure-regulated cool air for air conditioning. Suit at right is equipped with a standard self-contained gas mask with liquid air tank (in 25-lb. (11 kg) back-pack unit) and pressure regulated air supply. Unit maintains a constant internal temperature of 70 F (21 C) will enable a technician to live up to 2½ minutes in a flash fire (enough time to reach safety). Unit has a duration of 55 minutes, but could function as long as 1½ hours in emergency.

contained breathing apparatus are discussed under Self-Contained Breathing Devices, which follows this section.

There are no generally accepted specifications for such suits; therefore, considerable dependence must be placed upon the manufacturer. The material should have sufficient mechanical strength to resist rough handling and considerable abuse without tearing.

The hose line supplying the air should be connected to the suit itself, as well as to the helmet (Fig. 32), since it is not only extremely fatiguing but also dangerous to wear such a suit for a long period unless it is well ventilated.

Personal air conditioning devices utilizing a vortex tube are available for air supplied suits or hoods. These cooling devices are desirable to reduce fatigue where high ambient temperatures may be encountered (as in heat-protective clothing), or where body heat may build up (as under impermeable chemical protective clothing).

The vortex device (Fig. 17–33) works by taking an air stream under pressure and dividing it. One portion loses heat; the other gains heat. The cold portion passes into the suit or hood; the warm portion is vented to the atmosphere, or vice versa in cold weather.

## 3. Self-Contained Breathing Devices

When a person must work in an atmosphere immediately dangerous to life (IDLH), a self-contained breathing apparatus should be used. In an environment that contains a substance which is dangerously irritant or corrosive to the skin, a self-contained breathing device must be supplemented by impervious clothing.

Such devices afford complete respiratory protection in any toxic or oxygen-deficient atmosphere, regardless of the concentration of the contaminant. They also allow relative freedom of movement.

There are two main classes of self-contained breathing devices: (*a*) closed circuit (recirculating), and (*b*) open circuit (demand).

• There are two types of closed circuit apparatus generally available:

Self-generating type, in which oxygen-generating chemicals in a container are activiated by the moisture in the user's expired breath, and

Compressed air or liquid oxygen type, which employs a container of compressed or liquid oxygen (Fig. 17–34).

• The open circuit (demand) type of apparatus uses a container of compressed or liquid air, or a

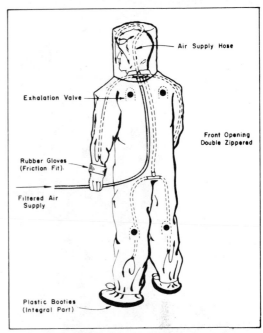

FIG. 17–32.—Diagram of air supplied suit for use in corrosive chemical atmospheres.

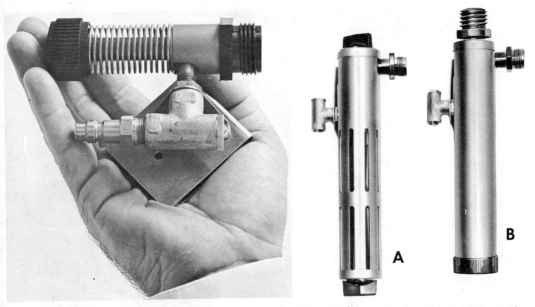

FIG. 17–33.—The vortex tube. Compressed air at 100 psig, 100 F (690 kPa, 37.8C) enters tube from T-shaped fitting at side; it is fed to nozzles and accelerates to sonic speed, creating cyclone spinning at 500,000 rpm. Major portion of air spirals inward, expanding and cooling to 40 F (4C) before it is ejected. Smaller portion of air churns down the tube, heats up to 270 F (132 C). In photograph at right, tube A is capable of providing either cool or hot air; tube B provides cool air only.

**511**

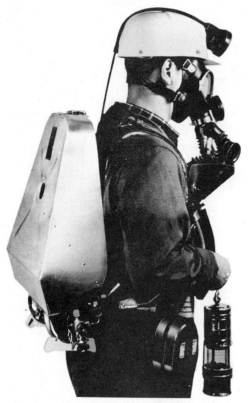

FIG. 17–34.—Compressed oxygen (cylinder) rebreathing apparatus.

retention is important as it permits fog-free lenses). The apparatus is light in weight and contains no intricate parts.

The quick-start canister, however, might act as an autoignition source to gases with an autoignition temperature of 600 F (315 C) or less. The apparatus produces more oxygen than the user requires, so venting must be done periodically. Some models do this automatically but with others it must be done by hand. The apparatus and canister should normally be stored at above-freezing temperatures and be completely started before being worn and used at subzero temperatures. Quick-start canisters are standard; these contain chemicals that quickly heat the canister to permit the apparatus to start quickly under low-temperature conditions.

A new canister should be used each time the apparatus is worn, for it is dangerous to enter a hazardous atmosphere (or even engage in a drill) with a previously opened canister. Used canisters should be promptly disposed of in accordance with instructions printed on them. Used canisters

container of compressed or liquid oxygen (Fig. 17–35).

When used in the conventional manner, no oxygen-supplying, self-contained breathing device should be used where the ambient pressure is more than two atmospheres, because of the danger of oxygen poisoning.

## Closed circuit apparatus

The self-generating (recirculating) apparatus consists of a chemical canister, a breathing bag that acts as a reservoir, a facepiece with tube assembly, and a relief valve and check valves to regulate flow in accordance with respiratory requirements. The chemical in the canister evolves oxygen when contacted by the moisture and carbon dioxide in the exhaled breath, and also retains the carbon dioxide and moisture (moisture

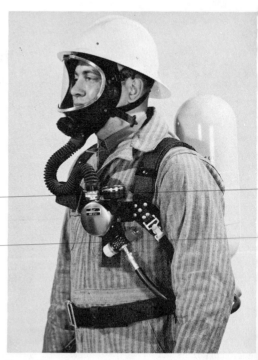

FIG. 17–35.—Compressed air (cylinder) nonrebreathing apparatus.

should be kept away from combustibles so that residual oxygen will not have a chance to activate them. Only copious amounts of clean water should be used to destroy a canister.

It is important that no one wear self-contained breathing apparatus unless he is physically fit and well trained. Physical fitness and training are essential because poor physical condition of users and lack of proper training have been responsible for injuries and deaths. After the initial training, workers should receive refresher training at least every six months in order to maintain efficiency.

The facepiece or mouthpiece and nose clip of a self-contained breathing apparatus should be carefully fitted to the wearer to ensure leak-proof protection against the hazardous atmosphere the person is to enter.

*Because of the extreme hazard no one wearing self-contained breathing apparatus should work in an irrespirable atmosphere unless other persons similarly equipped are in attendance, ready to give assistance.*

**The compressed or liquid oxygen (cylinder) recirculating apparatus** (Fig. 17–34). This equipment is supplied with either a full facepiece or a mouthpiece and nose clip. The seal around the facepiece must be kept absolutely tight.

Such equipment consists, essentially, of a high-pressure oxygen cylinder with reducing and regulating valves, a lung-governed admission valve which supplies oxygen from the cylinder only during inhalation, a carbon dioxide scrubber and cooler, and a reservoir breathing bag connected by tubes to the mouthpiece or facepiece. Check valves direct the flow through the circuit so that the exhaled oxygen is purified of carbon dioxide, and rebreathed from the bag, with replenishment from the cylinder as required. The liquid oxygen type operates similarly.

The rebreathing principle permits the most efficient utilization of the oxygen supply. The exhaled breath contains both oxygen and carbon dioxide because the body consumes only a small part of the inhaled oxygen.

Because this equipment is quite complicated to use and maintain, personnel should be thoroughly trained.

### Open circuit apparatus

**The compressed or liquid air (cylinder) open circuit (demand) apparatus** (Fig. 17–35) consists of a high-pressure cylinder of oxygen or air, a cylinder valve, a demand regulator, and a facepiece and tube assembly with an exhalation valve. To use, the wearer turns on the cylinder valve after carefully putting on the facepiece, inhales to draw oxygen or air through the demand regulator at breathing pressure to the facepiece, and then exhales through the exhalation valve in the facepiece to the atmosphere. This makes the apparatus relatively inefficient when compared with rebreathing apparatus.

Pressure demand types are available. These maintain a slight pressure in the mask or facepiece to prevent leakage of ambient atmosphere into the mask or facepiece because of improper fit.

Once a cylinder has been used for compressed air, it should not be refilled with oxygen because of the possibility of fire if oxygen comes in contact with even a trace of oil or grease.

### Training and Care

Once the respirator has been determined, the wearer must be trained in its use and care. This is important for every type respirator.

#### Training

For safe use of any respiratory protective device, it is essential that the user be properly instructed in its use. Supervisors as well as workers must be so instructed by competent persons.

OSHA requires that all employees be trained in the proper use of the device assigned to them. See 1910.134(b)(3) and (e)(5). Many companies have their employees sign a document attesting to their having completed a training session with the respiratory device.

Each respirator wearer should be given training which would include (a) an explanation of the respiratory hazard and what happens if the respirator is not used properly, (b) a discussion of what engineering and administrative controls are being used and why respirators still are needed for protection, (c) an explanation of why a particular type of respirator has been selected, (d) a discussion of the function, capabilities, and limitations of the selected respirator, (e) instruction in how to don the respiratory and to check its fit and operation, (f) instruction in the proper wearing of the respiratory, (g) instruction in respirator maintenance, and (h) instruction in recognizing and handling emergencies.

The instructor should be a qualified person, such as an industrial hygienist, safety pro-

**513**

fessional, or the respirator manufacturer's representative.

## Care of respiratory equipment

**Particulate filter and chemical cartridge types.** Maintenance is simplified by selection of respirators that can be easily cleaned, disinfected, and repaired.

If possible, particulate filter respirators which use cotton facelets should be selected because the facelets protect the facepiece from skin oils. Facelets are not approved for use on chemical cartridge or metal fume respirators. If the filters are likely to clog rapidly, a respirator which allows convenient, inexpensive, and frequent filter replacement should be chosen.

Supervisors should be responsible for making daily inspection, particularly of functional parts such as exhalation valves and filter elements. They should see that the edges of the valves are not curled and that valve seats are smooth and clean. Inhalation and exhalation valves should be replaced periodically.

In addition to the daily check, respirators should be inspected weekly by trained persons. During the weekly inspection, rubber parts should be stretched slightly for detection of fine cracks. The rubber should be worked occasionally to prevent setting (one of the causes of cracking), and the headband should be checked to be sure that the wearer has not stretched it in an attempt to secure a snug fit.

Sometimes, in an effort to reduce resistance to breathing, workers will punch holes in the filter, the rubber facepiece, or other parts. Underlying causes of this mistreatment should be discovered and corrected. For instance, it may be found that in the interest of economy, filters are allowed to become completely plugged before they are replaced.

In cleaning respirators, dirt and dust should first be blown from them by means of compressed air at not more than 10 to 20 psi (70 kPa to 140 kPa) of pressure, through a fixed nozzle directed towards an exhaust hood. The cleaners should wear dust-tight goggles. Dust filters should not be cleaned by brushing.

Then filters, screens, headbands, and cotton facelets should be removed. If the respirators are coated with paint or other foreign matter, they should be soaked for three hours in a cleaning solution of 1½ pounds (0.7 kg) of commercial alkaline base cleaner and 7 gal (26.5 liters) of water. Fresh paint can be wiped off with a clean rag moistened in alcohol. Thorough rinsing is always necessary before use.

Respirators having no visible accumulation of foreign matter should be scrubbed in warm, soapy water, rinsed, disinfected, then rinsed again and dried.

Knitted facelets should be washed in warm, soapy water, rinsed and dried before reuse. Dirty or oily elastic headbands should be washed in warm, soapy water and rinsed. The water should be warm to remove perspiration and hair oil from the elastic fabric.

Rubber parts should never be dried by direct application of heat or sunlight.

Employees should be instructed to wipe off oil, grease, and other harmful substances from headbands and other parts of the respirator as soon as they collect. They should be warned not to use solvents to clean plastic or rubber parts.

Most face and mouthpieces for respiratory protective devices are made from rubber or rubber-like compounds. Usually hand brushing or agitation in a washing machine, using detergent and warm water is sufficient to clean them.

Hypochlorite or quaternary ammonium compounds in the proper strength in aqueous solution can be used to disinfect the parts.

Ethylene oxide gas, handled under proper precautions, is sometimes used where large quantities of respirators must be disinfected.

All detergent should be rinsed from the device before disinfecting, except where combination detergent and quaternary ammonium compounds (that both clean and disinfect) are used.

After cleaning and disinfecting, the parts should be rinsed in clean water and dried quickly. It may also be desirable to rinse parts treated with quaternary ammonium compounds since their disinfecting properties continue and, except for rare cases, it will not produce a skin irritation.

Hot water, steam, solvents, and ultraviolet light should not be used to clean and disinfect rubber parts because they have a deteriorating effect.

Petroleum jelly should not be used to prevent skin irritation from rubber facepieces, for it is harmful to rubber. Disinfection and the use of clean cotton facelets will eliminate the need for a salve.

Respirators should be turned in at the end of each shift to be cleaned and repaired if necessary. They should be disinfected at least once a week

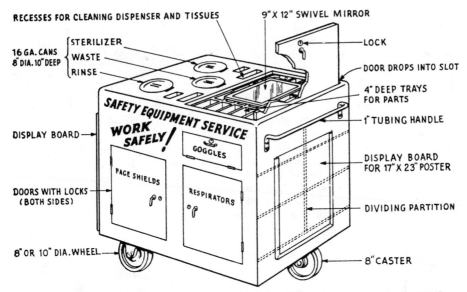

RECESSES FOR CLEANING DISPENSER AND TISSUES

9"X 12" SWIVEL MIRROR

16 GA. CANS
8" DIA.10" DEEP
{ STERILIZER
WASTE
RINSE

LOCK

DOOR DROPS INTO SLOT

4" DEEP TRAYS
FOR PARTS

1" TUBING HANDLE

DISPLAY BOARD

SAFETY EQUIPMENT SERVICE
WORK SAFELY!

GOGGLES

FACE SHIELDS

RESPIRATORS

DISPLAY BOARD
FOR 17" X 23" POSTER

DOORS WITH LOCKS
(BOTH SIDES)

DIVIDING PARTITION

8" OR 10" DIA. WHEEL

8" CASTER

FIG. 17–36.—Maintenance service provided by this type of equipment improves employee attitude toward the use of personal protective devices. The service cart may be made of plywood or steel. Dimensions may be 36 in. long, 36 in. high, and 30 in. wide (91 cm × 91 cm × 76 cm).

when retained by the same employees.

In some plants, maintenance service for respirators, as well as for other kinds of personal protective equipment, can be effectively provided by traveling service carts (Fig. 17–36).

Where a number of respirators are in regular use, a central station is often set up for their care and maintenance, as well as for the care and maintenance of other items of personal protective equipment. Each employee is then provided with two respirators and either a locker or a hook at the central station.

Some plants have found that if two respirators are assigned to each worker, equipment lasts more than twice as long. This plan is most desirable when cleaning cannot be done between shifts or before the next scheduled shift.

Under such a plan, marked respirators are turned in daily or weekly, depending upon use, for cleaning, disinfection, inspection, and repair. The worker then uses the second respirator until the first can be serviced.

Another plan is to keep quantities of disinfected respirators on hand for groups. This plan works where individual needs vary, but in such a plan the user is not so easily charged with responsibility. If the same respirator is used by several

persons, it is always best to clean and disinfect it after each use.

Respirators should be marked to indicate to whom they are assigned. The method of identification should be permanent enough so that the marking cannot be changed inadvertently or without effort.

Before being stored, a respirator should be carefully wiped with a damp cloth and dried. It should be stored without sharp folds or creases. It should never be hung by the elastic headband or put down in a position which will stretch the facepiece.

Since heat, air, light, and oil cause rubber to deteriorate, respirators should be stored in a cool, dry place and protected from light and air as much as possible. Wood, fiber, or metal cases are provided with many respirators. Respirators should be sealed in clean plastic bags.

Respirators should not be thrown into tool boxes or left on work benches where they may be exposed to dust and damage by oil or other harmful materials.

**Air line respirators.** Maintenance suggestions for filter respirators apply also to air line respirators. In addition, the latter should be inspected at

**515**

weekly or monthly intervals, depending on use. Pressure regulators, relief valves, air control valves, and demand (or pressure demand) regulators should be checked periodically for cleanliness and proper operation. Rubber (or other elastomer) and plastic parts (such as hoses, facepieces, and exhalation valves) should be checked regularly for deterioration caused by age, heat, ozone, or other deleterious action.

The pressure regulator, filter, hose, and facepiece should be checked for deterioration.

The air hose and attachments should be cleaned regularly to prevent accumulation of paint, oil, grease, or solvents which might harm the rubber or connections. Oil and grease should be removed with steam at no more than 5 psig (34.5 kPa) of pressure. The steam nozzle should not be held so close to the air hose as to "burn" it. Protective goggles and rubber gloves should be worn during cleaning operations.

**Gas masks.** Canisters should be stored and handled as directed by their manufacturer.

A canister with broken seals should not be kept in service for more than one year, regardless of how little it has been used. Although some depend on employees to record the length of time of canister use, an indicator is more reliable. A good rule to follow is that if there is any doubt, replace the canister.

### Lifelines, Lanyards and Safety Belts

Lifelines, safety belts, and associated equipment are often used in construction and general industry. While references to specific services and uses are made, reference should be made to both the OSHA General Industry Regulations and appropriate ANSI recommendations. (Linemen's body belts, pole straps, and safety ladder belts are not covered in this discussion.)

### Personal lifelines

Personal lifeline systems are usually rope systems that provide flexibility for worker freedom of movement, yet will arrest a fall and help absorb the shock. These systems always have some type of belt or harness that is worn around the waist to which a lanyard or rope-grabbing device is attached. Body belts should be used only where very short free falls of less than two feet (0.6 m) are anticipated. The safety belt D-ring should be arranged at the back of the worker. A body

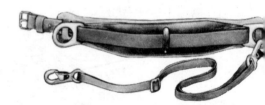

FIG. 17–37.—This ANSI Class I belt design (showing pad and lanyard) allows the wearer to use it as a tool belt or as a restraint in a hazardous work position.

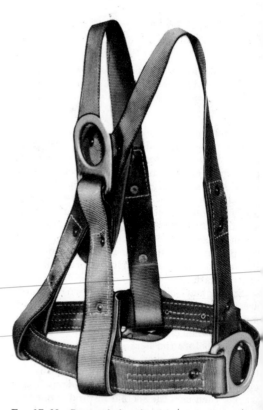

FIG. 17–38.—Retrieval chest harness (ANSI Class II) for lifting workers from enclosed places such as quarries, tanks, bins.

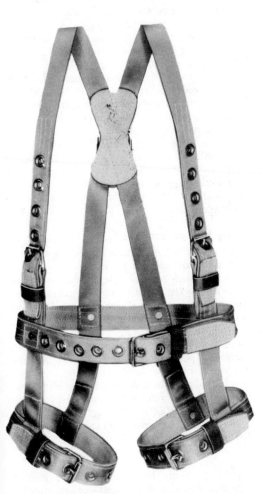

FIG. 17-39.—Full-support tower harness. ANSI Class III. Ideal for workers on elevated sites. Distributes fall impact over body.

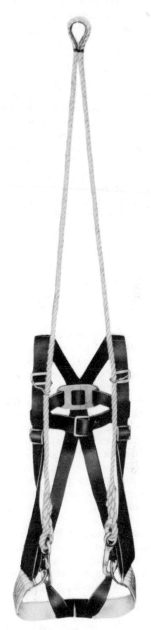

FIG. 17-40.—An ANSI Class IV harness.

harness should be used where longer free falls, up to six feet (1.8 m), are anticipated. A harness will spread the shock load over the shoulders, thighs, and seat area.

One particular body harness has pelvic and chest belts that work together to distribute impact force evenly and guard against slipping out of the harness at the end of the fall. The chest belt is worn loosely to allow freedom of breathing and movement; the pelvic belt should be adjusted to fit snugly. The two belts are attached by a strong web band at back, long enough to keep them independent of each other during normal work, but short enough for the pelvic belt to catch the chest belt in case of fall.

The lifeline is defined (in ANSI A10.14) as a horizontal line between two fixed anchorages, independent of the work surface, to which the lanyard is secured. The lifeline must be capable of supporting a dead weight of 5400 lb (2450 kg) per person, applied at the center of the lifeline. Lifelines are to be constructed of wire rope, at least 1/2 in. (12.5 mm) in diameter, and be attached to at least two fixed anchorages (ANSI A10.14).

Retracting lifelines are portable self-contained devices that are attached to a fixed anchorage point above the work area. The lifeline extends from the device and is connected to the user's safety belt. A constant tension is maintained up to the maximum extension, and the lifeline freely retracts when the user moves closer to the anchorage and pulls out as the worker moves away from it. In the event of a fall, one type of retracting lifeline uses a centrifugal mechanism which causes pawls to move outward, engaging a brake; another type uses a centrifugal mechanism which causes a lever to move outward, engaging a belt-locking system.

The lanyard is a short piece of flexible line used to secure the wearer of a safety belt or harness to a lifeline, dropline, or fixed anchorage. Lanyards may be constructed of any fibrous or metallic material meeting ANSI qualification criteria. A lanyard should have as little slack as possible to limit free fall distance. Shock-absorber-type lanyards are designed to absorb up to 80 percent of the stopping force of a regular lanyard and should be used where longer free falls are predicted. Lanyards should be spliced permanently to the safety belt, making it possible for manufacturers to certify that the combination meets ANSI drop test requirement.

Care should be taken to see that the lanyard is attached to a fixed anchorage by means that will not reduce its required strength. A knot will reduce the strength of a rope lanyard by at least 40 percent. (See Table 5–C on page 193 of the *Engineering and Technology* volume of this series.) The free ends of lanyards of materials must also be seared or otherwise tightened. In addition, wire rope or rope-covered wire lanyards must not be used where impact loads or electrical hazards are anticipated.

Lanyards and associated hardware also require attention as to construction and use. Lanyards must not be lengthened by connecting two snap hooks together and should be proportioned to minimize the possibility of accidental disengagement.

## Safety belt or harness

The safety belt or harness is used for securing, suspending, or retrieving a worker in or from a hazardous work area. This device can be secured around the waist, chest or a large portion (torso, thighs, chest, buttocks, and shoulders) of the body to distribute the stopping force.

Strength members of belts may be made of any material, *except leather*, that in turn will meet the minimum performance tests (ANSI A10.14). Hardware, buckles, hooks, and rings are also subject to determined specifications. The buckle must be the quick release type and must withstand a tensile test of 4000 lb (1815 kg) without failure.

Safety belts, harnesses, and lanyards are classified (see ANSI A10.14) according to their indended use as:

*Class I:* Body belts (work belts), used to restrain a person in a hazardous work position and to reduce the probability of falls (see Fig. 17–37).

*Class II:* Chest harnesses, used where there are only limited fall hazards (no vertical free-fall hazard) and for retrieval purposes, such as removal of a person from a tank or bin (see Fig. 17–38).

*Class III:* Body harnesses, used to arrest the most severe free falls (see Fig. 17–39).

*Class IV:* Suspension belts, independent work supports used to suspend or support the worker (see Fig. 17–40).

Belts and lanyards should always be scrutinized for weak points that may cause the piece to

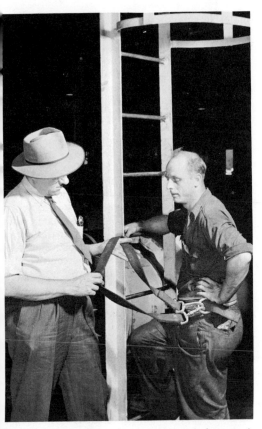

FIG. 17–41.—Competent belt inspection before use is never excessive caution.

A window cleaner's belt is subject to a moderate static load most of the time it is in use, as the worker leans back in the belt and is held in position by it while he works. It will, however, be subjected to a severe loading in case of a fall with only one terminal of the belt attached to the window anchor.

This is the most common kind of fall in window cleaning and also the most hazardous one with this type of belt, because the worker will slide to the end of the safety line, transmitting impact to the single window anchor which may, particularly in older buildings, be broken off or pulled out.

The amount of impact force developed in arresting a fall depends chiefly on three elements: the weight of the person, the distance of his fall, and the suddenness of his stopping. Of these three elements, the suddenness of his stopping is of far greater importance than the other two factors.

The maximum possible fall in a window cleaner's belt is limited to the length of the safety rope or strap, 8 ft (2.5 m). In other types, the fall may be much longer than the rope length. For example, the maximum fall in a construction worker's belt may be as much as twice the length of his lifeline in case he falls from above his lifeline anchorage. In all cases where the lifeline is attached to the support on which he is standing, the free fall will be usually the full length of the life line plus the distance from his feet to the D-ring of his belt. If at all possible, the wearer of the safety belt should not "tie off" below waist level.

## Construction

Belts should be scrutinized for weak points which might cause the belt to fail under a heavy impact (Fig. 17–41). For instance, the waist belt should always be inserted through the D-rings or other attaching devices and never riveted to them in such a way that the D-ring or lifeline could be separated from the belt through the failure of the rivets.

Buckles should hold securely without slippage or other failure, and this holding power should be achieved by only a single insertion of the strap through the buckle in the normal or natural way. If the buckle is of a type that requires that the free end of the webbing be turned back and inserted again through the buckle in order to achieve its full holding power, the management, through safety instruction and inspection, must make every effort to see that the workers always use this

fail under impact. The assemblies must be inspected according to the manufacturer's recommendations not less than twice annually. The date of each inspection is then recorded on an inspection tag that shall be permanently attached to the belt. Chest harness (Class II) and suspension belts (Class IV) must not be used for stopping falls and do not have to meet impact requirements. Belts and lanyards that have been subjected to impact loading shall be removed from service and destroyed.

## Window cleaner's belts

Employers of window washing personnel are required to provide safety equipment and devices conforming with the requirements of ANSI A39.1. Specified applications should be referenced to that standard.

method of fastening their belts; otherwise, the belt may slip under very minor strains. Where there is danger of falling into water or of being trapped by fire, a quick-release buckle should be used.

In general, webbing is the only for any safety belt which may be called upon to take impact loads. Webbing has three to four times as much resistance to impact loading as leather of the same size. Leather belts are used primarily for positioning. Webbing belts normally use friction buckles which avoid loss of strength at buckle holes.

An ordinary single-tongue buckle will cut through 1/4-in. (0.6 cm) thick leather strap of best commercial grade harness leather at a loading of 300 to 500 pounds (136. to 227 kg); in contrast, web belts can be obtained that possess strengths of more than 12,000 pounds (5440 kg).

The width of a leather strap does not materially affect its strength at the buckle. A leather belt 1/4 -in. thick and 1 in. (2.5 cm) wide has as much strength as a belt of the same strap 3 in. (7.6 cm) or 4 in. (10.2 cm) or even 10 in. (25.4 cm) wide. The only factors affecting the strength of such a belt are the quality of the leather, the thickness of the leather, the size of the metal tongue in the buckle, and the number of tongues in the buckle.

Leather requires special care and treatment to retain its strength; webbing does not. Leather stands ordinary abrasion well, but is easily cut. It is not easily attacked by chemicals, but is easily damaged by heat, dryness, or inadequate care and oiling.

No one but a leather expert can tell by visual inspection with any degree of accuracy the condition or strength of leather. Webbing, on the other hand, can be judged more accurately by visual inspection.

Cotton webbing is not seriously affected by dryness or moisture nor by heat, short of actual scorching or burning. Untreated cotton webbing should not, however, be long-subjected to moisture (which may promote mildew) or to corrosive chemicals unless the material has been prepared for such conditions.

There are several different materials and weaves used for webbing. The most common is cotton webbing, but synthetic fiber webbing such as nylon and Dacron are supplanting cotton because of their superior strength, mildew and moisture resistance. For some applications, namely chemical and oil work, webbing, coated or impregnated with plastic or neoprene rubber

materials, which are impervious to oils and acids are desirable. The most common weaves are the square or basket weave and the herringbone weave. For the same size and thickness, the herringbone weave usually has approximately twice the strength of the basket weave. One reason is that better yarn is used in the herringbone material, but most of the difference is due to the weave itself.

Under the stress of loading, herringbone weave webbing will elongate while basket weave webbing will not. However, the amount of elongation that occurs under loads common in this use will not significantly affect the fit of a safety belt nor will it provide adequate shock absorbency.

Herringbone weave webbing is much more soft and pliable, and looks weaker than the stiffer, harder basket weave. For this reason, some concerns hesitate to use this material until better acquainted with its real superiority.

If the only purpose of the belt is to stop a worker in case of a fall, then a waist belt with a single D-ring may be satisfactory. This single D-ring may be attached for positioning at any point on the belt, for the belt can be turned to different positions after being buckled on the wearer.

Where possible, a body harness is preferable for absorbing impact and keeping a person upright in case of a fall.

If a belt is to furnish support to a person while he is working, it should have adequate means for such support. A belt for a person who will lean back in it as he works on a sloping roof or hillside should have two D-rings, one on each side of the belt, (Fig. 17–42), to which a suitable lanyard can be attached and connected to a suitable anchorage.

If the belt is to be used much for supporting the entire weight of a person vertically while working, as in being raised and lowered along the wall of a building, a boatswain's suspension harness may be used. In this type of belt, one strap is used as a seat, sometimes with a board to make it more comfortable. Leg straps and a strap around the persons's waist prevent him from falling out of the seat.

An industrial belt used to hoist a person out of a tank is usually subjected only to a static load. Such a belt should be of either the shoulder harness, chest-waist, or parachute type with the D-ring so placed as to hold a person in a relatively erect position.

In a window cleaner's belt, separate ropes

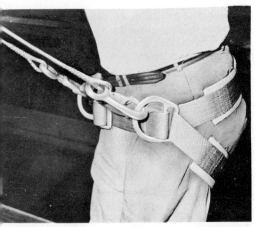

Fig. 17–42.—Multipurpose safety belt with two D-rings can be worn about the waist or slipped down around the buttocks for work on inclines.

should be used for the service and safety lines. The service rope, which supports the person while he works, must be shorter than the safety rope so that the former will be taut and the safety rope slack. Thus, all wear will be placed upon the service rope, and the safety rope will retain its full strength for use in stopping a fall.

The safety rope should contain a shock absorber which will reduce the loading in the event of a fall, thus relieving strain on the building anchor, waist belt, and person. There should be a device in the belt to release the service rope in case of a fall and bring into play the shock-absorbing safety rope.

## Belt Care

Dirt adhering to leather safety belts should be brushed off carefully so as not to scratch the leather. The belt should then be washed with warm water and either saddle soap or castile soap. After a rinse in clean, warm water, it should be dried at room temperature.

Before becoming completely dry, a leather belt should be oiled with neatsfoot, castor, soy bean, or a compound oil, *never a mineral oil.* A leather belt which has been unused and not oiled for a year or two is much weaker than one that has been regularly used and also adequately oiled over the same period. However, the unused belt will look newer and stronger.

Leather belts should not be exposed to exces-sive heat, such as from a radiator, because they may be permanently damaged by a temperature as low as 150 F (66 C). Any heat painful to a person will damage leather.

Cotton or linen webbing belts should be washed in soapy water, rinsed, and dried by moderate heat. They are not damaged by temperatures up to 212 F (100 C). If a belt is to be subjected to unusual conditions of use, the manufacturer should be consulted as to its care.

Synthetic fiber belts should not be exposed to excessive heat that might soften or melt the fibers, or to chemicals that might affect the composition of the fiber.

## Inspection and testing

Wearers of safety belts should inspect them before each use (Fig. 17–41). At least every one to three months they should be examined by a trained inspector. Leather belts especially must be watched for cuts or scratches on either side of the strap. A deep cut of any considerable length, crosswise to the belt, warrants discard. However, cuts running lengthwise do not seriously affect strength.

Fabric belts should be discarded if considerable portions of the outer fibers are cut or worn through. Again, leather belts alone should not be used for fall protection.

Belt hardware should be examined and worn parts replaced. Each belt rivet should be examined to be certain that it is secure. No rivet should be used in a web belt which may be subjected to impact loading.

Safety belts in service should not be tested. Any service test to prove whether the belt could take the maximum impact loading which might be required of it would very likely so damage the belt as to render it unsafe for use. Therefore, only sample belts and worn or doubtful belts should be tested, and these should always be tested to destruction to determine their safety. They should be kept as samples and used only to help judge the safety of other belts. Belts subjected to the maximum impact in an accidental fall should not be reused because the fittings might have been overstressed and weakened.

In judging the safety of a belt, the following vital, and to some extent conflicting, factors must be considered:

1. Sufficient strength to stop the wearer after a maximum free fall. The safety belt lanyard

should be a minimum of ¹/₂-in. (12.7 mm) nylon (or equivalent), with a maximum length ot provide for a fall of no greater than 6 ft (1.8 m). The rope shall have a minimum breaking strength of 5400 pounds (2450 kg).

2. A shock absorber to limit the impact loading and prevent injury to the wearer or failure of the anchorage, life line, or belt.

3. Short enough stopping distance to prevent the wearer from striking some dangerous obstruction before he stops.

4. Sufficient margin on all these factors, so far as possible, to cover all unknowns such as weight of the wearer, distance of his fall, his physical fitness, the distance to any damaging obstruction, variations in the strength or elasticity of materials, and deterioration of materials due to wear or other causes.

The primary caution regarding the use of safety belts, as with other personal protective equipment, is to see that they are worn and used correctly. A safety belt is worthless unless it is being worn at the time that a fall is possible. It should also be securely buckled and worn tightly enough to prevent any possibility of the man's slipping out of it.

## Lifelines

Lifelines should be secured above the point of operation to an anchorage or structural member capable of supporting a minimum dead weight of 5400 pounds (2450 kg).

For most lifelines, nylon rope of ¹/₂-in. (12.7 mm) diameter is recommended. Nylon is more resistant to wear or abrasion than is manila and is also more resistant to some chemicals. Ropes made of other synthetic fibers such as Dacron, polyethylene, and polypropylene have characteristics that make them very good performers in certain applications. In a lifeline where shock loading strength and high energy absorption is paramount, nylon is superior.

Knots reduce the strength of all ropes. (See Table 5–C in the *Engineering and Technology* volume of this series.) Tests have shown that manila lifelines of ¹/₂-in. diameter, when knotted around a bar or other anchorage, are not strong enough at the knots to be safe for general use unless a shock absorber of low load limit is used.

How much a knot reduces strength depends upon the type of knot or hitch used and the amount of moisture in the rope. Moisture increases the strength of a rope in a knot or around a sharp bend, and dryness greatly diminishes its strength at such points. In some cases, a knot will reduce the tensile strength of a rope to less than half of its breaking strength.

If rope is spliced into snaps and D-rings instead of knotted (Fig. 17–42), the splice will retain approximately 90 percent of the breaking strength of the rope. Breaking strength is always measured in a straight line pull on the rope. (See Chapter 5, "Ropes, Chains, and Slings" of the *Engineering and Technology* volume.)

Wire ropes should not be used as lifelines where a free fall is possible unless some shock-absorbing device is also used, because their rigidity greatly magnifies the impact loading. Also, wire ropes must not be used around electricity.

Lifelines should be tied to permit as little slack as possible, and thus stop a person with the minimum free fall. Special notice must be taken of the nearness of any beam or other obstruction which the worker might strike in case of a fall. Serious injury or death may result if the total free fall plus the total stretch or elongation of the lifeline and shock absorber will allow the worker to strike some damaging object before he is stopped.

If there is a long clear space in which a person may be stopped, then a low-limit shock absorber may be used with less discomfort to the worker. If this space is closely limited, a shorter stop is imperative, even though greater discomfort results.

Wire ropes should be kept clean and dry and should be frequently lubricated. Before use in acid atmospheres, they should be coated with oil. After such use, they should be thoroughly washed and again coated with oil.

Rope lines should be washed with mild soap and water and dried in circulating air. They should not be exposed to high temperatures.

If there has been wear or abrasion sufficient to reduce the diameter of the rope only slightly and give it a "smooth" appearance, with the high ridges worn down and the "valleys" partly filled with the vertical ends of broken and worn fibers, the rope should be discarded. Each long fiber will have been cut or broken many times, and the rope will have very little remaining strength.

Inner fibers should be examined for breaks, discoloration, or deterioration. Rope should be kept in open coils and never bent sharply.

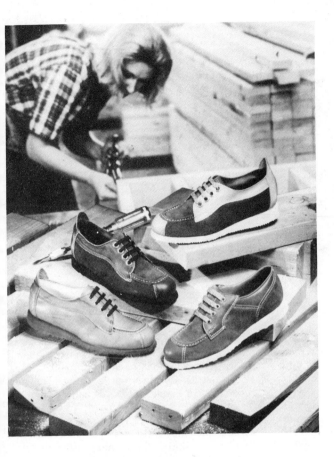

Fig. 17-43.—Protective footwear is also available in women's styles and sizes.

## Protective Footwear

As a guide to the selection of protective footwear, the Office of Technical Services of the Division of Safety, U.S. Department of Labor, has classified safety shoes into five principal types:

Safety-toe shoes

Conductive shoes

Foundry (molders) shoes

Explosives-operations (nonsparking) shoes

Electrical hazard shoes

Specifications for various kinds of protective footwear have been standarized by ANSI Z41.1, *Men's Safety-Toe Footwear.*° Safety-toe footwear has been divided into three classifications—75, 50, and 30—based on its ability to meet the minimum requirements for both compression and impact shown in Table 17-C.

Steel, reinforced plastics, and hard rubber are

### TABLE 17-C
### MINIMUM REQUIREMENTS
### OF AMERICAN STANDARD Z41.1

| Classi-fication | Compression (pounds) | Impact (pounds) | Clearance (inches) |
|---|---|---|---|
| 75 | 2500 | 75 | 16/32 |
| 50 | 1750 | 50 | 16/32 |
| 30 | 1000 | 30 | 16/32 |

1 lb mass = 0.45 kg
1 lb force (avoirdupois) = 4.4 newtons
1 in. = 2.54 centimeters

---

°The revised Z41.1 standard differentiates between men's and women's designs. (Note: Not yet published as of the date of this Manual's editing.)

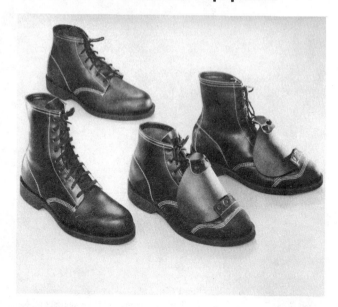

FIG. 17–44.—Typical safety shoes. On the left, are shown the regular safety toe shoe and on the right are the shoes with the metatarsal guard.

used for safety toes with the choice depending on the protective level desired and the shoe design. The test requirements are identical for both women's and men's shoes (see Fig. 17–43).

Toe boxes are used in shoes of various types such as conductive, spark resistant, molders, or nonconductive shoes. For work under wet conditions, rubber boots or rubber shoes may be obtained with a steel toe box to protect against impact. Puncture-resistant soles are another optional feature.

OSHA requires that the safety-toe shoe be used for work requiring the handling of heavy materials. Safety shoes also afford good protection against rolling objects, such as barrels, heavy pipe, rolls, or truck wheels, and against the hazard of accidentally kicking sharp objects.

The toe box adds a little to the weight and cost to the shoe. A well-made and properly fitted safety shoe is as comfortable. Comfort is an important factor in the wearing of any shoe, but particularly so when safety footwear is required. Great care should be exercised in selecting as well as fitting the correct type and size.

Many companies set up shoe departments, with the aid of shoe manufacturers, in their plants and provide trained employees to see that individuals are properly fitted with the correct types for the hazards involved. Some retail organizations provide the same type of service.

To protect feet, behind the toes, from impacts, integral metatarsal (or over-foot) guards should be worn in addition to safety-toe shoes (Figs. 17–44 and 17–45). Heavy-gage, flanged, and corrugated sheet metal footguards help protect the feet.

With the flanges resting upon a firm floor surface, they may resist an impact of at least 300 foot-pounds (400 joules) without sufficient deformation to damage the shoes underneath or injure the feet.

### Conductive shoes

Safety shoes, boots, and rubber overshoes may also be obtained with a conductive construction to allow a drain off of static charges, and with nonferrous construction to reduce the possibility of friction sparks in locations with a fire or explosion hazard. Initial and subsequent periodic tests should be made on conductive footwear in order to make sure that the maximum allowable resistance of 450,000 ohms is not exceeded. A special design is offered for use in munitions plants; see later discussion.

### Foundry shoes

Safety shoes of the "congress" or gaiter type are used in some plants where employees are exposed to splashes of molten metal. Having no fasteners,

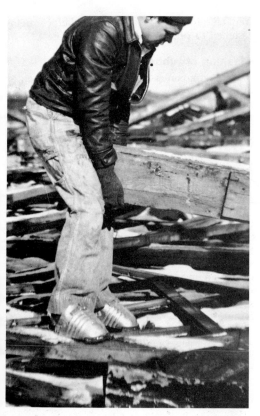

FIG. 17–45.—Metal instep guards protect this demolition worker.

such shoes are easily and rapidly removable in an emergency. Some National Safety Council members engaged in foundry and steel mill operations have reported that serious burns have occurred to workers who are unable to remove shoes of ordinary work type in an emergency. As in all such occupations, the tops of the shoes should be covered by the trouser leg, spats, or leggings, to keep out molten metal.

## Explosives-operations (nonsparking) shoes

Explosives-opeations shoes are used (a) in hazardous locations where the floors are non-conductive and grounded such as in the manufacture of certain explosive compounds, or (b) when cleaning tanks that have contained gasoline or other volatile hydrocarbons. These shoes have conductive soles, nonferrous eyelets and nails, and metal-

box toes are coated with a nonferrous metal.

### Electrical hazard shoes

Electrical hazard shoes are intended to minimize hazards resulting from contacts with electric current where the path of the current would be from the point of contact to the ground. No metal is used in construction, except for the box toe which is insulated from the rest of the shoe. If damp or badly worn, they cannot be depended on for protection.

### Special shoes

In some industries, such as construction, where there may exist an increased hazard from protruding nails, and where contact with energized electric equipment is remote, shoes or boots are equipped with flexible metal-reinforced soles or inner soles (Fig. 17–46).

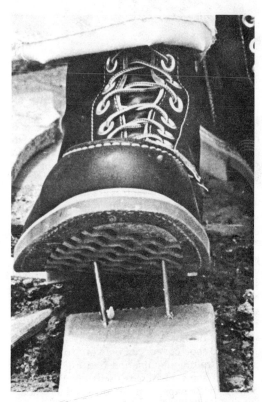

FIG. 17–46.—This type of foot protection is worn extensively in the construction industry. A flexible steel insole prevents the nail from puncturing the foot.

**525**

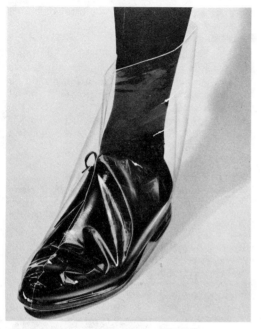

FIG. 17–47.—This polyethylene shoe cover is an example of footwear designed to protect the product—in the cleanroom. The cover fits either foot and is disposable.

Special shoes made with a stitched and cemented construction are available for electricians. These shoes serve as good insulators, so when they are repaired, avoid the use of nails which will destroy their insulating value.

For wet conditions such as are found in dairies and breweries, leather shoes with wood soles, or wood-soled sandals worn over shoes, are effective.

Wood soles provide good foot protection on jobs which require walking upon hot surfaces which are not hot enough to char the wood. Wood soles have been so generally used by men handling hot asphalt that they are sometimes called paver's sandals or paver's shoes. They are, however, equally satisfactory for other work which requires soles that do not conduct heat.

Plastic shoe covers can be worn to protect a product from contamination (see Fig. 17–47).

Where shower baths are used, many organizations provide paper slippers or wooden sandals for each individual, to reduce the possibility of foot infection. Paper slippers are discarded after a single use, while the sandals are disinfected at frequent intervals, particularly before being assigned to others.

## Cleaning of rubber boots

Some companies find it necessary for men on different shifts or jobs to wear the same pair of rubber boots. Where such conditions are encountered, great care should be exercised to disinfect boots afer each shift or job. First, the boots are washed inside and outside with a hose under water pressure. Then they are dipped into a tub containing a solution of 1 part sodium hypochlorite and 19 parts water. The hose is again used for rinsing, after which the boots are ready for drying. Other disinfecting agents can be used, but this one has been satisfactory and is easily obtainable.

One company has a drying rack consisting of a tank with low-pressure steam coils having upright steel-pipe boot holders which permit circulation of hot air inside the boots. After the boots are washed thoroughly and dipped in the disinfecting solution, they are completely dried in about 12 minutes.

If much work of this type is necessary, the rack with water jets could be rearranged so that a number of boots could be cleaned and rinsed at one time.

## Special Work Clothing

In our modern industrial environment, exposure to fire, extreme heat, molten metal, corrosive chemicals, cold temperature, body impact, cuts from materials which are handled, and other highly specialized hazards are often part of what is known as "job exposure."

Special protective clothing is available for all these hazards, however, to minimize their effect. Sample swatches of materials used can usually be obtained from the manufacturers for testing.

## Protection against heat and hot metal

**Leather clothing** is one of the more common forms of body protection gainst heat and splashes of hot metal. It also provides protection against limited impact forces and infrared and ultraviolet radiation.

The garments should be of good quality leather, solidly constructed, and provided with fastenings to prevent gaping during body movement. Fastenings should be so designed that the wearer can rapidly and easily remove the garment. There should be no turned-up cuffs or other

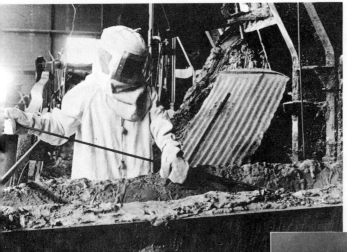

FIG. 17–48.—Open hearth worker opens tap hole. He is protected by long coat and hood made of asbestos-polyester cloth; gloves are sewn to cuffs of the coat.

projections to catch and hold hot metal. Pockets should have flaps which can be fastened shut.

For ordinary protection against hot metal, radiant heat, or flame hazards of somewhat more intensity than those represented by welding operations, asbestos and wool, as well as leather clothing is used. Specially treated asbestos clothing has been developed which is impervious to metal spash up to 3000 F (1650 C).

**Asbestos and wool garment** requirements are in general the same as those for leather, except that metal fastenings should be covered with flaps to keep them from becoming dangerously hot.

The most common types of asbestos clothing are the leggings and aprons usually worn by foundry personnel working with molten metal (Fig. 17–48). Such leggings should completely encircle the leg from knee to ankle, with a flare at the bottom to cover the instep. The design of the leggings should permit rapid removal in emergencies. There is no evidence that wearing asbestos equipment presents a health hazard.

The front part of the legging may be reinforced to provide impact protection when it is required. The most common material for this reinforcement is fiber board.

**Aluminized clothing.** Where people must work in extremely high temperatures up to

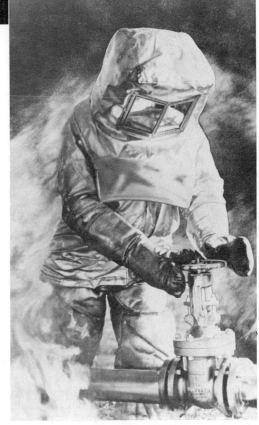

FIG. 17–49.—Demonstration of fire-entry suit. The material of suit is chemical resistant and will not burn, even in pure oxygen atmosphere.

**527**

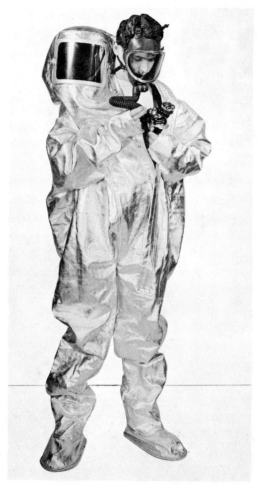

FIG. 17–50.—Fire-entry suit for use in entering a burning area. Note the self-contained breathing apparatus.

2000 F (1090 C) such as furnace and oven repair, coking, slagging, firefighting, and fire rescue work, aluminized fabrics are essential. The aluminized coating reflects much of the radiant heat and the underlying material insulates against the remainder. Some of these suits consist of separate units of trousers, coats, gloves, boots, and hoods. Others are one-piece from heat to foot. Some suits used in industrial operations are airfed to reduce heat and increase comfort.

Aluminized heat-resistant clothing generally falls into two classes:

- Emergency suits (Figs. 17–49 and –50) may b used where the temperatures may exceed 1000 ] (540 C), as in a kiln or furnace, or where men mus move through burning areas for firefighting o rescue operations. These suits are constructed o aluminized asbestos or glass fiber, with layers c quilted glass fibers and a wool lining on the inside

- Fire proximity suits (Fig. 17–51) are used in th proximity of high temperature, such as slagging coking, furnace repair work with hot ingots, an firefighting where the flame area is not entere These suits are seldom of one-piece constructio They depend primarily on the reflective ability c an aluminized coating on a base cloth of asbesto glass fiber, or synthetic fiber. *Never use fir proximity clothing where fire entry is require*

### Flame-retardant work clothes

Cotton work clothing can be protected agains flame or small sparks by flameproofing. One c the commercial preparations can be applied i

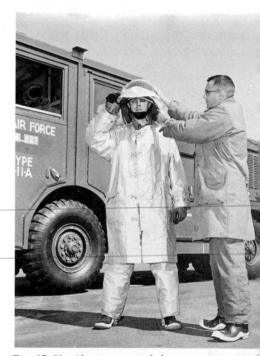

FIG. 17–51.—Aluminum-coated, heat-protective suit i used in fighting fires without entering the burning area Transparent face shield is metal coated to offer increase heat protection. Head fitting includes chin strap.

ordinary laundry machinery after the garment is washed. Treating the material will make it highly flame-resistant and will not add much to the weight or stiffness of the cloth.

These compounds are usually water soluble, and must be replaced after each laundering. An effective flameproofing solution can be made by dissolving 8 oz (227 g) of borax and 4 oz (113 g) of boric acid in 1 gal (3.8 liters) of hot water. If stiffening of the fabric is not objectionable, more durable flameproofing methods can be applied, some of which are resistant to both laundering and dry cleaning.

Durable flame-retardant work clothes are readily available. Cotton treated with tetrakis hydroxymethyl)-phosphonium chloride (THPC), developed by the U. S. Department of Agriculture Research Laboratories, gives good flame retardancy and will withstand many launderings. Nomex, a high-temperature nylon that chars rather than melts, is available for the most severe situations. Modacrylic fabrics that resemble cotton fabrics have permanent fire-retardant properties and are light in weight.

Flameproofed clothing should be marked or otherwise made distinctive to reduce the chance that untreated garments may be used by mistake.

## Cleaning of clothing

Manufacturer's recommendations should be followed in laundering and cleaning of clothes. Excessive water temperatures or use of certain washing preparations can cause deterioration of the fabric or affect its properties. Spot cleaning with organic solvents will soften or dissolve some synthetics. Chlorine bleaches will remove most flame retardent treatment from cotton.

Compressed air used for dusting of clothing must not exceed 30 psig (200 kPa) pressure. It is recommended that a vacuum system be used; this will prevent dust from being spread into the air where it could get into someone's eyes or lungs.

Many industrial laundries and industrial clothing rental agencies can advise on cleaning and maintenance of work clothing.

## Protection against impact and cuts

It is necessary to protect the body from cuts, bruises, and abrasions on most jobs where heavy, sharp, or rough material is handled. Special protectors have been devised for almost all parts of the body and are available from suppliers of safety equipment.

Pads of cushioned or padded duck will protect the shoulders and back from bruises when men carry heavy loads or objects with rough edges.

Aprons of padded leather, fabric, plastic, hard fiber, or metal will protect the abdomen against blows. Similar devices of metal, hard fiber, or leather with metal reinforcements provide protection against sharp blows with edged tools. For jobs requiring ease of movement, aprons may be split and equipped with fasteners to draw them snugly around the legs.

Guards of hard fiber or metal are also widely used to protect the shins against impact.

Knee pads should be worn by mold loftsmen and others whose task requires continual kneeling.

No one type of personal protective equipment for the extremities is suitable for the many different work situations involved in any business or industrial operation, from the laboratory to the loading dock.

Thus, proper protection for the hands, fingers, arms, and the skin must be selected on a job-rated basis.

The specific type of protection and its material depends upon: the type of material being handled; the work atmosphere.

Gloves. The material to be used for gloves depends largely upon what is being handled (Fig. 17–52). For most light work, a canvas glove is both satisfactory and cheap. For rough or abrasive material, leather or leather reinforced with metal stitching will be required. Leather reinforced by metal stitching or metal mesh also provides good protection from edged tools, as in butchering and similar occupations.

There are many plastic and plastic-coated gloves available. They are designed to give protection from a variety of hazards. Some surpass leather in wearing ability. Others have granules or rough materials incorporated in the plastic for better gripping ability. Some are disposable (Fig. 17–53).

Where the use of a complete glove is not necessary, finger stalls may be used. These are available in combinations of one or more fingers. Some of the more common materials used are asbestos, rubber, duck, leather, plastics, and metal mesh. The construction of the stall depends on the degree or type of hazard to be confronted.

Gloves should not be used while working on

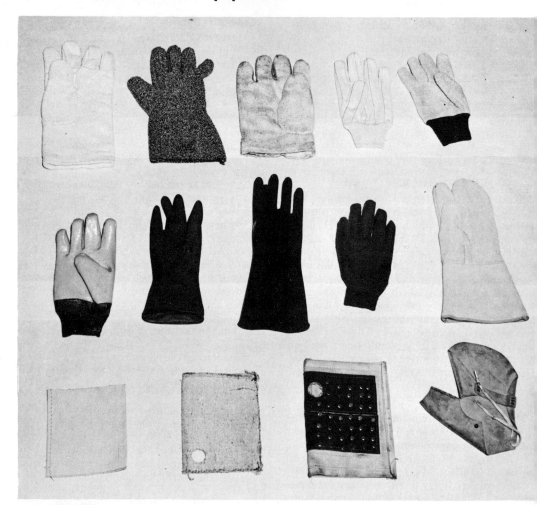

FIG. 17–52.—Pictured are various types of specialized hand protectors. *In the top row (l. to r.)* are asbestos, loop pile, and aluminized gloves, all heat resistant; 19-ounce cotton glove and loop pile glove are for general shop wear. *In the middle row* are plastic-dipped gloves for oily work, fine rubber gloves for protection against acids, etc., where finger dexterity is required, neoprene gauntlet for acid, caustic handling, neoprene and cork-dipped glove for slippery and oily jobs, and a chrome leather welder's glove for arc welding. *In the bottom row* are a neoprene sandwich palm pad for protection against sharp edges, asbestos palm pad for hot sharp edges, brass-studded palm pad for handling heavy material, and open-back leather palm pad for annealing operations.

moving machinery such as drills, saws, grinders, or other rotating and moving equipment that might catch the glove and pull it and the worker's hand into hazardous areas.

In addition to gloves—and the types are virtually countless—there also are available mittens (including one-finger and reversible types), pads, thumb guards, finger cots, wrist and forearm protectors, elbow guards, sleeves, and capes, all of varying materials and lengths.

**Hand leathers and arm protectors.** Where the problem is protection from heat or from extremely abrasive or splintery material, such as rough lumber, hand leathers or hand pads are likely to be more satisfactory than gloves, since

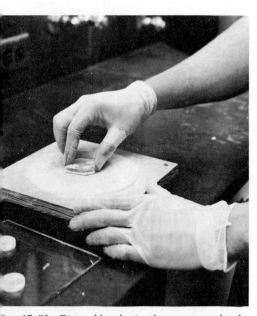

FIG. 17-53.—Disposable plastic gloves protect hands, maintain product purity. Although unit cost is low, replacement costs and accident frequency should be watched closely.

they can be made heavier and less flexible without discomfort.

Since hand leathers or pads are primarily for heavy materials handling, they should not be used around moving machinery. They should at all times be sufficiently loose to release the hands and fingers if caught on a rough edge or nail.

For protection against heat, hand and arm protectors should be of asbestos cloth or wool. Leather can be used, too, but will not stand a temperature over 150 F (65 C).

Wristlets or arm protectors may be obtained in any of the materials of which gloves are made.

## Impervious clothing

For protection against dusts, vapors, moisture, and corrosive liquids, there are many types of impervious materials available. These are fabricated into clothing of all descriptions, depending on the hazards involved. They range from aprons and bibs of sheet plastic, to garments which completely enclose the body from head to foot and contain their own air supply.

Materials used include natural rubber, olefin, synthetic rubber, neoprene, vinyl, polypropy-lene, and polyethylene films and fabrics coated with them. Natural rubber is not suited for use with oils, greases, and many organic solvents and chemicals. Make sure that the clothing selected will protect against the hazards involved.

Some synthetic fabrics used for regular work

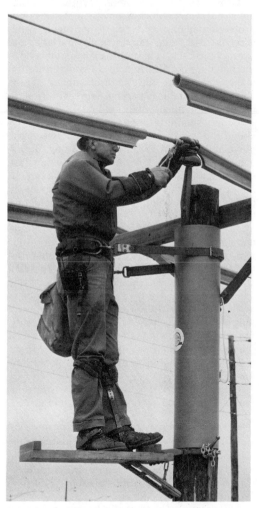

FIG. 17-54.—Protective equipment worn by this linemen includes electrical-style safety hat, rubber sleeves, rubber gloves with leather glove protectors, and safety belt. In order for personal protective equipment to be effective, it must be put on before a person reaches a place where he could contact energized lines or equipment, even by accident. Rules should require equipment to be worn when the work area is reached. (Note insulating line hose that covers the electrical conductors.)

**531**

clothing in chemical plants, where daily contact with acids and caustic solutions would cause rapid deterioration of regular cotton clothes, are not impervious and should not be used where impervious materials are indicated.

**Gloves** coated with rubber, synthetic elastomers, polyvinyl chloride, or other plastics offer protection against all types of petroleum products, caustic soda, tannic acid, muriatic and hydrochloric acid. They are also recommended in the handling of sulfuric acid. Less deterioration takes place than with natural rubber. These gloves are available in varying degrees of strength to meet individual conditions.

Gloves should be long enough to come well above the wrists, leaving no gaps between the glove and the coat or shirt sleeve. Long, flaring gauntlets should be avoided unless they are equipped with locking devices to assure a snug fit about the wrist. Such gauntlets are especially desirable when acids and other chemicals are being poured.

In this operation, the chemicals may splash, and unless precautions are taken, harmful results may occur. When caustic substances and harmful solvents are being poured from large to small containers, sleeves should be worn otside gauntlets.

In many operations, rubber gloves with extra long cuffs have been used to advantage. The cuffs of these gloves are made with a heavy ridge near the top edge, which, when turned back, forms a trough to catch liquids running down the wrist or forearm.

Gloves or mittens having metal parts or reinforcements should never be used around electrical apparatus.

Work by such perons as linemen (Fig. 17–54) and electricians on energized or high-voltage electric equipment requires specially made and tested rubber gloves. The requirements for electrician's rubber gloves are detailed in ANSI J6.6, *Rubber Insulating Gloves.*

Over-gloves of leather must be worn to protect the rubber gloves against wire punctures and cuts and to protect the rubber in the event of flash. Frequent testing and inspection of linemen's rubber gloves are essential, and those gloves failing to meet original specifications should be discarded.

Where acid may splash, rubber boots or rubber shoes also should be worn. The tops of the boots should be high enough to come beneath the

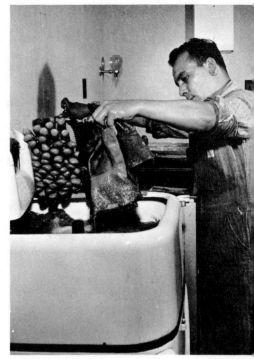

FIG. 17–55.—Laundering of gloves removes contaminants prolongs gloves life, sanitizes, and permits reissue.

edge of the apron. If shoes are worn, the top should come inside the legs of impervious trou sers. These precautions keep the liquid from draining off apron or trousers into the footwear

**Procedural setups.** When personal protective equipment is used in a corrosive atmosphere, a rigid procedure should be set up for taking care o it after use to prevent contact with contaminated parts. Before the equipment is removed, whethe or not it has come in contact with the corrosiv chemical, it should be thoroughly washed with hose stream. Gloves can be laundered to remov contaminants, prolong glove life, sanitize, an permit reissue (Fig. 17–55).

Boots, coats, aprons, and hats should then b removed, followed by removal of the gloves. Thi is the logical order of removal if the coat has bee properly put on with the sleeves outside the cuff of the gloves. Hands should be washed thoroughl before face shield and goggles are removed. Th hands and face should then be thoroughly washe

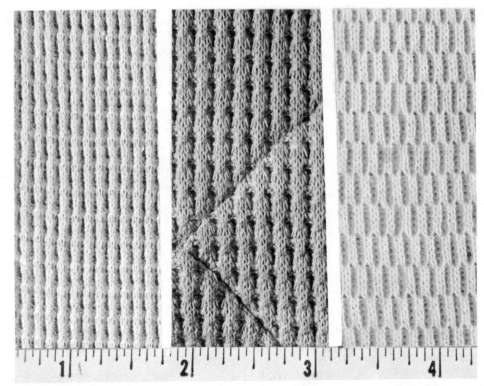

FIG. 17–56.—Various types of thermal knit cotton materials used for regular style cold weather underwear. Note the air pockets which give materials their insulating properties.

gain, but complete shower and change of clothing are much more desirable.

For protection against exposure to oil and the various other compounds which rapidly attack ordinary rubber, all the equipment discussed can also be obtained in plastic and synthetic rubbers.

### Women's clothing and protection

Women require practically the same safety features in protective clothing and equipment as men do, but styles of clothing may differ considerably in appearance.

It is desirable to have women wear the same type of dress, uniform, or smock. Skirts and loose, frilly clothing are easily caught in moving machinery. Where this danger is present, slacks and short-sleeved shirts are commonly worn. Tie strings for aprons should be a type that can be easily broken.

The possibility of serious scalp injury is present when women with long hair work near moving machinery. Hair covering is desirable for cleanliness, particularly in food products industries. Details on caps were given under Hair protection, earlier in this chapter.

Shoes with high or run-over heels, sneakers, and toeless shoes or sandals are not suitable for factory work, particularly where heavy materials or hot liquids are handled. Many companies require women employees to wear a medium or low heeled shoe. Safety shoes are also available in women's styles and their use should be encouraged where sharp or heavy objects are handled or where there is other danger of injury to the worker's toes.

Rings, bracelets, and earrings commonly cause accidents. Many companies prohibit jewelry or ornaments being worn on or near jobs involving moving machinery.

Rules on the use of protective equipment, such

**533**

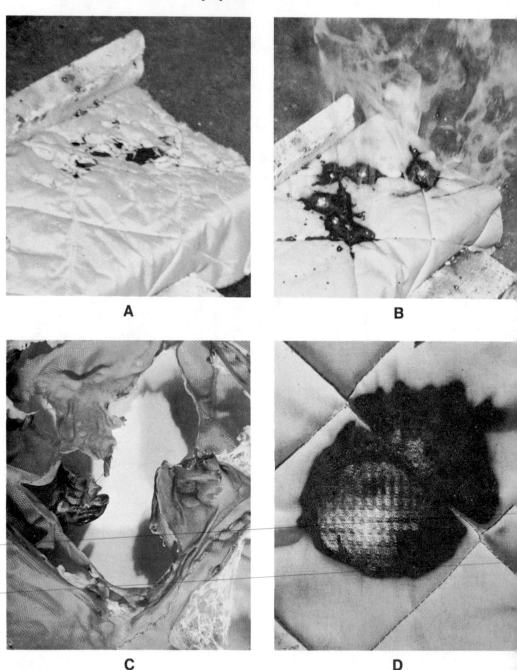

FIG. 17–57.—Demonstration of resistance to molten globules of welding metal by A—Regular thermal insulating underwear material; B—Fire-retardant material (note how fire-retardant material prevents burnthrough, even though it smokes); C—Melting nylon and polyester materials form a hot, pitchy mass; D—Fire-resistive material merely scorches, as shown in this closeup photograph.

as eye protective devices, face shields, and respiratory protective equipment, such as discussed previously in this chapter, should apply to both women and men.

## Cold weather clothing

In recent years thermal insulating underwear has become popular among outdoor workers because of its lightweight protection from the cold. Two types are generally available. One is a thermal knit cotton (Fig. 17–56) patterned after regular underwear. The other consists of quilted materials (Fig. 17–57). Dacron quilted between nylon is a common type of construction.

While this material does not catch fire any easier than cotton, once it starts burning, the nylon and Dacron melt, forming a hot plastic mass, not unlike hot pitch, which will adhere to skin and cause serious burns. Quilted insulating underwear is now available that has been made fire retardant to combat this danger.

A nylon material (called "Nomex"), that chars at a relatively high temperature and does not melt, is available. Glass fiber material is also available for special uses.

In order to get a good idea of how warmly to dress in cold weather, it is frequently not enough to look at only the thermometer. It may read 35 F (1.7 C), but if there is also a wind of 45 mph (72.4 km/h), it will feel like $-35$ F $(-37$ C). (See Fig. 16–5, in "Planning for Emergencies.")

## Special clothing

Safety experts have been very ingenious in developing many highly specialized types of clothing for protection against special hazards. A partial list includes such items as:

**High visibility and night hazard clothing** for construction, utility, and maintenance workers, police and firefighters whose work expose them to traffic hazards.

**Disposable clothing** made of plastic (Fig. 17–53) or reinforced paper is available for exposure to low level nuclear radiation, or for use in the drug and electronic industries where contamination may be a problem.

**Leaded clothing** of lead glass fiber cloth, leaded rubber or leaded plastic for laboratory workers and other personnel exposed to X rays or gamma radiation.

**Electromagnetic radiation suit,** which provides protection from the harmful biological effects of electromagnetic radiation found in high level radar fields and similar hazardous areas.

**Conductive clothing,** made of a conductive cloth, is available for use by linemen doing bare-hand work on extra-high voltage conductors. Such clothing keeps the worker at the proper potential.

For special applications, manufacturers have a vast number of materials they can draw upon to meet specific hazards.

## Acknowledgement

The following companies and sources cooperated in furnishing illustrations of personal protective equipment for use in this chapter:

Acme Protective Equipment Co.
American Industrial Hygiene Assn.
American Optical Co.
Armco Steel Corp.
Bausch & Lomb, Inc.
E. D. Bullard Co.
Caterpillar Tractor Co.
Chicago Eyeshield Co.
Curtis Safety Products Co.
David Clark Co., Inc.
Detroit, Mich., Division of Instruction
H. E. Douglas Engineering Sales Co.
E. I. du Pont de Nemours and Co., Inc.
Eastern Safety Equipment Co., Inc.
Ellwood Safety Appliance Co.
Encon Manufacturing Co.
Factory Stores
Ford Motor Co.
Fyrepel Products, Inc.
Humble Oil & Refining Co.
International Shoe Co.
Iron Age Shoe Co.
Jackson Products Co.
Kennedy Ingalls, Inc.
Klein Tools, Inc.
Lehigh Safety Shoes
Midwest Glove Co.
Mine Safety Appliance Co.
NASA, Mississippi Test Facility
Northern Illinois Gas Co.
Norton Company, Safety Products Div.
Owens-Corning Fiberglas

# 17—Personal Protective Equipment

Raybestos-Manhattan, Inc.
Redwing Shoe Co.
Rohr Aircraft Corp.
Rose Manufacturing Co.
W. H. Salisbury & Co.
Scott Aviation Corp.
Sigma Engineering Co.
Standard Safety Equipment Co.

Universal Safety Equipment Co.
Welsh Manufacturing Co.
Western Electric Co., Inc.
Westinghouse Electric Corp.
Wheeler Protective Apparel, Inc.
Willson Products Div., ESB Inc.
U.S. Industrial Chemicals Co.
U.S. Navy Electronics Laboratory

## References

American Conference of Governmental Industrial Hygienists, Cincinnati, Ohio 45201. *A Guide for Control of Laser Hazards,* 1976.

American National Standards Institute, 1430 Broadway, New York, N.Y. 10018.
*Identification of Air-Purifying Respirator Canisters and Cartridges,* K13.1.
*Men's Safety-Toe Footwear,* Z41.1.
*Method for Measurement of Real-Ear Protectors and Physical Attenuation of Garments,* S3.19.
*Practice for Occupational and Educational Eye and Face Protection,* Z87.1.
*Practices for Respiratory Protection,* Z49.1.
*Requirements for Construction and Care of Industrial Safety Belts, Harnesses, Lanyards, and Droplines,* A10.14.
*Safety Guide for Respiratory Protection Against Radon Daughters,* Z88.1.
*Safety in Welding and Cutting,* Z49.1.
*Safety Requirements for Industrial Head Protection,* Z89.1.
*Safety Requirements for Industrial Protective Helmets for Electrical Workers,* Z89.2.
*Safety Requirements for Window Cleaning,* A39.1.
*Standard for Safe Use of Lasers,* Z136.1.

American Society for Testing and Materials, 1916 Race St., Philadelphia, Pa. 19103.
*Standard Specification for Rubber Insulating Gloves,* D 120-70, ANSI J6.6.
*Standard Specification for Rubber Insulating Sleeves,* D 1051-70, ANSI J6.5.

Compressed Gas Association, 500 Fifth Ave., New York, N.Y. 10036.
*Commodity Specification for Air,* G-7.1.
*Oxygen,* C-4
*Oxygen-Deficient Atmospheres,* SB-2.

Mack Publishing Co., 208 Northampton St., Easton, Pa. 18042. *U.S. Pharmacopoeia.*

National Safety Council, 444 N. Michigan Ave., Chicago, Ill. 60611.
Industrial Data Sheets
*Flexible Insulated Protective Equipment for Electrical Workers,* 598.
*Industrial Skin Diseases,* 510.
*Respiratory Protective Equipment,* 444.
*Industrial Noise and Hearing Conservation.*
"Safety Award Clubs."
*Safety With the Laser,* NSNews Reprint No. 17.

Olishifski, Julian B., ed. *Fundamentals of Industrial Hygiene,* 2nd ed. Chicago, Ill., National Safety Council, 1979.

*Respiratory Protective Devices Manual.* Committee on Respirators, P.O. Box 453, Lansing, Mich. 48901.

U.S. Department of the Interior, Washington, D.C. 20240. 30 C.F.R. Chapter 1, Subchapter B, Respiratory Protective Devices, Tests for Permissibililty, Fees; Part 11. Note. The *Code of Federal Regulations* is available through the U.S. Government Printing Office, Washington, D.C. 20402. (See pages 56 and 57 in Chapter 2.)

U.S. Department of Human Resources, Public Health Service Center for Disease Control, National Institute for Occupational Safety and Health, Morgantown, W.Va. 26505. *NIOSH Certified Equipment.*

# Industrial Sanitation and Personnel Facilities

# Chapter
# 18

# 18—Industrial Sanitation and Personnel Facilities

A work environment should be kept clean and sanitary, and be well equipped for employee comfort and convenience. To achieve this, watch these five industrial health areas:

1. Potable water supply for drinking, washing, and food preparation;

2. Adequate disposal of sewage and garbage;

3. Adequate personal service facilities;

4. Sanitary food service; and

5. Satisfactory heating and ventilation.

These areas must be given the necessary attention if employees are to work efficiently, with the assurance that their health and welfare are well protected.

As with other industrial functions, maintaining a clean, sanitary work environment should rate a separately managed and comprehensive department if management and employees are to benefit fully. Sanitation, for example, must be properly managed and effectively integrated with production and maintenance if it is to be safe, efficient, orderly, and economical.

The general rules for sanitation include:

- Good housekeeping—as clean as the nature of the work allows

- Personal cleanliness

- A good inspection system

Where wet processes are used, drainage must be maintained.

The director or supervisor responsible for maintaining the work environment must be at a level high enough in the organization to permit him to sustain his function against the pressures exerted by other departments, and to provide surveillance of the entire company or plant environment, in order to keep it at an appropriate and balanced level of cleanliness and order.

Some firms are appointing a manager of environment and safety, who has additional product safety responsibility.

## Drinking Water

Most plants receive water for drinking, washing, and food preparation from a municipal supply. As delivered to the plant meter, this water most probably meets the requirements of the U.S. Public Health Service's *Drinking Water Stan-*

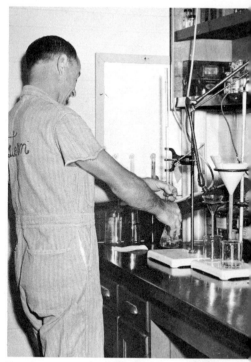

FIG. 18–1.—Periodic laboratory tests are needed to deter mine the quality of both source water and treated water

*Courtesy Olin Industries, Inc.*

*dards* or an equivalent local ordinance. Since it purity is controlled by local health officers, the municipal water supply can usually be considered safe.

### In-plant contamination

The fact that water is potable when delivered to the plant meter does not necessarily mean that i will be so when it is used, for there are many opportunities within a plant for water to become contaminated. If the requirements of America Standard and Sanitary Corporation's "Nationa Plumbing Code," or applicable local ordinance are followed, the chances for in-plant contamina tion of the potable water supply will be minimized.

One of the most common causes of contamina tion of the water supply is direct or indirect cross connection with a source of nonpotable water Before the "National Plumbing Code," there were cases of typhoid fever contracted from

rinking fountains with supply pipe lines con-
ected to septic pipes. Other common causes are
mproper maintenance of drinking and cooking
acilities and improper installation of plumbing
acilities, permitting back-siphonage of used
vater.

The integrity of the drinking water system
nust be maintained throughout the plant. If there
re piping systems containing water used for
ther purposes, such as sprinklers and fire
ydrants or manufacturing processes, each should
e clearly identified, particularly at outlets.
There should be no direct connection between
lrinking water and other water systems. Long
lead-end runs of pipe which cannot be flushed or
lrained and which might serve as a reservoir for
ontaminated water should also be eliminated.
The location of, and piping for, drinking water
hould be easily identified.

Nonpotable water may be used for cleaning
vork premises (other than food preparation and
ersonal service rooms), provided it does not
ontain concentrations of chemicals or fecal
oliform bacteria.

Where there is a possibility of misuse or cross
onnection of pipe lines, all nonpotable water
ines should be marked as being unsafe for drink-
ng, washing the person or utensils, or food areas,
ersonal service rooms, or clothes washing.

## Plumbing

Fixtures and faucets should be installed to
revent back-siphonage of contaminated water if
he pressure drops in the supply line. Faucets and
imilar outlets should be at least 1 in. (2.5 cm)
bove the floordrim of the receptacle below. To
revent backflow into the drinking water supply,
urge tanks and air gaps may also be required in
he drainage lines from process equipment.

Open joints in underground supply lines into
vhich ground water or water from leaky sewers
an seep are another common source of contami-
ation. This condition may arise where pipes are
ubject to vibration or corrosion and the joints
etween pipes open mechanically or the pipe
ections crack. Codes usually prohibit sewer and
lrinking water lines to be installed in the same
rench, unless the sewer line is placed at a much
reater depth and a certain horizontal offset is
rovided.

Frequently, contamination of the water sup-
ly results when a system is opened for repair for
he addition of new pipe and is not disinfected and
properly flushed with clean water before being
put back into service.

If the supply for sprinklers and fire hydrants is
the same as that for drinking water, hydrant drains
or "weeps" connected directly to sewer lines may
be a source of contamination. An open standpipe
or reservoir may also permit contamination.

Plastic pipe can be considered, but be sure to
check local code requirements. Unplasticized
PVC (polyvinyl chloride) is good for cold water
lines. Hot water up to 165 F (75 C) and 100 psi
(690 kPa) can usually be handled in pipe made of
chlorinated polyester or unplasticized PVC.

## Private water supplies

Industrial establishments in outlying districts
commonly supply and treat their own water from
private sources. Such installations should be
made and operated under the supervision of a
thoroughly trained and experienced sanitary engineer. The information in this and the next few
sections is not meant to substitute for such supervision. The USPHS *Manual of Individual Water
Supply Systems* should also be consulted for
methods of selecting, developing, and treating
private supplies.

All underground and surface waters to be used
for drinking purposes should be considered contaminated until proved otherwise. The water
supplied from private sources for the personal use
of plant personnel should meet the requirements
of the USPHS *Drinking Water Standards,* and
before it can meet these requirements, it will have
to be treated according to the degree of its
contamination. As a rule, ground water collected
from deep-drilled wells will be free of biological
contamination but may be contaminated by various mineral or chemical substances. In contrast,
surface water usually will be reasonably free of
mineral and chemical contamination but very
likely to have biological contamination.

Where there are several sources of water, the
final choice will be influenced by (a) the daily
water requirements, (b) the amount of treatment
which water from each source will need to make it
meet the purity standard, and (c) the potential
each source has for additional contamination.

The daily per-person water requirements of an
industrial plant can be estimated as follows: 15 to
20 gallons (55 to 75 liters) for drinking, lavatory,
and toilet usage; 20 to 25 gallons (75 to 95 liters)
per shower; and 5 to 10 gallons (20 to 40 liters) per
meal if food is prepared on the premises.

# 18—Industrial Sanitation and Personnel Facilities

TABLE 18–A

RECOMMENDED LIMITING CONCENTRATIONS OF CONTAMINANTS
IN DRINKING WATER

| Undesirable Substance | Concentrations above which water should not be used if other sources are available (mg/L) | Dangerous Substance | Concentrations above which water supply should be rejected (mg/L) |
|---|---|---|---|
| Alkyl benzene sulfonate | 0.5 | Arsenic | 0.05 |
| Arsenic | 0.01 | Barium | 1.0 |
| Chloride | 250. | Cadmium | 0.01 |
| Copper | 1. | Chromium |  |
| Carbon chloroform extract | 0.2 | (hexavalent) | 0.05 |
| | | Cyanide | 0.2 |
| Cyanide | 0.01 | Fluoride | See Table 18-B |
| Fluoride | See Table 18-B | Lead | 0.05 |
| Iron | 0.3 | Selenium | 0.01 |
| Manganese | 0.05 | Silver | 0.05 |
| Nitrate | 45. | | |
| Phenols | 0.001 | | |
| Sulfate | 250. | | |
| Total dissolved solids | 500. | | |
| Zinc | 5. | | |

*From* Drinking Water Standards, U.S. Public Health Service.

## Water quality

The water supply source must be evaluated on the basis of the chemical and biological contaminants it may contain. Table 18–A lists the limiting concentrations of two classes of contaminants: (*a*) those which usually have no toxicologic effect, but may give an undesirable taste or appearance to the water, and (*b*) those which constitute a health hazard and, if present, are grounds for rejecting the water supply. Standards under consideration for limiting mercury as a contaminant propose values between 0.002 and 0.005 mg/liter. (See EPA reference at end of chapter.) A limit of 0.5 mg/kg of fish is used currently.

Criteria for asbestos fibers, if present as a

TABLE 18–B

RECOMMENDED CONTROL LIMITS FOR FLUORIDE IN DRINKING WATER

| Max Daily Air Temperature Five-Year Annual Average (deg F) | Concentration (mg/L) | | |
|---|---|---|---|
| | Lower | Optimum | Upper |
| 50.0-53.7 | 0.9 | 1.2 | 1.7 |
| 53.8-58.3 | 0.8 | 1.1 | 1.5 |
| 58.4-63.8 | 0.8 | 1.0 | 1.3 |
| 63.9-70.6 | 0.7 | 0.9 | 1.2 |
| 70.7-79.2 | 0.7 | 0.8 | 1.0 |
| 79.3-90.5 | 0.6 | 0.7 | 0.8 |

*From* Drinking Water Standards, U.S. Public Health Service.

discharge from an industrial process in the surrounding area, may be less than those present in already treated or natural water. Information on proposed fibers testing and standards are available from the American Waterworks Assn.; see References.

Temperature criteria which affect the limiting concentrations of fluoride in drinking water are given in Table 18–B. Other factors influencing the limiting concentrations of these contaminants, particularly in combination with other substances, are given in the USPHS "Drinking Water Standards," published in Title 42-Public Health, *U.S. Code of Federal Regulations*, part 72. These standards also serve as a guide to radioactive substances in water supplies.

If the degree of contamination from the substances previously discussed is within recommended limits, the water supply source may be used, provided its bacteriological quality is acceptable. Standards for bacteriological quality are specified in the USPHS *Manual of Recommended Water-Sanitation Practice.*

The equipment necessary to treat water and make it potable depends on the degree of contamination and the likelihood that the source will become more heavily contaminated later. These factors can be evaluated only on the basis of a thorough sanitary survey of the water source. Such a survey will determine not only the type of treatment necessary, but also the nature and frequency of periodic laboratory tests of the source water and the treated water (Fig. 18–1).

## Wells

The safest source of water is often a drilled well whose intake is well below the water table. Such wells show a reliable yield and are reasonably free from bacterial contamination and finely suspended fibers. If both well and city water are used, there should be no cross-connection between the two systems. Be sure to check the local code.

The wellhead should be carefully located away from sewage lines, septic tanks, and sewage drainage fields or process waste disposal systems. The following distances are often considered adequate for separation: sewers, pit privies, and septic tanks, 50 ft (15 m); seepage pits and disposal fields, 100 ft (30 m); cesspools, 150 ft (45 m). Process waste disposal systems require special consideration. As soil and drainage conditions vary from one location to another, approval by local health authorities is recommended.

The USPHS *Manual of Individual Water Supply Systems* recommends that the casing for such wells be made of wrought iron or steel with threaded couplings or welded joints. "Stovepipe" or sheet metal casings are not recommended.

To prevent contamination of the underground water by seepage of surface waters, the space between the casing and the surrounding area should be sealed with a cement grout to a minimum depth of 10 ft (3 m) below the finished ground level or floor. As a further precaution, the casing should be grout-sealed to the lowest impervious stratum it passes through.

The well casing should extend 6 in. (15 cm) above the pump platform, which should be of reinforced, waterproof concrete at least 4 in. (10 cm) thick and continuous with the grout seal which surrounds the well casing. The platform should be designed so that water spilled at the wellhead will drain away from the casing. The joint between the casing and the concrete pump platform should be sealed with an asphalt caulking compound.

The top of the well casing should be at least 2 ft (60 cm) above the highest known floodwater mark. The pump should be self-priming and designed so that it makes a watertight seal with the well casing. The wellhead should not be covered over by paving or other material which would make access difficult.

Both submersible and turbine pumps must be considered. Submersibles are located in the well and do not require a pumphouse.

A safety factor is provided by two wells and two pumps. An automatic alternator can take effect if either unit fails.

### Disinfecting the water system

The pipes, reservoirs, standpipes, pump, and well casing of a new system should be thoroughly disinfected before being put into service. An old system carrying treated water for the first time following an extended outage should also be disinfected on the discharge side of the treatment plant, and a system which has been opened for repairs should be disinfected before being put back into service.

A drinking water system can be disinfected most easily by filling with water containing not less than 100 mg/liter of available chlorine. The solution should be allowed to remain for 24 hr in a new system or one which has not previously held treated waters. If the system has previously held treated water and is being put back into service following minor repairs, 12 hr will probably be sufficient.

To determine the success of the disinfecting job, the residual chlorine in the solution is measured at the end of the required time. Test kits for this purpose are available commercially and are easy to use. If tests show residual chlorine, the biological chlorine demand of the system has been met and the system can be connected to the drinking water supply, flushed out, and put into service. If no residual chlorine is present, the system should be drained and recharged with new disinfectant solution and the procedure repeated.

If the system contains a standpipe or reservoir, the disinfectant solution can be added through it. Otherwise, the solution can be supplied in a temporary reservoir on the supply side of the system pump and injected through it. A solution containing 500 mg/liter available chlorine, applied with a fog nozzle, will disinfect standpipes and covered reservoirs.

Underground water supplies may become contaminated while being developed. If so, they too will have to be disinfected as follows. After the 24-hr yield of the well has been determined, the test pump should be run to clear the well of turbidity. A chlorine solution should then be added to the well to make, with the 24-hr yield, a solution of 50 mg/liter. The permanent pumping equipment is then connected to the wellhead and operated until the discharge has a distinct odor of chlorine.

There are several methods for uniformly distributing the disinfecting solution. The well casing can be sealed and the solution injected under pressure, or the solution can be added from a hose or a small pipe at several levels beneath the surface of water in the well. The chlorine solution should remain in the well for 24 hours, as mentioned.

## Water purification

Of the several methods of water purification available, filtration and chemical disinfection are the most practical for industrial private water supplies.

**Filtration.** This method of water purification is used primarily to clarify turbid waters, but it may also serve to remove some bacterial contamination. Filtering plants are of two types: slow filters and rapid filters.

Slow sand filters will clarify turbid waters

when operated at a rate of 25 to 50 gallons per day per square foot (100 to 200 liters per day per square meter) of filter area. Such filters should be made with 0.25 to 0.35 mm sand and should be at least 20 in. (50 cm), but preferably 36 to 40 in. (90 to 100 cm), deep. During the operation of the filters, the film that accumulates on the surface of the sand must be kept below water level because this film increases the effectiveness of the filter.

Rapid sand filters, made with a uniform 0.4 to 0.5 mm sand with a depth of 30 in. (75 cm), will handle about 3000 gallons of turbid water a day per square foot (12,000 liters a day per square meter) of filter surface.

Both types of filters should be made under competent engineering supervision and operated under continuous inspection. Depending upon the water source, filters may require a presedimentation basin for preliminary treatment of the water. Filters should be provided in pairs so that one can be removed for cleaning and maintenance without disrupting the supply of filtered water.

**Disinfection.** Chlorine is the best available disinfecting agent for drinking water. It can be added to the water directly as a gas or as a soluble salt (calcium hypochlorite or chlorinated lime—refer to the Council's *Fundamentals of Industrial Hygiene*, for hazards of these chemicals). The free chlorine available from any of these materials makes them preferable to chloramine-B, which is frequently used as a disinfecting agent.

Small-capacity chlorinators, which inject gaseous chlorine into a water system, are available and easy to operate. Injection pumps that supply high concentration chlorine solutions to the system at a proper rate are preferable, however, because of the ease and safety of operation.

Standby equipment should be maintained at all chlorinating stations, together with an adequate supply of spare parts. Gas masks that are effective against chlorine and a small bottle of ammonia to test for leaks should be kept just outside of areas in which chlorine is stored or used. Masks should be inspected at regular intervals, and authorized employees should be trained in emergency procedures.

The chlorinator should be adjusted to leave a chlorine residue of about 0.2 mg/liter in the water after 20 minutes of contact between chlorine and the untreated water. Test kits are available that will measure residual chlorine rapidly.

Small quantities of water for emergency use may be disinfected in one of several ways. Commercial preparations should be used according to the manufacturer's instructions. Boiling water for five minutes, or adding four drops of household bleach (hypochlorite solution, 4 percent available chlorine) or two or three drops of common tincture of iodine to a quart of water and allowing it to stand for 30 minutes will also produce safe drinking water. Its flatness and medicinal taste can be partially removed if it is aerated after disinfection by being poured from one container to another.

## Water storage

Reservoirs or standpipes for treated water should be completely enclosed and located so that accidental contamination is impossible. The reservoir should be large enough to hold a 48-hour reserve supply of treated water. Vents should be fitted with screened downspouts well above flood level. Entrance manholes should be enclosed by watertight frames at least 6 in. (15 cm) higher than the surrounding surface and fitted with watertight covers extending at least 2 in. (5 cm) down the outside of the frames. When not in use, the cover should be closed and locked.

A reservoir permits full use of a smaller well and pump and still provides a buildup for peak demand. Quality of water is generally improved by aeration.

## Sewage, Waste, and Garbage Disposal

In some outlying districts and rural areas, industrial plants must provide their own sewage disposal systems. If there are state or local ordinances governing disposal, they must be adhered to. In addition, the recommendations given in the USPHS *Individual Sewage Disposal Systems* can be used as a guide for providing safe disposal of sanitary sewage from toilets, washrooms, showers, and kitchens. The disposal of process waste requires separate facilities. Many states and health departments require prior examination of all plans concerning disposal treatment.

Provisions should also be made for the storage and collection or disposal of garbage and refuse.

## Building drains and sewers

The in-plant sanitary sewage collection system should conform to local codes, and the recommendations of American Standard and Sanitary

Corporation's "National Plumbing Code" should also be considered.

Every fixture should be properly trapped and vented by means of drain(s) and stack(s) serving it, to prevent the discharge of sewer gases into the building and to assure proper draining. Traps and especially grease interceptors (such as those placed in waste pipes serving the plant cafeteria and kitchen) and interceptors designed to collect other particulate foreign materials should be of adequate size, located for easy access, and should be cleaned periodically. Be sure not to (a) install a type trap that is prohibited by the local code, or (b) place a trap in a prohibited location.

The building drain and sewer should be constructed of extra-heavy cast iron, bell-and-spigot pipe with drainage fittings. This material is less susceptible to clogging and much easier to clean out than pipes made from other materials, and it provides good "insurance" when installed under floors which would be expensive to tear up. Lead or other suitable material should be used for joints. The sewer should be tight under a 10-ft (3 m) head of water.

A cleanout should be provided where the building drain passes through the building wall, and at other selected places as the code requires. Check local codes for trap size, and permitted locations, and whether a strainer is required. In some areas, codes call for installation of backwater valves to prevent backup in the sewer line. These should be located where they are accessible for inspection and cleaning.

## Septic tanks

The main function of a septic tank is to separate solid from liquid wastes. It serves a secondary purpose of permitting aerobic bacteria to convert some solid waste matter into liquid waste.

The effluent from the dosing chamber of the septic tank should pass through a tight sewer over as short a distance as possible to the disposal field. The distribution box or boxes, which are the first unit of the disposal field, equalize the flow of liquid waste through the disposal field lines and serve as an inspection point where the quality of the effluent may be checked. Sludge must not be carried into the disposal field because it will clog the absorption system.

The disposal field should have enough discharge lines to permit the daily liquid waste to be absorbed and disposed of by aerobic bacteria. The number of lines and the length of each are based on the permeability of the soil to the liquid.

A septic tank should be located at least 50 ft (15 m) from any drinking water source. Surface drainage from the area around the septic tank should not be permitted to reach the water sources. The tank itself should be located well below neighboring water sources.

Details of construction and maintenance of septic tanks and disposal fields are given in two USPHS publications: *Individual Sewage Disposal Systems* and *Manual of Septic Tank Practice*. Compact sewage treatment plants for populations of 50 to 500 persons are available commercially. If required, they can be specified with a grinder and chlorination apparatus.

The disposal field should be at least 100 ft (30 m) from any water supply, 50 ft from any stream, and 10 ft from any building or property line. A minimum distance of 50 ft between a disposal field and the head of a deep well is acceptable if the well has a watertight casing extending downward at least 50 ft.

A detailed map should be made of the sewage disposal system, showing the location of septic tanks, distribution boxes, and tile fields. The area covering the disposal field should be kept free from vehicular traffic. Sodium and potassium hydroxides and similar "conditioning" agents, as well as brine discharges, should not be emptied into the sewage disposal system or building drains. If they are, a clogged and useless disposal field may be the result. Frequent monitoring of the effluent of the absorption field to assure the proper function of the system should be done.

## Garbage disposal

Companies and plants that have food services for their employees must provide for proper disposal of food wastes and refuse. There are several methods of disposal—local ordinances should be followed in each case.

Many plants collect garbage and store it for later pickup and disposal by municipal or private collection services. Large outside metal storage receptacles and compactors should be fenced in or covered and locked to prevent children from entering and playing in them.

Garbage and refuse containers should be metal or plastic with tight-fitting covers to prevent the entry of insects or rodents. Containers should be easy to clean and handle, and washed with detergent-deodorant solutions. The use of plastic or polyethelene bags or liners is desirable. The liner and contents can be removed easily and will help keep garbage containers clean. Garbage containers in the plant should be located so that employees will not throw food waste in waste baskets or other unsuitable receptacles. Collections should be frequent enough to prevent undue accumulation of garbage.

Discharge of ground food waste into the municipal sewage system is an acceptable method of disposal in many localities. Installation of food waste disposers in the plant kitchen can provide a convenient, efficient way of eliminating the need for garbage storage and collection. Disposers should be located, grounded, and installed according to approved plumbing practices and local code requirements.

Kitchen employees should be instructed to use nonmetallic tampers, keep silverware out of the disposer, and clean the trap metal catcher daily. The disposer should be stopped and the power disconnected before any attempt to clean or clear it is made.

## Insect and rodent control

The bacterial problem is often the limiting factor for securing good sanitary procedures. We must recognize other potential biological hazards, the flying, leaping, crawling vermin, such as insects and rodents, which create esthetic and microbial problems.

In plants where insect or rodent infestation is a problem, it is always best to employ a professional exterminator. The hazard of poisonous chemicals and preparations should not be risked by personnel with little or no previous experience in exterminating.

Communication with all plant departments, food vendors, and others concerned should be set up well in advance of the exterminator's visit. Outside signs may provide an extra warning to neighboring plants or residents, to protect pets from exposure.

To protect the workplace against entrance of vermin, wire mesh and metal screens can be used near the base of foundations. See Hopkins and Schulze (References) for ideas.

## Refuse collection

Hazards in refuse collection vary with the type of equipment used and the various conditions surrounding the operation. A frequent cause of accidents involve packing blades which cause partial loss of fingers, hands, arms, and feet. Other

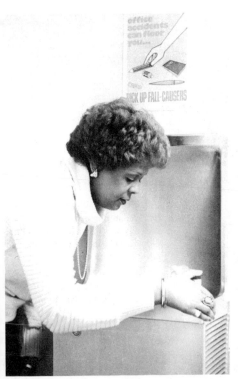

Fɪɢ. 18–2.—Fountains should be conveniently located so that employees can maintain their daily water intake. A safety poster can be located nearby the fountain.

hazards arise from "booby traps" unwittingly laid by companies whom they serve—loose broken glass in a refuse container, lightweight trash cans filled with heavy objects (like chunks of concrete), heavy objects concealed by paper or other trash, hose or other obstacles strewn along the pathway to a rubbish can. Containers that are rusted through or that have unserviceable handles increase the risk of job injury.

The incident rate for refuse collection for those units reporting injuries for 1978 to the National Safety Council, is 38.7. This compares to about 7.8 for the 1979 all-industry average.

Cuts, lacerations, and punctures accounted for about 14 percent of the lost-time injuries; this compares favorably to industry in general where 17 percent of the workers suffered such injuries. Wearing heavy work gloves minimizes these types of injuries.

Refer to the booklet, "Operation Responsible—Safe Refuse Collection," published by Envi-

ronmental Protection Agency (see References).

## Personal Service Facilities

Drinking fountains, washrooms, locker rooms, showers, and toilets—personal service facilities that contribute to employee comfort—should be conveniently located. These facilities make up an essential part of the occupational health program in most industries.

### Drinking fountains

Sanitary drinking fountains, one to about every 50 people, should be installed at convenient places throughout an industrial plant, in accordance with American National Standard A112, *Specifications for Drinking Fountains*, and local code requirements. The fountain should have an angle jet and a lip guard (Fig. 18–2). A waste can may be located at each fountain. It is important that the stream projector cannot be flooded or submerged in the event of stoppage, and that the stream be directed and projected so that it cannot be contaminated by the user. In dusty areas, fountains should be covered.

The water temperature should be 50 to 55 F (10 to 13 C) for heavy manual labor, or 45 F (7 C) for less-active office work. If ice is used, it should be in a separate compartment, without direct contact between the water and the ice.

Where city water is available on construction work, a water line can be extended to upper floors as the building is erected. A standard drinking fountain can be installed on each floor.

On some types of work, such as highway, pipeline, power line construction, and timber clearing, the drinking water source is so remote that it is impractical to pipe water to the job. Some companies have successfully solved this problem by using portable drinking fountains. These fountains have an insulated tank equipped with an angle jet drinking nozzle. The tank has an air pump and pressure release valve so that it can be pumped up to the necessary operating pressure. Containers should be kept scrupulously clean and should be sterilized daily with steam, boiling water, or chlorine solution.

Under no circumstances should use of a common drinking cup or ladle be permitted. If drinking cups are required, they should be single-service paper cups kept in a sanitary container at the drinking faucet, with a receptacle provided for disposal.

**545**

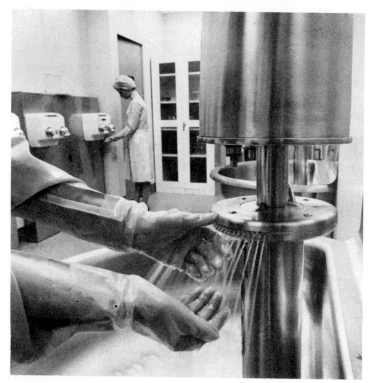

FIG. 18–3.—Employees "prep" before entering critical super-clean areas by washing hands and rubber gloves, then drying them under air dryers in order to prevent lint and dust contamination.

*Courtesy Western Electric Company, Allentown, Pa., plant.*

American National Standard A117.1, *Specifications for Making Buildings and Facilities Accessible to, and Usable by, the Physically Handicapped*, section 5.7, mentions modifications necessary for use by the handicapped.

Drinking fountains are usually not permitted to be installed in any toilet room. Bubblers are usually not permitted by codes to be installed as an integral part of—or connected to—another fixture, such as a lavatory or sink.

Carafes (vacuum-type bottles) that are frequently used in private offices are a potential source of bacterial contamination. They should be rinsed and refilled daily and cleaned periodically, using a sanitizer such as a cationic quaternary ammonium germicide.

## Salt tablets

On extremely hot, heavy jobs, it may be advisable to provide extra salt. Use of plain salt tablets is not recommended because of the heavy strain they place on body systems.

Automatic water salinators can be installed in drinking fountains located in extremely hot work areas. These salinators add salt to the drinking water in such small quantities that no significant salt taste is perceptable, and the strain on the body systems is minimal.

Buffered fruit-flavored drinks also aid in maintaining body fluid balance.

Some workers may be on salt-restricted diets, but they will have already been warned about their own salt requirements and are not likely to be doing heavy work. Other persons are nauseated by fairly high salt concentrations. This condition can be avoided by the use of enteric-coated salt tablets which prevent dissolving of the salt in the stomach, by the use of impregnated tablets which dissolve slowly in the stomach, or to some extent by the use of salt tablets containing dextrose.

Diabetics should be warned about tablets containing dextrose and, if necessary, should be provided with tablets without the sugar.

A doctor should supervise the choice and use of any salt-replenishing method.

## Washrooms and locker rooms

ANSI Z4.1, *Requirements for Sanitation in Places of Employment,* serves as a guide to the types and sizes of washroom, locker rooms, and accessories.

A large, single washroom and locker room for each sex may be sufficient for a compact plant or establishment employing fewer than 500 people. Washrooms in a large one-story plant generally are scattered throughout the building. If the plant consists of a series of separate buildings with only a few people working in each, all the facilities may be placed in a centralized building. This arrangement has been successful in such establishments as chemical plants, oil refineries, and railroad yards.

If the plant is relatively small, it is advisable to have the dressing rooms, lockers, and washrooms near the entrance. In a larger plant it is better to have these facilities in a single building centrally located or in several buildings near the work areas. In some industries, washing facilities are also used to prevent product contamination (Fig. 18-3).

**All washing facilities** should be maintained in a sanitary condition. Each lavatory should have hot and cold water, or at least must have tepid running water, and hand soap or similar cleansing agent.

Waterless skin cleansers are not substitutes for soap and water, but are convenient for special use or where water is scarce.

One or more of the following means of drying hands and/or face must be convenient to the lavatories—individual paper or cloth handtowels or sections, clean individual sections of continuous cloth toweling, or warm air blowers.

Common-use towels should not be permitted. Paper towels should be soft enough not to cause irritation. They should be kept in a covered container with a disposal receptacle nearby.

Hot air hand driers should be well secured either to the floor or the wall to prevent loosening of the fixtures or the electric element. The equipment must be grounded and permanently installed without extension cords or plugs. Blowers must provide air at not less than 90 F (32 C), nor more than 140 F (60 C).

For industrial occupancies of up to 100 employees, one lavatory for each 10 employees is recommended; for more than 100 employees, one lavatory for each additional 15 employees is considered adequate. In industries where workers need additional washing time, one lavatory for every five employees is recommended.

Circular wash basins (Fig. 18-4) of stainless steel, stoneware, enameled iron, or other materials impervious to moisture permit a number of persons to wash at the same time by means of center water sprays which are continuous or are controlled by a treadle. These basins are easily kept clean and sterile. Their construction prevents splashing and spilling of water.

To eliminate standing water, which can transmit disease from one employee to another, lavatories should have no stoppers. A mixing faucet or a spray will permit employees to wash in a flowing stream with controlled temperature. Knee-actuated water controls are available.

Wherever practicable, a thermostatic control should be installed in the hot water supply system in order to keep temperature below 140 F. Injecting live steam into tanks or lines of a cold water system (to make warm water) is dangerous, since failure of pressure in such a system could release steam through the taps.

A regular maintenance program for equipment should be in effect, and employees should be requested to report defective equipment. Broken faucets and valve handles may cause serious cuts or lacerations. Handles should be made of metal, not a breakable material, such as porcelain. If leaky faucets are repaired at once, employees will not develop the bad habit of turning valves off too tightly.

The proper type of soap is important, not only for ordinary hygiene, but as a protection against dermatitis caused by the cleaning agent. The soap used should have no free alkali and should have a pH less than 10.5. It should be free of mineral abrasives. Individually dispensed paste, liquid, or powder (not bar soap) for common use should be provided. Liquid or powdered soaps are preferable, because they lend themselves to ready dispensing and are also an aid to housekeeping.

The practice of removing paint, dye, and other stains with solvents or other chemicals, and especially the practice of removing grease from the hands with naphthas, should be strongly discouraged. Solvents may cause a severe skin irritation.

Protective or barrier creams, if properly used and reapplied frequently, provide limited protection against irritants to the hands and arms. There are four common types of creams; no one cream is

**547**

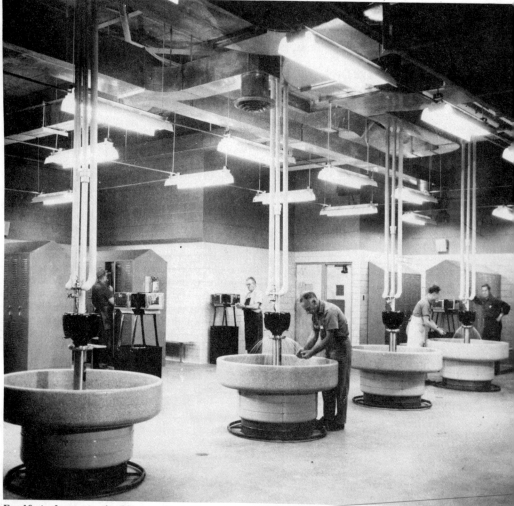

Fig. 18–4.—Lavatories should be supplied with running water at a controlled temperature. A sufficient number of wash-up facilities should be available. In a multiple-use lavatory, 24 in. (60 cm) of a wash sink or 20 in. (50 cm) of a circular basin when provided with water outlets for each space, shall be considered equivalent to one lavatory.

effective against all irritants. Repeated washing to remove the barrier cream is one principle benefit from its use.

**Lockers** should be perforated for ventilation and be large enough to permit clothing to be hung up to dry. If the clothing may be heavy or wet, it is highly desirable to provide forced circulation of hot air through the base of the lockers and out through the top, or to provide hangers on elevat-

ing chains so that the work clothing may be dried between shifts.

Lockers should have sloped tops to prevent material from being stored on the tops (see Fig 18–4). The multiple legs of lockers are serious impediments to floor cleaning; lockers should be placed on metal frames with a minimum of floor supports. They should be anchored together to prevent their being overturned.

Persons working with highly toxic materials

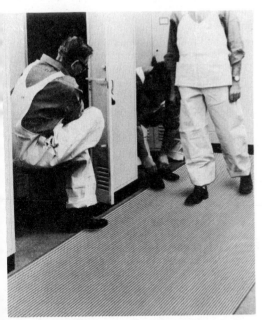

FIG. 18–5.—Flooring material should be selected for durability and sanitation and should minimize the hazard of slips and falls.

*Courtesy Samuel Furiness Mat Company, Inc.*

that are dusty or which may otherwise contaminate the clothing should have separate lockers for work clothing and street clothing. These lockers should preferably be in rooms on opposite sides of the shower room so employees will have to pass through the shower room when changing from work clothing to street clothing, and back.

Benches in front of the lockers should be permanently fastened to the locker base, preferably on a hinged support so that they can be turned up against the faces of the lockers while the aisles are swept. The benches should be checked at regular intervals and kept in repair, free from splinters, breaks, and other imperfections.

**Floors.** Washrooms and locker rooms should be well ventilated, kept warm and comfortable, and at 50 percent relative humidity. The heating equipment should be so installed as to protect against burns and should comply with state codes.

The floors of washrooms and locker rooms should be of nonabsorbent material such as glazed brick, tile, or concrete. The floor material should

be continued up into the walls as a cove for at least 6 in. (15 cm) before there is a joint. The walls should then be connected to the floor cove with a tight joint and should be impervious to water to a height of at least 5 ft (1.5 m).

Flooring material should be selected for durability and sanitation and to minimize the hazard of slipping and falling (Fig. 18–5). Terrazzo, tile, marble, and polished concrete floor surfaces are particularly hazardous when wet. For safety with such floors, a rigid cleaning and mopping schedule must be maintained to keep them dry when they are in use.

Concrete floors can be made much less hazardous by covering the surface with a finishing layer of abrasive grain concrete. Abrasive strips may be helpful on old concrete floors, which have been worn smooth. Ceramic tiles with a nonskid, nonabsorbent, and watertight surface, are also available. Mats can also be used.

A floor should frequently be inspected for watertightness. Leaky floors cause damage to joists and other structural members of the building, and, if organic materials collect in them, may attract vermin. Worn wood or concrete floors may be covered with a plastic material to obtain a watertight surface.

### Showers

Showers should be installed in establishments in which workers become dirty or wet with perspiration, or are exposed to dust or vapors. The showers should be as close to the job as possible, preferably in a separate room adjacent to the dressing and locker rooms. Workers exposed to high temperature who come off the job wet with perspiration should not be exposed to cold weather in going to the shower room and change house.

One shower should be provided for each ten employees of each sex, who are required to shower during the same shift. Each shower should be supplied with hot and cold water through a mixing fixture that the user can regulate. The maximum temperature of the hot water should be automatically maintained at 140 F (60 C).

Deluge showers, eyewash fountains, and similar installations for emergency use are discussed in Chapter 19, "Occupational Health Services."

Body soap or other appropriate cleaning agents, convenient to the showers, should be provided, and also hot and cold water feeding a common discharge line. Employees who use showers should be provided with individual clean towels.

When employees are required by a particular standard to wear protective clothing because of possible contamination with toxic material, change rooms should be equipped with storage facilities for street clothes. As discussed earlier under Lockers, separate storage should be provided for protective clothing.

Where clothes are provided by the employer, and become wet, or are washed between shifts, provision should be made to make sure that the clothing is dry before reuse.

The floor of the shower room and of the individual compartments should be made of non-skid material to provide good footing when it is wet. Either abrasive grain concrete or concrete with a wood-float finish is a satisfactory surface.

Existing floors which were made smooth or which have become smooth through long wear can be given a nonskid surface. Concrete floors should be scrubbed thoroughly with an abrasive pad using a synthetic detergent. Strips of abrasive material can be applied to other types of floors to provide a nonslip surface. The floor throughout the shower room area should slope toward drains, preferably at the back of the shower stalls. Curbs around the individual shower stalls are not necessary if the floor is properly sloped. They are a tripping hazard and, if used, should be dyed or painted a contrasting color.

Wood mats should not be used on shower room floors because of the tripping hazard and the probable exposure to splinters and loose joining members.

The pans of antiseptic solution commonly seen at the entrance of shower stalls or shower rooms are useless for killing organisms and a nuisance to keep clean.

As an item of general sanitation, shower rooms and stalls should be well ventilated and adequately lighted to prevent the formation of mold. The floor of the shower should be mopped daily with detergent, hot water and disinfectant to combat athlete's foot (fungus and ringworm infection). A foot-actuated spray can aid in controlling athlete's foot.

## Toilets

Wall-hung, elongated-bowl flush toilets with open-front seats should be provided according to the number of employees (Table 18–C). If persons other than employees are allowed to use toilet

### TABLE 18–C

### MINIMUM TOILET FACILITIES

| Number of Employees | Minimum Number of Water Closets* |
|---|---|
| 1 to 15 | 1 |
| 16 to 35 | 2 |
| 36 to 55 | 3 |
| 56 to 80 | 4 |
| 81 to 110 | 5 |
| 111 to 150 | 6 |
| More than 150 | One additional fixture for each additional 40 employees. |

* Where toilet facilities will not be used by women, urinals may be provided instead of water closets, except that the number of water closets in such case shall not be reduced to less than ⅔ of the minimum specified.

*From* OSHA Regulations, § 1910.141(c)(1).

facilities, their number should be increased accordingly. Paper holders must be provided for every water closet. For each three toilet facilities, there should be at least one lavatory in the toilet room or adjacent to it.

Wall-hung units are easier to keep sanitary and to clean under. Codes prohibit any type that is not thoroughly washed at each discharge or that might permit siphonage of bowl contents back into the tank. Water supplied to tanks must have vacuum breakers or have a positive air gap between the top of water in the tank and the water supply inlet.

Toilets should be placed not more than 200 ft (60 m) from any work place. In multistory buildings, toilets should be not more than one floor above or below the work area. With toilets and lavatories at various points throughout the plant, the main locker room and shower room can be closed for cleaning during the work period, an advantage for the janitorial crew.

Toilet rooms and washrooms for women sometimes have an attendant on duty during use. Washroom attendants should not attempt to give first aid to women who become ill at work. Such aid is best given by the plant nurse or physician. Some states also require that women work no more than a certain distance from a woman's rest room. This should be checked during design tages. Some states also require cots to be installed.

Ventilation is required for toilet rooms. If natural ventilation is relied upon, there should be windows or skylights having a ventilation area of 5 sq ft (0.5 m²) for a room with one toilet, with an additional square foot (0.1 m²) of window ventilation space for each additional toilet. If this amount of window space cannot be provided, forced ventilation should be supplied at a rate of three to four air changes per hour in the room.

Because windows and skylights generally do not afford sufficient light, light fixtures should be installed in all toilet rooms and washrooms. Switches, for the lights or for electric driers or other equipment, should be located so that they cannot be operated by persons who are at the same time in contact with piping or other grounded conductors.

Individual wall-hung urinals should be provided in the men's room. These may be substituted to the extent of one-third or less of the number of stools specified. Trough urinals are poor substitutes for individual fixtures and are prohibited in many states. Approved urinals must have all surfaces which are subject to soiling accessible for cleaning. Integral screens over the discharge openings are the major cause of chronic toilet room odors because the decomposing soil under the screen cannot be removed by any practicable method. Blow-down washout urinals are the only acceptable type. Floor-type urinals, in which the drain pipe becomes chronically offensive, and wall-hung urinals with integral screens should be replaced by the approved sanitary type (blow-down washout), thus making room deodorants unnecessary.

Employees should be prohibited from lunching in toilet rooms, or in process areas where toxic or noxious materials are present. The habit of some workers to heat foods in molten lead reservoirs or other process heating equipment can be dangerous to their health and should be prohibited. This prohibition naturally implies the provision of proper lunchrooms or other eating facilities outside the toilet rooms or process areas.

Covered receptacles should be provided in plant lunchrooms for disposal of waste food and papers, and employees should be prohibited from disposing of such refuse in the toilet rooms. If cups of coffee or other drinks are carried from the lunchroom, they should be in covered containers or on trays to prevent spillage which might create unsanitary or slippery conditions.

Privies are unsatisfactory, but where no other method is feasible, privies and chemical closets should be approved by health authorities having jurisdiction, or conform to USPHS *Individual Sewage Disposal Systems*. Portable toilets are also available. These are often necessary on construction jobs. The supplier can provide waste removal and maintenance.

## Janitorial service

As a part of an overall, managed plant sanitation function, a minimum, daily janitorial service should be provided for all personal service facilities. When properly designed, washrooms, shower rooms, and toilets can be thoroughly cleaned with little personal involvement in the process. Floors and fixtures should be mopped and cleaned with detergent and hot water, at least once daily. A sanitizing cleaner should be used as often as necessary. The occasional use of an acid-type cleaner may be necessary on toilet bowls and urinals.

Rubber gloves and goggles should be worn and the fixtures thoroughly flushed following use.

When floors are being mopped, the area should be blocked off by signs reading CAUTION—WET FLOOR, as a precaution against possible slipping accidents.

This subject is also covered in Chapter 2, "Construction and Maintenance of Plant Facilities," in the *Engineering and Technology* volume.

## Food Service

### Nutrition

Nutrition, another factor in industrial health and safety, concerns the medical and safety departments of any company or plant. If a survey of the food service establishments in the neighborhood shows that they cannot supply the nutritional needs of employees, then the plant is justified in establishing its own food service. With care and thought, adequate, balanced in-plant meals can be provided. Food must also be properly prepared and attractively served, with strict adherence to sanitary practices.

The company nurse, working with the company or visiting physician, can provide employees with leaflets on better nutrition. The Council on Foods of the American Medical Association, and the American Dietetic Association (see References) have many excellent articles and materials

**551**

## TABLE 18-D

### MINIMUM FLOOR SPACE IN EATING AREAS

| Number of People | Sq Ft per Person |
|---|---|
| 25 or less ........................ | 13 |
| 26 through 74.................... | 12 |
| 75 through 149.................. | 11 |
| 150 and over.................... | 10 |

*From American National Standard Z4.1*

available. A good breakfast, high in protein for "timed energy release" during the day, contributes to less fatigue and, consequently, less chance of accidents.

Workers usually need additional nutrition during the first half of a shift. Low blood sugar tends to be a health and accident hazard. A survey of vending machines will show that about two out of three food snack items are overbalanced in sweets. Overeating of sweets can contribute to low blood sugar. Snacks that contain higher protein, such as peanuts, meat sticks, and peanut butter foods, are desirable. Brown sugar rolls and buns, raisins, and sandwiches made of protein-rich breads are helpful.

Some organizations have dietitians review their food service menus and even talk to employees.

## Types of service

There are five main types of industrial food service:

1. Cafeterias preparing and serving hot meals

2. Canteens or lunchrooms serving sandwiches, other packaged foods, hot and cold beverages, and a few hot foods

3. Mobile canteens that move through the work areas, dispensing hot and cold foods and beverages from insulated containers

4. Box lunch service

5. Vending machines

Even using a mobile canteen to provide a midshift snack adds considerably to the nutrition of the average worker. If lunches are also served, the mobile canteen should carry both hot and cold

foods and beverages.

The central cafeteria with a kitchen where full meals can be prepared and served is often the most satisfactory form of food service. In large plants, it may be economical to supply several cafeterias from a central kitchen.

**Vending machines and microwave ovens.** Self-service vending machines offer a wide variety of packaged, ready-to-eat foods. Some machines have ovens that let the user quick cook his meal. Two important safety and health precautions should be followed in the use of microwave ovens. (See Fig. 15–12.)

1. All repairs should be made by manufacturer' trained repair personnel.

2. Persons with pacemaker heart units should be warned against coming too close to microwave ovens.

Details are given in the Council's *Fundamentals of Industrial Hygiene*.

Proper installation and maintenance of food heating and refrigeration systems is important. Normal sanitary precautions of course apply to vending machines. Can openers in safe working order, sufficient utensils, and adequate waste disposal facilities, in both kitchens and eating areas, are other necessary provisions of a self service operation.

## Eating areas

The cafeteria or lunchroom should be clean and attractive to encourage employees to eat away from their work area. Refrigerators for the storage of lunches will also help convince employees that they should eat in the proper area.

Minimum floor spaces for the number of people using the eating area at one time are given in Table 18–D. Where space is limited, lunch periods should be staggered so that employees do not have to eat on the job.

## Kitchens

When a cafeteria kitchen is set up, the same attention should be paid to proper equipment and working conditions as would be in any other part of the plant. Food equipment should be of types approved by the National Sanitation Foundation. The layout should conform with public health food service codes, and be such that the various operations are segregated, with adequate walk-

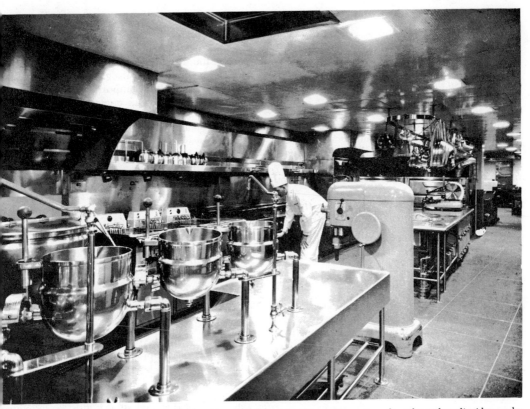

FIG. 18-6.—The modern industrial kitchen should include fire protection equipment, such as the carbon dioxide nozzles over the deep fat friers (at left) in this installation. Also note racks for hand tools.

*Courtesy Walter Kiddle and Co.*

ways from point to point about the kitchen.

Floors should be made of impervious, water-resistant, nonskid material to minimize the hazard of slips and falls if water or grease should be spilled on them, as often happens in a busy kitchen.

Ranges and other heat-producing equipment should be hooded and ventilated to carry away heat, combustion products, and vapors. Since these ventilating systems get very greasy, the duct work should be easily available for cleaning. They should be made of heavy gage steel so any fire can be self-contained.

Sprinkler systems and portable extinguishers should be installed for fire protection (Fig. 18-6). (See Chapter 17, "Fire Protection," in the *Engineering and Technology* volume.) A fire blanket should be located near the ranges or in areas where clothing may be ignited.

Easily changeable racks for handtools, such as knives, cleavers, and saws, and storage racks or cabinets for utensils should be provided in convenient places.

### Controlling contamination of foods

Incorporated communities have detailed sanitary regulations for the installation and operation of industrial food service facilities. Regulations of the local authority having jurisdiction should be followed in detail. In unincorporated areas with no local authority, the state code or the recommendations of the USPHS *Food Service Sanitation Manual* should be followed.

Perishable food and drinks, particularly custard-filled and cream-filled pastry, milk and milk products, egg products, fish, meat, shellfish, gravies, poultry, stuffing, sauces, dressings, and salads containing meat, should be kept at or below 40 F (4 C) except while being prepared or served. If foods of this kind have been permitted to stand for some time at room temperature after preparation, reheating them is not a sufficient protection against bacterial poisoning.

The types of bacteria (staphylococcus) which may infect these foods produce a toxin that is not destroyed by normal cooking temperatures. If the bacteria have grown in the food during room temperature storage, they will be killed by reheating, but the toxin will remain and food poisoning will result.

To prevent bacterial food poisoning, the following suggestions are made.

1. Keep perishable foods under refrigeration until they are to be used.

2. Keep hot foods hot (160 F, 70 C, or above) and cold foods chilled (40 F or below).

3. Remove leftover foods from food-warming devices immediately after the last feeding period. Never hold hot foods in warmers from one meal to the next, or for several hours before a dinner is served.

4. Place leftover food under refrigeration as quickly as possible.

5. Instruct employees who handle food and utensils that they must wash their hands thoroughly with soap and water after using the restrooms and before handling foods.

6. Eliminate flies, roaches, rodents, and other pests that may transmit disease. Consult a professional exterminator if necessary.

7. Never use galvanized or cadmium-plated containers for storage of moist or acid foods.

8. Consult your local health authorities if you have questions on sanitation.

9. Employees with open infections or communicable diseases should not handle food.

As a further precaution against the transfer of infections, no first aid material should be permitted in the kitchen. All conditions requiring first aid should be seen immediately by the company or plant nurse or the physician, and the individual should continue on the job only at the doctor's discretion.

To prevent cross infections in large dining rooms, the proper cleaning, sanitizing, and storing of containers, utensils, glassware, dishes, and silverware are highly important.

Use of single-service containers and utensils however, can eliminate washing and handling.

It is generally easier to sanitize utensils by machine washing than it is by hand washing if the machine is kept clean and in top operating condition. In either case, one of the main requirements in maintaining adequate sanitation is proper training of employees.

Utensils should be carefully scraped and preferably pre-rinsed before being put into the detergent solution. They should be thoroughly washed with soap or a detergent, and well rinsed by a method which will destroy bacteria.

For thorough machine washing, the utensils must be stacked in the trays loosely enough so that the cleansing agent gets to every part; the concentration of detergent in the wash water and the wash water temperature must be maintained. The wash water must be changed before it becomes excessively dirty. Spray nozzles in the dish washing machine must be cleaned daily to maintain proper flow and distribution.

Requirements for washing by hand are the same, except that each utensil must be individually scrubbed in all parts rather than simply stacked in a tray.

For rinsing, the cleaned utensils may be immersed in clean hot water at 170 F (77 C) for one-half minute. One problem is that of maintaining the temperature of the rinse water over long sessions of dishwashing, since a large volume of fresh hot water is required for this method. Water heaters should be of adequate size. Less water, however, will be needed if a chemical sterilizing agent is used. Hypochlorite solutions at a concentration of at least 50 ppm of available chlorine for an immersion time of one minute at 75 F (24 C) will provide adequate sterilization. Cationic quaternary ammonium germicides are also suitable.

When the utensils have been properly cleaned, they should be stored and handled so as to prevent contamination by the handler's fingers and from ordinary dust and dirt or from leakage from overhead pipes.

# References

American Dietetic Association, 430 N. Michigan Ave., Chicago, Ill. 60611.

American Medical Association, Council on Foods, 535 N. Dearborn St., Chicago, Ill. 60610.

American Public Health Assn., 1015 18th Street, Washington, D.C. 20036. *Standard Methods for the Examination of Water and Wastewater.*

American National Standards Institute, 1430 Broadway, New York, N.Y. 10018.
*Air Gaps in Plumbing Systems,* A112.1.2.
*Drinking Fountains and Mechanically Refrigerated Drinking Water Coolers,* A112.11.1.
"Gas-Burning Appliances," Z21 Series.
*Minimum Requirements for Non-Sewered Disposal Systems,* Z4.3.
*Minimum Requirements for Sanitation in Temporary Labor Camps,* Z4.4.
*National Electrical Code,* C1.
"Pipe Flanges and Fittings," B16 Series.
*Requirements for Sanitation in Places of Employment,* Z4.1.
*Specification for Acrylonitrile-Butadiene-Styrene(ABS) Plastic Drain, Waste, and Vent Pipe and Fittings,* ANSI/ASTM D2661.
*Specifications for Cast Iron Soil Pipe and Fittings.* A74.
*Specifications for Making Buildings and Facilities Accessible to, and Usable by, the Physically Handicapped,* A117.1.
*Threaded Cast-Iron Pipe for Drainage, Vent, and Waste Services,* A40.5

American Standard and Sanitary Corp., 40 W. 40th St., New York, N.Y. 10018. *National Plumbing Code.*

American Waterworks Association, 6666 W. Quincy Ave., Denver, Colo. 80235.

Environmental Management Association, 1710 Drew St., Clearwater, Fla. 33515.

Hopkins and Schulze, *The Practice of Sanitation,* 4th ed. Baltimore, Md., Williams & Wilkins, 1970.

National Institute for the Foodservice Industry, 20 N. Wacker Drive, Chicago, Ill. 60606. *Applied Foodservice Sanitation,* 2nd ed. 1978.

National Restaurant Association, One IBM Plaza, Chicago, Ill. 60611. "A Safety Self-Inspection Program for Food-Service Operators."

National Safety Council, 444 N. Michigan Ave., Chicago, Ill. 60611.
*Fundamentals of Industrial Hygiene,* 2nd ed. 1979.
Industrial Data Sheets
*Dusts, Fumes, and Mists in Industry,* No. 531.
*Industrial Skin Diseases,* No. 510.
*Refuse Collection in Municipalities,* No. 618.
Public Employee Safety Guides
*Refuse Collection.*
*Water Department.*

National Sanitation Foundation, 3475 Plymouth Rd., Ann Arbor, Mich. 48106.

Public Health Service, U.S. Department of Health and Human Services, Washington, D.C. 20234.
*Drinking Water Standards,* Publication No. 956.
*Food Service Sanitation Manual,* Publication No. FDA 78-2081.
*Individual Sewage Disposal Systems,* Reprint No. 2461.
*Inspection Report for Food-Service Establishments,* Publication No. FD 2420.
*Manual of Individual Water Supply Systems,* Publication No. 24.
*Manual of Recommended Water-Sanitation Practice,* Publication No. 525.
*Manual of Septic Tank Practice,* Publication No. 526.
*Vending of Foods and Beverages—A Sanitation Ordinance and Code,* Publication No. FDA 78-2091.

U.S. Environmental Protection Agency, Water Supply Program Div., Washington, D.C. 20460.
*Manual for Evaluating Public Drinking Water Supply.*
"Operation Responsible—Safe Refuse Collection." Available through National Audio-visual Center, General Services Administration, Washington, D.C. 20409.

# 18—Industrial Sanitation and Personnel Facilities

*Water Quality Criteria*, Report No. 3A. Sacramento, Calif., Dept. of General Services, Office of Procurement—Stores, Documents Section, 1015 North Highland, Sacramento, Calif. 95662.

*Water Treatment for Industrial and Public Supply.* Department of Trade and Industry, Control office of Information, London, England. 1971.

Williams, Roger J. *Nutrition Against Disease.* New York, Pitman Publishing Co., 1971; reprint ed., New York, Bantam Books, Inc., 1973.

# Occupational
# Health
# Services

# Chapter
# 19

# 19—Occupational Health Services

Occupational health services may range from the truly elaborate to the bare minimum required by OSHA. One establishment may have a full-time staff of physicians, nurses, and technicians, housed in a model dispensary; another may have only the required first aid kit with an adequately trained person to render first aid. There are, of course, many intermediate stages.

Modern occupational health programs, regardless of size, ideally are composed of elements and services designed to maintain the health of the work force, to prevent or control occupational and nonoccupational diseases and accidents, and to prevent and reduce disability and the resulting lost time. A good program should provide for the following:

1. Maintenance of healthful environment

2. Health examinations

3. Diagnosis and treatment

4. Immunization programs

5. Medical records

6. Health education and counseling

7. Open communication between plant or company physician and personal physician

Any treatment of ill or injured persons has a bearing on the practice of medicine. All states, therefore, regulate medical and nursing practice to curb the activities of persons who are not properly trained and licensed. Ideally, all the services related to health, injuries, first aid, and medication of any kind should be under the *supervision* of a licensed physician.

## Occupational Health

Occupational health programs are concerned with all aspects of a worker's health and his relationship with his environment.

The American Medical Association's Council on Occupational Health's official guides to occupational health programs, *Scope, Objectives and Functions of Occupational Health Programs* and *Guide to Small Plant Occupational Health Programs*, state that the basic objectives of a good occupational health program should be:

1. "To protect employees against health hazards in their work environment

2. "To facilitate placement and ensure the suita-

bility of individuals according to their physical capacities, mental abilities, and emotional makeup in work that they can perform with an acceptable degree of efficiency and without endangering their own health and safety or that of their fellow employees

3. "To assure adequate medical care and rehabilitation of the occupationally injured

4. "To encourage personal health maintenance

"The achievement of these objectives benefits both employees and employers by improving health, morale, and productivity."

If an industrial worker is to perform his tasks safely and efficiently, he must be in good health. It is not uncommon for a worker to have lower personal efficiency and increased accident susceptibility when feeling below par because of a nonoccupational illness, sometimes aggravated by self-diagnosis and self-medication.

Application of occupational health principles also helps to assure that workers are placed in jobs according to their physical capacities, mental abilities, and emotional makeup. This phase of medical-safety teamwork is also effective in the proper placement of severely handicapped workers (see Chapter 20). It also assures continuing medical care and rehabilitation of occupationally ill and injured workers.

There is a relationship between accident prevention and occupational health. For example, some industrial chemcials present a variety of serious hazards to health, property, and/or the environment when improperly handled. Depending on conditions, the vapor from a chemical can ignite or explode; it can cause dizziness or death when inhaled, or dermatitis after contact. (For details on the effects of specific chemicals, see National Safety Council's *Fundamentals of Industrial Hygiene.*)

The safety professional has ably demonstrated his ability to reduce accidental injury frequency by control of many phases of the industrial environment, through education of the worker, and by improved supervisory techniques. A large part of the remainder of the problem rests within the physical and emotional characteristics of individual workers. Here lies the key to variations in job attitude, productivity, safety, and absence for personal health reasons.

The services and skills of several additional professions are also frequently needed if maxi-

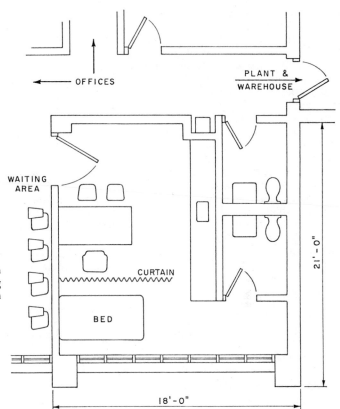

OFFICES

PLANT &
WAREHOUSE

WAITING
AREA

CURTAIN

BED

21'-0"

18'-0"

ɪɢ. 19–1.—The floor plan for a health
ervice office. The office has a waiting
oom, a treatment room, and a consultation
oom.

num results are to be attained.

Medicine plays an important role, with physicians being specially trained in industrial and
preventive medicine. They are assisted by specialists in orthopedic surgery, ophthalmology,
radiology, surgery, dermatology, and psychiatry,
to name a few.

• Nursing in an occupational health service
requires a specialized knowledge not only of good
basic nursing procedures and health maintenance,
but also of the legal, economic, social, and labor
laws that form the parameters within which the
nurse practices. Often, the nurse is the only full-
time medically oriented employee in a company
or plant.

• The industrial hygienist, a professional development of this technological age, serves as the
analytical preventive engineering arm of occupational medicine by applying specialized knowl-

edge to the recognition, evaluation, and control of
health hazards in the work environment. For
additional details, see the Council's *Fundamentals of Industrial Hygiene.* (See References.)

• Other phases of occupational health may use
the expertise of the industrial dentist, the sanitary
engineer, the public health expert, the psychia-
trist, the podiatrist, and the psychologist.

Working both individually and collectively,
these specialists have helped to improve the
occupational health and safety record of many
industries. In some companies, the application of
these talents is so well organized and effective in
the anticipation and correction of hazards that the
employee is unquestionably safer and healthier at
work than he is at home. In fact, the work
environment is so well controlled, in many cases,
that the problem now is how to get the worker to
avoid the hazards of home life, recreation, and

**559**

travel so that he will be able to return to work each day safe and sound.

Occupational health services of a company should be involved in the off-the-job safety program without being obviously intrusive. The personnel of the medical department can be influential in extending this program beyond the facility to include the employee and his family's off-the-job activities. The health and well-being of the employee's family has a direct bearing on his efficiency and safety on the job. If the employee is injured off-the-job, he is as much a loss to the operation as if he were injured on the job.

Some insurance carriers offer a consulting service which will help organizations set up an occupational health program suitable for their needs. The consultants usually know who the doctors and clinics are that would be available for this kind of service. The basic work, however, has to be done by the organization desiring to set up a program.

The justification for these services lies in their accomplishments. Prevention is not only better than cure—it is easier and less expensive. Off-the-job safety programs and activities can benefit a company, plant, or shop of any size.

## Employee health services

Although good industrial medicine can be practiced in any logical location in the plant that is clean and private, experience indicates that the medical unit commands respect only if careful attention is paid to suitable and efficient housing, appearance, and equipment. The entire unit should be painted in light colors and be kept spotlessly clean. The dispensary should have hot and cold running water and be adequately heated, ventilated, and illuminated. Proximity to toilet facilities is necessary. Suitable provision should be made for men and women, if both are employed.

**Health service office (dispensary).** A minimum of three rooms, consisting of a waiting room, a treatment room, and a room for consultation or for making physical examinations, is recommended (Fig. 19-1). Rooms for special purposes can be added according to the needs and size of the company. New employees who are waiting for physical examinations should not mingle with injured workers.

The surgical treatment room should be large enough to treat more than one person at a time—small dressing booths can be arranged to give some degree of privacy.

## First aid

Good administration of first aid is an important part of every safety program. It is recommended that a first aid facility of some sort be set up in all establishments regardless of size. This may range from a deluxe first aid kit to a well-staffed first aid and medical facility, depending on the size of the establishment.

First aid kits and supplies should be kept in a central location so that they are readily accessible to the establishment or department. Under no circumstances should medical supplies be spread about the plant for self-administration by employees. Where there is no nurse in charge, a supervisory employee for each shift should be delegated the responsibility for all medical supplies.

A careful record should be kept of each administration of first aid and an injury investigation report sent to the injured person's supervisor at the time first aid is administered.

Establishments that do not have a full-time medical doctor should maintain good liaison with a physician, or physicians, designated to handle plant injuries. The physician should be invited to the plant occasionally to evaluate the quality of first aid procedure, to make recommendations for improvement, and occasionally to tour the establishment. The company-designated physician (or physicians) should be well aware of the type of work done so he may better evaluate information given him by patients. The physician or nurse or supervisor designated should routinely inspect first aid supplies, stretchers, and stretcher locations.

**Definition and limitations.** In many small organizations and in field operations, it is neither practical nor justifiable to have qualified professional medical personnel available. In such cases the best arrangement is to use suitable first aid attendants who follow procedures and treatments outlined by a doctor. However, a doctor should be available on an on-call or referral basis to take care of serious injuries.

It should be noted that in some jurisdictions injured employees have their choice of a physician. In such cases, the employer should comply with this request, if possible.

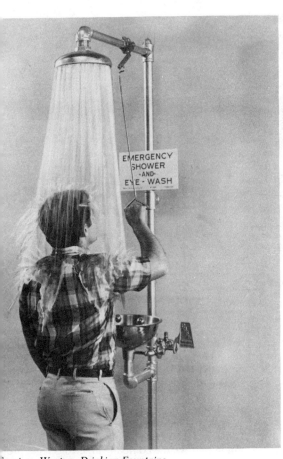

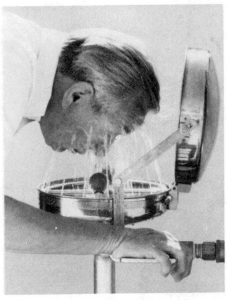

Fig. 19–2.—The emergency shower and eye wash should be well identified. Harmful chemicals are quickly washed away and clothing fires doused immediately by the drenching action of the shower (*left*). First aid treatment to the eye must be prompt and consists of prolonged irrigation of the exposed eye with low-pressure water.

There are two kinds of first aid treatment.

One is emergency treatment. According to the American Red Cross first aid textbook, "First aid is the immediate, temporary treatment given in the case of accident or sudden illness before the services of a physician can be secured." Proper first aid measures reduce suffering and place the injured person in a physician's hands in a better condition to receive subsequent treatment.

The other kind of first aid is the prompt attention given to injuries, such as cuts, scratches, bruises, and burns, which are usually so minor that the injured person would not ordinarily seek medical attention.

Under OSHA recordkeeping procedures, first aid is defined as a one-time treatment plus any followup visit for observation of minor scratches, cuts, burns, splinters, and the like that do not ordinarily require medical care.

The requirement that all employees report for treatment immediately upon being injured, regardless of the extent of the injury, has resulted in much headway in the reduction of infection and disability, and also in the avoidance of false claims of injury and disability.

A first aid program should include:

1. Properly trained and designated first aid personnel on every shift

2. A first aid unit and supplies, or first aid kit

3. A first aid manual

**561**

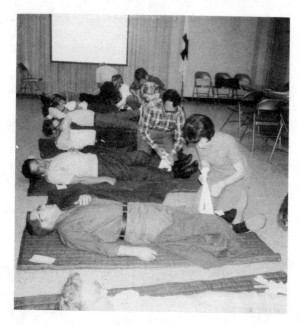

Fig. 19–3.—Demonstration and practice play an important role in first aid training. This is part of the American Red Cross multimedia system.

*Courtesy Shell Pipeline Corp., Houston, Texas.*

4. Posted instructions for calling a physician and notifying the hospital that the patient is en route

5. Posted method for transporting ill or injured employees and instructions for calling an ambulance or rescue squad

6. An adequate first aid record system

First aid procedures, approved by the consulting physician, should embrace the type of medication, if any, to be used on minor injuries, such as cuts and burns. These are two examples where there is often considerable difference of opinion regarding proper treatment. In areas where chemicals are stored, handled, or used, emergency flood showers and eye-wash fountains (Fig. 19–2) should be available. They should be well identified.

The equipment and supplies should be in accordance with the recommendations of the physician, and service should be rendered only as covered by written standard procedures, signed and dated by him. If it is intended to furnish temporary relief for minor nonoccupational ailments, such as colds and headache, the physician should specify the procedures to be followed. The limitations of first aid must be thoroughly understood.

The majority of states have medical practice acts under which a person is limited to a certain definite procedure when attending anyone who is sick or injured—except, of course, under the direct supervision of a physician. It is important, therefore, that anyone who is responsible for first aid have a full understanding of the limits which restrict the work. Since improper treatment might involve the company in serious legal problems, the first aid attendant should be duly qualified and certified by the Bureau of Mines or the American Red Cross. These certificates must be renewed at specific intervals.

**First aid training.** The American Red Cross first aid textbook and the United States Bureau of Mines manual of first aid instruction are recommended for the teaching of first aid. It is often found that accidents occur less frequently and, as a rule, are less severe among persons trained in first aid work. It is therefore advisable that as many industrial workers as possible be given this training (see Fig. 19–3).

The National Safety Council publishes posters and pamphlets that can be used for training employees.

Another valuable reference is *Emergency Care of the Sick and Injured*, by the Committee on

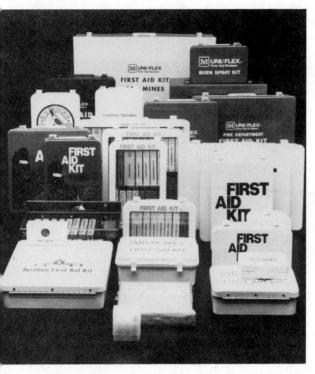

Fig. 19-4.—First aid kits can be obtained for special purposes.

Trauma, American College of Surgeons. (See References.)

**First aid room.** It is always advisable to set aside a room at a convenient location for the sole purpose of administering first aid. It upsets morale to administer treatments in public as injured persons prefer privacy. Furthermore, the person administering first aid should have a proper place to work.

The environment of a good first aid room should be similar to that of the dispensary. The room should be equipped with the following items:

1. Examining table

2. Cot for emergency cases, enclosed by movable curtain

3. Dustproof cabinet for supplies

4. Waste receptacle

5. Small table

6. Chair with arms, and one without arms

7. Magnifying light on a stand

8. Dispensers for soap, towels, cleansing tissues and paper cups

9. Wheel chair

10. Stretcher

11. Blankets

12. Bulletin board on which are posted all important telephone numbers for emergencies

Oxygen is of great benefit in the treatment of many cases requiring first aid. Where oxygen is being administered, smoking should be prohibited because of the danger of fire or explosion. Any type of resuscitating device should only be used by trained persons.

**First aid kits.** There are many types of first aid kits; they are designed to fill every need, depending on the type of accident that might occur (Fig. 19-4). Commercial or cabinet-type first aid kits, as well as unit-type kits, must meet OSHA requirements.

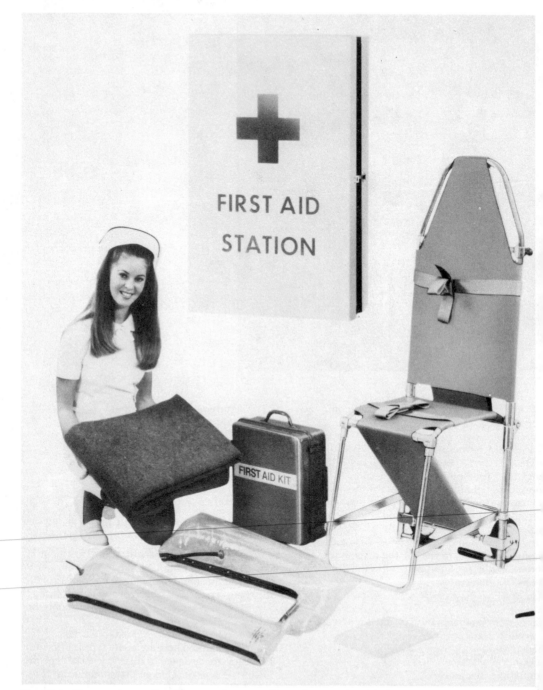

FIG. 19–5.—For areas that are distant from a well-equipped first aid room, a "trunk kit." as shown here, can be useful. *Courtesy Ferno-Washington Inc.*

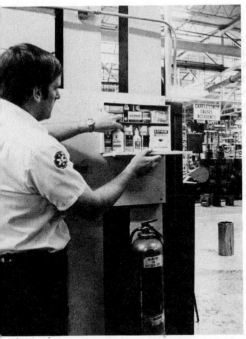

FIG. 19-6.—First aid kits should be well-distributed throughout a plant. They should be supervised by a trained person so employees do not try to "doctor" themselves.

Kits vary in size from the pocket model to what amounts to a portable first aid room. The size and contents depend on the intended use and the types of injuries that are anticipated. For example, "personal kits" contain only essential articles for the immediate treatment of injuries. Departmental kits are larger—they are planned to cover a group of workers and the quantity of material depends on the size of the working force. "Trunk kits" are the most complete (Fig. 19-5)—they can be carried easily to the accident site, or can be stored near working areas that are distant from well-equipped emergency first aid rooms. Although the kit can include such bulky items as a wash basin, blankets, splints, and stretchers, it can be carried easily by two persons.

Distribution of first aid kits throughout the plant seems to work to best advantage when supervised properly (Fig. 19-6). Each kit is the responsibility of a single, trained individual who should understand that he is to care for the most trivial injuries only or to render only temporary treatment for more serious cases. It is believed that with this system, many slight scratches and cuts are given attention which they would otherwise not receive.

In industrial organizations such as mining companies and public utilities, where activities are widely scattered, the use of first aid kits and some self-medication by employees may be necessary. Under these circumstances, however, it is better if first aid service can be controlled by having the attendant in charge properly instructed in first aid and by seeing that the service as a whole has medical supervision.

The maintenance and use of all first aid kits should be under the supervision of medical personnel, and contain the materials approved by the consultant physician. A member of the medical services group should be assigned to inspect all first aid materials regularly, and to submit a report of their content level and serviceability.

Maintenance of quantities of materials in the first aid kit is facilitated if each kit contains a list showing the original contents and the minimum quantities below which new materials should be ordered. All bottles or other containers should be clearly labeled.

Recommended materials for first aid kits are listed in the American Red Cross and the U.S. Bureau of Mines first aid textbooks. Suggestions are also available from the American Medical Association, the American Petroleum Institute, and from manufacturers of first aid materials.

**Stretchers.** Inadequate facilities for transporting a seriously injured person from the scene of the accident to a first aid room or a hospital can add to the seriousness of the injury and may be the determining factor between life and death.

The stretcher provides the most acceptable method of hand transportation and it can be used as a temporary cot at the scene of the accident, during transit in a vehicle, and at the first aid room or dispensary.

There are several types of stretchers. The ordinary army type is commonly used, and is satisfactory. However, when it is necessary to hoist or lower the injured person out of awkward places, use of a specially shaped stretcher to which the patient may be strapped and thus kept in an immovable position is better. A lightweight stretcher is shown in Fig. 19-5.

Stretchers should be located conveniently near all places where employees are exposed to serious hazards. It is customary to keep stretchers, blan-

**565**

kets, and splints in cabinets that are marked and placed to stand out among everything surrounding them. Stretchers should be kept clean; should not be exposed to destructive vapors or fumes, dust, or other substances; should be protected against mechanical damage; and should be ready for use at all times. If the stretcher is of a type that will deteriorate, it should be tested periodically for durability and for strength.

## Medical Services

The medical department should be easily accessible to and near the greatest number of employees so that distance does not become a barrier against the immediate reporting of all minor injuries for treatment. If possible, it should also be connected with the employment and safety departments, facilitating prompt physical examinations of applicants, the mutual use of clerical service, and the interchange of ideas and plans relative to employment, accident, and health problems. Another location that should be considered is near the entrance to the plant so that an ambulance can be brought to the door, if necessary; or so injured workers, who are off duty but under treatment, may come and go through a separate entrance.

The medical department should be in a place of greatest safety in case of a major company or plant disaster that might otherwise destroy first aid or dispensary facilities.

### The industrial physician

Physicians in industry may be employed on a number of different stations, at the same time (part time at each), dependent upon such considerations as the number of employees, the hazards in the operations, and the type and extent of the occupational health program. Arrangements may be made for full-time, part-time, on-call, or consulting service.

● If the service of a full-time physician is warranted, one should be employed. Some large organizations employ a full-time medical director on their headquarters staff, with part-time physicians serving their decentralized operations.

● Some physicians devote a scheduled number of hours, either daily or weekly, to the medical service needs of a company, yet they are available at other times for emergencies. Others arrange their service by telephone on the basis of current

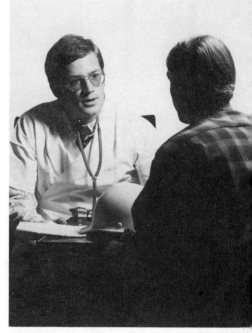

Fig. 19–7.—The industrial physician can provide eme gency medical care for employees who are injured or wh become ill on the job.

needs of the company—when job applican require examination, injured employees nee medical care, or other medical problems aris

● The on-call physician arrangement is mo often used by companies (or establishments) hav ing fewer than 500 employees, a low incidence o accidental injuries, or a minimum program o health services for employees. The on-call physi cian is usually located nearby and is available i emergencies. He cares for most injuries no requiring hospitalization and for those case requiring hospitalization that fall within his com petence. He often uses specialists as consultant

Frequently, the on-call physician has a simil arrangement with a number of companies in th vicinity—a particularly convenient system wit the small-plant or small-company clusters, suc as in industrial parks.

It is not unusual to find physicians specializin in the care of industrial injuries and diseases, an providing occupational medical services in som manufacturing centers.

A physician who has a consulting service is not usually called in except for diagnosis and treatment of serious injuries, illnesses, toxicological problems, and special kinds of injuries or disorders (such as eye injuries) that require the services of a specialist.

State and local health departments often supply, without charge, medical, nursing, and engineering consultation, as well as make industrial hygiene and radiological surveys to industries within their areas. Many insurance and private consulting companies also provide this type of service to their clients.

**Duties of the industrial physician.** An effective medical service program should be planned by the medical department head (usually a physician), with the approval of management. Full support of management can only be obtained when management is sympathetic to a cause that reflects management's policies. Only then is it possible to establish and maintain an adequate professional staff and facilities for examinations, emergency cases, and storage of records.

The industrial physician must be given enough authority so that workers will respect his judgment and follow his instructions on personal health and safety. He should be familiar with all jobs, materials, and processes that are used within the company where he is working. An occasional inspection trip will help him keep abreast of what is going on. This inventory of hazards will help the physician suggest to the safety professional those potentially harmful environments from which the employees should be protected.

The physician should be involved in other company services that relate to health of workers, such as food service, welfare service, safety program, sanitation, and mental health. He can also initiate and be responsible for sponsorship of company-wide immunization programs (against tetanus, polio, or flu) as well as for blood donor and chest X-ray programs.

Maintenance of the true physician-patient relationship (with fairness to both employee and employer) is essential to the success of any occupational health program—for example, worker patients should receive the same courtesy and professional honesty as do private patients. The first meeting of physician and employee usually occurs at the introductory physical examination and this meeting may be followed by subsequent examinations. The examining physician in his professional discretion should acquaint the examinee with the results of these examinations and, if necessary, refer him to his own personal physician for correction of defects.

The industrial physician should provide emergency medical care for all employees who are injured or become ill on the job, and he should arrange for the necessary followup treatment of employees suffering from occupational disease or injuries (Fig. 19–7). The treatment of employee injuries or diseases not industrially induced is the function of private medical practice. Therefore, the industrial physician should abstain from rendering such services except when independent facilities are not readily available, or the ailment or discomfort is so minor that the employee would ordinarily not seek medical attention, or the rendering of such service would enable an employee to complete a shift.

The industrial physician should not devote time or facilities to diagnose or treat dependents of employees. Instead, health education programs should be promoted for employees and their families so that they will be encouraged to seek proper private consultation.

Medical and surgical management in every case of industrial injury or disease should aim to restore the disabled worker to his former earning power and occupation as completely as possible and without unnecessary delay. To help achieve this, concise, dependable medical reports should be promptly submitted to those agencies entitled to them. In the same way, equitable administration of workers' compensation rests on medical testimony which adheres closely to reasonable scientific deductions regarding the injury or its possible consequences.

Maintenance of necessary records and reports is the responsibility of the industrial physician. These records act as a guide to management, and keep both management and employees informed as to the success of the program. Records and reports are necessary to direct and evaluate preventive medical and safety engineering techniques, to chart progress in the reduction of accidents, and to meet the recordkeeping requirements of the Williams-Steiger Occupational Safety and Health Act of 1970 (see Medical records later in this section, and also refer back to Chapter 2, "Federal Legislation," and Chapter 6, "Accident Records and Incidence Rates").

The physician is also responsible for properly instructing nurses and paramedical personnel and

**567**

# 19—Occupational Health Services

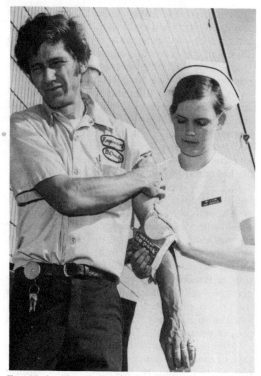

FIG. 19-8.—The occupational health nurse can provide initial health care in case of injury or illness.

*Courtesy of Kwik Kold*

directing their activities. Their duties, therefore, should be described in clear, concisely written directives, a copy of which should be posted in the medical department. There must be no delegation of any services that require expert medical attention.

## The occupational health nurse

Occupational health nursing is a specialized branch of the nursing profession. The position requires a registered professional nurse, who is licensed in the state where employed. In addition, it is desirable that the occupational health nurse have some knowledge of workers' compensation laws, insurance, health and safety laws, occupational diseases, sanitation, first aid, and record-keeping.

The occupational health nurse contributes the most when he works with the company physician who provides him with written directives that

have been discussed between them, so they ar mutually understood and agreed upon.

Working with the physician, the occupationa health nurse can provide a variety of nursin services, such as initial care for injuries (Fig. 19-8 or illnesses, counseling, health education, consu tation about sanitary standards, and referral t community health agencies. He also can partic pate in programs to evaluate employee healtl such as health examinations, or to prevent diseas such as immunizations.

Working with the physician, the plant nurs can perform excellent employee health educatio services in the distribution of literature on hear care, weight control, cancer and tuberculosi prevention, and the prevention and treatment c venereal disease.

When the physician is only at the establish ment part time, the nurse works with the safet director in planning and conducting acciden prevention programs.

The occupational health nurse must maintai a confidential professional relationship with th employees in conformity with legal and ethic codes. The nurse may not divulge informatio contained in individual employee health record unless the employee gives his signed permissior the medical files should be accessible only t medical personnel.

It must be clear that establishment of medic. diagnosis and definition of treatment are th functions of the physician. The nurse is not substitute for the physician. Each has a legall defined area of practice and responsibility. T have an effective medical program, a compan should have the services of a physician and nurse.

## Physical examination program

Supervision of the health status of workers b qualified medical personnel is essential if an occupational health program is to obtain maxi mum benefits for both employer and employee Therefore, a program of physical examinatio should be established. The examining physicia should discuss all significant findings with th worker. However, good judgment should be use to prevent the raising of unnecessary fears, whil emphasizing the importance of obtaining ade quate personal medical care. A transcript of th data may be supplied to the worker's persona physician or for an insurance company with th consent of the employee. Courts, workers' com ensation commissions, or health authorities may request this information by legal means, but employee consent is a more agreeable method. Certainly the confidential character of health examination records should be observed.

The employer should be informed of a potentially harmful work environment detected through examination of persons subjected to it, because OSHA requires employers to keep accurate records of employee exposure to potentially toxic materials or harmful physical agents.

**Scope of the examination.** It is impossible to set forth what constitutes a complete examination, or even a suitable examination, because physicians have different opinions regarding the relative values of various test procedures, based on their own training and experience. Therefore, the scope of a physical examination should be determined by the company physician, who is familiar with the operations involved—the nature of the industry, its inherent hazards, the variations in jobs, in physical demands, and in health exposures are determinants. The values of different test procedures and their cost in time and dollars must be assayed. Perhaps examinations should be different in scope for different jobs. For example, the physical condition of the iron-worker to be engaged in construction of the skyscraper is a far different problem from that of the sedentary seamstress, yet there are basic physical examination considerations applicable to each.

The various kinds of examinations may be classified as follows—preplacement, periodic, transfer, promotion, special, and termination.

**Preplacement examinations.** The preplacement examination is made to determine and record the physical condition of the prospective worker so that he can be assigned to a suitable job in accordance with his mental ability and physical capacity, and in which his disabilities, if any, will not affect his personal efficiency, safety, and health, or the safety of others. The applicant (or his personal physician, on the applicant's approval) should be advised of conditions that need attention. Medical department followup may be necessary.

It must be a paramount principle that the purpose of the program is selection *and* placement—not merely selection of the physically perfect and rejection of all others.

From the public and occupational health standpoint, the only bar to immediate employment in nonhazardous occupations should be communicable disease, progressively incapacitating injury or disease, or incapacitating mental illness. It is obvious that communicable diseases must be controlled, and this may involve the assistance of public health officials. One of the values of an examination program is the detection of disease in its early stages, when it is most amenable to treatment. Applicants with incipient but still nondisabling disorders can often be employed while being treated by their personal physicians. Many applicants with incapacitating injury or disease can improve their employability and job opportunities after being assisted by rehabilitation agencies. (See details in the next chapter, "The Handicapped Worker.")

A significant percentage of persons have mental illness or emotional disturbance that impairs judgment or prevents them from performing normal work. These aberrations vary in degree and can be serious enough to bar employment. The trained physician can frequently detect them during the preplacement examination.

It is not the function, however, of the physician to inform the applicant whether he is to be employed. This is the prerogative and duty of management, as there are other factors in addition to physical qualifications that bear upon suitability for employment.

**Periodic examinations** of all employees may be on a required or voluntary basis.

A required program should be applied to workers who are exposed to health-hazardous processes or materials, or whose work involves responsibility for the safety of others, such as vehicle operators. Substances like lead or carbon tetrachloride that are capable of causing occupational disease are usually subjected to process controls that will keep the workers safe from poisoning; however, caution dictates the advisability of periodic examination of such workers, to be certain that the engineering and hygiene controls are effective and continue to be so. This procedure also enables early detection of the hypersusceptible individual, and the worker whose personal unsafe practices defeat the control measures.

Frequency of the examination must vary in accordance with the quality of the engineering control, the nature of the exposure (this is influenced by the rapidity of the action of the hazard-

# 19—Occupational Health Services

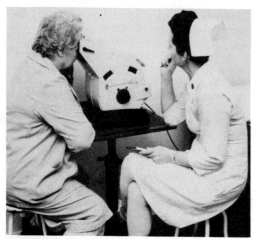

FIG. 19–9.—A typical device for testing vision.

*Courtesy of Titmus Optical Co.*

ous substance on the human body), and the findings on each examination. Thus, exposures to some substances might justify examinations or laboratory tests on a weekly basis, others monthly or quarterly, whereas annually or biennially may be adequate in some dust exposures.

In many cases, laboratory tests of blood or urine will suffice as the major portion of a periodic examination program, with complete examinations being made less frequently. The type of special examination (laboratory, X ray, etc.) necessary for any exposure and the interpretation of the results are decisions requiring the most expert medical personnel.

**Special examinations.** Employees having on-the-job difficulties that may be health related are often benefited by special examinations. Job transfer may also require medical evaluation.

Many organizations find it worthwhile to make "return to work" examinations of employees who have been absent more than a specified number of days as a result of a nonoccupational illness or injury. This is done to control communicable disease, as well as to determine suitability for return to work. There is a wide difference in the actual effects of the same disease on different persons, and an even greater divergence of personality reaction to the disorder. One person will go to bed at the first sign of discomfort, whereas another must be truly overwhelmed before he

will fail to report for work.

When an employee returns to work followin serious injury, either occupational or nonoccupa tional, a new evaluation of physical capacitie may be necessary. Also the application of rehabi itation procedures may reduce the disability an improve the range of employability.

**Exit examinations.** Upon termination o employment of workers, some organizatior make examinations and record the findings, pa ticularly where operations involve definite expc sure to health hazardous substances, such as lea benzene (benzol), silica, and asbestos dust, or t harmful noise.

**Laboratory tests.** Urine and blood tests are good investment in detecting liver and kidne disease, diabetes, anemia, to name the mor common ones. Where there is to be an exposure t toxic substances, appropriate laboratory test may be indispensable.

**X-ray tests.** A record of the condition of th lungs as shown by X ray is desirable for ever applicant. Those who will be engaged in a dust trade should have periodic chest X rays. Every ) ray should be carefully identified with date an name and each should be compared with previou X-ray photographs.

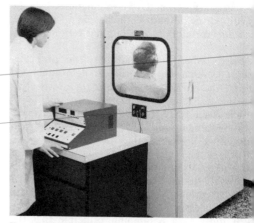

FIG. 19–10.—A hearing test using an automatic audiome ter being performed in a booth to ensure a quiet environ ment without distractions.

*Courtesy of Environmental Technology Corp.*

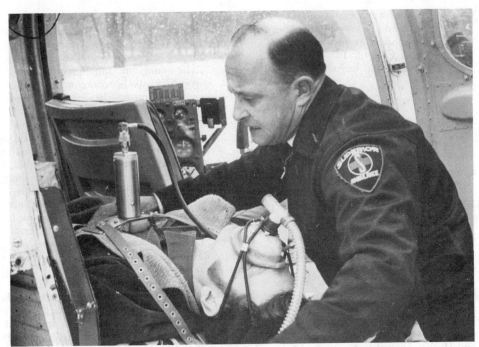

FIG. 19–11.—In cases where speed is essential, a helicopter can be used for transfer.

X-ray screening tests, as part of the preplacement medical examination are of no significant value in predicting the onset of back pain or injury. They are indeed an unnecessary expense as well as exposing the person to needless X-ray radiation.

**Vision tests.** In recent years, special devices have been developed for routine testing of several aspects of vision (Fig. 19–9). Near, as well as far, vision should be recorded. The old method of testing only distance vision at 20 ft (6 m) is inadequate. Failure to compare the visual requirements of a job with the visual abilities of employees may result in employees becoming easily fatigued, inefficient, and involved in an accident.

If facilities are not available at the establishment, arrangements can be made with outside doctors for annual eye examinations and fitting prescription safety glasses if needed.

If the job demands it, color vision should also be tested.

**Hearing tests.** Workers who are to be exposed to hazardous noise levels should be examined for hearing acuity before placement to determine prior hearing loss, if any, and periodically thereafter to detect early loss due to noise. Personal protective devices can reduce noise reaching the auditory nerve, but wisdom dictates the value of tests and records. The audiometer is the accepted method of testing (Fig. 19–10). A special booth will usually be required to administer these tests.

**Health history.** Some doctors think that a carefully taken personal health and occupational history gives clues to the areas of examination which warrant extra-careful study. A nurse or other specially trained person can secure basic data from the examinee, such as height, weight, age, and the history. Nurses may also assist in other portions of the examination when specially trained and authorized to do so.

### Emergency medical planning

The industrial physician, nurse, and safety professional should confer with management to plan for emergency handling of large numbers of seriously injured employees in the event of disas-

**571**

ter, such as explosion, fire, or other catastrophe. These plans should be coordinated with community plans for such events. See "Planning for Emergencies," Chapter 16.

Procedures should include the following:

1. Selection, training, and supervision of auxiliary nursing and other personnel

2. Transportation and caring for the injured (Fig. 19–11)

3. Transfer of seriously injured to hospitals

4. Coordination of these plans with the safety department, guards, police, road patrols, fire departments, and other interested community groups.

## Medical records

Employers are required under OSHA to maintain accurate records and make periodic reports of work-related deaths, injuries, and illnesses. See Chapter 6, "Accident Records and Incidence Rates."

A final standard, effective August 1980, permits both the worker and the Occupational Safety and Health Administration access to employer-maintained medical and toxic exposure records.

The standard, which also specifies conditions under which access is allowed, applies to all employers in general industry, maritime, and construction whose employees are exposed to toxic substances or harmful physical agents.

According to the regulation, exposure records include records of the employee's past or present exposure to toxic substances or harmful physical agents, exposure records of other employees with past or present job duties or working conditions related to those of the employee, records containing exposure information concerning the employee's working conditions, and material safety data sheets.

Medical records contain an employee's medical history, examination and test results, medical opinions and diagnoses, descriptions or treatments and prescriptions, and employee medical complaints. Exposure records must be maintained for 30 years and medical records for the duration of employment plus 30 years under the new standard.

Industrial medical records also provide data for use in job placement, in establishing health standards, in health maintenance, in treatment and rehabilitation, in workers' compensation

cases, in epidemiologic studies, and in helping management with program evaluation and improvement. These data are collected in the history interview, from the preplacement examination and any subsequent examinations, and from all visits the worker makes to the dispensary or first aid room—they establish a medical profile of each worker.

The key to accurate diagnosis and treatment often lies in the adequacy and completeness of this medical profile; therefore, its maintenance is a professional responsibility. Further, to make a complete history, medical records should include absences caused by illness or off-the-job injury. Thus record keeping, nonoccupational as well as occupational, often uncovers chronic or recurrent conditions where treatment (referral to family doctors) and preventive measures pay dividends, assist in absenteeism control, and reduce accident rates.

Maintenance of health records, however, should not be so laborious a task that the occupational health nurse (or first aid attendant) becomes a file clerk. It is important that the recording forms and filing systems be simple so that they are usable by and interpretable by a physician, nurse, or first aid attendant.

Descriptions and illustrations of medical record forms are shown in Parts 1, 2, and 3 of AMA's *Guide to Development of an Industrial Medical Records System* (see References). The forms can be modified by the medical director to suit the specific industry. Basically, the information should be important and useful, easily and accurately obtained, and the yield should justify the cost.

Although the employer should know the individual's limitations from a placement standpoint, only persons who have a need to know should have access to the records. These records are confidential.

If a company does not have a resident medical director or nurse, its medical records are usually filed in the personnel department.

Reports to the insurance company and to the state authorities, as well as compensation payments, should, of course, be attended to promptly.

## Neck or wrist tags for medic alert

A universal symbol for emergency medical identification has been developed by the American Medical Association (Fig. 19–12). The object

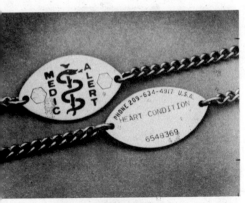

G. 19–12.—Persons with a physical condition for which ergency care may be needed should wear an identifica- n tag that provides a general indication of the problem d a phone number that can be reached for more details in se the victim is unable to supply them.

urtesy Medic Alert Foundation, Turlock, Calif.

the symbol is to identify its wearer immediately a person with a physical condition requiring ecial attention. If the wearer is unconscious or herwise unable to communicate, the symbol ill indicate that there are vital medical facts to found on a health information card in the arer's purse, wallet, or elsewhere. A telephone mber is given on the identification tag for taining more detailed information. These tails should be known by anyone before tempting to help an individual struck down by accident or sudden illness. (See Medic Alert undation and Emergency Medical Identifica- n in References.)

Another type of identification device is a card medallion that contains a microfilm record of e person's problem. (See Lens-Card System and edical History Inc. in References.)

## Special Problems

### ealth problems of women

There is no reliable evidence to support the ew that women are more susceptible than men occupational health hazards, except during regnancy.

Some companies used to dismiss women on arning of their pregnancy. As a result, many omen concealed their condition until it became vious, frequently until the last half of the

pregnancy. This policy can work to the disadvantage of both employee and company inasmuch as the early months of the pregnancy present the greatest danger. It is desirable that women who work during this time be under medical department supervision. The woman should consult her own doctor who should, in turn, report her condition to the plant or company physician so that he may determine the advisability of her continuing to work.

Chemical substances, such as carbon monoxide, chloroform, phosphorus, and mercury, may produce harmful effects on the fetus and lead to abortion. Ionizing radiation and biological agents are also of potential harm.

Pregnancy limits the ability of women to do physical work, since a pregnant woman tires more readily, has poorer balance, and is unable to respond normally to the physiological demands of strenuous physical work.

### Placement of women

State or provincial and federal laws and regulations governing employment of women in industry should be studied carefully before female employees are placed, and these should be rechecked before women are transferred to other types of work or are placed on different shifts.

The examining physician, at the time of employment, should furnish enough information to help place the applicant most advantageously from the standpoint of her health and safety. Periodic examinations and medical histories have indicated that properly trained women are capable of performing safely most types of work.

Methods for the prevention of industrial accidents among women are the same as those for men. However, when women are placed on machine jobs, it is important that adjustments be made at all points of operation because adjustments that do not consider that people are of different sizes can result in accidents. For example, machine guards may have to be set so that smaller hands cannot enter the openings. Height of benches, distance away from parts, and foot or hand controls should be adjusted to conform to those with generally shorter stature and reach. For some jobs, low platforms may be provided. Smaller hand tools may also be advisable. Some jobs may need to be broken down into simpler operations or mechanical aids may need to be provided.

More details are provided in Chapter 10,

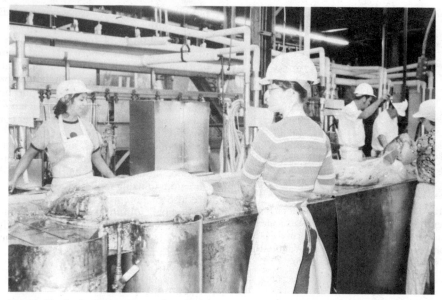

FIG. 19–13.—In the U.S., women make up about 44 percent of the work force. Although women can apply and be considered for performing any job, there are some extremely important physiological elements of concern for the safety and health status for women of child-bearing age.

*Courtesy Monford of Colorado, Greely, Colo.*

"Human Factors Engineering," and in the Council's book, *Fundamentals of Industrial Hygiene* (see References).

## Alcohol and drug control

Alcoholism and drug abuse problems are important, and it is essential that the physician as well as the employer have a good understanding of the potential for helping many of these persons in the work setting. Alcoholism and drug abuse continue to be among the nation's leading illnesses.

The combination of alcohol and drugs can produce a variety of effects that may severely impair a worker. Concentrations of alcohol and drugs remain in the blood stream much longer than most users realize, and the effects of this combination may arise unexpectedly.

Dependence on alcohol or other drugs is a major contributor to deterioration of family life, impaired job performance, morale and disciplinary problems, increased insurance rates, occupational accidents, increased absenteeism, and the rising crime rate. These illnesses know no boundaries. There is no "generation gap" among abusers—all races are susceptible, and socioeconomic status provides no barrier.

It is estimated that one out of every ten U.S. workers may have a drinking problem, resulting in an estimated $125 billion-a-year drain on the economy; but fewer than 10 percent of those who have drinking problems actually receive any treatment.

Managers and supervisors should be alert employees whose work and performance are deteriorating because of an alcohol problem. These employees should be referred as speedily possible for medical care.

Every time an applicant or employee visits physician or nurse, there should be some health education and/or counseling given. Medical departments in industry provide an ideal opportunity for these services, which constitute an asset for the employees and for the employer as well. Employers are paying an increasing part of the costs for health care for employees and their dependents. It is economically important for the employer that his employees have an entry into the health care system when needed and, further, that the proper care is obtained.

# References

American Association of Occupational Health Nurses, Inc., New York, N.Y.
> *Guide for the Development of Functions and Responsibilities in Occupational Health Nursing,* Copyright 1973; Revised, 1975, 1977.
> *Guide for the Preparation of Manual of Policies and Procedures,* Copyright 1969, 1977.
> *Standards for Evaluating an Occupational Health Nursing Service,* Copyright 1965; Revised, 1975, 1977.

American College of Surgeons, Committee on Trauma. *Emergency Care of the Sick and Injured.* Philadelphia, Pa., W.B. Saunders Company.

American Conference of Governmental Industrial Hygienists. *Guide to Health Records for Health Services in Small Industries.* Cincinnati, Ohio, ACGIH.

American Medical Association, Dept. of Occupational Medicine, 535 N. Dearborn St., Chicago, Ill. 60610
> *Guide to Developing an Industrial Disaster Medical Service.*
> *Guide to the Development of an Industrial Medical Records System.*
> *Guide to Small Plant Occupational Health Programs.*
> *Guiding Principles of Medical Examinations in Industry.*
> *The Legal Scope of Industrial Nursing Practice.*
> *Occupational Health Services for Women Employees.*
> *Scope, Objectives, and Functions of Occupational Health Programs.*

Bond, M.B. "Occupational Medical Services for Small Employee Units," *Rocky Mt. Med. J.* 68:31-36.

Brown, M.L. "The Occupational Health Nurse: A New Perspective." *Occupational Medicine—Principles and Practical Applications.* Chicago, Ill., Year Book Medical Publishers, Inc. 1975.

——.*Occupational Health Nursing.* New York, N.Y., Springer Publishing Company, Inc., 1956.

Burkeen, O.F. "The Nurse and Industrial Hygiene." *Occupational Health Nursing,* April 1976, pp. 7-10.

*Emergency Care and Transportation of the Sick and Injured,* Committee on Injuries, American Academy of Orthopedic Surgeons. Menasha, Wis., George Banta Co., Inc., 1971.

Emergency Medical Identification, American Medical Association, 535 N. Dearborn St., Chicago, Ill. 60610.

*Emergency Removal of Patients and First Aid Firefighting in Hospitals,* 3rd ed. Chicago, Ill., National Safety Council, 1974.

*A Guide for Establishing an Occupational Health Nursing Service.* New York, N.Y., American Association of Occupational Health Nurses, Inc., 1977.

Lens-Card Systems, Inc., 2817 Regal Road, Plano, Texas 75075.

Medic Alert Foundation, Turlock, Calif. 95380.

Medical History Inc., 521 Fifth Ave., New York, N.Y. 10017.

Murphy, A.J. "The Identity of the Nurse in an Industrial Hearing Conservation Program." *Occupational Health Nursing,* May 1969, pp. 32-36.

Olishifski, Julian B., ed. *Fundamentals of Industrial Hygiene,* 2nd ed. Chicago, Ill., National Safety Council, 1979.

————."Guidelines for Alcohol and Drug Abuse Programs," NSNews Reprint No. 111.17-93. Chicago, Ill., National Safety Council.

Onyett, H.P. "The Nurse's Role In Industry." *Safety Newsletter.* Chicago, Ill., National Safety Council, March 1974.

Popiel, E.S. "Principles and Concepts of Occupational Health Nursing." *Occupational Health Nursing,* September 1973. pp. 23-25.

# The
# Handicapped
# Worker

# Chapter
# 20

Today, almost every worker with some type of physical or mental impairment can qualify for some job. Industry and government surveys made during the past two decades prove that it is good business to hire the handicapped. They excel in promptness; they can produce as well as the nonhandicapped; their turnover rate is lower.

In addition, the law requires "affirmative action" for the hiring, upgrading, promotion, award of tenure, demotion, transfer, layoff, termination, right of return from layoff, and rehiring of qualified handicapped individuals. The law also requires that an employer provide "reasonable accommodation" for the handicapped when necessary.

If the employer denies a handicapped individual a specific job, the burden of proof is upon management to show that the person is unqualified for one of the following reasons:

● The job would put the handicapped individual in an unsafe situation, or

● Other employees would be placed in an unsafe situation if the handicapped person were put in the job, or

● The job requirements cannot be met by an individual with certain physical or mental limitations,

● And (for all above) accommodation cannot reasonably be accomplished.

"Affirmative action programs," including those for hiring the handicapped, are usually the responsibility of personnel other than the safety professional. The safety professional, however, should be a key resource person to such personnel and must play a critical role in job placement of the handicapped. Safety evaluations for the handicapped worker must include access to and exit from the work place as well as safety at the job.

This chapter has been included in this latest edition of the Manual to assist in the safe and productive placement of handicapped individuals in the work force. The professional and legal responsibilities are spelled out, and "how to do it" information is given.

## History and the Law

In the 1940's, the hiring of the handicapped in industry was given special attention by a number of large companies that realized that hiring the handicapped was just good business practice.

Although some companies employed handicapped workers prior to the 1940's, three events occurred in that decade that stimulated these programs and caused other companies to initiate hire-the-handicapped programs.

● The first event was World War II. Many handicapped individuals were hired to help fill the jobs vacated by employees who left for military service.

● The second contributing event was the restoration of World War II's wounded. For example, International Harvester Company undertook an affirmative action program, in the early 1940's, to help each Harvester handicapped veteran to become an employable person. Some other companies established similar programs. (See Fig 20–1.)

● The third event was a study published in the late 1940's by the U. S. Department of Labor. This study debunked the myths that handicapped workers were less productive, suffered more accidents, and lost more time from work than nonhandicapped workers. The Department of Labor found that handicapped workers were as productive as nonhandicapped workers, had lower frequency and severity rates due to lost-time injuries and were absent from work only one more day per year than their fellow workers. In studying over 11,000 handicapped workers for almost two years, the study's authors did not find a single disabling injury to a handicapped worker or to a fellow worker that was caused by the handicap.

Du Pont conducted a study in 1958 and updated it in the early 1970's. The later Du Pont study of more than 1000 of its handicapped workers revealed that 96 percent of them rated average or better on safety performance; 91 percent rated average or better on job performance; 93 percent rated average or better on turnover; and 79 percent rated average or better on attendance. After a decade or more of direct experience in hiring the handicapped, the personnel files of many companies held indisputable proof of their programs' worth.

## Occupational Safety and Health Act of 1970 (OSHAct)

The Occupational Safety and Health Act of 1970 has no special standards pertaining to handicapped employees nor does OSHA maintain any separate statistics on these workers. In fact, the

(Section 503) and recipients of federal assistance programs (Section 504). Therefore, all employers who do work for the federal government, and/or receive funds from the government, are subject to this law.

• Section 503 of the Act requires employers to take "affirmative action" to recruit, hire, and advance qualified handicapped individuals. The law applies only to employers who have federal government contracts or subcontracts of $2500 or more. Those holding contracts or subcontracts of $50,000 or more, with at least 50 employees, must prepare and maintain (review and update annually), at each establishment, an affirmative action program. The program, which sets forth the employer's policies, practices, and procedures regarding handicapped workers, must be available for inspection by job applicants and employees. This Section is enforced by the Office of Federal Contract Compliance Programs, which has issued extensive implementing regulations.

• Section 504 of the Act forbids acts of discrimination against qualified handicapped persons in employment. This pertains to employers who are recipients of federal funds. This Section is enforced by each department or agency that provides federal funds.

• In the Rehabilitation Act Amendments of 1974, Congress amended, and thus broadened, the definition of "handicapped individual" for purposes of Section 504. With this amended definition, it became clear that Section 504 was intended to forbid discrimination against all handicapped individuals, regardless of their need for or ability to benefit from vocational rehabilitation services. Thus, Section 504 reflects a national commitment to end discrimination on the basis of handicap and establishes a mandate to bring handicapped persons into the mainstream of American life.

• U. S. Department of Labor regulations (41 CFR 60-741), as last amended, became effective February 12, 1980, and were established to assure compliance with Section 503 of the Act. Department of Education regulations (34 CFR 104), effective May 4, 1980, were implemented to enforce the requirements of Section 504. Other federal departments and agencies also have issued regulations similar to those of the Department of Education, indicated above. For example, the U.S. Department of Labor has issued regulations (29 CFR 32), effective November 6, 1980, which

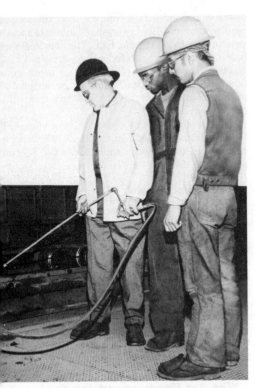

FIG. 20–1.—After losing his leg in combat in 1944, Felix "Phil" Sitkowski returned to U.S. Steel South Works, in South Chicago, as a clerk. Later, he applied for and was promoted to field lubricating analyst, his prosthesis allowing him to use ladders for making inspections. He is shown at left, with two of the eight millwright helpers that he supervises; Sitkowski's crew is responsible for the smooth operation of equipment at two ore-unloading docks and a sintering plant.

*Courtesy U.S. Steel South Works.*

requirements of some OSHA standards may be detrimental to certain types of handicapped employees and must be considered when placing such employees in jobs where these standards apply. (Refer to Job Placement section of this chapter.)

## Rehabilitation Act of 1973

The federal Vocational Rehabilitation Act of 1973 (Public Law 93-112), commonly referred to as the Rehabilitation Act, is the first major civil rights law protecting the rights of the handicapped. This law applies to federal contractors

**579**

# 20—The Handicapped Worker

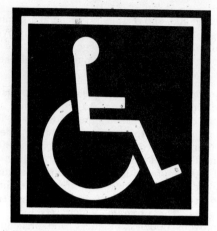

Fig. 20–2.—International symbol designates access for the handicapped. Symbol is in white on a blue background.

*Courtesy American National Standards Institute.*

implement Section 504 of the Act for the department. All of these regulations require contractors and/or recipients of funds to make "reasonable accommodations" when necessary in employing the handicapped.

All records pertaining to compliance with the Act, including employment records plus complaints and actions taken as a result of them, must be maintained by the employer for at least one year. Failure to maintain complete and accurate records or failure to update annually the affirmative action program may result in the imposition of "appropriate sanctions" against the employer. The employer must permit access, during normal business hours, to its place(s) of business, its books, records, and accounts pertinent to compliance with the Act, and all rules and regulations promulgated (pertaining to the Act) for the purposes of complaint investigations, and investigations of performance concerning affirmative action.

## Vietnam Era Veterans' Readjustment Assistance Act of 1974

This Act (Public Law 93-508), effective December 3, 1974, is the amended version of the 1972 Act (Public Law 92-540). Section 402 of the Act provides a legal incentive for America's

business and industry to employ and advance in employment disabled veterans of all wars and al veterans of the Vietnam Era. The law require that all employers with federal government contracts or subcontracts of $10,000 or more mus take "affirmative action" (similar to Section 50: of the Rehabilitation Act of 1973) to accomplisl this endeavor.

U.S. Department of Labor regulations (41 CFF 60-250) last amended February 12, 1980, wer established to assure compliance with Section 402 of the Act.

## State and local laws

All 50 states and many local governments have now adopted building codes or legislation requiring barrier-free design or removal of barriers to the handicapped person's mobility. Many of these codes require any "public" building or facility to be barrier free if the public is invited to use it for "any normal purpose." This is defined as shopping, employment, recreation, lodging, or services.

If accessible facilities are to be identified, then the international symbol of accessibility shall be used. (See Fig. 20–2.)

## Who Are Handicapped Job-Seekers?

The law defines three basic types of handicapped persons seeking employment—the handicapped individual, the disabled veteran, and the qualified handicapped individual.

## 'Handicapped individual'

The Rehabilitation Act of 1973, as amended, defines a "handicapped individual" as any person who:

1. Has a physical or mental impairment that *substantially limits* one or more of the person's major "life activities," such as:

   Ambulation
   Communication
   Education
   Employment
   Housing
   Self-care
   Socialization
   Transportation
   Vocational training

2. Has a record of such impairment, or

3. Is regarded as having such an impairment.

The term "substantially limits," as used above, has to do with the degree to which the disability affects employability. A handicapped worker having a hard time getting a job or getting ahead on the job because of a disability would be considered "substantially limited."

The handicapped definition adopted by the federal government is broad. All of the traditional conditions are covered: loss of hearing and sight, the physically disabled in wheelchairs or using crutches or braces, etc. Also included are other conditions such as mental retardation, stroke effects, epilepsy, muscular dystrophy, arthritic conditions, asthma and diabetes. In addition, regulations enacted in April 1977 also include, for the first time, those over 65, alcoholics and drug addicts.

This broad definition extends the traditional idea that the handicapped are only those in wheelchairs or using crutches. Actually, this group represents only 2 to 5 percent of the general population. The 1973 federal definition covers an estimated 32 to 45 percent of the general population.

Some examples:

- A blind person or a paraplegic person would have "an impairment substantially limiting one or more of his major life's activities." So would a mentally retarded person.

- A person who had been in a mental hospital and had been rehabilitated would have "a record of such impairment," even though he now is mentally sound. So would a person with a history of heart condition or cancer.

- A person who people "think" is handicapped—for example a person who might seem mentally retarded but isn't—would be "regarded as having such an impairment."

### 'Disabled veteran'

A disabled vetaran is a "handicapped individual" who:

1. Is entitled to disability compensation under laws administered by the Veterans Administration for disability rated at 30 percent or more; or,

2. Was discharged or released from active duty due to a disability incurred or aggravated in the line of duty.

Veterans with nonservice-connected disabilities are not considered "disabled veterans" but may still qualify as a "handicapped individual" under Sections 503 and 504 of the Rehabilitation Act of 1973.

The Vietnam War had the highest proportion of disabled service personnel of any war in history. A disabled veteran of the Vietnam Era is a person who was discharged or released from active duty for a service-connected disability if any part of such duty was performed between August 5, 1964, and May 7, 1975.

### 'Qualified handicapped individual'

Is every handicapped person covered by the Rehabilitation Act of 1973? No. There is another crucial word: "qualified." A person must be capable of performing a particular job—with reasonable accommodation to his handicap.

Is every disabled veteran (of any war) and Vietnam Era disabled veteran covered by either the Rehabilitation Act of 1973 or the Vietnam Era Veterans' Readjustment Assistance Act of 1974? No. The veteran also must be "qualified" for the job. That is, the veteran must be capable of performing a particular job, with reasonable accommodation to his disability.

### Reasonable Accommodation

An employer shall make "reasonable accommodation" to the known physical or mental limitations of an otherwise qualified handicapped applicant or employee unless the employer can demonstrate that the accommodation would impose an "undue hardship" on him. The employer may not deny any employment opportunity to a qualified handicapped employee or applicant if the basis for the denial is only because there is a need to make a reasonable accommodation.

"Undue hardship" is determined by considering the following factors:

1. The overall size of the employer's operation with respect to number of employees, number and type of facilities, and size of budget;

2. The type of the employer's operation, including the composition and structure of his workforce; and

3. The nature and cost of the accommodation needed.

Reasonable accommodation may include:

1. Making facilities used by employees readily accessible to and usable by handicapped persons, and

2. Job restructuring, part-time or modified work schedules, acquisition or modification of equipment or devices, the provision of readers or interpreters, and other similar actions.

### Examples

Reasonable accommodation is demonstrated in these three examples:

• A construction equipment salesman, whose job description required him to climb onto the equipment and demonstrate its operation during sales presentations, was given a desk job after he suffered the amputation of his arm during an off-the-job motor vehicle accident. Although his prosthetic device enabled him to operate the equipment controls, the employer had considerable concern about the man's ability to climb on and off the equipment using the prosthetic device. This resulted in the job change. Upon enactment of the Rehabilitation Act of 1973, and its amendments, his employer reinstated the man as a salesman making a reasonable accommodation for his handicap. The accommodation consisted of providing him with a portable climbing device that enabled him to safely get on and off the equipment.

• A fork lift (powered industrial truck) mechanic became blind in one eye due to a nonindustrial health problem. Since his job description required the mechanic to test drive each fork lift truck after completing maintainance or repair on it and since the employer's standard safety policy required that all drivers of powered industrial trucks must have binocular vision (use of both eyes), the employer at first was going to switch the man to another job, which unfortunately would have lowered his earnings. Upon reviewing the requirements of the Rehabilitation Act of 1973, however, the employer provided the mechanic with a reasonable accommodation. The accommodation consisted of altering this mechanic's specific job description eliminating the requirement for him to test drive the vehicles and broadening the job description of the other mechanics to include the

test driving of any vehicle repaired by the handicapped mechanic.

• A handicapped individual working for an electrical applicance firm was provided with a reasonable accommodation to assemble small parts. The accommodation consisted of minor readjustments of the work bench so as to accommodate the handicapped individual in a wheel chair.

The following example was considered to be unreasonable accommodation.

• An example of an unreasonable requirement would be the need to completely redesign or alter the circuitry and/or operating levers of a machine in order to accommodate a physically handicapped individual.

### Accomodation is not new

Accommodations may include modifications of equipment or facilities and/or process or job description alterations.

Accommodation in employment is not a novel concept. The first application of a machinery guard or a ventilating fan were innovations which in essence were job accommodations. Also, the first hod carrier who lacquered and reinforced his bowler as a hard hat made a job accommodation. Job placement of employees based on medical examinations, either as a new-hire or upon return to work after recovery from illness or injury, is, again, an application of accommodation. This experience is common to every employer.

The safety professional is routinely involved in evaluating accommodations for employees to reduce or eliminate hazards. This professional, therefore, is preeminently qualified for assignments in evaluating reasonable accommodations of the work place, its procedures and access, for the physical or mental limitations of a handicapped worker.

Job safety analysis and safe work procedures are a means of eliminating or reducing work hazards to minimize worker risk. They are directly transferable to the process of accommodation. Training in safe work procedures will be important in accommodating the job for the handicapped.

### Role of the Safety Professional

Since "affirmative action programs" required by the government usually come under the responsibility of the EEO (Equal Employment Opportunity) manager or coordinator (or labor affairs personnel) in most companies, the placement of qualified handicapped individuals is normally under their overall jurisdiction.

The safety professional, nonetheless, should be a key resource person available to those responsible for implementing government and company requirements for job placement of qualified handicapped individuals. This professional should be consulted before such placement is made and used to evaluate any proposed reasonable accommodation. The following is an example of some of the typical responsibilities of the safety professional in relation to handicapped employees.

## General Responsibilities

• Maintain close liaison with EEO manager/coordinator, plus the medical and employment departments to effectively place individuals.

• Increase emphasis in the area of employment, promotions, transfers, and selection of handicapped employees for training programs may require a job hazard analysis of an existing occupation.

• Make safety evaluations pertaining to recommendations for the modification of machine tools, established processes and procedures, existing facilities and the working environment when provisions are to be made to reasonably accommodate a handicapped employee.

• Closely cooperate, as needed, with the plant or building engineer or mechanical engineer plus the planning, production and maintenance departments when evaluating an "accommodation" for a handicapped employee.

## Specific responsibilities

• Review the company's affirmative action program for general background knowledge.

• Establish specific communication channels, pertaining to handicapped employees, with:

a. *EEO Manager/Coordinator.* Let this person know you are part of the team and are ready *when necessary* to evaluate a job.

b. *Medical department.* Let them know you will be requesting their help when evaluating a job.

c. *Employment department.* Let them know you are ready when necessary to assist them in safety evaluation of jobs, and remind them of basic safety considerations such as:

1. Don't place a coronary worker in a job with great stress.

2. Don't place a person with a back problem in a job requiring heavy lifting.

3. There is *no* requirement to place a handicapped employee in a job that would be unsafe for that person or cause a hazard to others.

NOTE: Individual judgments are based on a physician's evaluation with input from the safety professional.

d. *Plant and mechanical engineers.* Since "reasonable accommodation" does not necessarily mean reinstalling machines, but rather could mean minor relocating of a machine's controls so that a handicapped employee could properly operate them, advise the engineers you will evaluate any safety aspects of such an accommodation. Also advise them that you are available for safety evaluations when they design "reasonable accommodations" into future facilities such as:

1. Ramps for wheelchairs

2. Wider door passages for wheelchairs

3. Grab bars in accessible washroom facilities

4. Braille numbers on elevators (Fig. 20–3)

5. Easy access to company facilities such as lunchrooms

6. Elimination of curbed cross walks

e. *Production and maintenance departments.*

1. Since "reasonable accommodations" also refer to job restructuring and modifications, tell the production and maintenance departments you will help by evaluating the safety aspects of such changes.

2. When they strike out any job specification which would arbitrarily, without business justification, screen out handicapped individuals, you will be available if a safety evaluation is needed.

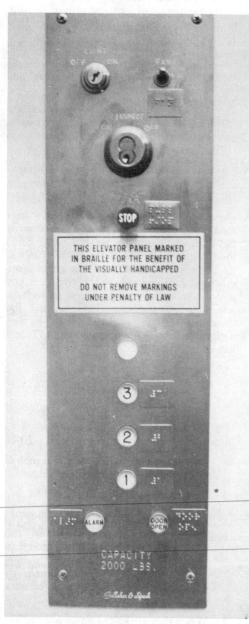

FIG. 20–3.—"Reasonable Accommodation" for the handicapped includes marking elevator buttons in braille.

*Courtesy Governors State University, Park Forest South, Ill.*

- Refer all safety complaints (or hazards noted), involving a handicapped employee, to the EEO manager/coordinator.

- Conduct a safety evaluation of a handicapped employee (in relation to the specific job or prospective job), and perform an entire job hazard analysis if needed.

- Conduct a safety evalation whenever a "reasonable accommodation" is being *planned* for a handicapped employee.

- Coordinate with both the EEO manager/coordinator and the employment department to make sure that no handicapped employee is scheduled for a training program that will provide qualification for a new job position until a safety evaluation of the employee in relation to the position has been completed, and produced favorable results.

- Evaluate if reported harassment of a handicapped employee is safety related. For example, name calling would not normally involve the safety of the employee but pranks by other employees could jeopardize the safety of the handicapped employee.

- Refer all questions about interpretation of the government requirements to personnel responsible for implementing the affirmative action program (usually the EEO manager/coordinator) or to the appropriate attorney.

The evaluation form (Fig. 20–4) may be helpful to the safety professional when performing a safety evaluation for a handicapped employee, especially if a "reasonable accommodation" is involved. Supporting material (memos, blueprints, photos, etc.) can be attached to the form to provide detailed information on why certain decisions were made.

It is recommended that such evaluations be kept for at least one year after the employee leaves the company. Records should be destroyed only after approval from the EEO manager/coordinator or other personnel responsible for the government-required "affirmative action programs."

## Insurance Considerations

There has been a general misconception of the effect of employment of handicapped workers upon insurance rates. It has been thought by many

## HANDICAPPED EMPLOYEE SAFETY EVALUATION

Applicant: ☐

Employee: ☐ _____
                    (Last Name          First Name          M.I.)          (Clock No.)

Handicap: _____

Evaluation of          ☐ Current job          ☐ Prospective job

Job Title: _____

Job Description (primary duties): _____

_____

_____

Hazards to This Employee:
(State "none" if none)          _____

_____

Hazards to Other Employees:
(State "none" if none)          _____

_____

Proposed "reasonable accommodation" (if any): _____

_____

CONCLUSION   (Based on all known factors at this time):

☐ Job is safe for this employee:

    ☐ as is          ☐ with proposed "reasonable accommodation"

☐ Job is unsafe for this employee:

    ☐ as is          ☐ with proposed "reasonable accommodation"

☐ No hazard to other employees:

    ☐ as is          ☐ only with proposed "reasonable accommodation"

☐ Hazard to other employees:

    ☐ as is          ☐ with proposed "reasonable accommodation"

| Location: | Safety Supervisor (Print Name) |
|-----------|-------------------------------|
| Date: | Safety Supervisor (Signature) |

NOTE:  Complete two copies of this form and give one copy to local EEO manager/coordinator. Second copy is for the safety file.

FIG. 20–4.

585

that companies issuing worker's compensation insurance coverage increase the premiums where the physically handicapped are employed. This is not true. Rates are based on experience by the class of industry and modified in most cases by the individual plant experience. There is no indication that losses are increased when the physically handicapped are properly placed.

## Job Placement

When properly placed and trained, and competing on an equal basis, the handicapped usually equal or excel nonhandicapped workers in production and safety; and their attendance and labor turnover records are usually superior to those of the able-bodied.

### General concepts

To place a handicapped worker properly, the following requirements should be observed, where applicable, after receiving a physician's evaluation of the individual.

- Worker should meet physical qualifications of the job. For example, a person on crutches should not be placed in a job requiring heavy lifting, carrying heavy weights, or extensive walking.

- Worker should not be a personal hazard. For example, a person subject to dizzy spells should not work on a ladder or scaffold or around moving machinery, where injury or death could occur.

- Worker should not be a hazard to others. For example, an epileptic should not drive a bus or operate an overhead crane, because the individual may have an attack while working, lose control, and cause injury to himself and to others.

- Task should not aggravate the degree of disability. For example, a person with heart trouble should not be placed on a job that requires considerable stair climbing, running, heavy lifting, or other strenuous tasks. A person with skin disease should not be exposed to skin irritants.

- To obtain valuable input, a conference with the handicapped individual should be held before job placement is made.

What proper placement does, then, is match the worker to the job on the basis of his ability to meet the qualifications of the job. (See Fig. 20–5.) When this is done, the impairment disappears as a job factor. Moreover, it should be realized that

most disabled persons have more ability than disability, because few jobs actually require all of a handicapped worker's ability.

It is important to remember that each impairment may impose limitations on the activities in which the individual may engage and the working conditions and accident and health hazards to which this person may be exposed.

### OSHA obstacles

The safety professional should be aware that there are certain OSHA safety standards which, although promulgated for the protection of the average employee, may be detrimental to handicapped employees. Some examples are:

- Standards referring to storage of flammable and combustible liquids, § 1910.106 (d) (6) (iii), include a requirement for a curb to capture spilled liquids. This would be a barrier for some handicapped individuals.

- The "Means of Egress" standards, § 1910.37, are based on the ability of an individual to move 100 feet (30 m) in 30 seconds. Perhaps some handicapped employees cannot move that fast.

- Respirators are required by the standards, for example, § 1910.134, for certain jobs. Some handicapped individuals may have a physical impairment which can be affected by restricted breathing. If there is some indication of this problem, such employees must not wear a respirator until it is determined by a physician that it can be worn safely. This may preclude the individual from performing a specific job where a respirator is necessary.

- The Permissible Exposure Levels (PELs) listed in the OSHA "Air Contaminants" standards, § 1910.1000, are based on the susceptibility, of persons with normal breathing capacities, to such contaminants. Some handicapped individuals do not have normal breathing capacities.

The safety professional must take into consideration whether or not a handicapped individual would be adversely affected by safety standards which apply to the job being evaluated.

## Analysis of the Job

Each job must be evaluated to make sure that the handicapped individual being considered for that job can do it safely. The following areas

## PHYSICAL DEMANDS FORM

Job Title ...Linotype Operator... Occupational Code. 4-44.110

Dictionary Title. LINOTYPE OPERATOR.

Firm Name & Address

Industry ............... Industrial Code.

Branch ............... Department

Company Officer ............... Analyst ...Wetzel... Date

### PHYSICAL ACTIVITIES

| | |
|---|---|
| x 1 Walking | 61 Throwing |
| 2 Jumping | x17 Pushing |
| 3 Running | x18 Pulling |
| 4 Balancing | x19 Handling |
| 5 Climbing | x20 Fingering |
| 6 Crawling | 21 Feeling |
| 7 Standing | 22 Talking |
| 8 Turning | 23 Hearing |
| 9 Stooping | x24 Seeing |
| 10 Crouching | 25 Color Vision |
| 11 Kneeling | 26 Depth Perception |
| 12 Sitting | 27 Working Speed |
| x13 Reaching | 28 |
| x14 Lifting | 29 |
| x15 Carrying | 30 |

### WORKING CONDITIONS

| | |
|---|---|
| x51 Inside | 66 Mechanical Hazards |
| 52 Outside | 67 Moving Objects |
| 53 Hot | 68 Cramped Quarters |
| 54 Cold | 69 High Places |
| 55 Sudden Temp. Changes | 70 Exposure to Burns |
| 56 Humid | 71 Electrical Hazards |
| 57 Dry | 72 Explosives |
| 58 Wet | 73 Radiant Energy |
| 59 Dusty | 74 Toxic Conditions |
| 60 Dirty | 75 Working With Others |
| 61 Odors | x76 Working Around Others |
| x62 Noisy | 77 Working Alone |
| 63 Adequate Lighting | 78 |
| 64 Adequate Ventilation | 79 |
| 65 Vibration | 80 |

### DETAILS OF PHYSICAL ACTIVITIES:

Sits at linotype machine most of the day, reads copy, and fingers keyboard to set lines of type. Periodically walks short distances, reaches for, lifts and carries matrices, galleys of type, and pigs of type metal. Reaches for, handles, pushes, and pulls handwheels and levers and fingers gages, stops, and micrometer in setting up machine.

---

## PHYSICAL CAPACITIES FORM

Leg Amputation 5" below knee

Artificial leg—good fitting

Name ............... Sex M  Age 31  Height 5'9½" Weight 155

### PHYSICAL ACTIVITIES

| | |
|---|---|
| √ 1 Walking | 16 Throwing |
| 2 Jumping | √17 Pushing |
| 3 Running | √18 Pulling |
| √ 4 Balancing | 19 Handling |
| √ 5 Climbing | 20 Fingering |
| 6 Crawling | 21 Feeling |
| √ 7 Standing | 22 Talking |
| 8 Turning | 23 Hearing |
| 9 Stooping | 24 Seeing |
| 10 Crouching | 25 Color Vision |
| √11 Kneeling | 26 Depth Perception |
| 12 Sitting | 27 Working Speed |
| 13 Reaching | 28 |
| √14 Lifting | 29 |
| 15 Carrying | 30 |

### WORKING CONDITIONS

| | |
|---|---|
| 51 Inside | √66 Mechanical Hazards |
| 52 Outside | √67 Moving Objects |
| 53 Hot | 0.68 Cramped Quarters |
| 54 Cold | 69 High Places |
| 55 Sudden Temp. Changes | 70 Exposure to Burns |
| √56 Humid | 71 Electrical Hazards |
| 57 Dry | 72 Explosives |
| √58 Wet | 73 Radiant Energy |
| 59 Dusty | 74 Toxic Conditions |
| 60 Dirty | 75 Working With Others |
| 61 Odors | 76 Working Around Others |
| 62 Noisy | 77 Working Alone |
| 63 Adequate Lighting | 78 |
| 64 Adequate Ventilation | 79 |
| 65 Vibration | 80 |

Blank Space = Full Capacity    √ = Partial Capacity:  0 = No Capacity

May work ...... hours per day ...... days per week.   (If TB., cardiac or other disability requiring limited working hours.)

May lift or carry up to ...**.. pounds.

Details of limitations for specific physical activities Should not be required to walk, balance, climb, stand, kneel for prolonged periods of time.

**Should not lift heavy weights continuously.

Should not carry long distances.

FIG. 20-5.—Sample of an employment service form used in matching workers to jobs.

should be taken into account when making the analysis; they have been adapted from the Seventh Edition of this Manual.

## Physical classification

The labor market simply cannot supply all "physically perfect" workers. In fact, the percentage of workers in perfect health is relatively low—the working population now includes more persons with disabilities than ever before. Advances in medical science now prolong the lives of many who would have died of war injuries, or of illnesses, such as smallpox, tuberculosis, diabetes, and heart disease. Accidents in industry, in traffic, and in the home continue to increase the number of handicapped persons. Also the definition of "handicapped" has been broadened, as discussed earlier in this chapter.

Because of proximity to the problem and ability to make regular plant inspections, the company's physician should have a better understanding of the job requirements than other physicians. Therefore, it is the physician's responsibility to provide management with clear evaluations of the employability, limited employability, or nonemployability of applicants for jobs.

Many systems of classification are now in use:

• Generally, however, these systems use broad statements, such as "physically fit for any work"; "defect that limits applicant to certain jobs" (the defect may or may not be correctable, but may require medical supervision); and "defect that requires medical attention and is presently handicapping." This last statement disqualifies a person for any type of employment.

• Another method provides a greater range in expression of limiting factors, allowing more alternatives for the individual case.

• Yet another method, which approaches the ultimate in functional evaluation of the individual, appraises capacities on a form with the identical terminology used in evaluating the physical or functional factors and working conditions of jobs. (See Fig. 20–6.) This effective method of presenting information from a physical examination clearly indicates the specific work capability and limitations of the individual. Thus the medical report is more meaningful to the placement manager because the examining physician, then, is responsible for determining the occupational significance of physical disorders. This now makes proper analysis of each job important.

## Job appraisal

Employers must be aware of the physical requirements of jobs and the accident and health hazards involved. Each job-appraisal factor has a direct relationship that makes it either definitely unsuitable or potentially undesirable for one or more types of disability. The factors to be considered in job appraisal are physical requirements, working conditions, health hazards, and accident hazards.

**Physical requirements** include agility, strength, exertion, vision, hearing, talking, sitting, standing, walking, running, climbing, crawling, kneeling, squatting, stooping, twisting, lifting, and handling. They should be evaluated according to quality of ability and duration of activity. For example, a job involving a considerable amount of stair climbing is unsuitable for workers with heart disease, respiratory diseases, obesity, or lower limb orthopedic disorders. However, some of these people may tolerate a small amount of stair climbing.

**Working conditions** include indoors, outdoors, excessive heat or cold, excessive humidity or dryness, wetness, sudden temperature changes, ventilation, lighting, noise, whether the work is performed alone, near others, with others, or as shift work or piece work. Some of these conditions could have a harmful influence upon certain disabilities. For example, work in excessive heat is generally unsuitable for persons who have had malaria, or for those with high blood pressure, heart disease, skin disease, the aged, and the obese.

**Health hazards** include air pressure extremes; radiant energy (ultraviolet, infrared, radium emanations, and X rays); silica, asbestos, dusts, and skin irritants; respiratory irritants; systemic poisons; and asphyxiants. These hazards have serious effects and can aggravate a preexisting bodily defect. For example, a job might involve exposure to respiratory irritants of insignificant quantities to a normal person; yet this condition might aggravate the disability of a person who has chronic bronchitis. (These were discussed in the previous section, Job Placement.)

## JOB ANALYSIS
## FOR PHYSICAL FITNESS REQUIREMENTS

TITLE OF POSITION | GRADE

NAME AND LOCATION OF ESTABLISHMENT | AGENCY

Does establishment have medical supervision ☐ Yes ☐ No
Is there an industrial safety branch ☐ Yes ☐ No

*Refer to the manual for job analyses before using this form. Check all functional and working condition factors as well as acceptable disabilities whenever appropriate.*

## I. FUNCTIONAL FACTORS
**L - Little   M - Moderate   G - Great   O - None**

| Hands - Fingers | L | M | G | O | Arms | L | M | G | O | Legs - Feet | L | M | G | O | Body - Trunk | L | M | G | O |
|---|---|---|---|---|---|---|---|---|---|---|---|---|---|---|---|---|---|---|---|
| 1. Reaching | | | | | 8. Reaching | | | | | 14. Walking or running | | | | | 22. Sitting | | | | |
| 2. Pushing or pulling | | | | | 9. Lifting | | | | | 15. Standing | | | | | 23. Bending | | | | |
| 3. Handling | | | | | 10. Pushing or pulling | | | | | 16. Sitting | | | | | 24. Reaching | | | | |
| 4. Fingering | | | | | 11. Carrying | | | | | 17. Carrying | | | | | 25. Lifting | | | | |
| 5. Climbing | | | | | 12. Climbing | | | | | 18. Climbing | | | | | 26. Carrying | | | | |
| 6. Throwing | | | | | 13. Throwing | | | | | 19. Jumping | | | | | 27. Jumping | | | | |
| 7. Touching | | | | | **Eyes** | | | | | 20. Turning | | | | | 28. Turning | | | | |
| | | | | | 30. Near vision | | | | | 21. Lifting | | | | | | | | | |
| **Voice** | | | | | 31. Far vision | | | | | **Ears** | | | | | | | | | |
| 29. Talking | | | | | 32. Color vision | | | | | 33. Hearing | | | | | | | | | |

## II. WORKING CONDITION FACTORS

| | | | | | | | | | | | | | | | | | | | |
|---|---|---|---|---|---|---|---|---|---|---|---|---|---|---|---|---|---|---|---|
| 34. Inside | | | | | 41. High humidity | | | | | 48. Odors | | | | | 55. Toxic conditions | | | | |
| 35. Outside | | | | | 42. Low humidity | | | | | 49. Body injuries | | | | | 56. Infections | | | | |
| 36. High elevations | | | | | 43. Wetness | | | | | 50. Burns | | | | | 57. Dust | | | | |
| 37. Cramped body positions | | | | | 44. Air pressure | | | | | 51. Electrical hazards | | | | | 58. Silica dust | | | | |
| 38. High temperature | | | | | 45. Noise | | | | | 52. Explosives | | | | | 59. Moving objects | | | | |
| 39. Low temperature | | | | | 46. Vibration | | | | | 53. Slippery surfaces | | | | | 60. Working with others | | | | |
| 40. Sudden temperature changes | | | | | 47. Oily | | | | | 54. Radiant energy | | | | | | | | | |

## III. ACCEPTABLE DISABILITIES          *Check appropriate square if acceptable*
**A - Amputation   D - Disability   Y - Yes   N - No**

| Hands - Fingers | A | D | Arms | A | D | Legs - Feet | A | D | Body - Trunk | | D |
|---|---|---|---|---|---|---|---|---|---|---|---|
| 1 or 2 on primary hand | | | 1 Arm | | | 1 Leg (high) | | | 1 Hip | | |
| 1 or 2 on secondary hand | | | 2 Arms | | | 2 Legs (high) | | | 2 Hips | | |
| More than 2 on primary hand | | | None | | ☐ | 1 Leg (low) | | | 1 Shoulder | | |
| More than 2 on secondary hand | | | | | | 2 Legs (low) | | | 2 Shoulders | | |
| 1 Hand | | | | | | 1 Foot | | | Back | | |
| 2 Hands | ☐ | | | | | 2 Feet | | | None | ☐ | |
| None | ☐ | | | | | None | ☐ | | | | |

| Eyes | Y | N | Ears | Y | N | | | | Tuberculosis | Y | N |
|---|---|---|---|---|---|---|---|---|---|---|---|
| Blind | | | Deaf | | | Cardio - Vascular | Y | N | Minimal (healed, stable or arrested) | | |
| Industrially blind | | | Hard of hearing, 1 ear | | | Moderate tension | | | Moderate (healed, stable or arrested) | | |
| Blind one eye | | | Hard of hearing, 2 ears | | | High tension | | | Far advanced (healed, stable or arrested) | | |
| Color blind | | | Hearing aid acceptable | | | Organic heart disease compensated | | | Collapse therapy | | |
| Color blind for shades | | | | | | | | | | | |

FIG. 20-6.—Sample of form used when analyzing jobs for fitness requirements.

589

# 20—The Handicapped Worker

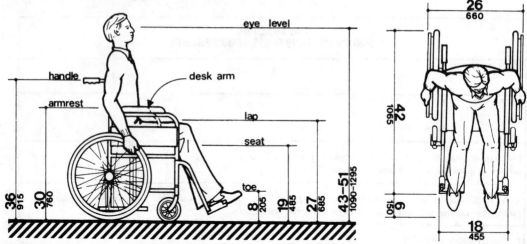

FIG. 20–7a.—Dimensions of adult-sized wheelchairs. (Foot-rests may extend further for very large people.) Dimensions in this figure and Figs. 20–7c and –8b are in inches and millimeters.

*Courtesy American National Standards Institute.*

**Accident hazards** include danger of falls from elevations, work on moving surfaces, slipping and tripping hazards, exposure to vehicles or moving objects, falling objects from overhead, foot injuries, eye injuries, cuts and abrasions, burns, mechanical and electrical hazards, and fire and explosion hazards. These hazards could have an unfavorable relationship to the disability of the handicapped person. For example, a job that may involve foot injury hazards is unsuitable for the diabetic because of his susceptibility to gangrene of the feet, slow healing of wounds, and union of fractures.

## Access to Facilities

Safety considerations for hiring the handicapped begin at the very first step in the employment process, and at the very beginning of the work day for the handicapped employee. Is there reasonable access to the reception area, applicant-processing area, or work situation for the handicapped? Curbs and stairs could present barriers to paraplegics or quadriplegics in wheelchairs, increasing their chances of accidents due to falls.

### Access to and from work station

Can handicapped applicants safely proceed to where they must go to complete an application? If employed, can such handicapped individuals safely proceed to their work stations? Access and safety are interdependent factors which need to be reconciled when employing handicapped people. Traditionally, the accessibility of premises has been the principal factor restricting work for the disabled.

The crux of the safety problem is means of escape in an emergency; considerations of this problem frequently restrict, or deny, the freedom of handicapped people to use premises as they would wish. However, in many establishments where persons with mobility handicaps are employed, routines to develop a means of escape have been worked out satisfactorily by the employer. Thus, effective safety management of the handicapped in many firms is already well established and provides a freedom of movement which is entirely compatible with principles of general safety. These measures include supervised use of the elevator for means of escape (which is discussed later), designated staff to assist in an emergency, strategic ramping of entrances/exits, and alarm systems suitable for the blind and deaf.

In practice, for most firms that employ disabled people (wheelchair users in particular), the need for adjusting safety procedures from the already established pattern is not evident. There is an important exception that concerns the development and use of the elevator as a means of escape.

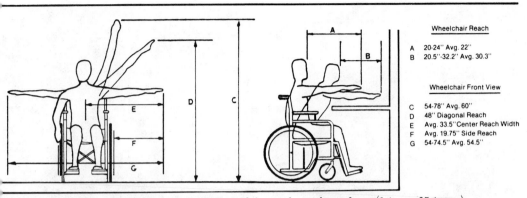

**Wheelchair Reach**

A  20-24" Avg. 22"
B  20.5"-32.2" Avg. 30.3"

**Wheelchair Front View**

C  54-78" Avg. 60"
D  48" Diagonal Reach
E  Avg. 33.5" Center Reach Width
F  Avg. 19.75" Side Reach
G  54-74.5" Avg. 54.5"

FIG. 20-7b.—Maximum design reach from wheelhair—*left*: to sides; *right*: to front. (1 in. = 25.4 mm.)

*Courtesy State Board for Barrier-Free Design, Columbia, S.C. Used with permission.*

# HUMAN FUNCTIONING DIMENSIONS

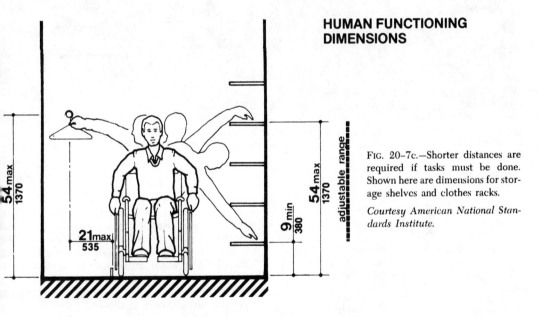

FIG. 20-7c.—Shorter distances are required if tasks must be done. Shown here are dimensions for storage shelves and clothes racks.

*Courtesy American National Standards Institute.*

Historically, and for compelling reasons, the elevator is not part of a fire escape route. There are some fairly simple refinements that can be made, such as protected circuitry, installation of a fireman's switch, and supervised use, which together may allow elevators to be used for the purposes of evacuating people who are not able to use the stairs.

In the absence of these possibilities, many disabled would be denied access to their places of employment. It is suggested that employers dis-cuss this with fire prevention specialists and check state or provincial and local codes and regulations.

## General access

Do not overlook washroom and restroom facilities, width of doors, height of plumbing fixtures, etc. These and related questions require careful analysis by the safety professional.

With a minimum of expenditures, improvements and special considerations made for the

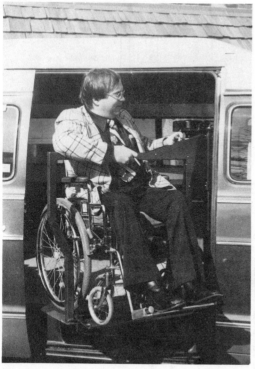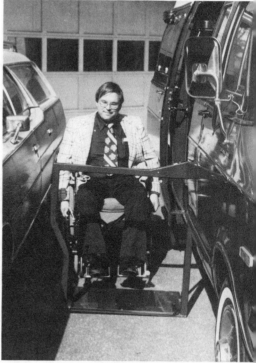

Fig. 20–8a.—Access aisle adjacent to normal-width parking space is required for wheelchair clearance. Shown here is a chair lift that swings along side of van. For return, a locking outside control box opens sliding doors, lets the user control the lift. .

*Courtesy ABC Enterprises, Inc.*

handicapped also can benefit all employees, safety professionals point out.

- For instance, ramps created for wheelchairs are safer than steps—but only if the slope is correct, and if such ramps are kept free of mud, snow, and ice.

- Good housekeeping, with unobstructed and distinctively marked aisles, not only creates a safer workplace, but also improves traffic patterns and eliminates hazards.

### Wheelchair Checklist

The space requirements of the average wheelchair are as follows: most wheelchairs are 36 in. high, 26 in. wide, and 42 in. long. (See Fig. 20–7a.) They require at least $60 \times 60$ in. to make a 180 or 360 degree turn. However, $60 \times 78$ in. is preferred to make a smoother U-turn.

People who use wheelchairs are usually able to stretch their arms 48 in. on the diagonal and extend their arms 64½ in. straight out. The average reach directly upward is 60 in. (See Fig 20–7a.) The usual maximum downward reach from the chair is 10 in. (See Fig. 20–7b.) Shorter distances may be needed, however, to accomplish certain tasks. (See Fig. 20–7c.)

### Access to buildings

Eight-feet-wide parking spaces, adjacent to a five-feet-wide access aisle, should be reserved for automobiles driven by handicapped personnel and visitors. (See Fig. 20–8a.) Two accessible parking spaces, however, may share a common access aisle. (See Fig. 20–8b.) Wheelchairs require room to be removed and replaced in an auto and also for riding between aisles.

At least one accessible route and entrance to

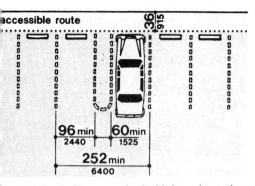

**36**
**915**

| 96 min | 60 min |
|--------|--------|
| 2440 | 1525 |

**252 min**
**6400**

FIG. 20–8b.—Parking spaces for disabled people can share a common passenger loading (access) aisle. Aisle shall be part of the accessible route to the building or facility entrance. Overhangs from parked vehicles must not reduce the clear width of the accessible route, which must be the shortest possible to the entrance.

*Courtesy American National Standards Institute.*

the building must be provided. The entrance width should be 32 in. (80 cm) and if a ramp leads to the entrance, it should be at least 36 in. (90 cm) wide. The ramp should be a maximum of 30 ft (9 m) long with an open, level area of at least 5 ft (1.5 m) at the bottom. Physically handicapped employees (and visitors) using wheelchairs, crutches, or canes can then move in and out of the building completely on their own.

Revolving doors are taboo for anyone in a wheelchair as well as for most people using crutches, wearing a leg cast, or even carrying bulky packages. These people need entry doors that are preferably of the time-delay type. When a knob is necessary, it should be 36 in. from the floor. It is better, however, to have a verticle grab handle on the door.

### Interior access

Both entry and interior doors should be 32 in. wide. Interior doors should open by means of a single effort and have thresholds as nearly level with the floor as possible.

To make a 180 or 360 degree turn, persons in wheelchairs need an open area of 60 in. (1.5 m) in a typical building corridor.

Restrooms should have at least one stall wide enough for wheelchair entry, that has grab bars and other fixtures no higher than 36 in. above floor level. (See Fig. 20–9.) The grab bars should

preferably be at 33 in. (83 cm).

Controls, switches, fire alarms, and other devices to be used by the handicapped individual must be within reach of the wheelchair user.

### Office accommodations

Desk tops should be 28 in. (70 cm) from the floor to accommodate wheelchairs. Metal desks usually have adjustable feet that can be raised to the maximum. If more room should be needed, the desk can be raised further with additional blocks.

Chairs can be of a regular height, but they should also be sturdy and have arms to enable handicapped people to lift themselves up more easily. Although some individuals need a chair that will not easily move so they can stand without the chair sliding out from under them, casters placed on the bottom of chairs may be desirable for other handicapped workers. Casters make for easier mobility and, if necessary, allow the chair occupant to pull himself from one piece of furniture to another, thereby avoiding constant movement to and from the chair.

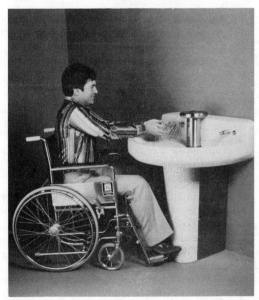

FIG. 20–9.—Semicircular washstand no higher than 3 ft (0.9 m) permits those confined to wheelchairs to have ready access.

*Courtesy Bradley Corp.*

Business machines should be placed, if possible, in such a way so as not to become a barrier and obstruct traffic.

The following accommodations may sometimes apply, depending upon the individual handicapped worker and the job requirements:

• Files should be placed so drawers can be reached from both the front or side. This eliminates awkward reaches from those who must use crutches, a cane, or a wheelchair.

• If books, reports, or other bulky objects must be carried from place to place, a shopping-type cart on wheels should be kept handy so the materials can be loaded on to it and pushed.

• Venetian blind, window shade, and drapery cords should be long enough to be reached easily.

## Sources of Help

The overall goal of all employers should be to hire qualified handicapped individuals and place them in safe available occupations. One of the basic goals of the safety professional is to assist the employer in this worthwhile endeavor.

The following list includes government and private agencies that can help achieve this goal

Alabama Institute for the Deaf and Blind, Talladega, Ala. 35160.

George Washington University, Job Development Laboratory, Rehabilitation Research and Training Center, 2300 I St., NW., Washington D.C. 20037.

Mainstream, Inc., 1200 15th St., NW., Washington, D.C. 20005.

The National Institute for Rehabilitation Engineering, Pompton Lakes, N.J. 07442.

Paralyzed Veterans of America, 7 Mill St., Wilton, N.H. 03086.

President's Committee on Employment of the Handicapped, Washington, D.C. 20210.

The Rehabilitation Institute of Chicago, 345 E Superior St., Chicago, Ill. 60611.

## References

American National Standards Institute, 1430 Broadway, New York, N.Y. 10018. *Specifications for Making Buildings and Facilities Accessible to and Usable by Physically Handicapped People*, A117.1.

Brooks, Wayne T. "Supervising Handicapped Workers for Safety." *Transactions of the National Safety Congress—Industrial Subject Sessions*, 1978.

Moscato, Richard F. "Hire the Handicapped—Role of the Safety Supervisor." Chicago, Ill., International Harvester Co.

President's Committee on Employment of the Handicapped, Washington, D.C. 20210.
"Affirmative Action To Employ Handicapped People—A Pocket Guide."
"Affirmative Action To Employ Disabled Veterans and Veterans of the Vietnam Era—A Pocket Guide."

Superintendent of Documents, U.S. Government Printing Office, Washington, D.C. 20402.
Occupational Safety and Health Act of 1970 (P.L. 91-596).
*Occupational Safety and Health Act Regulations*, Title 29, CFR, Chapter XVII, Part 1910.
Rehabilitation Act of 1973 (P.L. 93-112).
Rehabilitation Act Amendments of 1974 (P.L. 93-516).
Vietnam Era Veterans' Readjustment Assistance Act of 1974 (P.L. 93-508), Section 402.

U.S. Department of Human Resources, Washington, D.C. 20202. "Nondiscrimination on the Basis of Handicap in Programs and Activities Receiving or Benefiting from Federal Financial Assistance" (45 CFR 84).

U.S. Department of Labor, Employment Standards Administration, Office of Federal Contract Compliance Programs, Washington, D.C. 20212. "Affirmative Action Obligations of Contractors and Subcontractors for Handicapped Workers" (41 CFR 60-741).

Woodward, Robert E. "Industry Unlocks Its Doors to the Handicapped." *Plant Facilities*, Vol. II, No. 2 (February 1979).

————.*Comprehensive Barrier-Free Design Standard Manual.* Columbia, S.C., State Board for Barrier-Free Design, P.O. Box 11954. 1979.

# Nonemployee Accident Prevention

# Chapter
# 21

# 21—Nonemployee Accident Prevention

Evidence of good management is found not only in the conduct of the routine operation of a successful business, but in other areas which have a direct bearing on the public relations between the management, personnel, and customers.

The nonemployee accident exposure affects not only nonemployees, but also the employees and the quality of the product or service they sell. Operations stop (or at least slow down) whenever there is a bad accident, no matter who had it, or who is involved. With the increasing legislation concerning consumer product safety (see the following chapter) and greater cost of claims, more attention must be given to this area of business loss.

Today, there are more businesses and people involved in serving and selling to the public than there are those engaged in making the products that are sold. Just look at the types of businesses, specialty shops, department stores, shopping center complexes, restaurants, fast-food service operations, hotels and motels, automotive service and dealerships, hardware building supply stores, amusement parks, banks and office buildings, to name a few, that all serve the public. The main "franchise" businesses, basically, provide services and market products to their patrons. Patrons, guests, or visitors are the source of nonemployee injuries.

These service and selling operations must provide a constant surveillance of patron activities. They cannot control the public's personal activity or habits (such as smoking). The business owner or manager does not have the degree of discipline or control over patrons that he has over the actions of his employees.

The inebriated guest or patron of a hotel, motel, or store can be a threat when he improperly disposes of smoking materials or his instability contributes to slips, falls, or other problems. Children can also be a problem in the business environment.

Loss control plans must recognize the possibility of nonemployee accidents. These unplanned events can be minor or catastrophic; businesses that invite customers on their premises must provide extensive plans to protect nonemployees. A firm can be liable for damage or for injuries from the minute someone enters the property (including the parking lot). A firm can be liable for the actions of its employees that result in damage or personal injury when that employee is sent off the company property on business.

## The Legal Side of Nonoccupational Injuries

Customer or product claim cases often wind up in a courtroom. The legal terminology and aspects of the law that deal with accident claims, in situations in which one is likely to become involved, include the following definitions and explanations. They are not intended to be all-inclusive, but to provide a quick review of some of the principal considerations.

TORT. A private or civil wrong or injury—a violation of a right not arising out of a contract. It may be either (a) a direct invasion of some legal right of the individual, (b) the infraction of some public duty by which special damage accrues to the individual, or (c) the violation of some private obligation by which like damage accrues to the individual. Torts deal with negligence, accidents, trespass, assault, battery, seduction, deceit, conspiracy, malicious persecution, and many others.

NEGLIGENCE. Failure to exercise that degree of care which an ordinarily careful and prudent person ("reasonable man") would exercise under similar circumstances. To establish a proper claim of negligence, however, there must be (a) a legal duty to use care, (b) a breach of that duty, and (c) injury or damage.

DEGREE OF CARE. The degree of attention, caution, concern, diligence, discretion, prudence or watchfulness depends upon the circumstances. For example, a high degree of care is demanded from people who invite others onto their premises, by formal, verbal, or implied invitation. All sales and service enterprises must exercise a high degree of care for the safety of their patrons. As long as a business is open, it assumes a responsibility to its clientele.

INVITEE. One whose presence on the premise is upon the invitation of another, such as a patron at a sports stadium or a person who visits an exhibition hall even though no admission is charged.

LICENSEES. Licensees are neither "invitees" nor "trespassers." They have not been specifically invited to enter upon the property but they have a reasonable excuse (by permission or by operation of the law) for being there. These could be vendors, delivery personnel, people visiting executives and purchasing agents for business purposes, and the like. Policemen and firefighters who enter property in the course of their duties have sometimes been held by the courts to be invitees (patrons) and sometimes licensees (nonpatrons).

CONTRIBUTORY NEGLIGENCE. Not every injury gives rise to a claim for damages. If a defendant can prove that the plaintiff (claimant) contributed to the injury by not exercising ordinary care, the resultant damages may be considerably reduced or negated. If it can be proven that the plaintiff was even only slightly negligent in a manner that contributed to the harm or damage, he might not be allowed to collect damages.

This points up the importance of a proper accident investigation procedure; this can strengthen a company's ability to reduce the overall cost of doing business and help prevent future incidents of contributory negligence.

ASSUMPTION OF RISK. The claimant cannot collect damages when the law presumes he was aware of peril or danger, yet was willing to proceed with his original intention and undertake his action. "That to which a person assents is not regarded by law as an injury." For example, a skier who falls while descending a slope is said to assume the normal risks that can happen when participating in this sport, unless there was special negligence in the design or maintenance of the slope and its environment, since there is no assumption of risk when the owner or operator is negligent. However, an injury involving a chair lift or tow rope could be of a mechanical nature and could be costly.

HOLD-HARMLESS. A clause in a contract agreeing for one party to assume all liabilities or losses or expenses involved, thus reimbursing the other party held liable. For example, a department store may have a hold-harmless agreement with a manufacturer who supplies it with a particular type of merchandise. Should a claim for injury arise out of the use of that product by a consumer, the manufacturer would reimburse the store, should it be held liable, and will pay for legal and other expenses incurred by the store in defending itself. Even though the consumer purchased the item from the department store, a hold-harmless agreement may relieve the store of the financial effect of direct liability.

ATTRACTIVE NUISANCE. Liability growing out of a dangerous condition, generally to children. It excuses trespassing and penalizes for failure to keep children away or for failure to protect or eliminate a hazard that may reasonably be expected to attract them to premises.

BURDEN OF PROOF. The injured party must prove his injury or damage and its causal relation to the event or item that resulted in the accident. The defense, on the other hand, is not liable if it is without fault. Proof must be established by facts, *not* opinion, suspicion, rumor, hearsay, gossip, or emotional reaction. Proof is the conclusion drawn from the evidence.

Honest and sincere witnesses convey different impressions from the same evidence attested to by dishonest witnesses. Thus we see how important promptness is when assembling and preserving the evidence. Signed statements taken shortly after the accident or an all-important photograph can often make the big difference. In liability claims, the burden of proof rests upon the plaintiff (claimant).

This chapter cannot begin to cover all possible nonemployee involvements. Instead it will describe prominent ways that nonemployees can get hurt. Accident prevention techniques will necessarily be broad and varied. It will be up to each safety professional, regardless of title or business, to examine his own operations in light of these guidelines.

## Problem Areas of Accidents

When starting a nonemployee accident prevention program, go back over the records of past nonemployee injuries to identify accident trouble spots, so that the hazards at these locations can be mitigated. Next, pick general accident trouble spots, such as those due to lighting, interior design, and traffic flow (to name a few), and do the same thing. Change facilities and/or operations so that both employees and nonemployees are given a safe business environment.

The following paragraphs review some of the major problem areas and discuss typical accidents occurring in modern business facilities.

### Glazing

Modern design of office buildings, stores, and manufacturing operations often specifies the extensive use of glass in doors, show windows, panels, and enclosures. Often such areas provide a confusing pattern, especially to the first-time

**597**

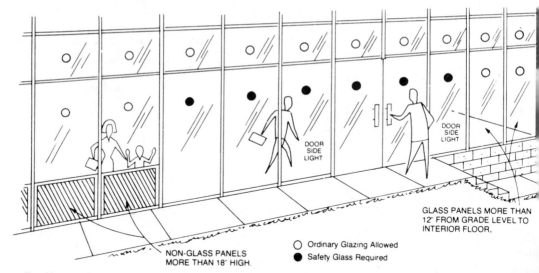

FIG. 21.1.—In this example of a commercial installation, doors and panels marked with a solid black circle must be made ⟨ safety glass; ordinary glazing is allowed for the other panels. Doors and panels with black dots should also be marke⟨

*Courtesy PPG Industries, Inc.*

visitor or patron.

Unmarked glass panels and doors can cause severe injuries and cuts. Be sure to follow recommended practices and standards for glazing and strength of glass. Safety glass and marked identification of doors and panels (see Fig. 21–1) is required by law in some states. The U.S. Consumer Product Safety Commission has regulations affecting glazing (Title 16—*Code of Federal Regulations*, Chapter II; see References).

Some plastics have similar advantages as glass for glazing, but without the hazard of damage or injury. In fact, some plastics have higher impact resistance; but, conversely, plastic glazing tends to scratch or be more easily abraded than glass. Plastic, however, is harder to break than glass if escape through a window is necessary.

A few precautions will allow the continued enjoyment of the beauty of glass and lessen the chances for injury:

1. Make glass doors more visible to adults and children by placing decals or pressure-sensitive tape at their respective eye levels. Sandblasted or etched designs will serve the same purpose.

2. Decals or pressure tapes will also prevent glass

panels from appearing to be doorways. A⟨ attractive and tall plant, placed in the center ⟨ the panel, will also identify the true purpose ⟨ the panel.

3. Installing safety bars reduces the size of th⟨ open glass areas and lessens the chance of gla⟨ breakage. The bars should be at the doo⟨ handle level on sliding doors and should be o⟨ both sides of a swinging door.

4. Keep doorways and areas that are close to gla⟨ panels clear of tripping hazards, such as scatt⟨ rugs and toys. Indeed, this is a good rule for a⟨ areas of occupancy.

5. Enforce no horseplay, no running rules esp⟨ cially where there is a glass hazard.

**Parking lots**

Most every shopping or business center has ⟨ parking lot for patron use; usually these are of th⟨ self-service type. Bicycles, mopeds, an⟨ motorcycles also require parking facilities. We⟨ designed, self-service parking lots are attractiv⟨ to customers and employees, and they nearl⟨ eliminate parking damage to cars. (See Fig. 21-2⟨

Problems in parking lots depend to som⟨

xtent on how the lots are used. Self-service parking lots for employees in industrial plants, for instance, usually differ somewhat from public lots found at shopping centers, theaters, stadiums, stores, schools, restaurants, or motels. Public lots usually have a more steady flow of traffic, but they may have children present or be obstructed by shopping carts. More important, they handle a greater variety of drivers who are less experienced with the layout of the lot.

Some public parking lots, however, at places such as theaters, sports arenas, and schools, frequently present the combined hazards of both extreme traffic fluctuation and great variations in skill and alertness among drivers who use the lot.

Easy-to-use layout, adequate signs, and conspicuous markings help produce a safe, attractive parking lot. They are the first step in reducing hazards which may be imposed by disadvantageous location or property configuration.

Enclosing the parking lot with a curb or fence so that cars cannot enter or leave traffic unexpectedly at any point will reduce accidents in the area more than any other single safety measure. Parking lots should have separate, well-marked entrances and exits, placed so that they favor right-hand turns. Single lane entrances should be at least 15 ft (4.5 m) wide; exits should be at least 10 ft (3 m) wide. Where entrance and exit must be combined, the double-lane drive should have at least 26 ft (8 m) of usable width. If the double-lane combination is necessary, it should have median curbs or strips to positively control the flow of traffic.

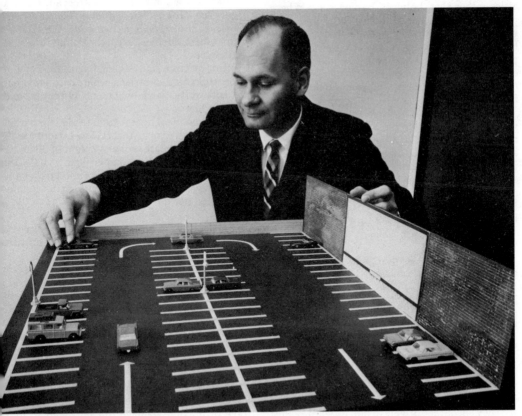

Fig. 21-2.—Well-marked parking stalls, entrances, and exits encourage safe parking and traffic flow. *Courtesy 3M Company.*

In general, entrances and exits should be:

- At least 50 ft (15 m) from intersections;

- Away from heavily traveled highways or streets;

- Well marked and well illuninated;

- As few in number as possible.

Pedestrian traffic must be considered in parking lots. Stairways and ramps for them should be constructed in accordance with ANSI Standard A64.1. They should be well marked, well illuminated, and provided with handrails. The needs of handicapped must also be considered in the design of the lot and in the walkway to the building. See Chapter 20, "The Handicapped Worker."

Parking aisles should be perpendicular to the buildings, so that pedestrians will walk down the aisles rather than between parked cars. Where possible, marked lanes, islands, or raised sidewalks should be provided between rows, particularly where there are heavy concentrations of pedestrian traffic. These walks should be wide enough so that car bumpers overhanging them do not restrict pedestrians who are walking to or from their cars.

Angle parking has both advantages and disadvantages. The smaller the angle, the fewer the number of cars that can be parked in the same area. Aisle widths can be narrower, but traffic is usually restricted to one way. On the other hand, angle parking is easier for customers and it does not require a lot of room for sharp turns.

The area allowed per car in parking lots varies from 200 to more than 300 sq ft (18.5-28m²), if aisles are included.

**Parking stalls.** The design of parking stalls depends on (a) the size and shape of the lot; (b) the traffic pattern in the lot; and (c) the type of driver and pedestrian in the lot. (See Fig. 20–8 on pp. 592-593 for stall dimensions for the handicapped.)

- Bumpers on stalls have these advantages:

1. They prevent drivers from driving forward through facing stalls and proceeding in the wrong direction in one-way aisles.

2. They encourage drivers to pull forward against the bumper, thereby preventing rear overhang which might reduce aisle width.

3. They break up huge expanses of open lo which tempt drivers to cut across aisles an endanger pedestrians and other drivers.

4. They block cars from accidentally rollin down inclines or running through walkwa areas.

- Stall bumpers also have some disadvantages

1. They may require maintenance.

2. They may interfere with drainage or snov removal.

3. They may cause pedestrians to trip and fall

4. They may restrict some desirable flexibility o traffic flow.

**Signs and lighting.** Traffic signs in parking lot should conform to recommended standards, an they should be similar to other street and highwa signs (see *Manual on Uniform Traffic Contro Devices for Streets and Highways*, U.S. Depart ment of Commerce, Bureau of Public Roads; se References.)

Stop or Yield signs should be installed at main crosswalks for pedestrians, where exits cross pub lic sidewalks, and where exits enter main thoroughfares.

The amount of light recommended for parking at night usually ranges from 0.5 to 1.0 foot candle (decalux) per square foot at a height of 36 in. (0.9 m). Lights are usually mounted 30 to 35 ft (9-10m high on poles that have bases protected against impact by cars. A well-lit parking lot reduce accidents and discourages crime.

**Supervision.** The third factor necessary i preventing parking lot accidents is effectiv supervision.

Traffic control in public lots is not always easy The shopping center caters to the public, and i must weigh the possibility of claims against the affect of control enforcement on public relations Good traffic flow controls can be built into the lo however, and these may be the most effectiv controls. In many areas, police have no jurisdic tion on privately owned parking lots.

**Design.** Built-in bumps on lot surfaces hav been used to deter speeding, but their disadvan tage of possible damage to cars seems to make their use questionable. Another device is to keep straight lanes short and to provide sharp curve which reduce speed.

Parking lot operators should definitely try to control unauthorized use of lots. Weekend parking, scooter races, games, and other unauthorized activity should be forbidden, and local police or company security police should check parking areas after hours. If lots cannot be fenced in or if entrances cannot be protected against unauthorized entry, prominent warning signs will help minimize the risks of unauthorized use and vandalism.

Whenever possible there should be close cooperation between local traffic authorities and those responsible for the supervision of lots. Cooperation must be developed with police and sheriff's departments responsible for traffic control and crime prevention, and also with fire departments which must have access to fire hydrants in a lot and to buildings served by the lot. Zoning boards are also interested in problems connected with parking lots.

**Shopping carts.** Ideally, shopping carts should be kept out of parking lots. Customers might bring their cars to a loading point where an attendant would put their goods in the car, or an attendant might wheel the cart to the car, unload it, and bring the cart back.

If shopping carts are permitted in the parking lot, they should be frequently collected and termporarily stored in a space allocated for them. Carts should not be left to accumulate in stalls, or worse still, in heavily trafficked aisles. Cart-collecting areas should be well marked and well illuminated. Preferably, they should be separated from traffic by barriers or bumpers in the pavement. Customers should be encouraged by signs and access lanes to leave carts in such areas.

The hazard of carts rolling into traffic lanes can be controlled by low curbs or a shallow depression which will prevent uncontrolled rolling.

People who supervise the lot should check that children do not play with the empty carts or use them as scooters and racers.

**Other vehicles.** The use of the bicycle, moped, and motor cycle as a commuting vehicle is increasing. More people would use these vehicles if the (a) routes were safer and (b) secure parking would be available. Current parking facilities are not generally adequate for these vehicles. The bicycle, moped, or motorcycle operator, like the motorist, likes to park near his destination. In parking, there are two major problems (a) convenience and (b) security.

Storage of a bicycle is fairly easy. Twelve to 15 bicycles can be stored in the space it takes to park one car. A lesser number of mopeds or motorcycles will also fit in the same area.

The problem of security is more difficult, however.

There are three basic types of bicycle parking facilities in current use.

First, the common bicycle rack, which comes in many types and shapes and requires chaining or clamping the bike to the rack. Unless the bicycle frame and both wheels are locked, the operator can lose part of his bike.

Second, a hitching post that has a chain secured to lock the bike.

Third, a key-operated locker much like baggage lockers used in stations and airports. These are totally closed to both view and weather. Weather protection is also of concern, especially for all-day parking.

Moped owners and motorcyclists face most of same convenience, security, and weather problems as a bicyclist.

### Entrances to the building

This discussion taken from *Loss Control—A Safety Guidebook for Trades and Services*, by George J. Matwes and Helen Matwes. Copyright © 1973 by Litton Educational Publishing, Inc. Reprinted with permission of Van Nostrand Reinhold Company.

Entrances to department stores and office buildings must be of number and size to meet all building codes. Revolving doors should have governors that limit their speed to 12 rpm. All worn weatherstripping should be replaced. Sidewalks and driveways should be kept in good repair in order to avoid tripping and falling hazards. Entrance lighting should be a minimum of ten footcandles.

In order to provide passage from the sidewalk to the customer's car, it is customary in shopping centers to construct a ramp. The best type of ramp is an indented ramp; one that is acually cut into the sidewalk itself with an easy slope. This type should have rails on each side to prevent someone from falling into one of the recessed sides if they are sufficiently deep enough to be a hazard. The ramp should not be painted, because paint seals

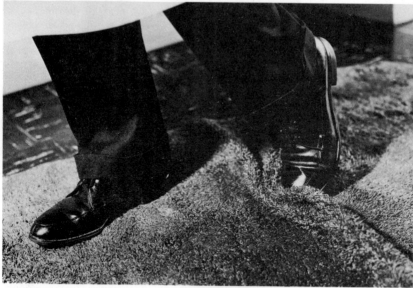

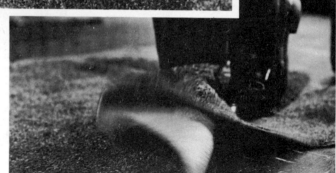

FIG. 21–3.—Cotton and other fabric mats used in entrances are useful for absorbing moisture and dust, but require constant watching to minimize tripping hazards.

*Above:* The first person's toe or heel will catch in the mat.

*Right:* The next person will either trip on the raised portion or dislodge it further, building up the hazard. The remedy is to lay the mat flat and fasten it securely.

the concrete surface to the point where it becomes excessively slippery.

Entrances to buildings are of considerable importance from a safety viewpoint. Often the entrance and exit doors are of the automatic type that are activated by anyone stepping onto a carpet. Actually each door has two carpets. One on the sidewalk and one on the floor on the inside of the door. For the "in" door, the outside carpet when stepped on activates the door inward. The carpet on the inside of the door acts as a safety mat, i.e., should anyone, even a child, step onto the safety mat, it will automatically deactivate the outside carpet thereby eliminating the possibility of the door swinging inward and striking the person on the other side. The same principle, in reverse, applies to the "out" door.

The sidewalk carpet installation in front of the entrance door is usually flanked by two handrails to avoid activation when someone is merely walking by.

Where there are glass-enclosed vestibules, decals should be applied to alert people against walking into glass panels, as discussed earlier.

## Walking surfaces

Slips and falls are the most likely source of nonemployee injuries. These injuries can occur almost everywhere at any time. There are few surfaces that can be ignored and the dangerous ones include everything from asphalt roads, concrete walks, wooden, tiled or rug-covered floors, and special surfaces on stairs and conveyances (moving sidewalks, escalators, elevators), to

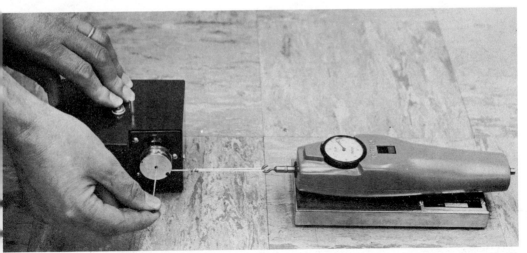

FIG. 21–4.—Slipometers, ranging from the motorized type (shown here) to a simple spring scale and heavy block pulled by hand, can be used to gage the slipperiness of floors.

*Courtesy Liberty Mutual Insurance Company.*

bridges and catwalks.

The natural properties of any surface can be changed substantially when people track in mud, snow, dirt, and moisture on their shoes, boots, and galoshes. Moisture-absorbant mats, runners, or rugs designed to reduce such hazards and floor maintenance themselves require special attention to eliminate the hazard of torn or curled-up floor coverings. (See Fig. 21–3.) Floors, stairs, and other walking surfaces should be kept nonslippery, clear, and in good repair.

Slipmeters developed by testing agencies and insurance companies measure the slipperiness of floors. One type of instrument (see Fig. 21–4) is mounted on three leather "feet." It is pulled across the floor by a motorized winch; the dial on top measures the intensity of the pull required to start moving it. This is converted into a "slip index." The slip index, or coefficient of friction (0.5-.6 is ideal), is very important, but not foolproof. Floor slipperiness, however, may increase because of moisture, oil, grease, foreign or waste materials, and incorrect cleaning or waxing.

Falls on floors occur in various ways and from various causes. A person may slip and thus lose traction, or he may trip over an open drawer, box in the aisle, or other object. The primary mechanical causes of falls on floors are: unobserved, misplaced, or poorly designed movable equip-

ment, fixtures, or displays; poor housekeeping; and defective equipment. The condition of shoes or type of footwear soles and heels are likely to be major contributing factors.

Inadequate illumination can also be a cause of falls. Light values at floor level should be uniform with no glare or shadows. Also, there should be no violent contrasts in light levels between floor areas, such as from bright sunlight outside the entrance to a dimly lit lounge or restaurant.

Some other causal factors are patron-related: age, illness, emotional disturbances, fatigue, lack of familiarity with the environment, and poor vision; these cannot be readily identified. It thus becomes doubly important to make the walking surface as safe as possible. Mirrors and other distracting decorations should not be placed in areas visible from steps or from approaches to steps or escalators.

**Types of floor surfaces.** A wide variety of floor surfaces are available. In office buildings, hotels, mercantile, and similar establishments, it is common to find masonry (terrazzo, cement, or quarry tile) floors at entrances, in lobbies, on stairways, and sometimes extensively throughout the ground floor and in upper floor corridors. Decorative materials such as terrazzo, marble, and ceramic tile are most often used for interiors

**603**

TABLE 21-A

PHYSICAL PROPERTIES OF FLOOR FINISHES

| Types of Finish | Resistance to | | | | Quality of | | |
|---|---|---|---|---|---|---|---|
| | Abrasion | Impact | Indentation | Slipperiness | Warmth | Quietness | Ease of Cleaning |
| Portland cement concrete *in situ* | VG - P | G - P | VG | G - F | P | P | F |
| Portland cement concrete precast | VG - G | G - F | VG | G - F | P | P | F |
| High-alumina cement concrete *in situ* | VG - P | G - P | VG | G - F | P | P | F |
| Magnesite | G - F | G - F | G | F | F | F | G |
| Latex-cement | G - F | G - F | F | G | F | F | G - F |
| Resin emulsion cement | G - F | G - F | F | G | F | F | G - F |
| Bitumen emulsion cement | G - F | G - F | F - P | G | F | F | F |
| Pitch mastic | G - F | G - F | F - P | G - F | F | F | G |
| Wood block (hardwood) | VG - F | VG - F | F - P | G - F | F | F | G |
| Mastic asphalt | VG - F | VG - F | VG - F | VG | G | G | G - F |
| Wood block (softwood) | F - P | F - P | F | VG | G | G | G - F |
| Metal tiles | VG | VG | VG | F | P | P | G - F |
| Clay tiles and bricks | VG - G | VG - F | VG | G - F | P | P | VG |
| Epoxy resin compositions | VG | VG | VG | VG | F | F | VG |

Code: VG—Very Good; G—Good; F—Fair; P—Poor; VP—Very Poor.

while concrete and granite are generally considered more practical for exterior use. Details are in Tables 21–A and B.

In other public areas in these buildings, the base floor, usually of concrete or wood, is generally surfaced with one or more of the popular resilient floor covering materials. Carpeting is commonly used on limited areas in the department, furniture, specialty, and similar stores and in hotels. Elsewhere, asphalt, linoleum, rubber, or plastic in either sheet or tile form, will usually be found. Obviously, safety, initial cost, durability and maintenance costs are some factors which govern the choice of floor covering.

Most flooring materials, whether of wood, masonry, or the resilient types, are reasonably slip resistant in their original untreated condition. Exceptions will be found among some of the masonry materials. A highly polished marble, terrazzo, or ceramic tile may be used to achieve an ornamental effect. These highly polished surfaces can be slippery when dry. Their slipperiness will be greatly increased by moisture, by improper surface treating preparations, and by improper cleaning materials and methods. Unless a non-slip material is added to the aggregate during construction, the only preparation which should be used on such floors is a penetrating sealer of the slip-resistant type.

**Floor coverings and mats.** Reduce the possibility of slips and falls by using good carpeting, bound edging, and flush floor-level mats and runners (see Fig. 21–5). If material such as an extruded metal runner is used to provide self cleaning removal of snow, ice, or mud at entryways, it should be flush and not present a tripping hazard. Care also in the use of rubber mats, rug runners, and the like must be taken to prevent them from becoming tripping hazards. Oftentimes the edges become rumpled (Fig 21–3), corners and ends are torn or do not lie flat and excess wear can cause tears. Mats and runners

(*Text continues on page 608.*)

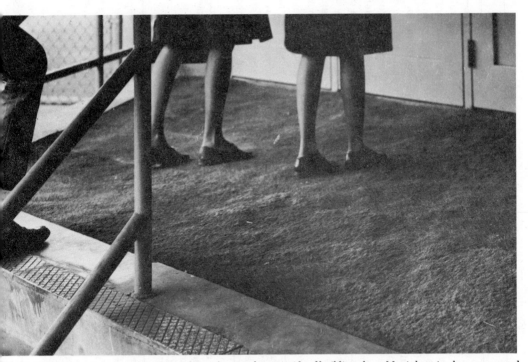

FIG. 21–5a.—Recessed coconut-fiber mat reduces slipping, keeps inside of building clean. Mat is kept in place year-round and is vacuumed about twice a week. Each year it is taken up and thoroughly cleaned.

*Courtesy Kingsport Press, Inc.*

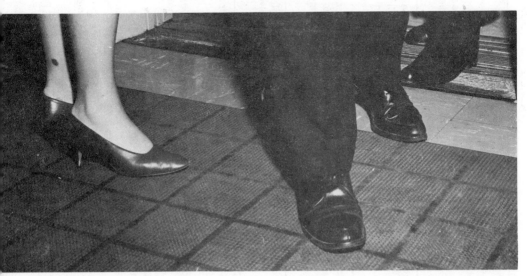

FIG. 21–5b.—A heavyweight rubber or plastic mat with a nubby finish or raised design and beveled edges tends to lie flat and in place. Rotating the mat distributes the wear and minimizes "bald" spots in high-traffic locations such as this.

## TABLE 21-B   GUIDE TO FLOOR MATERIALS AND SURFACINGS

| Floor types* | Characteristics | Use of Abrasives | Dressing Materials |
|---|---|---|---|
| Asphalt tile | Composed of blended asphaltic and/or resinous thermoplastic binders, asbestos fibers and/or other inert filler materials, and pigments. | Abrasive materials of various types may be used to reduce slipperiness of floors. Colloidal silica** can be incorporated in wax and synthetic resin floor coatings. | **Wax or wax-base products**—For most purposes, wax has several advantages. This is especially true of Carnauba wax, an ingredient generally used in so-called wax products. This wax, a Brazilian palm tree product, dries in place with a very hard and glossy finish, but with a characteristically slippery surface. Because of its many good qualities, it is widely used as a base for floor surface preparations, both in paste and emulsion forms. Other waxes, notably petroleum wax and beeswax, have their place in floor dressing formulas; they are softer and less slippery than Carnauba, but are still slippery to a degree depending on the formulation. |
| Linoleum | Cork dust, wood flour, or both, held together by binders consisting of linseed oil or resins and gum. Pigments are added for color. | | |
| Rubber | Vulcanized, natural, synthetic, or combination rubber compound cured to a sufficient density to prevent creeping under heavy foot traffic. | Slip-resistant except when wet. | |
| Vinyls | Composed of inert, nonflammable, nontoxic resins compounded with other filler and stabilizing ingredients. | Adhesive fabric with ingrained abrasives can be used. They are patterned in strips, tiles, and cleats. | **Slip-resistant sealant** will typically improve slip-resistant quality if renewed periodically. |
| Terrazzo | Consists of marble or granite chips mixed with a cement matrix. | Silicon carbide or aluminum oxide can be included in mix when floor is laid. Also an abrasive-reinforced plastic coating can be painted on. | |
| Concrete | Made of portland cement mixed with sand, gravel, and water and then poured. | | |
| Mastic | Like asphalt tile in composition but is heated on the job and troweled onto the floor to form a seamless flooring. Such floors are often used over concrete to give a new durable, resilient surface. | (Same as asphalt tile) | **Synthetic resins**—These preparations, known as "synthetics," "resins," or "polishes," are intended to supply the desirably characteristics of wax without producing the same degree of surface slipperiness. They include soaps, oils, resins, gums, and other ingredients, compounded in the various ways to produce the desired result. |

|  |  | |  |
|---|---|---|---|
| Wood | May be either soft or hard, in a variety of thicknesses and designs. | Metallic particles and artificial abrasives in varnish or paint give good non-slip qualities to various floors. | **Other materials**—Paint products (paint, enamel, shellac, varnish, plastic) are semipermanent finishes used principally on wood and concrete floors. They do no materially increase the slipperiness of the base. |
| Cork tile | Made of molded and compressed ground cork bark with natural resins of the cork to bind the mass together when heat cured under pressure. | (Same as asphalt tile) | |
| Steel | Iron containing carbon in any amount up to about 1.7 percent as an alloying constituent, and malleable when used under suitable conditions. | Surface can be touched up with an arc welding electrode so the shape of raised places on the surface resembles angle worms. Also an abrasive-reinforced plastic coating can be painted on to any desired thickness, dries hard as cement and has a sand-paper like finish. If a temporary non-skid surface is needed two uses of mats can be employed: (*a*) flexible rubber mats made from old automobile tires; (*b*) rubber or vinyl runners. | |
| Clay and Quarry tile | Kiln-dried clay products are similar to bricks and are extensively used in areas requiring wet cleaning. | Typically resistant to abrasives. | May be treated by etching. May be formulated as nonslip by adding carborundum or aluminum oxide when mixing the clay before kilning. |

*Floors and stairways should be designed to have slip-resistant sufaces insofar as possible; adhesive carborundum strips may be used on stair treads or ramps and at critical concrete areas. Etching with mild hydrochloric (muriatic) acid solution will lessen slip problems.

**Colloidal silica is an opalescent, acqueous solution containing 30 percent amorphous silicon dioxide and a small amount of alkali as a stabilizer.

should be replaced at the first sign of such unsafe condition.

Floor mats, runners and carpeting are often used in places other than building and store entrances such as around swimming pools, in shower stalls, around drinking fountains and vending machines, on boat decks, and in garages, factories, and other areas where water, oil, food, waste, and other material on the floor might make it slippery.

Definite procedures should be set up for placing, cleaning, removing, and storing mats. Those who put mats in place during inclement weather should have clear-cut instructions as to where and when mats should be put down and removed. Failure to get the mats down promptly and close enough to the door may result in slippery entrance-ways and in water and dirt being carried beyond the entrance-way to create a hazard and maintenance problem in another location.

Definite procedures for inspecting and checking the condition of mats and for maintaining them in safe condition should be followed.

Stair rails, treads, and surfaces should be in good repair and checked frequently for defects. Nothing should be stored on the stairways and landings that can contribute to falls. See also Chapter 15, "Office Safety."

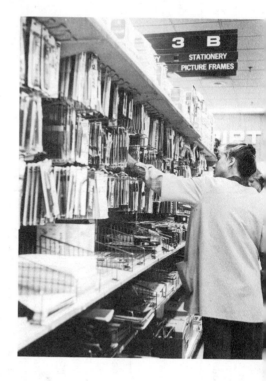

## Merchandise Displays

This section was adapted from *Loss Control—A Safety Guidebook for Trades and Services*, by George J. Matwes and Helen Matwes. Copyright © 1973 by Litton Educational Publishing, Inc. Reprinted with permission of Van Nostrand Reinhold Company.

Displays must be constructed in such a manner as to prevent the dislodging of breakables and other articles that could strike, injure, or trip the customer. Sharp or broken edges of displays and counters should be made smooth, noncutting, and unlikely to catch on the passersby.

Marketing people in some stores (like supermarkets) try to stack as much merchandise as possible on a display table for its obvious eye appeal. However, as happens with too much of a good thing, the tendency is to get carried away by enthusiasm. As a result these displays are allowed to be stacked so high as to be impractical for the shopper to reach for an item without making himself vulnerable to a cascade of boxes, cans, bottles, or whatever else is being displayed on the shelf or table.

The average woman shopper is five foot four inches (1.6 m). If heavy juice cans or glass bottles or jars are permitted to be stacked on the top tiers of shelves or displays, it is quite obvious why accidents stemming from these causes occur. An added dimension to the self-defeating practice of too high stacking is that by requiring the customer to reach so far up, it may be necessary for the customer to step up onto a lower shelf to reach the product. Shelves should be stacked evenly by layers (Fig. 21-6, center). It is advisable to place heavy items on the lower shelves and lighter items on the top shelves.

With the proliferation of nonfood accessories such as hardware items, notions, kitchen equipment, etc., which are often carded and hung on pegboard panels, it is recommended that the panels or sections be adequately recessed to accommodate the extended J-hooks (with minimum J-radius of 1m.). Keep in mind that the shopper will be bending over to reach a lower item and the hooks above should not be extended

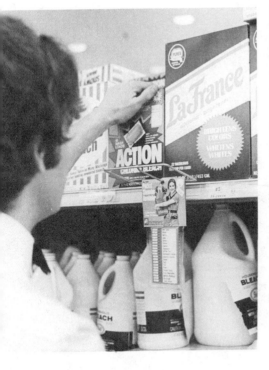

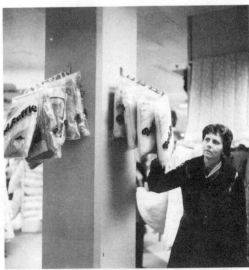

FIG. 21–6.—Point-of-purchase display hangers must be located in such a way that the human eye cannot reach them (such as shown *at left* where both the upper and lower shelves project beyond the hangers). Shelf hangers must be safeguarded if they project into the aisle (*at left*). Locating projections above eye level is another safe method (*above*).

out so far as to cause contact with a person's eyes or face. Specially safeguarded extenders are available (Fig. 21–6, center).

**Display platforms** should be of color(s) or lighting that contrast with the floor or carpet and should not obstruct aisles (Fig. 21–7). Corners of platforms should be rounded or clipped. Displays and manikins should be at least 6 in. (15 cm) off the floor so that they will not be tipped over. The display or the manikin should be fastened to this base.

Floor displays should be at least 3 ft (0.9 m) high to be seen and not become a tripping hazard. They should not be at the ends of the aisles where shopping carts can dislodge them.

**Hanging displays** should be at a safe height. If hooks are installed at 90-degree points around a column, approximately 18 in. (50 cm) down from the ceiling. This then becomes part of the fixturing and allows for easy change of seasonal displays. It can also eliminate the need for taping, stapling, and other makeshift methods that are

not always safe.

There should be a duplex electrical receptacle 18 in. from the ceiling on certain columns, as well as an outlet 12 to 18 in. from the floor.

If displays are to be hung from the ceiling, make sure that ceilings are structurally sound and that all code requirements have been met.

All electrical and mechanical display elements should have adequate protective features.

Merchandise that has sharp or cutting edges should not be in open displays unless the edges are covered or otherwise protected. Protective sleeves or plastic coatings or covers serve to protect the edges from customer handling.

### Housekeeping

In mercantile establishments, it is estimated that fixtures, displays, and other portable equipment are involved in over 40 percent of customer falls. It is essential that management provide safe equipment and that the accident control program place particular emphasis on safe placement and use of that equipment.

**609**

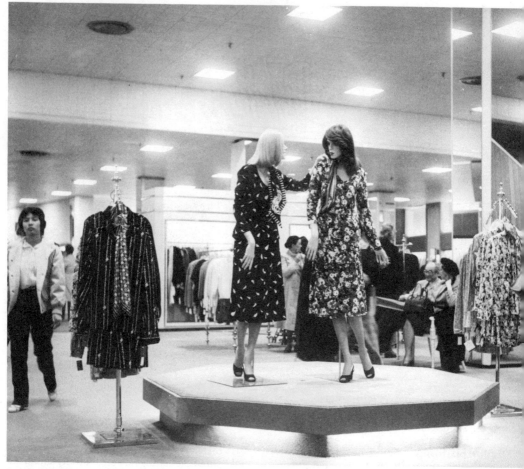

FIG. 21-7.—Display platform should contrast with the floor or carpet; manikins should be securely fastened so they canno tip.

Dress racks and stock trucks should be removed from the sales area and returned to the stock room as soon as they have been emptied.

All electrical wiring and extension cords for store machines, displays, special decorations, and the like should be designed so as not to lie on the floor. Where necessary, wires or cords may be installed in low-profile channels.

Poor housekeeping accounts for one-third or more of all customer falls. Each employee should be made to realize that it is part of his responsibility to maintain good housekeeping in the work area, to report promptly unsafe floor conditions, such as tears in carpets and holes in the floors. He should wipe up spills immediately, or else barri cade them until the hazard can be removed. A special warning sign can be used (see Fig. 21-8)

## Escalators, Elevators, and Stairways

Many business establishments move people vertically by escalators, elevators, stairways, and ramps.

Escalators can be operated from a low of 70 feet per minute (fpm) to a speed of 125 fpm (0.36- 0.64 m/s). The average recommended speed is 90 fpm (0.46 m/s). A 4 ft (1.2 m) wide escalator can move 4000 to 8000 passengers per hour. Faster or

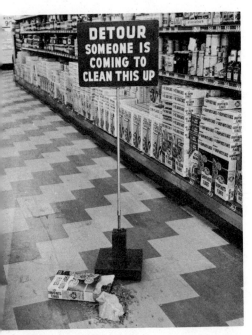

slower operation often is a source of injury to the young or the elderly.

See also the discussion in Chapter 7, "Plant Railways and Elevators," in the *Engineering and Technology* volume.

## Escalators

Accidents may occur when passengers are entering or leaving escalators or while they are riding them. Common encumbrances that may cause accidents are:

1. Unsafe floor conditions and poor housekeeping at landings

2. Sales counters, manikins, display bases, and similar units hampering the movement of passengers

3. Lights or spotlights facing passengers as they step on or off at landings

4. Mirrors near escalator landings causing passengers to misjudge their step and stumble

5. Merchandise signs or displays distracting rid-

ers, causing them to bump into one another or to fall

6. Failure of passengers to step on the center of a step tread causing them to fall; possibly against others

7. Overshoes, particularly the thin plastic type, sneakers, or other objects catching in the comb-plate when pressed against a riser, or catching at the side of the moving steps

8. A passenger "riding" his hand on the handrail beyond the combplate and back into the handrail return may receive an injury if his fingers run into the handrail guard

9. A passenger (or object) that accidentally presses the emergency STOP button, if it is not protected against accidental contact, and causing the escalator to halt unexpectedly

10. Personal injury to a child and to other passengers resulting from a package, stroller, or other conveyance placed on the escalator which may jam between the balustrades or slip from the grasp of the person trying to hold it.

11. Falls, lacerations, and amputations resulting when toes, fingers, or other parts of the body become involved with the moving parts of the escalator. (This might occur if patrons are barefooted, as they may be in tropical areas.)

12. A passenger who walks or runs up or down a moving escalator may fall or jostle others, causing them to fall.

13. Children sitting on escalator steps.

14. A passenger who fails to hold onto a moving handrail is more likely to stumble or fall.

**Escalator standards and regulations.** When installing or modifying escalators, check local and state ordinances. Also refer to National Safety council Data Sheet No. 516, *Escalators.* The American National Standard A17.1, *Safety Code for Elevators, Dumbwaiters. Escalators, and Moving Walks,* is known as the Elevator Code. Some of its important points are:

• Hand and finger guards are to be protected at the point where the handrail enters the balustrade.

• Prominent signs recommending PLEASE HOLD

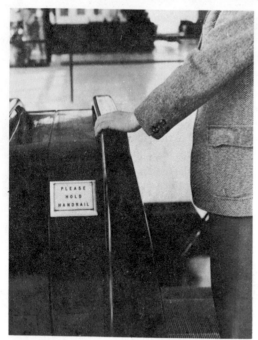

FIG. 21–9.—Close-up of escalator entrance shows PLEASE HOLD HANDRAIL sign that is placed conspicuously on the balustrade.

HANDRAIL (or equivalent message) should be displayed (see Fig. 21–9).

• Comb plates with broken teeth should be replaced immediately.

• Strollers, carts, and the like must be prohibited on escalators.

The Elevator Code also states that balustrades must be provided with handrails moving in the same direction and substantially at the same speed as the steps.

City, state or provincial, and local code requirements also should be followed.

*Inspections.* Examine all escalators from landing to landing every day. This includes riding them before store opening to find out if any visual- or sound-indicated defects exist.

• Once a week, inspect for the following:

Step treads and comb plates should not have any broken treads or fingers.

Examine handrails for damage.

Check balustrades for loose or missing screws and for damaged or misaligned trim

• Semiannually, inspect:

Step chain switches

Governor

Top and bottom oil pans

Skirt clearances

Step treads and risers

Steps

Machine brake

Skirt switch

Handrail brushes

*Start and stop controls.* Escalators should have an emergency STOP button or switch accessibly located at the top and the bottom landing. These must stop, but not start the escalator. Placemen

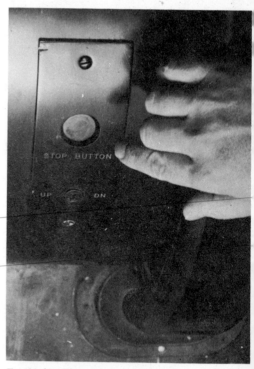

FIG. 21–10.—Those who are authorized to stop escalators should know the location of STOP buttons and the safe procedures for handling emergencies. Note the close fitting guards where the handrail enters the balustrade

of a STOP button at the base of a newel (Fig. 21–10), with either recessed design or provision of a cover, will help protect the button from being activated unnecessarily. All employees should be trained in the location and use of emergency switches.

## Elevators

Some business establishments have elevators in addition to escalators for customers. Often, elevators are self-operating. One of the most common accidents is a customer being struck by an elevator door.

**Inspections.** A logbook containing the following information should be kept:

Day, month, year, and time of inspection

Observations by mechanics or inspectors

All breakdowns, including causes and corrective action(s)

Entries should be initialed and dated.

City, state or provincial, and local codes should be followed. American National Standard A17.1, the Elevator Code referred to under Escalators, should be used.

At least every three years, all elevators should have a balance test and a contract load test. Make any required adjustments.

Once a year, hand test the following controls:

Governors

Governor cable grip jaws

Gripping jaws of car and counterweight

Releasing carrier

Cutoff switches

Tail rope and/or trip rod drums

Safety rails

Spot check automatic elevators at the start of each day for level floor stops, brakes, and other mechanical operations. Test the alarm bell to hear that it rings and that its signal registers in the maintenance department.

See Chapter 7, "Plant Railways and Elevators," in the *Engineering and Technology* volume.

## Stairways

Because stairways figure so prominently in emergency egress from buildings, they are covered in detail in the National Fire Protection Association's publication *Life Safety Code*, NFPA 101, Chapter 5, "Means of Egress." Also

covered in this chapter are ramps, exit passageways, smokeproof towers, outside stairs, fire escape stairs and ladders, illumination, exit marking, and escalators and moving walks. Only inside stairways are included in the following discussion, however.

The typical stair accident occurs when the victim slips while descending a stairway. The fall victim tends to look at the treads a great deal less than other people do; apparently, some people look at other things beside the stair tread. See the U.S. Department of Commerce study "Guidelines to Stair Safety" (listed in References at the end of this chapter).

The major areas of concern are listed next, along with corrective actions.

• Stairway use should be minimized by posting signs directing people to the escalators and elevators. Stairs place an unusual burden on people, different than walking on level surfaces. Exits to and from stairs should never be chained or otherwise locked in such a way that the stairs cannot be used in an emergency.

• Treads and handrails should be highlighted so they are immediately and easily distinguished from the riser and wall surfaces. Adequate lighting is essential; NFPA specifies a minimum of one foot-candle (decalux), measured at the floor. Arrange lights so they do not create glare surfaces or temporarily "blind" stair users; lights should be arranged so that the failure of one unit will not leave any area in darkness. If one side of the stairwell is open to adjoining space, it is a good idea to close off that view to prevent distraction that results in falls.

• The edge of the step or tread (nosing) should be easy to see. If possible, use carpeting to contrast between the approach to the steps and the stairs themselves. If not, special nosing may be installed to provide definition between the steps. Nosings must be securely fastened. Uncarpeted stairs should be edgemarked.

• A continuous handrail must be provided; see details on page 426. The railing should preferably be of a lighter color, because people seem to be more inclined to use a lighter colored railing than a dark one that looks dirty and greasy. The railing should be kept clean. The handrail should extend to the top and bottom of the staircase so that it may be grasped before stepping on the first step or leaving the last step of the flight. Be sure that the railing does not extend into a passageway in such a way as to create a hazard.

• Stair treads should give good traction and be stable. Outdoor stairs need extra slip resistance and should have adequate water runoffs that lead away from other walking surfaces.

• Worn or defective treads or other parts should be replaced immediately.

• Stairs should be clear of obstructions. Sharp ends of handrails and guardrails should be removed or covered to prevent injury. Glass areas adjacent to stair landings or at either end of the stairway should be clearly marked and protected to prevent people from walking through them. Fixtures that project into the stairway should be moved.

## Protection Against Fire, Explosion, and Smoke

If fire breaks out or an explosion occurs, the quick and orderly evacuation of the premises will protect all persons including visitors. All evacuation plans should be based on the premise that visitors will be on the property for the first time. Such persons should be protected by ample and special direction signs, even though location of exits might be a well established and known fact to regular employees.

Businesses that generally attract large numbers of customers, guests, or patrons should provide well marked exits, emergency lighting (see Fig. 21-11), and ample direction signs inscribed to direct people to safe exits.

Dense, penetrating smoke can be as deadly as the heat or flame of a fire. Lungs can be seared quickly.

Enclosed stair wells provide the best fire escape routes. Doors to such stair wells must never be obstructed, locked, or propped open.

To help evacuate a building, a public address system, manned by a qualified and trained person, can be used to direct the evacuation and issue life-saving instructions.

Usually the early detection of a fire and the use of a good evacuation plan can prevent panic and personal injuries. More details are given later in this chapter and in Chapter 16, "Planning for Emergencies."

Design and installation of a fire-detection and suppression system for life safety should be considered by every business. Architects should be

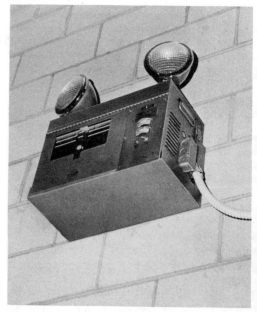

FIG. 21-11.—This emergency lighting unit is positioned at a stair landing to afford proper illumination during a power failure.

held accountable for proper design for new construction, especially in the high-rise buildings.

### Fire detection

Properly engineered fire detection systems are sound investments. But the best installation is useless if there is no response to the alarm. Systems should have a direct connection to the local fire department or to some alarm center.

**The four stages of fire.** Fire is a chemical combustion process created by the rapid combination of fuel, oxygen, and heat. A full discussion is found in Chapter 17, "Fire Protection," in the companion volume *Engineering and Technology*.

Most fires develop in four distinct stages and detectors are available for each.

• INCIPIENT STAGE. No visible smoke, flame, or significant heat is developed, but a significant amount of combustion particles are generated over a period of time. These particles, created by chemical decomposition, have weight and mass, but are too small to be visible to the human eye. They behave according to gas laws and quickly ise to the ceiling. Ionization detectors respond to hese particles.

• SMOLDERING STAGE. As the incipient condition continues, the quality of combustion particles ncreases to the point where they become visi-le—this is called "smoke." There is still no flame or significant heat developed. Photoelectric letectors "see" visible smoke.

FLAME STAGE. As the fire condition develops urther, the point of ignition occurs and flames tart. The level of visible smoke decreases and the eat level increases. Infrared energy is given off; this can be picked up by infrared detectors.

• HEAT STAGE. At this point, large amounts of heat, flame, smoke and toxic gases are produced. This stage develops very quickly, usually in seconds. Thermal detectors respond to heat energy.

**Burning plastics.** It should be noted at this point that some fuels such as plastic waste recep-tacles can produce a great deal of toxic smoke when they burn. Therefore nontoxic and noncom-bustible materials (such as metal cans) might be used.

For example, polyvinyl chloride (PVC) in a single foot of one-inch size PVC rigid non-metal-lic conduit involved in a fire:

1. Can produce a sufficiently heavy, dense smoke to obscure 3500 cu ft (100m$^3$) of space, and

2. Can generate enough hydrogen chloride to provide a lethal concentration of HCl in approximately 1650 cu ft (45 m$^3$) of space.

**Engineering and control procedures.** The best fire detection system is only as good as its weakest component. The services of a fire protec-tion consultant should be obtained in engineering the system and establishing the control proce-dures. Here are four steps to consider.

1. Select the proper type detector(s) for the hazard areas. For example, a computer area may involve ionization or combination detec-tors. A warehouse may have infrared and ionization detectors. In low-risk areas, thermal detectors or combinations of detectors may be used.

2. Determine the spacing and locations of detec-tors to provide the earliest possible warning.

3. Select the best control system arrangement to provide fast identification of the exact source of alarm initiation.

4. Assure notification of responsible authorities who can immediately respond to the alarm and can take appropriate action. Every detection system must have an alarm signal transmitted to a point of constant supervision. If this cannot be assured at the premises, the signal must be transmitted to a central station, fire department, or other reporting source to assure prompt response.

## Response methods

Early warning systems are as important during hours of occupancy as they are when the premises are vacant.

When detection pinpoints a trouble spot, immediate response by a responsible trained com-pany representative is all important. Shaving seconds and minutes can mean the difference between lives lost or saved, and fire confined or allowed to spread out of control.

Here are some systems that are used.

**Twenty-four hour supervisory service.** If the installation has 24-hours-a-day, seven-days-a-week supervision at some point in the building, or complex of buildings, then it is recommended that alarm, trouble, and zone signals be indicated at this location.

**Less than 24 hour supervisory service.** For periods when the installation does not have responsible personnel to respond to the alarm, then a backup annunciation system should be provided. The National Fire Protection Associa-tion recommends that this be done with a connec-tion to a central station supervisor's service or other service.

Such systems should include the means of initiating fire and trouble signals to the central station transmitter equipment. In the case of a trouble signal, the station can immediately dis-patch a representative to investigate the trouble and notify proper representatives of the property under surveillance.

**If central station tie-in is not available.** In areas where no central station supervision is available, the local fire or police department may accept a remote fire alarm panel to be installed at

**615**

## EVACUATION PREPAREDNESS
## CHECKLIST

All questions in this checklist should be answered with "yes," "no," "NA" (not applicable), or "U" (undetermined.) For all answers that are not "yes," or "NA," the specific areas needing correction, the persons responsible, etc., should be noted.

### Floor Diagrams

Are floor plans prominently posted on each floor?

Is each plan legible?

Does the plan indicate every emergency exit on the floor?

Is a person looking at the plan, properly oriented by an "X" (that is, "you are here now").

Are room number identifications for the floor as well as compass directions given?

Are directions to stairwells clearly indicated?

Are local and familiar terms used on the diagram to define directions to emergency exit stairwells? For example, are particular areas identified, such as mail room, cafeteria, personnel department, wash rooms?

### Exit paths to stairwells

If color coding of pillars and doors, or stripes and markings on floors are used, are they properly explained?

Is additional clarification needed?

Are paths to exits relatively straight and clear of all obstructions?

Are proper instructions posted at changes of direction en route to an emergency exit?

Are overpressure systems and venting systems operative?

### Elevators

Are signs prominently posted at and on elevators warning of the possible dangers in use of elevators during fire and emergency evacuation situations?

Do these signs indicate the direction of emergency exit stairwells which are available for use?

### Elderly and physically handicapped

Are there elderly or physically handicapped persons who will need assistance during a fire and emergency evacuation of premises?

What provision is made for their removal during an emergency?

Who will assist? How will the handicapped be moved?

### Emergency exit doors

Are all emergency exits properly identified?

Are exit door location signs adequately and reliably illuminated?

Do exit doors open easily and swing in proper direction (open out)?

Are any exit doors blocked, chained, locked, partially blocked, obstructed by cabinets, coat racks, umbrella stands, packages, etc.?

Note: Blockage must be prohibited and removed immediately.

Are all exit doors self-closing?

Are there complete closures of each door?

Are all exit doors kept closed, or are they occasionally propped open for convenience or to allow for ventilation?

Note: This practice must be prohibited.

### Emergency stairwells

Are stair treads and risers in good condition?

Are stairwells free of mops, pails, brooms, rags, packages, barrels, or any other obstructing material?

Are all stairwells equipped with proper handrails?

Does each emergency stairwell go directly to the grade floor exit level without interruption?

Does the stairwell terminate at some interim point in the building?

If so, are there clear directions at that point which show the way to completion of exit?

Is there provision for directing occupants to refuge areas out of and away from the building when they reach the ground floor?

Are directions provided where evacuees can congregate for a "head count" during and after the evacuation has been complete?

Is there adequate lighting in the stairwell?

Source: *National Safety Council Industrial Data Sheet 656*, Evacuation System for High-Rise Buildings.

heir headquarters or firehouse.

If central station or telephone-leased line tie-
n is not available. If none of the foregoing
possibilities is available, then consideration
should be given to the use of qualified and
licensed telephone answering services. Automatic dialing units connected to responsible officials of the property is another alternative.

**High-rise building fire and evacuation
controls**

Just what is a high-rise building? The General
Services Administration, at a conference in War-
renton, Virginia, in April of 1971, established four
basic criteria to designate a high-rise. First, the
size of the building made personnel evacuation
impossible or not practical. Second, part or most

of the building was beyond the reach of fire
department aerial equipment. Third, any fire
within the building must be attacked from within
because of building height. Fourth, the building
had the potential for "stack effect."

The huge high-rise megastructures now building or already constructed all have one thing in
common—they are intended to house people. As
buildings go higher, the population density per
square foot of ground area increases, which poses
a whole new set of problems concerning the
health, safety, and welfare of their occupants.
Actually, each building is a sealed life-support
system. Present engineering approaches facilitate
heating and cooling but are extremely wasteful of
energy. They are more airtight than ever, thus
there is increasing danger from smoke and toxic
combustion by-products.

Regarding most fire department aerial equipment, most ladders are limited to a height of approximately 85 ft (26 m). This means that a building higher than about 8 to 10 stories cannot be served by this equipment.

From a height standpoint and also due to increased floor areas, fires must be fought from within the building. This can be accomplished by automatic sprinklers, hose standpipes, and portable extinguishers, as well as hose lines from the building exterior.

An evacuation checklist is given in Fig. 21-12.

**Stack effect.** Every building has its own peculiarities for creation of a "stack effect," among them being structure configuration, height, number and size of openings, wind velocities, temperature extremes, number and location of mail chute openings, and elevator shafts. All of these factors create varying air flows which tend to accelerate and intensify an interior fire. Unprotected air conditioning systems are an open invitation to catastrophe. If there is no automatic smoke and heat detection, no automatic fan shutdown, and no automatic fire dampers, smoke and toxic fumes would be quickly drawn into the exhaust or return air duct system and promptly distributed to all other floors and areas of the building served by the air conditioning system.

The National Fire Protection Association recognizes this potential and in its Standard No. 90A, *Installation of Air Conditioning and Ventilating Systems*, states that in systems of over 15,000 cfm (7 m³/s) capacity, smoke detectors *shall* be installed in the main supply duct downstream of the filters. These detectors shall automatically shut down fans and close smoke dampers to stop the recirculation of the smoke—or they may incorporate automatic exhaust.

Considering evacuation, it must be assumed that children and elderly and handicapped people will be involved and cannot move promptly. In addition, some people are psychologically prone to panic in a fire situation. The quantity and size of staircases will undoubtedly prohibit complete evacuation. Tests conducted in Canada indicate that based on an occupant load of 240 persons per floor, total evacuation of an 11-story building can take up to 6½ minutes, while an 18-story building can take up to 7½ minutes. Exits are just not designed to handle all occupants simultaneously.

Most codes do not consider elevators to be an exit component and prohibit their use during fire emergencies. But codes generally also require that one or more elevators be designed and equipped for firefighters. Key operations shall transfer automatic elevator operation to manual and bring the elevator to the street floor for use by the fire service. The elevator shall be situated as to be readily accessible by the fire department.

Many elevators use capacitance-type call buttons, which may bring them to a stop on the fire-involved floor, from which they cannot move because smoke interrupts the light beam that keeps the doors open. Other possibilities include the inadvertent arrival of the elevator at the fire-involved floor by a passenger not knowing the fire exists and wishing to get off, and also the possibility of a person pushing the call button in the elevator lobby and then, in panic, using the staircase for exit. With problems of this magnitude, it can be assumed that complete evacuation is impossible.

## Crowd and panic control

Any commercial establishment may be faced with an unruly crowd as a result of an emergency, a panic, or even a planned demonstration. Self-interest dictates that a preplanned scheme be worked out to protect the facility and its employees, as well as patrons and bystanders. Different measures are needed depending on whether the panic occurs in the building or outside of it. Actually, it be be only an above-average size group of shoppers who are waiting to be admitted. For shoppers, it would be good to have directional signs displayed at many areas in the building. Exit signs are especially important. But these alone do not reduce the higher risk potential inherent when a great number of people are gathered, such as at sports events, entertainments, schools, and other places.

In almost every emergency, there could be panic. However, it is best to try to prevent panic from starting. Employees need periodic drills and practice in handling emergency situations with customers, some of whom may be confused and others who may be handicapped. The threat of unusual occurrence (such as riot, bomb threat, and the like) cannot be overlooked and plans must be made to handle such a possibility.

High-rise buildings pose new and special problems but other public places such as theaters and other amusement and recreation facilities must also provide well-planned emergency procedures lures. Panic and the press of frantic, hysterical people have caused wholesale destruction of life in many emergencies. Often times, such losses could have been prevented. Strict observance to building and fire codes can do much to eliminate physical hazards and "death traps" through improper design and installation of facilities.

Civil strife and sabotage are covered in Chapter 16, "Planning for Emergencies." Demonstrations are covered next.

**Demonstrations.** Here are suggestions of what to do in the event of demonstrations. The procedure concerns store activities, but is easily adapted to the needs of any establishment. These suggestions are taken from *Loss Control—A Safety Guidebook for Trades and Services,* by George J. Matwes and Helen Matwes. Copyright © 1973 by Litton Educational Publishing, Inc. Reprinted with permission of Van Nostrand Reinhold Company.

• *Demonstration outside of store building.* Advise employees to call Security and/or management. Security should telephone police, advise them of the situation, and follow their instructions.

Arrange for two key personnel to assume previously assigned positions at all store entrances and other key points; they should know Security's telephone number in order to relay information and receive instructions. They should never leave their assigned post unless relieved or advised accordingly. Caution them to remain calm and not to interfere with the entrance or egress of customers or employees.

Those employed in portable, high-valued merchandise departments (diamonds, furs, etc.), should arrange to have such merchandise placed in an assigned secure area. Those employees working in departments selling firearms, knives, axes, straight razors, bows and arrows, even meat cutlery, should have them removed from the selling floor to a secure area. Proceed with "business as usual" in all other departments.

Because rumors can create panic situations or problems among employees and customers present, it is recommended that all employees be advised of two or three emergency interior telephone numbers, to verify information and squelch rumors.

• *Demonstration moving into store.* (People carrying signs, groups linking arms across aisles and taunting employees, fights between individuals.)

1. Advise all employees to avoid any comments, antagonisms, or physical contact with marchers, to answer all queries courteously, and above all to keep calm.

2. In areas where demonstrations are taking place, have employees suspend selling, lock their registers, remain in their areas as calm as possible, and await further instructions from their supervisors.

3. In areas where "business as usual" is being maintained, arrange for frequent cash pickups.

4. Key personnel and employees should take their assigned places, as discussed above.

5. In the event such a demonstration turns into group looting or group "hit and run" stealing, employees should not attempt to make any apprehensions. Security personnel will follow previous orders for such conditions as advised by management.

Remember, personal safety is more important than property protection.

**Panic** is one of the most serious situations that can grip people; through panic, they may take irrational means for self-preservation. Often panic leads to injury of many persons who might otherwise have been saved. An evacuation plan, well rehearsed with supervisors and employees, is needed for every business. (A good discussion of panic and techniques for handling it is given in the National Safety Council's publication *Supervisors Guide to Human Relations.*)

## Self-service operations

The best-known self-service operation is the self-service gasoline station. Here, a customer puts the gasoline in his vehicle without any employee assistance. The employee merely sees that the customer observes the safety rules and follows the prescribed procedure, usually posted on the pump housing or on a nearby sign.

All states require that the vehicle engine be turned off and that there be no smoking or open lights.

## Evacuation of the handicapped

The problem of evacuation of handicapped persons from hotels, stores, and other facilities is an added problem to both management and the safety professional. Communication, especially, is a problem. Special written instructions can be given to people with an auditory impairment; verbal instructions can be given the blind.

More details on how to help the handicapped are given in Chapter 20, "The Handicapped Worker."

## Transportation

Some businesses by their very nature have special, and often prominent accident control problems. A majority of their loss control efforts must be directed at protecting the nonemployee from harm.

All types of transportation—from commercial airlines, railroads, marine, and buses to local transit, taxi, and school bus operations—must be vitally concerned with prevention of injury through accidents. Not only is maintenance and operation of the vehicle or unit itself involved, but the problem also extends into areas around it, such as terminals, stations, school bus loading areas, and the like.

**Courtesy cars.** When transporation is provided by a business for customer courtesy and convenience (such as a hotel or motel courtesy car or bus), the same concern and precautions used in commercial operations should be considered. These include providing the safest vehicle, maintained in proper working condition (meeting all local, state or provincial, and federal requirements), and operated by a professional who is trained and skilled in all elements of operating the vehicle.

**Company-owned vehicles.** Another source of damage and injury claims arises out of the operation of company motor vehicles by employees. Chances are that one out of every four drivers will have a collision in any given year. This probability makes the occurrence of such liability accidents a constant threat and often a very real dollar drain for insurance protection and claim settlement. The question of liability resulting from an employee's use of his own car on company business must also be considered.

## Protect Attractive Nuisances

The natural curiosity of human beings often brings grief to themselves and trouble to others. There are many opportunities for every business to be involved in losses caused by the public curiosity. Some examples follow.

Any unattended vehicle and machine that is left in an operable condition is attractive to the young (and the so-called "young in heart"). Unauthorized use of vehicles or machines should be discouraged by use of "tamper-proof" locks. Watchmen and security guards should be employed if necessary.

Frequently, partially finished road repairs or other construction can "booby trap" a vehicle. So, also, can unprotected and unbarricaded hazards, especially in adverse weather or in storms. American National Standard D6.1, *Manual on Uniform Traffic Control Devices for Streets and Highways*, should be referred to.

Many contractors or builders provide special but safe, observation facilities for public "sidewalk superintendents." Local authorities and insurance engineers should be consulted for regulations and control measures.

### Swimming pools

Swimming pools are a part of many hotels and motels and public areas (Fig. 21–13). Some causes of pool accidents are inadequacy or lack of protective barriers around pools, absence of lifeguards or qualified adult supervision, disregard for the rules of good pool conduct, and the failure to teach youngsters drowning-prevention knowledge.

Pool requirements should include these precautions.

1. Pools must be screened, fenced, or otherwise enclosed in order to control admittance. A tamper-proof lock should be provided. A pool alarm may provide additional protection.

2. Basic lifesaving equipment should be available. This should include a lightweight but strong pole with blunt ends at least 12 ft (3.7 m) long, or a ring buoy to which a long throwing rope has been attached.

3. Someone should be in charge of pool operation; this person should be familiar with swimming pool management. A lifeguard should be on duty whenever the pool is in use.

4. A telephone should be handy, such as in the bathhouse or changing room. Emergency telephone numbers should be on hand—the nearest available physician, ambulance service, hospital, police, and the fire and/or rescue unit.

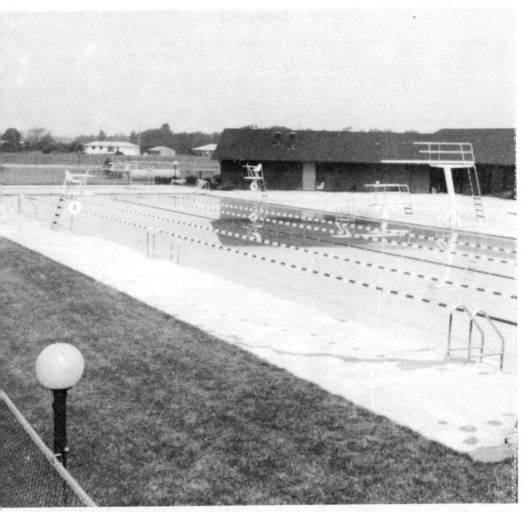

FIG. 21–13.—Basic lifesaving equipment must be available at every pool. Shown here at each lifesaving platform are ring buoys with throwing rope attached.

*Courtesy National Spa and Pool Institute.*

5. Decks around the pool should be kept clear of debris. Allow no breakable bottles in the area. Make sure all cups and dishes used at poolside are unbreakable. Litter baskets should be provided. Defective matting must be replaced.

6. Electrical equipment used for the pool must conform to local regulations and/or the latest *National Electrical Code* requirements. Any electrical applicance used near the pool must be protected by a ground fault circuit interrupter.

7. No one should be allowed in the pool during a thunderstorm.

8. All pool appliances and equipment should be maintained properly. Periodic safety checks should be made.

9. Sensible pool rules should be established and enforced. These rules should be posted.

# 21—Nonemployee Accident Prevention

## References

American National Standards Institute, 1430 Broadway, New York, N.Y. 10018.
*Manual on Uniform Traffic Control Devices for Streets and Highways*, D6.1.
*Requirements for Fixed Industrial Stairs*, A64.1.
*Safety Code for Elevators, Dumbwaiters, Escalators, and Moving Walks*, A17.1.
*Specifications for Making Buildings and Facilities Accessible to, and Usable by, the Physically Handicapped*, A117.1.

Hannaford, Earle S. *Supervisors Guide to Human Relations*, 2nd ed. Chicago, Ill., National Safety Council, 1976.

Matwes, George J., and Matwes, Helen. *Loss Control: A Safety Guidebook for Trades and Services*. New York, N.Y., Van Nostrand Reinhold Co., 1973.

National Fire Protection Association, 470 Atlantic Ave., Boston, Mass. 02210.
*Auxiliary Protective Signaling Systems*, NFPA 72B.
*Installation of Air Conditioning and Ventilating Systems*, NFPA 90A.
*Life Safety Code*, NFPA 101.
*Local Protective Signaling Systems*, NFPA 72A.
*National Electrical Code*, NFPA 70.
*Proprietary Protective Signaling Systems*, NFPA 72D.
*Remote Station Protective Signaling Systems*, NFPA 72C.
*Central Station Protective Signaling Systems*, NFPA 71.

National Safety Council, 444 North Michigan Ave., Chicago, Ill. 60611.
Industrial Data Sheets
    *Carbon Monoxide*, 415.
    *Escalators*, 516.
    *Evacuation System for High-Rise Buildings*, 656.
    *Falls on Floors*, 495.
    *Fire Prevention in Stores*, 549.
    *Floor Mats and Runners*, 595.
    *Sidewalk Sheds*, 368.
National Safety News Reprints
*Supervisors Guide to Human Relations.*

National Spa and Pool Institute, 2000 K Street NW., Washington, D.C. 20006.
"Tips and Information."
"Minimum Standards for Public Swimming Pools."

"Property Conservation Engineering and Management." *Record*, 50:3 (May-June 1973). Factory Mutual System, Norwood, Mass. 02062.

Superintendent of Documents, U.S. Government Printing Office, Washington, D.C. 20402. Commercial Practices, Title 16, *Code of Federal Regulations*, Chapter II—Consumer Product Safety Commission.

# Product Safety
# and Liability
# Prevention

# Chapter
# 22

Injuries resulting from the use (or often the misuse) of products are the basis for an ever-increasing number of product liability lawsuits, which are costing industry millions of dollars each year. It is obvious that the manufacturer must defend himself, and in the best way possible—by manufacturing a reasonably safe and reliable product, and (if necessary) providing instructions for its proper use. The key to achieving a reasonably safe and reliable product and, at the same time, reducing the product liability exposure is—"built-in" *product safety*. Product safety can be designed and built into the product through the establishment and auditing of an appropriate product safety and liability prevention program.

From the start, a product safety and liability prevention program must be designed to encompass all product management personnel and product manufacturing processes in order to determine what actions are necessary to produce a safe product and a reduced product liability potential.

To carry out the establishment and auditing of a product safety and liability prevention program, two functions are of prime importance:

The selection of a program coordinator

The selection of a program auditor.

### Establishing and Coordinating the Program

Regardless of a company's size, the establishment and coordination of a satisfactory product safety and liability prevention (PS&LP) program requires a comprehensive systems analysis of all of the various facets of operation and production, from the design stage through manufacturing, quality control, and shipping. To keep all these strings organized and to make certain that they all pull together, someone must be selected to coordinate the program, either individually or with the assistance of a committee.

### Program coordinator

The success of any PS&LP program depends upon all departments within an organization working together, effectively coordinated by an appropriately qualified and specifically designated individual, either alone or as chairman of a committee. This individual must exert stringent and continuous control over all phases of product development from initial product design through eventual product sale and distribution.

It is not critically important what the coordinator's primary function is within the organization. What is important is the PS&LP coordinator's level of authority. Can the coordinator take needed action without having to go through several supervisory levels? That is, does the coordinator have rapid access to top-level management? Within reason, is the coordinator permitted to implement his plans or suggestions?

If the business organization has a PS&LP committee to coordinate program activities, the head of the committee must have a similar level of authority and committee members should have the authority to speak for their respective departments.

**Responsibilities.** A program coordinator must have enough authority to take any required action, and should also have the responsibilities shown below:

Function in a staff capacity to corporate management

Assist in setting general PS&LP program policy

Recommend special action regarding:

    Product recall

    Field modification

    Product redesign

    Special analyses

Conduct and/or review complaint, incident, or accident analyses

Coordinate appropriate PS&LP program documentation

Assure the adequate flow of both verbal and written information

Develop sources of readily available product safety and liability prevention data for use by operating personnel

Maintain liaison with business, professional, and governmental organizations on all matters pertinent to product safety and liability prevention

Conduct PS&LP program audits, where appropriate.

**Ground rules.** The following ground rules must also be clearly defined by management if the PS&LP program coordinator is to be effective.

• The purpose of the PS&LP program coordinator

or must be clearly defined.

The authority and responsibilities of the
PS&LP program coordinator must be clearly
specified by top management and understood by
the PS&LP program coordinator.

As previously noted, a PS&LP program will
involve most of the departments in a company
and will require the application of many diverse
disciplines. Consequently, *coordination* must be
provided by the PS&LP program coordinator in
order to assure a thorough and systematic
approach by the company to the implementation
of a PS&LP program.

**Committee coordination.** Whenever a
PS&LP program committee is used, the size of the
group must be maintained within manageable
limits (generally no more than five or six members). In a large corporation, it may be more
desirable to appoint a small corporate committee
or individual corporate coordinator and also
appoint a separate program coordinator in each
corporate division or department.

A committee's makeup will vary as determined by the business organization. However,
key members of the committee will almost always
represent the following departments:

Design or engineering

Manufacturing

Quality control

Service, marketing, or installation

Legal.

In addition, sales, advertising, insurance, personnel, public relations, plant safety, and
purchasing department representatives should be
designated and be prepared to serve as consultants to the PS&LP program committee when the
expertise of these various departments is
required.

**Program auditor**

The program auditor is the single most important factor in a successful product safety and
liability prevention program.

Because the program auditor's role is so important, discussion of his responsibilities in the evaluation of all facets of the PS&LP program is the
main topic of this chapter.

Although the program auditor can be a private
consultant or an insurance company product

safety or loss control specialist, a company's
PS&LP program will probably be most effective
if the program auditor is a member of company
management. If possible, the program auditor
should not be the same individual as the program
coordinator—in order to maintain objectivity.

The program auditor's main duty is to evaluate
the adequacy of the organization's PS&LP program activities in relation to its actual and potential exposures, which determine what the
organization should be doing to prevent eventual
product-related losses; for example, the comparison of what the organization *is* doing against what
it *should be* doing to control product liability
exposures.

**Improve program effectiveness.** When auditing the organization's product management control system, the program auditor should strive to
make the company's program most effective.
This can be accomplished by doing the following:

• Determine the organization's potential product liability exposures.

• Determine the organization's PS&LP program
deficiencies (for example, evaluation of the
organization's ability to control those product
liability exposures that are found).

• Develop concise, realistic, corrective procedures to minimize product liability exposures.

• Get management to implement the proposed
corrective measures (to reduce losses, improve
good records, improve the level of product control, comply with government regulations, for
example).

• Transmit all product safety and liability prevention program audit information to management for review.

Product safety and liability prevention program audits may also be successfully conducted in
situations where the organization does not have a
formal program, as long as the program auditor's
knowledge of product management control practices is satisfactory.

The adequacy of the coordination should be
measured by the program auditor as each departmental activity is evaluated through observation
and questioning during the PS&LP program
audit.

**Systems analysis.** A business organization's

PS&LP program philosophy must be one of continuous overview or systems analysis of the entire product management control system. In performing the systems analysis, the PS&LP program auditor must:

• Evaluate management's commitment to product safety and liability prevention.

• Determine the effectiveness of the organization's PS&LP program coordinator as being the most tangible indicator of management's interest in manufacturing a safe, reliable product. Depending on the organization, there may be no need for a PS&LP committee and there may be no full-time PS&LP program coordinator. What must be determined is whether someone, regardless of title, has really been assigned the *responsibility* for coordinating all activities associated with the manufacture of safe, reliable products.

• Evaluate the PS&LP program coordinator's effectiveness in coordinating all activities associated with the manufacture of safe, reliable products.

**Duties.** The PS&LP program auditor must determine the business organization's ability to manufacture safe, reliable products and must evaluate how adequate its capabilities are for controlling existing products exposures, eliminating potential exposures, and determining uncontrollable exposures.

In addition to seeking purely quantitative responses, the program auditor must also be receptive to broad generalized impressions that may be gained during the course of evaluating the organization's product safety and liability prevention program activities.

For example, the program auditor should:

• Be alert for obvious deficiencies that reflect unconcern on the part of management

• Watch to see, when a deficiency is noted and "on-the-spot" corrective action is needed, whether the organization is honestly interested in manufacturing a safe, reliable product. Remember, actions speak louder than words. At the very least, when a deficiency is noted, responsible management should determine the cause of the problem and indicate what corrective action will be taken.

• Substantiate the organization's actual performance with regard to each deficiency or problem noted by preparing and submitting an appropriate report. Recommendations can be made as required.

• Discuss apparant deficiencies with responsible management personnel to be certain that all the facts have been given. Often as a result of making deficiencies known to responsible management personnel, additional information is forthcoming which can cause the program auditor to modify previous conclusion.

• Be aware of oversolicitous members of management who may be attempting to hide deficiencies

• Ask for substantiating documentation of actions taken, particularly if the response received are not always direct.

• Consider a failure to receive the undivided attention of responsible management during the course of the audit as an indication of a lack of concern for product safety and liability prevention on their part.

• Consider the possibility, when unable to elicit information from responsible management in response to specific questions, that the organization is deficient in the areas questioned and so note in the PS&LP program audit report.

The function of the PS&LP program auditor is to interview all key management personnel, to observe the actual manufacturing operation, and to investigate, question, and verify performance.

## How To Do a PS&LP Program Audit

The information contained in this section constitutes the heart of this chapter. Application of this information will enable the program auditor to evaluate comprehensively and accurately the PS&LP program activities and effectively achieve the goals of every product safety and liability prevention audit. The major goal of such an audit is to reduce substantially the causes of product liability exposure. Some of the principal ones are as follows:

Product designs not being reasonably safe (failure to review product design safety)

Inadequate manufacturing and quality control procedures

Inadequate preparation and review of warning and instructions

Misleading representation of product or services.

If uncorrected (and sometimes even if they are corrected), these causes may be the basis for several different types of product liability losses, such as:

Bodily injury

Property damage

Business interruption

Loss of income

Extra expenses.

Consequently, the purpose of a product safety and liability prevention program is to develop a means to perform (a) an evaluation and elimination of the accident potential of the product(s) manufactured, distributed, and retailed, and (b) an evaluation and increased ability to control effectively the accident potential through good management techniques (good hazard preventive procedures).

## Preliminary procedures

The following preliminary activities must be performed by the program auditor before beginning the formal audit. They are intended to facilitate and enhance the subsequent performance of the PS&LP program audit.

Clearly explain the purpose of the audit to top management.

Arrange mutually agreeable audit dates with involved members of management.

Clearly define how the operational plan (schedule) of the audit will involve members of management.

Review appropriate PS&LP program-related documentation.

Review appropriate product-related procedures.

Review appropriate product-related technical and standards information.

Acquire all the necessary product-related printed instructional and precautionary materials.

If these preliminary PS&LP program audit procedures are carried out, the program auditor will usually receive complete cooperation from the other involved management personnel, thus enhancing his potential for developing all information required to accurately evaluate product safety and liability prevention program activities.

Carrying out the objective of the product safety and liability prevention program entails following a procedure of checks and audits in each of the major departments of the manufacturing organization. In order to get the most from the procedure, it is necessary to have the total cooperation of management in general and the safety professional in particular. (More about the role of the safety person later.)

## Management commitment

The spark that initiates the PS&LP program and the catalyst that provides the impetus and continuity to its effectiveness is the wholehearted commitment and support of company management.

Just as with a safety program, management must have a written policy recognizing its responsibilities to provide support, to set basic objectives, and to establish priorities for a product safety and liability prevention program within the organization. Some evidence of management's commitment to product safety and liability prevention might include:

Evidence of shop conversations on the subject

A posted letter or bulletin

Evidence of specific meeting(s)

The distribution of brochures

A special mailing to employees

A formal statement of management policy on the subject

Use of a PS&LP program coordinator/committee

Use of a PS&LP program auditor.

Wholehearted management support has to be given to the product safety and liability prevention program in order for it to succeed. All key people within the business organization must be told by management that they have an important role to play in the program and that they must commit the time and effort required to make sure the program is successful. In short, management must clearly communicate to all employees by word and deed that the control of product losses is a key company objective.

Ideally, the chief executive officer should provide a clearly written policy with respect to the company's commitment to product safety and liability prevention. It should be widely and effectively distributed to management, all company departments, and to each employee.

As noted above, management's commitment to PS&LP does not necessarily have to be in the form of a written policy. However, there should be some tangible indication that top management is truly committed to product safety and liability prevention and that employees have been advised, or there should be an indication by employees in the performance of their daily activities that show they are aware (regardless of how they have been made aware) that top management is sincerely interested in manufacturing safe and reliable products.

### Role of the safety professional

The significance of the role played by the safety professional in a company's product safety and liability prevention program will likely vary inversely in proportion to the size of the company. However, in all cases the safety professional plays a vital role in the implementation of a successful product safety and liability prevention program. In a small to medium-sized company it is entirely possible that the safety professional, because of his broad experience in areas of safety technology, will be selected by top management as either product safety and liability prevention program coordinator or auditor. However, as the company product line increases, it is more likely that top management will select the head of the engineering or design department for this assignment with the safety professional as his assistant.

Regardless of the specific assignment of the safety professional within a company's product safety and liability prevention program, the PS&LP auditor should evaluate the company's safety professional to determine if he is, in fact, adequately contributing to the company's overall product safety and liability prevention program.

Here's a description of the contributions the safety professional can make.

• The safety professional, because of his knowledge of plant operations and general safety expertise, can evaluate and offer comments on the company's product safety and liability prevention program.

• The safety professional, because of his experience with respect to safety training programs, can evaluate and comment on the product safety-related training programs developed by those involved in the company's product safety and liability prevention program.

• The safety professional, because of his experience with respect to accident investigation techniques, can assist those individuals who will be performing product accident investigations for the company.

• Members of the safety department can provide product safety surveillance in production areas. This helps to prevent errors and resultant product-related accidents. These individuals should be advised that all product safety-related complaints or problems uncovered as a result of their surveillance must be discussed with the plant engineer and the production department and formally documented, with a copy of the documentation sent to the product safety and liability prevention program coordinator.

• Because of its past experience in developing and implementing employee safety programs, the safety department often is aware not only of potential product hazards but also of ways in which customers may misuse those products. Therefore, a knowledgeable safety department representative should be used as a consultant to the team performing design reviews, hazard analyses, and safety audits.

### Departmental Audits

#### Engineering or design department functions

The primary function of the engineering or design department should be to design reliable products that can be used with reasonable safety. It is more practical and usually much less costly for the manufacturer to build reliability and safety into the product than to suffer the consequences of catastrophic product liability losses. Products should be reasonably safe during (a) normal use, (b) normal service, maintenance, and adjustment, (c) "foreseeable uses" that the manufacturer did not intend, and (d) reasonably foreseeable "misuses." The courts are saying today that a manufacturer has the responsibility of making sure that his products are safe for any reasonable foreseeable use or misuse to which the customer might put them.

The engineering or design department may be the most critical area within the PS&LP program activity; consequently, the program auditor should check the following:

Does the organization evaluate product hazard prior to production?

anyone within the organization formally assigned this responsibility?

there a formal written or prepared design review procedure, even if it is not referred to as such?

At certain predetermined points in the manufacture of all complex products, tests or inspections of the products are made to determine compliance with the manufacturing requirements. Why? Because it has been found that problems detected at predetermined points in the process can be corrected more quickly and economically than problems that are detected after manufacture. This is true of all complex processes including the product engineering design process.

At predetermined points in the design process, the design should be checked for compliance with its requirements, the objective being to make sure that the optimum product design is achieved.

The appropriate check for the product engineering design process is called the *formal design review*.

**Formal design review.** The formal design review (FDR) is a scheduled systematic review and evaluation of the product design by personnel not directly associated with the product's development but who, as a group, are knowledgeable in and have a responsibility for all elements of the product throughout its life cycle, including design, manufacture, packaging, transportation, installation, use and maintenance, and final disposal.

It is the exception when one person has expertise in "all elements of the design," such as performance, total product costs, safety, reliability, producibility, environmental effects, maintainability, serviceability, life cycle costs, human factors, customer's needs and reasonable expectations, pertinent legislation (enacted and pending), pertinent litigation involving personal injury, property damage, and environmental damage, etc. Expertise in these elements should exist, however, within the organization.

The organization's engineering or design department manager should be responsible for making full use of all available talent and experience in the performance of a formal design review. The formal design review should be held before the initial design is formulated.

The primary purpose of the FDR should be to review the individual requirements in the product design specification for *validity, accuracy,* and *completeness.* No new design should be started without a design specification that clearly defines the requirements the product must meet. Some of the items that should be considered and reviewed (as appropriate) during the FDR include:

Identification of the ultimate customer

The customer's needs and his reasonable expectations of the product

Function to be performed by the product

Design constraints, i.e., size, weight, power requirements

Pertinent federal, state or provincial, local and industry standards concerning safety, reliability, environmental effects, quality, and the like

Total anticipated product cost (including installation, maintenance, etc.)

Conditions of use and possible misuse (safety, reliability, and environmental requirements)

Pertinent information documentation associated with the total life cycle (design, manufacture, packaging, transportation, installation, use and maintenance, and final disposal) of earlier models of the products under design or of similar products

Pertinent legislation (enacted and pending) that may place constraints on the product design — safety, reliability, environmental requirements

Pertinent litigation involving personal injury, property damage, and environmental damage which could place constraints on the product design

Schedule requirements

Design alternatives

Critical parts to be used in the assembly

High-risk areas (including product liability, safety, and environmental problems) for documented trade-off studies

Make-or-buy considerations

Test and inspection considerations

Documentation required

Establishment of relative rank of importance of all the requirements of the product design (to be

## RESPONSIBILITIES OF DESIGN REVIEW TEAM MEMBERS

| Functional Expertise | Responsibilities |
|---|---|
| Design engineering (not associated with the unit under review) | Constructively reviews adequacy of design to meet all requirements of the design specification |
| Reliability/Maintainability engineering | Evaluates design for optimum reliability/maintainability consistent with goals |
| Quality control | Makes sure that adequate controls to assure required quality can be economically established and that requirements are clearly stated in drawings and specifications |
| Manufacturing engineering | Makes sure that the design is producible at minimum cost and on schedule |
| Field service engineering | Makes sure that installation, maintenance, and operating considerations are included in the design |
| Purchasing | Assumes that acceptable parts and materials are available to meet cost and delivery schedules |
| Tooling | Evaluates design in terms of the tooling costs required to satisfy tolerance and functional requirements |
| Line manufacturing | Ensures that the final design is producible |
| Packing and shipping | Assures that the product is capable of being handled and shipped without damage or other ill effects |
| Marketing | Assures that requirements of customers are realistic and fully understood by all parties and that any tradeoffs made during the design cycle will still result in an acceptable product |
| Consultants or specialists for components, human factors, value engineering, as required | Evaluate design for compliance with goals of performance, cost, and schedule |
| Consultants and specialists, from research, engineering, manufacturing, legal, patents, the corporate design center, and other divisions as appropriate | Evaluate design for compliance with legislation, litigation, safety, standards, environmental effects, performance, cost, schedule, patent requirements |

Fig. 22-1.

used in trade-off studies).

In general, the participants in a design review meeting should be people who are knowledgeable in their area of expertise. The number of participants in a session should be kept to a minimum consistent with the skills and experiences needed to adequately review the subject design. Depending on the product design and the type of review, the engineering or design manager should be sure that the participants encompass the functional expertise shown in Fig. 22–1.

A key member of the company top management should assign clear responsibility to the engineering or design department head, or his representative, for design review. The engineering or design department head, in turn, should assign the responsibility of coordinating the design reviews for a given product to some person other than the design engineer assigned to the product. This person should act as chairman of the review team. It is the chairman's responsibility to call design review meetings at the appropriate point in the product design and development program, to prepare an agenda for each meeting, to conduct the design review, and to follow up on recommendations that were approved during the design review meetings.

**Codes and standards.** The PS&LP program auditor must determine whether products conform to all applicable safety standards (state, or provincial, federal codes and regulations, testing or inspection laboratory requirements, industry standards, technical society standards, machine safeguarding standards, etc.). These standards, in most cases, should be considered as being the minimum for safety and reliability. In some cases, where no applicable formal standards apply, he should determine whether or not in-house design standards are being used and, if so, what criteria are used before a decision is made as to the adequacy of the standard. Prior to each survey, the program auditor should become familiar with the applicable standards.

**Human factors.** The PS&LP program auditor must determine whether or not human factors have been considered in the design of the products. (See description in Chapter 10, "Human Factors Engineering.") Some of the human factors which should be considered are the physical, educational, and mental limitations of people

who may use these products, and the natural tendency of people to use products for purposes other than that for which they were designed. What the program auditor also tries to find out is whether or not consideration has been given to the proclivity of customers to use products in ways for which they were not designed to be used but which might *not* be considered "unreasonable" by a court of law.

**Critical parts evaluation.** To the PS&LP program auditor, *critical parts or components* are defined as those "whose failure could cause serious bodily injury, property damage, business interruption, or serious degradation of product performance." An individual organization, however, may have different criteria for defining a critical part, such as one that is unusually expensive, difficult to acquire, or requires lengthy order lead time. When analyzing critical parts, the program auditor must be certain that both he and company personnel use the appropriate definition.

The program auditor must also determine whether the products are being analyzed for critical parts or components. If so, are the critical items receiving any special attention? Have they been field tested and designed to outlast the product itself? If this is impractical, is a special effort made to warn customers and users of the product of the possible hazards of critical-part failure? Has any effort been made to instruct customers and users in inspection techniques to detect impending failures? Have maintenance procedures been outlined for critical parts or components on the product itself and in operating and maintenance instructions? Has careful consideration been given to the expected life of the product?

All parts or components must have a life expectancy that is compatible with the life expectancy of other parts and of the total product. A part or component whose life expectancy is shorter or not compatible with that of the remainder of the product should be considered "critical" because of the possibility of its being the basis for a product liability lawsuit, necessitating an expensive product recall, or field-modification program.

Some methods of evaluating a product for critical parts are:

System safety analysis (See Chapter 4, "Acquiring

# 22—Product Safety and Liability Prevention

Hazard Information," for details.)

Failure mode and effect analysis

Fault tree analysis

Reliability analysis

Review of failure experience of similar parts or components

In-house product testing to gain critical part experience

Field testing of products under harsher conditions than they can be expected to undergo in actual use.

**Packaging, handling, and shipping.** The PS&LP program auditor must determine whether the products have been adequately analyzed with regard to the packaging necessary to prevent deterioration, corrosion, or damage. Requirements for packaging must cover conditions affecting the product while at the manufacturing site, during transit, and under normal conditions of storage by the customer. Packaging methods should be established by the organization for each individual product. Product packages should be marked to indicate special requirements—Do NOT STORE IN HOT AREAS, THIS END UP, USE NO HOOKS.

When the maintenance of a specific internal or external environment is required, that environment should be specified both in the packaging instructions and on the exterior of the package. The nature of the materials used in packaging the product should be such that there are no hazards present when the product is unpacked by the customer. When the product is to be installed by the customer, installation instructions stressing safe installation methods and pointing out all hazardous conditions should be provided.

Special containers and transportation vehicles should be used as necessary to prevent damage. The following should also be provided:

Adequate means for safely picking up and moving products

Labels depicting safe lifting points on either the product itself or the product cartons, or boxes

Product packaging that is designed to resist tipping over in handling.

If the products are subject to deterioration or corrosion during storage, the products must be clean and have preservative applied by such methods as required to preclude damage during subsequent storage and handling, shipping, etc.

There should be a plan for protecting stored products against loss, deterioration, and damage. Procedures must be developed (if not already in use) to provide the required protection, perform the necessary preventive maintenance, and accomplish the necessary storage inspections as a function of required storage time.

A program should be in force for the control and inspection of products shipped. The program should make sure that:

Products have been subjected to and have satisfactorily passed the required preshipping inspections and tests

Products have been preserved and packaged in accordance with required specifications and procedures

Products and packages are identified and marked in accordance with required specifications and procedures

Products are accompanied by required shipping and technical documents, such as handling instructions, operating manuals, installation manuals, reports, drawings, and parts lists.

The program auditor must also carefully evaluate shipping procedures because a product shipped without proper instructions or with hidden damage may cause an accident when used. The reason for selecting the packaging material, cartons, and carrier should be based not only on economies, but also on the need for delivering product in perfect condition to the distributor or customer.

The product, as shipped, must agree with the purchase order. All appropriate labels, manuals, warnings, and descriptive materials must be included and should be checked by the organization at the time of shipping.

**Warning labels.** It is not enough for an organization to design and make a satisfactory product; it also has the responsibility to label its product correctly and to warn potential consumers and/or users of any dangers involved. The duty of a manufacturer to label his products and warn of any danger is increasingly becoming the basis for

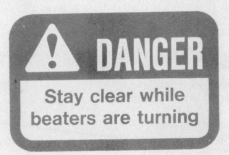

**Agricultural**

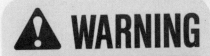

**Industrial**

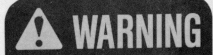

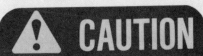

FIG. 22–2.—Not only must instructions accompany a product, but also very clear and specific warnings of inherent dangers of possible misuse should be conspicuously placed on the product.

*Courtesy Deere & Company.*

HAZARDS:

Highly Toxic by Inhalation

Highly Toxic by Absorption

**DANGER! MAY BE FATAL IF INHALED OR ABSORBED THROUGH SKIN**

Do not breathe (dust, vapor, mist, gas).*
Do not get in eyes, on skin, on clothing.
Keep container closed.
Use only with adequate ventilation.
Wash thoroughly after handling.

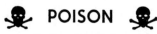 **POISON**

**Call a Physician**

**FIRST AID: If inhaled,** remove to fresh air. If not breathing give artificial respiration, preferably mouth-to-mouth. If breathing is difficult, give oxygen.

**In case of contact,** immediately flush eyes or skin with plenty of water for at least 15 minutes while removing contaminated clothing and shoes. Wash clothing before re-use. (Discard contaminated shoes.)

*Select applicable word or words in parentheses.

FIG. 22–3.—Typical label recommended for use with hazardous industrial chemicals spells out specific hazards and precautions to take.

*Courtesy American National Standards Institute.*

product liability lawsuits. This is especially true in chemical, drug, and food cases.

The program auditor must carefully examine the product instructions and labeling to be sure they conform to pertinent regulations and recent court decisions affecting a company's field of operations.

The basic rule, as stated in *Restatement of Torts* Second Series (see References), No. 388, is that "a manufacturer or supplier must exercise reasonable care to inform its consumers of a product's dangerous condition or the facts which make it likely to be dangerous if he knows or has reason to know that the product is likely to be dangerous for the use for which it is supplied and has no reason to believe that those for whose use the product is supplied will realize its dangerous condition."

Generally, a manufacturer has no duty to warn its consumers of the danger if such a danger is known. However, duty to warn and the adequacy of warning is a jury question and their interpretation of "duty" and "adequacy" will vary as a function of the circumstances of product use.

Usually, common dangers that are obvious do not require a warning; however, the manufacturer must exercise caution in these matters. For example, adults may be aware that furniture polish would be dangerous if swallowed but it does not follow that a child would also know this fact. Consequently, the manufacturer is required to instruct that such products be kept out of the reach of children.

There is a distinct difference between *warnings* and *directions*. In general, *directions* are designed to ensure effective usage of the product but say nothing about the dangers of misuse. *Warnings*, on the other hand, specifically refer to afe usage and must tell about the dangers of misuse. In general, the courts have tended to find that insufficient warning is the same as no warning. Therefore, a company must not only give clear and easily interpreted instructions on how to use the product, but must also give very clear and specific warnings of any inherent dangers or possible misuses which could result in injury. (See Figs. 22-2 and -3.)

The courts have consistently held that a manufacturer has a duty to warn with respect to any *reasonably foreseeable* use by a user or consumer and that for a warning to be considered adequate it must advise the user of the following:

The hazards involved in the product's use

How to avoid these hazards

The possible consequences resulting from a failure to heed warnings.

In labeling a product, it is impossible for the manufacturer to list all the things the product should not be used for, yet this lack could form the basis for a successful product liability suit. To minimize this possibility, labels should:

Have clear and specific instructions for using the product

Comply with all applicable standards and regulations (Department of Transportation, Federal Hazardous Substances Labeling Act, *American National Standard for the Precautionary Labeling of Hazardous Industrial Chemicals,* Z129.1)

Cover specific misuses

Be conspicuously placed

Be difficult to remove

Be as simple and easy to understand as is humanly possible. (One of the greatest problems in labeling is assuming a knowledge of the product's use on the part of the customer. When a product possesses inherently dangerous characteristics, the label must be worded in language appropriate to the degree of danger involved.)

Have suitable symbols (skull and crossbones, see Fig. 22-3 for example) and/or warnings in appropriate foreign languages if the product is known to be used in communities where English is not the mother tongue.

Instruction manuals that accompany the product should repeat hazard warnings as well as how the hazards may be lessened or avoided. In addition, instructions should be given on how to inspect the product upon receipt and how to assemble, install, and inspect it periodically. If the manuals include trouble-shooting hints, the dangers involved should be explained; that is, use of unauthorized parts, do not remove back panel, high voltage hazards, to name a few, as well as comments pertaining to the preventive maintenance program required.

Finally, the program auditor must determine whether or not sales brochures and product advertising should be reviewed by the engineering or design department to be sure the product's capabilities are depicted accurately and show only safe operating and maintenance procedures.

Conversely, the program auditor must also determine whether all warning labels, hazards, and/or instructions developed by the engineering or design department have been reviewed by the company's legal counsel to make sure that product users are receiving adequate instructions for use, warnings about potential product hazards, and instructions on proper product use and maintenance.

### Manufacturing department

After a reasonably safe and reliable product has been designed, the manufacturing department must turn the design specifications into a finished product. If this is not done satisfactorily, manufacturing errors could result in an unsafe and possibly unreliable product.

The manufacturing department can contribute to a company's overall PS&LP program in many ways. The most important are listed here. By evaluating each of the following (as it applies to a particular situation), the program auditor can effectively measure the manufacturing department's contribution.

• Motivate manufacturing employees by taking steps to make sure that each employee understands that he is making a vital contribution to a quality product.

• Instill each employee with pride in his work and in the company's product by:

    Using up-to-date manufacturing equipment

**635**

Keeping the plant's manufacturing capacity within bounds

Providing adequate room in which to work

Avoiding cramped working conditions

Keeping the work place clean and well lit

Implementing good equipment maintenance practices.

• Provide standardized foreman-supervised on-the-job training procedures.

• Implement zero defects or error-free performance or other error-elimination programs.

• Design a program or procedure to identify and eliminate all production trouble spots. (This should be accomplished in conjunction with the inspection and testing personnel of the quality control department.) (See Chapters 3 and 4 for techniques to reduce hazardous situations; quality control is discussed in the next section of this chapter.)

• Avoid unauthorized deviations from design specifications and work procedures.

• Participate in safety audits on new product designs. (This is often accomplished in the course of serving on the company's PS&LP committee, if one exists.)

Sometimes product specifications are not realistic for the machines and equipment that the company actually has in the shop. When this occurs, the production department must advise the engineering department that there is a problem. No attempt should be made to maintain cost or schedules, at the expense of deviating from the specifications, without consulting the engineering department. If deviations are necessary or unavoidable, they should be made only with the approval of the pertinent department.

**Recordkeeping.** Manufacturing records should be kept for the life of all the products and particularly for their critical parts or components. These records are absolutely necessary for the success of product recall or field-modification programs and for defense in product liability suits. Records on critical components should be complete enough to identify the batch or lot of raw material (or the supplier) from which they came or were made and the finished products in

which they were used.

**Discontinued products.** Another important area of manufacturing department exposure is the existence of discontinued products and the development of new products or product lines. If the company has discontinued products over the years or is likely to develop new products in the foreseeable future, consideration must be given to the reason these steps have been or will be taken. Some of these reasons might be as follows:

Lack of profit opportunity

Inability to acquire a competitive share of the market

Normal progression of technology

Unsolvable problems involving maintenance, service, warranty, engineering, and design

Innovative results of research and development

Progressive management policy that seeks new product lines internally or by acquisition.

The program auditor must evaluate these reasons and determine whether the existence of discontinued products (products on the market but no longer being manufactured) or the likelihood of new products being manufactured by the company will result in an undesirable product loss exposure situation.

## Service department

Most companies provide service functions to their customers, either directly through the dealer or distributor or by use of subcontractors to fulfill servicing contracts. Consequently, a company's product liability exposure may be significantly increased because the company may have extended its exposure beyond the confines of its manufacturing facility.

The PS&LP program auditor must carefully evaluate the company's service department controls in order to determine accurately not only the adequacy of these controls and their contribution to the company's PS&LP program activities, but also the adequacy of the company's use of the information feedback of its service department.

In many companies (depending upon the type of product), service department personnel are required to maintain close contact with customers. Consequently, they, more than any other employees, are familiar with the customers. They are most likely to hear any customer complaints eactions, and compliments to the company's products. They see product misuses and usually have some knowledge of incidents and accidents which have occurred. In fact, service department personnel are often the first to hear of product accidents.

In view of the service department's unique and advantageous position, the company should attempt to get the greatest PS&LP benefits to be derived from the service department by requiring their personnel to:

Use a check-off or report form when making a customer service call in order to determine if the company's product and safety devices are in good operating condition and are being used properly. Serial number, date serviced, reason for service, and specific service provided should be entered in the report. (When applicable, the company's service representative should have written comments on any unsafe conditions caused by customer misuse and/or use of the product. Also, any suggestions made to the customer to correct unsafe practices and conditions should be written into the report.)

Ask the customer to sign the report form. A copy of the report should then be forwarded to the company's legal department. A report of this type will prove useful in the event of an accident at a later date and any subsequent product liability claims involving the serviced product.

• Report customer complaints to the engineering or design or quality control departments.

Report product incidents and accidents to the company's PS&LP coordinator.

• Investigate product incidents and accidents at the request of the PS&LP coordinator.

• Participate in safety audits on new product designs. (This is very often accomplished in the course of serving on the company's PS&LP committee, if one exists.)

• Review formally all service contracts, if any, to make sure that they are realistic with respect to the company's being able to satisfactorily comply therewith.

• Increase the capability and efficiency of the service department by providing formal, documented training to all service personnel.

If the company does not service its products directly but subcontracts its service work to local contractors or uses its dealers to provide service, then the PS&LP program auditor must evaluate:

• Whether or not selected subcontractors are sufficiently familiar with the company's products to service them adequately

• Whether the company provides any service training to subcontractors, dealers, or distributors

• Whether the company's service instructions will provide sufficient guidance, in lieu of formal training, to anyone providing service for its products.

**Installation.** The company has the responsibility to inform its customers regarding the safe use, maintenance, service, installation, and other applications of its products. If a company's product is such that it is intended for installation by the customer, the company's installation instruction manual must be comprehensively prepared in a language that the typical customer will understand. If it is not intended that the customer perform his own installation work, he must be warned in no uncertain terms of the hazards of doing so and the consequences of improper installation.

In general, installation instructions should cover the following topics, if applicable.

Electrical connections

Siting of the equipment

Unpacking instructions

Procedures for safe handling

Safe assembly procedures

Warnings and cautions

Assembly diagrams

Initial startup procedures

Prestartup tests

Specification of items not furnished by the manufacturer but necessary for proper and safe installation (anchor bolts, brackets, fuses, etc.)

Applicable codes.

Warnings in the installation instructions, when necessary, should be conspicuous and complete. Any foreseeable dangers, even those that seem remote, should also be noted because the company may be held liable for injuries resulting from the installation of its products if adequate installation instructions have not been provided.

# 22—Product Safety and Liability Prevention

(See examples in Warning Labels, on pages 632-635.)

Installation agreements must be reviewed by the company to ensure that they are realistic in terms of the company's ability to fulfill them.

**Repair.** The repair function is oftentimes an overlooked source of product liability exposure. Consequently, the PS&LP program auditor must consider the following in any evaluation.

• Does the company repair its own products and also others? If so, the company has considerably increased its product liability exposure. This is particularly true when repairing the products of others, because it may be accepting the other manufacturer's product liability exposure as a function of the type and quality of repair performed.

• Where does the company perform its repair work? In its own shop or at the customer's location?

• Does the company use its dealers/distributors to repair its products? If so, are dealers/distributors adequately trained to perform satisfactorily, either by the company or by virtue of experience?

• Does the company prepare and retain detailed product repair records?

• Does the company provide a repair warranty? If so, it should be examined to determine whether it is realistic and what, if any, liability the company has incurred therefrom.

**Maintenance.** Great care should go into developing manuals pertaining to maintenance, installation, assembly, operation, and parts. The maintenance manual should clearly describe procedures for reducing wear and tear on the product, and should indicate how often parts should be inspected, serviced, or replaced. The maintenance manual should cite the product's limitations, warn of hazards that may be encountered during disassembly and maintenance, and stress the danger of not following the printed manual procedures. The consequences of product misuse or failure to maintain the product should be emphasized.

To guard against misstatements regarding function, use, maintenance, installation, etc., the company should have all of its manuals reviewed by its legal staff before they are published.

As in the case of service, installation, and repair, if the company uses subcontractors, dealers, or distributors to provide product maintenance service to its customers, their training and capability to provide this service must be evaluated. In addition, if the company has maintenance contracts, they must be reviewed to make sure that they are realistic in terms of the company's ability to fulfill them.

## Legal department

The legal department in any organization should play a significant role in both the prevention and defense of product liability cases. Too often, companies only use their legal department in those situations when product safety problems or product liability litigation is imminent. They very often fail to recognize the importance of having legal personnel become involved in the day-to-day aspects of product safety and liability prevention.

The legal department should be assigned the following responsibilities in order to maximize its contribution to the company's PS&LP program activities.

**Legal advisors.** Legal personnel should act as legal advisors to the PS&LP coordinator. As such they are responsible for formally advising the company's key management personnel, for example, on the impact upon the company of the current legal situation pertinent to:

The theory of negligence

The theory of strict liability

Foreseeable uses and misuses of the company's products

Express and implied warranties

Appropriate record retention activities

Recent legal decisions and current legal trends affecting the company's products, including product situations encountered by and product losses incurred by competitors.

**Legal review for potential liability.** The company's legal personnel should review all product related literature prior to its release to make sure that it is reasonable, accurately describes the product, and does not incur any undesired or unanticiapted legal liability as a result of its use. Examples are:

**638**

Advertising and product sales brochures

Instruction manuals (including warning labels, decals, and the like)

Disclaimers

Hold-harmless agreements

Warranties/guarantees

Vendors' endorsements

Any other product-related contractual obligations incurred by the company.

**Legal coordination.** The company's legal personnel should be capable of providing product-related legal coordination of:

• All product accident investigations including working with the insurance carrier. (Depending upon the company, this may be the responsibility of the insurance department.)

• All product claims defenses (including acquisition of both internal and external expert witnesses).

The program auditor should be prepared to evaluate the adequacy of the legal department's contribution to the company's PS&LP program, based upon the above criteria.

## Marketing department

Unfortunately, after a "reasonably" safe product has been designed and manufactured, product claims may be unnecessarily incurred by the manner in which the product was represented to customers and users. Customers often must rely on the company's sales personnel, advertising and sales brochures, and operating, service, and maintenance instructions for their knowledge of the product's capabilities and hazards.

Consequently, if the customer is led to believe that the product has capabilities it does not possess or if the instructions do not adequately warn of the product's hazards, an injured customer may have legal cause for action where none existed before. Therefore, the PS&LP program auditor must review the company's advertising and sales materials and evaluate whether:

They are clear and accurate

They overstate the product's capabilities

They encourage the customer to believe the product has uses for which it was not designed or intended

The product can safely do all that the company's advertising and sales material says it can

Only safe operating procedures are depicted

The company's product is illustrated only with safety devices in place

They have been reviewed and approved by the engineering or design and legal departments with regard to accuracy and potential legal liability exposures

The use of broad, absolute descriptive terms, such as "moisture-proof," "absolutely safe," "tamper-proof," "completely nontoxic," and the like, may very often be legally interpreted as an unjustified overstatement of a product's capabilities and may lead to an unwarranted sense of assurance on the part of the product user. Instead, terms such as *moisture-resistant, tamper-resistant,* and *nontoxic* are more appropriate for use in sales and advertising literature because they more clearly define the product's actual capabilities. Furthermore, these are terms that can be defended more easily in a court of law, if the need arises. The company should not advertise "safety" components or attributes in its products; instead, it should be stated that the particular component or attribute is intended to reduce, control, or minimize the hazard involved in the use of the product.

Warranties and disclaimers developed by the company must also be reviewed by the program auditor to determine whether they are:

Reasonable and practical for the uses intended

Included with each of the company's products

Clear and concise

Prominently displayed and easily recognizable by the customer or product user

Thoroughly reviewed by the company's legal department or legal counsel.

Disclaimers of liability should never be considered as a substitute for proper product design. Further, there are two important limitations to all disclaimers:

1. If a disclaimer is "unconscionable" (unreasonable, unfair, impractical, unscrupulous, etc.), no court will enforce it.

2. Some federal statutes impose criminal liability on a seller for failure to give warning of known hazards, regardless of any effort to disclaim liability.

Another important duty of the marketing department that must be verified by the program auditor is the retention (for the life of the product) of sales and distribution records that can be used to identify purchasers. These records are essential if product recall or field-modification programs are to have any chance of success. In addition, these records should indicate, whenever possible, the use to which the company's products will be put, particularly when the company is selling to subcontractors or assemblers.

The company must also be able to verify that its sales personnel and dealers have been instructed to accurately describe the capabilities of the products they are selling or distributing and thus avoid incurring undesired implied and/or expressed warranties; for example, sales personnel must be instructed not to exaggerate the capabilities of the company's products.

The PS&LP program auditor must review the manner in which the company's products are marketed. In other words, are they distributed and sold through dealers, direct sales, or manufacturing representatives, or other marketing channels? This review must be made in order to evaluate properly whether or not the company's advertising and sales literature, warranties and disclaimers, sales record retention activities, and advertising sales personnel training procedures are effective as a function of the type of product marketing techniques used by the company.

Finally, the program auditor must very accurately determine whether the company's marketing activities include the leasing or renting of its products to dealers, distributors, contractors, or customers. If so, it must be recognized that it is generally quite difficult for a company to maintain satisfactory control over the maintenance and repair procedures used in conjunction with leased or rented products unless it carefully plans to do so. Further, the quality of a company's maintenance, service, repair, and operating instructions becomes more significant than it would normally. Not only does a company's product liability exposure increase greatly because of the added difficulty in maintaining control over maintenance and repair procedures, but it is also extremely difficult to defend a product-related loss resulting from a product lease or rental situation unless the company can prove that the lessee or renter was adequately informed as to how to maintain, repair, use, and service the product being leased or rented.

## Purchasing department

Although some companies are not large enough to have a formal purchasing department, every company has someone responsible for acquiring the raw materials and components needed for the manufacture of the product.

This is a very significant activity with respect to the company's product liability potential. Consequently, the PS&LP program auditor must give careful consideration to the company's purchasing activities and determine whether or not the company is performing acceptably in this area.

For instance, the purchasing department or agent should:

• Become familiar with all material specifications set by the engineering, design, and manufacturing departments.

• Always purchase quality raw materials, parts, and components that meet the specifications set by the cognizant departments.

• Evaluate, in conjunction with the company's quality control department, the capabilities and reliability of suppliers, using vendor rating systems, and compile a list of approved suppliers.

• Set up and comply with mutually agreed upon raw material delivery schedules in conjunction with material specifications prescribed by the engineering or design departments.

• Refrain from any deviation from material specifications without the written permission of the engineering or design departments.

• Obtain raw material and component lab reports, mill certifications, certificates of manufacture, and other pertinent documents from suppliers.

• Incorporate, whenever possible, appropriately worded hold-harmless agreements (developed in concert with the company's legal department or counsel) into purchase orders to suppliers. In addition, hold-harmless agreements should not be accepted from suppliers or customers, unless approved by the legal department.

• Refrain from providing vendor's endorsements to anyone associated with the company unless absolutely necessary to the maintenance of a ormal business environment. (This restriction also applies to anyone else representing the company.)

Determine whether or not the company is engaged in the importing of parts, components, or products. If so, this may represent an uncontrollable exposure. When the foreign supplier does not have a United States affiliation, the company, in the case of a products liability loss, may be considered the manufacturer rather than the middleman, thus greatly increasing the company's potential exposure.

The documentation associated with the above purchasing responsibilities is of critical importance. However, in a loss situation, even with the required documentation, the company may still be in an undesirable position from a product-liability point of view.

## Personnel department

The job qualifications and work attitudes of the company's employees have a considerable influence on the quality of its products. Employees who lack proper job skills or who are not interested in their work greatly increase the possibility of defective products.

It is essential that the company's personnel department be diligent (a) in the selecting, training, and placement of new and transferred employees, and (b) that they continually seek to upgrade the morale and performance goals of those already employed.

The responsibilities assigned to the company's personnel department must be evaluated by the PS&LP program auditor to determine whether they are being performed satisfactorily. Among the responsibilities that may be assigned to the personnel department (depending on the individual company) are the following:

- Assisting in the various departments within the company's operation in setting up job classifications by (a) instituting job analyses (see discussions in Chapter 5 and Chapter 9), and (b) establishing specifications for each position level

- Actively screening prospective employees to determine their suitability for available positions

- Developing an internal employee promotion procedure

- Assisting in the development of educational and training programs to upgrade employee skills and subsequently improve employee performance

- Encouraging employees to seek company-reimbursed outside training or certificated courses, where appropriate

- Assisting in the development of employee motivational programs (zero defects, for example) in order to instill the individual employee with pride in his work, thus reducing work errors

- Instilling a sense of employment stability within the company by hiring and promoting according to carefully prepared job specifications.

With regard to personnel turnover, the program auditor should be aware of several possible situations.

If the company's lower-level employee turnover rate is excessive (more than 20 percent per year), this may indicate that the nature of the work involved is highly seasonal, the company's business situation has become very cyclical, i.e., good times—hire, bad times—fire, or, for some reason, employee morale is low and working conditions are undesirable.

Under any of these circumstances, the company's employee-selection procedure is unlikely to be satisfactory because of the constant need for lower-level personnel. Consequently, the one problem (working conditions) contributes to the magnitude of a second problem (hiring practices) and vice versa.

If there is an unusual turnover (in excess of 10 percent per year) in the company's medium- to high-level personnel, this may be indicative of a recent reorganization, recent takeover, impending takeover, poor business position, etc., with all the attendant turmoil, dissension, and possible lack of attention to, or concern for, required PS&LP activities.

If a union contract is due for renegotiation, the company's past labor-negotiating experience should be evaluated.

## Insurance department

The company's insurance department or specialist is too often considered only as the department which buys insurance and reports claims to the insurance company. In reality, because of its experience in handling product claims, the insurance department usually has a background of valuable knowledge and experience with respect to the factors that generate product liability lawsuits. Consequently, the insurance department should be used as an information clearing house by the company in conjunction with the PS&LP program coordinator.

The program auditor should be aware of the ways in which the insurance department can assist the company in the development and implementation of the PS&LP program activities. These various ways include:

• The capability to evaluate the company's product liability situation and make an intelligent selection and acquisition of product liability insurance coverage that will adequately protect the company's business interests. (Product liability is one of the fastest growing areas of risk in business and industry today. Therefore, the insurance department should have a formal program for periodically reviewing and adjusting the company's product liability policy coverage.

• The ability to prepare cost studies for the PS&LP program auditor and company management, which define the impact of product liability losses on profits. This information should be incorporated into a cost allocation system so the product liability losses can be recorded and tallied directly against the responsible department or group.

• Using the expertise of the insurance carrier.

Because of its knowledge of past accidents, claims, handling procedures, policy provisions, and limits, the insurance department should participate with the program coordinator in the analysis of potential product liability exposure from existing products, new products, and products from recently acquired or to-be-acquired companies. In addition, the department should be included in the review of all sales and advertising literature before it is released.

The insurance department usually reports liability claims to the insurance carrier as well as coordinates any investigation with the carrier. There are occasions when the insurance department will coordinate the legal defense (if one is necessary), between the legal department and insurance carrier. Depending upon the company, the legal department may perform these functions instead.

### Safety department

The safety professional generally plays an important role in a company's PS&LP program activities as described near the beginning of the chapter.

### Public relations department

Although a public relations department, like the safety department, generally plays a smaller role in a company's PS&LP program activities than many of the other departments, the program auditor should not overlook it in the overall evaluation of a company's PS&LP program.

Product accidents, product recalls, or product field-modification programs may not go entirely unnoticed by the news media and may require statements by the company for publication. If these statements are skillfully prepared from a public relations standpoint, they may help prevent unfavorable publicity. In fact, the correct handling of publicity on product accidents, product recall, or product field-modification programs can be skillfully used by the public relations department to display to the public the company's ostensibly diligent efforts to design, manufacture, and sell a safe, reliable product.

The public relations department should also be capable of generating favorable product-related publicity for media consumption in those instances wherein the company has legitimately incorporated advances in the state-of-the-art of product safety into its products.

### Quality Control and Testing Program

Quality control refers generally to action taken throughout manufacturing to detect and prevent product deficiencies and product hazards. Because of the extensive discussion of this subject that follows, quality control is being handled as a separate subject, even though it is one of the company departments that should be checked out by the program auditor.

The term *quality control* refers broadly to that function of company's management where calculated actions are taken to assure that manufactured, assembled, fabricated, etc., products conform to design or engineering requirements. At one time, the terms "quality control" and "statistical quality control" were considered synonymous because statistical techniques were considered to be the major tools of quality conol. Over the years quality control has taken on a larger meaning to include whatever actions are necessary to assure that products conform to design and other requirements and achieve customer acceptance and satisfaction.

Before discussing the fundamentals of quality control and their application to the evaluation of a company's quality control activities, it must be pointed out that quality control policy, department organization, function, and responsibility will vary according to a company's size, management policy and organization, type of product, plant location(s), number of plants, economic resources, and other variables.

## Evaluating the system

When evaluating the company's quality control system, the important points to determine are:

**Is the quality control system adequate** to carry out the company's quality objectives? The program auditor must determine if the company's quality control system is satisfactory as a function of the company's products and their attendant exposures. The lack of one or more functions or an incomplete function does not necessarily mean that the system is inadequate. A necessary function may be included as part of a subsequent function or may not be required because of the type of product, manufacturing process, company size, etc.

**Does the system function as planned?** To answer this question, the program auditor must go beyond the quality control manual and review the actual implementation or functioning of the system.

When performing an audit, the PS&LP program auditor must ask: How? Why? When? Where? What? Who? Then, follow through with "Explain how it works." "Let's see examples." "Show me the records."

Asking these questions may indicate that the company has instituted a quality control program, but it does not prove, however, that the system has actually been installed throughout the plant, nor that it is functioning as planned.

The program auditor must see evidence of the implementation and functioning of the system. To get a true picture of the system, the system's paper work, procedures, instructions, and records must be reviewed and specific items followed

---

### FUNCTIONS OF A COMPREHENSIVE QUALITY CONTROL/ASSURANCE PROGRAM

The basic quality control/assurance functions that must be evaluated by the PS&LP program auditor are as follows:

Organization and manuals

Engineering/product design coordination

Evaluation and control of suppliers/vendors

Evaluation of manufacturing (in-process and final assembly) quality

Evaluation of special process control

Evaluation of measuring equipment calibration system

Sample inspection evaluation

Evaluation of nonconforming material procedures

Evaluation of material status/storage system

Evaluation of error analysis and corrective action system

Evaluation of product preservation, packaging, and shipping procedures

Evaluation of record retention system

Evaluation of training procedures

Summary of quality control system evaluation

Evaluation of testing system.

Fig. 22-4.

---

through the complete program. (See Fig. 22-4.)

The program auditor should spend some time with the QC shop personnel, if possible. These individuals can expound on the "cons" as well as the "pros" of the system, thus providing information that is relevant to the system's weaknesses not otherwise obtainable.

## Manuals

One of the most important requirements for effective operation of a quality control program is positive interest and concern, which starts at the

**643**

top level of management. In most instances, quality control responsibilities must be delegated, and the assignment of responsibility and authority should be clearly defined throughout all levels of management, supervision, and operation.

There should be a quality control manual, the form and content of which will vary according to a company's requirements. The manual is usually divided into two sections: policy and procedures.

- Policy:

States company quality control policy and objectives

Establishes organizational responsibilities

Establishes systems for implementing quality control policy

- Procedures:

States operational responsibilities

Gives detailed operating instructions.

The policy section of the manual is general in nature, while the procedures section contains the daily detailed operations of the quality control department.

## Engineering and product design coordination

The quality control department can, by looking at things from a different viewpoint, assist the engineering or design department in its research, development, design, and specifications functions.

Quality control normally is not involved in engineering or design or research unless it has accumulated beneficial data. Quality control assists by performing such functions as inspection testing, recording, maintenance, equipment calibration, and data accumulation.

The major areas where quality control and engineering or design are closely related are:

- *Design review.* Review of engineering design to verify that the product can be produced and inspected from data given, that data given cannot be misunderstood or misinterpreted, and that tolerances are realistic for part to properly function.

- *Specification review.* Review of specifications to verify that data given is complete, usable, and cannot be misunderstood or misinterpreted, and

that tolerances, if applicable, are realistic. While performing this review, quality control should introduce necessary quality control requirements.

- *Change-control system.* A company producing a product must have a change-control system because nothing remains unchanged indefinitely. Regardless of who initiates the change, quality control must verify that it has been incorporated as specified.

## Evaluation and control of suppliers

It is just as important to control the quality of purchased materials and services as it is to establish and enforce such controls internally. The degree and extent of the quality controls established for a supplier will depend on the complexity and quantity of the supplier's product and its quality history. The most effective requirement is to choose suppliers who can maintain adequate quality. Another vital factor is open, active, and adequate flow of information between the company and its suppliers.

The control of suppliers and verification of procedures used to assure that the purchased raw materials, parts, assemblies, services, and other items conform to predetermined criteria can be done in several ways. The typical system includes

**Supplier planning.** It is vital to furnish suppliers with detailed requirements to avoid misunderstanding or misinterpretation. The three areas involved in this planning are:

- *Purchasing instructions.* Instructions to the purchasing department must include configuration data to which the item must be made, quality requirements to which the supplier must conform, and general data considering supplier control (those manufacturing, processing, and servicing suppliers authorized by quality control to perform work).

- *Supplier instructions.* The purchasing department must pass along to the supplier the configuration data, quality requirements, and supplier control data it receives from quality control.

- *Inspection instructions.* The instructions must indicate what inspection is to be made at the source and at what stage, and what inspection should be made by the receiving inspection personnel.

**Supplier surveillance.** The object of surveillance is to determine which suppliers consistently produce quality work and reward them with prompt payment and new orders. The supplier with an effective quality control system permits the company to reduce or eliminate its inspection. The various methods of maintaining surveillance are:

• *Quality control surveys.* Before placing purchase orders, quality control personnel should survey the manufacturing facilities to determine the adequacy of the supplier's quality control system.

• *Engineering-approved sources.* Based on successful test data, engineering will specify a particular product from a specific source and prohibit the substitution of a similar ("or equal") product from another source.

• *Source and receiving inspection.* Results of inspection by source or receiving inspection personnel immediately indicates the effectiveness of the supplier's quality control system.

• *Resident representatives.* Because of a large volume of orders placed with one supplier, some companies will keep a representative at the supplier's plant to monitor the quality control system.

• *Performance records.* The company accumulates data from source and receiving inspection areas to measure the effectiveness of the supplier's quality control system over a specified time period.

**Source and receiving inspection.** An inspection of the submitted product is made to determine whether or not it conforms to established requirements.

**Records.** Records should relate to supplier quality, including planning instructions, supplier surveillance data, and inspection results.

## Manufacturing (in-process and final assembly) quality

Quality control of items produced "in plant" is accomplished by planning, inspection, process control, and equipment calibration. (The latter two functions will be discussed in separate sections because they assure that items produced conform to the predetermined criteria.)

**Manufacturing planning.** Planning in advance of production assures uniformity of product and manufacturing instructions. It normally is a joint effort of the manufacturing department and quality control department. The manufacturing personnel initiate the internal paperwork, including all data necessary to produce the product. Quality control personnel review the paperwork to confirm that the data conforms to established parameters, and includes quality requirements.

**Manufacturing work instructions.** All work affecting quality should be supported by documented "how to" work instructions appropriate to the nature of the work, the situation under which the work is to be done, and the skill level of the personnel doing the work. Each instruction must also include quantitative and qualitative means for determining that each operation has been done satisfactorily. The depth of detail will depend upon the skill level of the worker and upon the complexity of the task.

The instructions to production personnel should specify in detail the steps necessary to produce the products.

**Inspection instructions.** Instructions must be given to inspection personnel to assist them in making sure that products conform to design parameters.

**Manufacturing inspection.** The inspection of the product determines whether or not it conforms to established requirements. It usually includes one or more of the following general methods:

Visual inspection
Dimensional inspection
Hardness testing
Functional testing (See Fig. 22–5.)
Nondestructive testing (NDT)
Chemical/metallurgical testing.

When inspection of a product is conducted on an in-process basis and not upon completion of all operations, the inspection must not be conducted until it has been determined that all previous inspections have been made as required and the product up to this point is acceptable.

**Records.** Records of the manufacturing operations, including incoming materials, assemblies or

```
┌─────────────────────────────────────────┐
│            TESTING CATEGORIES            │
│                                          │
│  Acceptance testing                      │
│     Raw materials                        │
│     Intermediate products                │
│     Discrete item components             │
│                                          │
│  Conformance testing                     │
│     Dimensions                           │
│     Physical and chemical characteristics│
│                                          │
│  Control testing                         │
│     Tools                                │
│     Jigs and fixtures                    │
│     Machinery                            │
│     Processes                            │
│     Test equipment                       │
│                                          │
│  Assurance testing                       │
│     Processes                            │
│     Products                             │
│                                          │
│  Performance testing                     │
│     Life tests                           │
│     Endurance tests                      │
│     Guarantee and warranty tests         │
│     Strength of materials tests          │
│     Comparison tests                     │
│     Overstress tests                     │
└─────────────────────────────────────────┘
```

Fig. 22–5.

processes, and final inspection results, should be maintained.

### Special process control

Processes used by manufacturing to change the physical, mechanical, chemical, or dimensional characteristics to make a product include, but are not limited to, the following:

Heat treating

Plating

Fusion welding

Stamping and forming

Batch mixing

Chemical mixing

Adhesive bonding.

Because processes greatly influence the fitness for use of the completed product, it is imperative that they be positively, yet economically controlled. A hundred-percent inspection is not feasible because it might require destructive testing to determine conformance. The processes, therefore, require controls that monitor the processes and assure that similarly processed items will be of the desired quality.

Processes are controlled as follows:

• Quality control reviews and approves the manufacturing procedures, detailed instructions, setup procedures, and controls.

• Quality control conducts audits periodically to verify that manufacturing is processing the work in accordance with established procedure.

• Quality control uses various methods to control the processes to assure that completed products comply with processing end requirements.

### Calibration of measuring equipment

Measuring and process control equipment and instruments used to assure that manufactured products and processes conform to specified requirements must be calibrated periodically. In other words, any equipment used, either directly or indirectly, to measure, control, or record should be calibrated against certified standards so that the equipment may be adjusted, replaced, or repaired before it becomes inaccurate.

Some typical measuring devices are:

| | |
|---|---|
| Micrometers | Pressure-measuring devices |
| Calipers | Temperature gages |
| Surface plates | Voltmeters |
| Hardness testers | Ammeters |
| Tensile testers | Recording instruments |
| Level indicators | Electronic gages. |

Equipment subject to periodic calibration should include equipment used by quality control personnel, devices used by manufacturing personnel in controlling an operation, and personally owned equipment where personnel provide their own measuring equipment.

### Sample inspection evaluation

A sample inspection is used by quality control to ascertain the quality of a lot without inspecting all items in the lot. It can be very beneficial if used correctly, but the converse is true if it is not used correctly.

Even when a hundred-percent inspection is performed under the most favorable conditions, it is only 85-90 percent effective because of human nd other error. A sampling inspection is not necessarily one hundred percent effective, but it an approach that level. The sampling disadvantage, which is far outweighed by its advantages, is hat occasionally the sample gathering procedure or a lot does not give a true picture of the lot quality—good lots can be rejected or bad lots can be accepted. The goal, however, is to make the acceptance of good lots much more likely than he acceptance of bad lots.

The level of quality desired in a sampling plan s normally expressed as an *AQL value* (acceptable quality level) and also referred to as the *quality index*. The standard definition of AQL is *a nominal value expressed in terms of percent defective or defects per hundred units, whichever s applicable.*

The most widely used standard sampling tables are those issued by the U.S. Government and contained in Military Standard, Mil-Std-105, 'Sampling Procedures and Tables for Inspection by Attributes."°

Sampling records, showing, at least part number, lot quantity, sample size, AQL value, and inspection results, should be maintained.

## Nonconforming material procedures

The term *nonconforming material* is usually applied to products that are rejected because they do not meet established requirements. Raw material, parts, components, subassemblies, and assemblies become nonconforming material at whatever manufacturing stage they become discrepant.

The company should have a system to control nonconforming material. It should include the following:

• *Identification.* The status of all nonconforming material must be immediately identified and clearly labeled with a tag, form, or other marking so that it is readily seen. A nonconforming material record showing the discrepancies in detail should be kept.

• *Segregation.* After identification, all nonconforming material should be separated from acceptable material and placed in a segregated area pending disposition. When nonconforming material cannot practically be moved to the segregated area, only the nonconforming material record should be sent to that area.

• *Disposition.* Disposition of nonconforming material must be made by authorized personnel. As a minimum, the engineering or design department and quality control department representatives usually are authorized. In some instances, other department representatives may be authorized to act in conjunction with the authorized engineering or design and quality control personnel, or the customer may specify that disposition of nonconforming material must have his approval.

• *Reinspection.* Nonconforming material that has been marked for rework or repair must be inspected afterwards to assure that it conforms to both the disposition and original parameters before being accepted.

• *Customer notification.* The system for handling nonconforming material must include procedures for submitting, when required, the discrepant material and proposed disposition to the customer for approval. The customer may or may not approve the disposition.

• *Supplier reporting.* The nonconforming material system must include procedures for subcontractors to report nonconforming material to the company. The company will decide on the disposition of the material and send the supplier a copy of its report.

• *Records.* Records of all nonconforming discrepancies, dispositions, and results of reinspection must be maintained.

## Material status and storage

The company must have a tangible means of knowing at all times whether a product (or lot) has not been inspected, has been inspected and approved, or has been inspected and rejected. All raw materials, components, subassemblies, assemblies, and end products should bear identification of process, inspection, and test status.

The material storage function involves the temporary holding of raw materials and recently purchased or in-process parts and assemblies. Stores personnel must have a control system that tells the *status* and the *condition* of stored raw materials, components, and products at all times.

The program auditor must evaluate the effec-

---

° Military Standards are available through the Regional Offices of the U.S. General Services Administration.

tiveness of the controls used by the company to make sure that the stock on hand is the stock ordered, and that the system used to identify the materials in the storeroom is adequate.

The program auditor should also verify that all stock is segregated into specific areas such as "Material awaiting receiving inspection or test sample results," "Accepted materials," and "Rejected materials." The program auditor should also determine which employees are authorized to withdraw material and he should specifically note whether any rejected material is likely to get into the production cycle at this point.

All stored material should be controlled by a material identification system comprised of color coding, tagging, or material stamping. When material is either lying on the ground, in the aisles, in the wrong racks, or in a congested condition, there is a strong likelihood that inadequate control and identification procedures are being used.

## Error analysis and corrective action systems

The error analysis and corrective action system is a followup of the nonconforming material system. The objective of this system is to use the discrepancies reported in the nonconforming material system to perform the following:

Analyze manufacturing errors

Initiate corrective action requests to the party responsible for the errors, evaluate responses, and determine the effectiveness of the action taken

Analyze manufacturing rejection rate and report to management the dollar losses due to scrappage, rework/repair, and reinspection costs.

The company must be aggressive in the pursuit of its problems and in establishing permanent corrective actions if it is to achieve a high level of product quality.

## Product preservation, packaging, and shipping

When a completed product is released to a customer, quality control is responsible for the following:

The product conforms to the purchase order requirements

The product is properly preserved.

The product is adequately packaged to prevent shipping or handling damage.

Warnings and required special instructions are on the package

Shipping papers, parts lists, manuals, warranty certification, and other required data are included in the shipment.

Records of products shipped, identification data if any, to whom shipped, and other pertinent data are maintained.

## Recordkeeping systems

Records are the backbone of a quality control program because they reflect the history of the product. Good records indicate that the company's quality control system is functioning as planned, substantiate that a product was inspected, and often provide the actual inspection findings. To repeat what has been said before—records are vital in the defense of a product liability lawsuit.

Good quality control records also contribute to product traceability and should include:

Lists of raw materials from which products are produced

Inspection results for purchased and manufactured products

Inspection results from each inspection station

Special processes control data

Calibration data

Sample inspection data

Nonconforming material data

Error analysis and corrective action data

Shipping data.

These records should be stored in metal cabinets in a low hazard area for the life of the product.

## Evaluation of training procedures

The program auditor must evaluate the type and quality of training offered to quality control department personnel. General checkpoints are listed here:

- Internal or external
    Supervisor/management led

On site

Union-sponsored

Incentive to train

Mandatory or voluntary training requirement

Reimbursement program for externally sponsored courses

Recordkeeping

Curricula

Attendees

Dates of attendance.

## Quality control system evaluation

This section shows a great many ways in which the contribution of the company's quality control program to its overall PS&LP program can be measured by the program auditor. Program details are discussed later in this chapter. The most important of these contributions would include:

Assistance in the production of quality products while also acting as an effective check against defective products leaving the company's facility. (To be effective, the quality control activity must have authority to prevent the unapproved use and distribution of raw materials and/or finished products that do not meet prescribed quality control standards.)

Preparation of cost studies on scrap, repair, and defective products and components.

Preparation and use of a quality control program manual appropriate for the needs of the company.

Assignment of special quality requirements for critical parts.

Existence of a program or procedures designed to identify and eliminate all production trouble spots. This should be accomplished in conjunction with manufacturing personnel.

Working with the engineering or design department to set minimum acceptable product standards of quality.

The independence and status of the company's QC department/group/activity. (The QC department should report at the same level as the manufacturing, engineering or design, and marketing departments and should operate on a budget that is its own. The head of the company's QC activity should participate in top management meetings and decision making.)

• Maintenance of quality control records for the life of the company's product, particularly for critical parts and components.

• Participation in safety audits on new product designs. (This is very often accomplished in the course of serving on the company's PS&LP committee, if one exists.)

• Existence of a means of segregating and controlling rejected parts, materials, components and products.

• Existence and supervision of a National Bureau of Standards-based program for the calibration of test instruments to required accuracy.

### Evaluation of testing program

It is the function of the Quality Control Department, using a number of internal testing procedures, to assure that desired product quality levels are achieved and maintained, and that scrap and rework are kept to a minimum by the manufacturing department. External testing procedures using the services of independent testing laboratories will be treated separately in a subsequent section.

When setting up a satisfactory testing program, the company must determine the types of testing required as a function of the product(s) involved. Types of testing that can be selected appear in the categories shown in Fig. 22–5.

**Acceptance and conformance.** The primary interest is in whether or not the products or components being tested meet given specifications.

• *Control testing.* The interest is in whether the methods, machines, equipment or processes being used by the company are adequate to perform their intended objectives.

• *Assurance testing.* The concern is with the quality (usually expressed as a percentage) of product output which fully meets the company's advertised specifications or marketing claims.

• *Performance testing.* It is necessary for the company to determine what the products begin tested will actually do as compared with a specification, a desired level of performance, or some alternative product.

The company is usually most active or involved in the acceptance, conformance, and performance testing areas. In a satisfactory testing environment, the PS&LP program auditor should see the following evidences of test planning:

The names of the tests

Statements of the test purposes and objectives

Descriptions of the sample sizes required, if appropriate

Descriptions of the sampling methods to be used, if appropriate

Descriptions of any special test sample preparation required

Specifications for the test equipment and ancillary materials needed

Definition of the details of the test methods to be employed

Definition of the measurements to be made and the data to be recorded

Specifications for the methods of data analysis to be utilized

Specifications for test reporting procedures and formats

Specifications for the actions to be taken depending upon any of several outcomes—pass, fail, or indeterminate.

The company *must* have a plan of action to implement test results. If the company's testing activities are to be worth anything, management must take action based upon the results of the product tests.

Once a product has been manufactured, the company should be interested in testing the product's actual performance characteristics against design objectives, and, for product safety and liability prevention considerations, against advertising and sales claims.

Further, under guarantee or warranty policies, the company should also be interested in estimating the percentage of products that will probably fail prior to the expiration of the guarantee or warranty period in order to estimate the probable costs of such policies.

Any company should have an awareness of and be able to effectively use simple testing concepts to enhance product performance and safety. This

should subsequently reduce the company's potential products liability exposure.

## Functional Activity Audits

Most of the remainder of this chapter is devoted to a discussion of three interrelated activities recordkeeping, field-information systems, and independent testing. These important activities are referred to as "functional" to differentiate them from the "departmental" categorization previously used (design, quality control, insurance, and the others).

The term "functional" implies that these are activities that, if properly accomplished (from PS&LP program standpoint), must be performed by several or possibly all of the departments within a company, rather than just one department.

### Recordkeeping

In today's products liability environment, company must not only manufacture and market safe, reliable products, but it must also be able to prove in court, if the need arises, that the products it manufactures are safe.

Complete, accurate records can be extremely convincing in a court of law. Consequently records should be retained pertinent to all phases of a company's manufacturing, distributing, importing, etc., activities, from the procurement of raw materials and components, through production and testing, to the marketing and distribution of the finished products.

In addition to their usefulness in demonstrating to courts and juries that a company manufactures safe, reliable products, comprehensive PS&LP program records also permit a company to readily identify and locate products that its data collection and analysis system indicates may have reached the customer in a defective condition. Should a product recall or field-modification program become necessary, comprehensive PS&LP program records can result in successful implementation.

There are two factors which can significantly affect the form and content (types and quantity of records retained, period of retention, etc.) of company's recordkeeping program.

**Federal regulations.** A company should be aware of federal regulations that will have an effect on recordkeeping requirements.

Some of the more important federal regula-ons that a company must consider in the development of an appropriate PS&LP recordkeeping system are:

Consumer Product Safety Act (PL 92-573)
Federal Hazardous Substances Act (15 USC 1261)
Federal Food, Drug and Cosmetic Act (21 USC 321)
Poison Prevention Packaging Act (PL 91-601)
Occupational Safety and Health Act (PL 91-596)
Child Protection and Toy Act (PL 91-113)
Magnuson-Moss Warranty-Federal Trade Commission Improvement Act (PL 93-637).

Manufacturers, distributors, importers, and retailers of products must establish and maintain such records and reports as may be prescribed by pertinent federal regulations for the purpose of implementing or determining compliance to them. For example, if the CPSC (Consumer Product Safety Commission) judges a product as being hazardous, a company may be ordered to provide public notice of the hazard. In addition, the company may be ordered to take remedial action, such as repair, modification, or replacement, and in extreme cases, conduct a complete product recall. Consequently, a company's recordkeeping system must be comprehensive enough to enable it to implement effectively whatever remedial action either it or a federal regulatory agency deems appropriate.

### Internal PS&LP program requirements

A company must maintain all pertinent information related to the design, manufacture, marketing, testing, and sales of its products. Of particular value are those records that document design decisions, since faulty design is an almost universal allegation in product liability lawsuits. It is an especially effective defense to be able to introduce evidence proving that a certain design or material was chosen with the safety of the consumer in mind. Also, records of why certain production techniques were chosen, such as having a part forged rather than cast, should be retained. Records can also establish the testing to which a product was subjected and the reasons for modifications and improvements. When a hazard cannot be eliminated, a company's records should show conclusively why it cannot.

All tests, analyses, quality control procedures, lot numbers, serial numbers, and shipping procedures must be recorded and retained on file for the life of the product plus approximately ten years. (This is the probable maximum statute of limitations time period allowed in conjunction with proposed tort reform statutes.)

All of the aforementioned requirements are directed towards documenting the fact that a company is genuinely concerned with the quality of its products and the safety of those who ultimately use them.

In the legal course of product liability cases, both sides employ the "discovery" process. Thus, the plaintiff's attorney may search the defendant's records for evidence; the "Fifth Amendment" does not apply to corporations. On the other side, a company's defense attorney will collect all evidence of the accident and use his client's file of documents and thus, hopefully, will be able to substantiate inconsistencies in the alleged chain of causation.

Both sides present their cases through testimony by witnesses and experts. An important factor in the verdict and the size of the award (if any) may be the court's perception of a company's attitude and concern for safety. Evidence of precautions and due care presented in trial may give the court a favorable impression. Therefore, an important means of product liability protection, in the absence of a fault-proof product, is a complete, up-to-date set of records that can establish the care taken by a company to market safe, reliable products.

For a tabulation of those general types of records a company should retain to enable it to prove its product's safety in a court of law and implement a successful product recall or field modification program, if need be, refer to Fig. 22–6.

The PS&LP program auditor must bear in mind that the records that should be kept by a company are determined by the company's size, product, and organizational structure.

It is a difficult problem for a company to determine what records should be retained and for how long. Product defects may be alleged many years after manufacture or sale.

Generally speaking, unless a company can accurately define the "life" of its product, it should be prepared to retain all PS&LP records in perpetuity. If this creates record storage or maintenance difficulties, a company should use a microfilm recordkeeping system. The PS&LP program coordinator must make sure that a company's key personnel fully understand why

### SCOPE OF RECORDKEEPING REQUIRED for a
### Product Recall or Field-Modification Program

*Administrative Records*
  Asset/Investment
  Acquisitions, Mergers, etc.
  Certificates of Incorporation
  Contracts and Agreements
  Corporate Policies and Procedures
  Deeds and Titles
  Government Regulations
  Government Standards
  Government Specifications
  Insurance Claims
  Insurance Policies
  Insurance Schedules
  Product Recall Plan
  Product Safety and Liability Prevention
    Program Plan

*Marketing Records*
  Distribution Data
  Installation, Inspection, and Servicing
    Reports (Field-Failure Reports)
  Advertising Literature and Publications
  Orders Completed
  Product Safety and Liability Prevention
    Literature
  Returned Goods Records and Reports
  Sales Records
  Complaint/Incident/Accident Records

*Engineering, QC, and Production Records*
  Design Data (Including Acceptance and
    Rejection Reports)
  Drawings (Product Blueprints and
    Schematics)
  Product and/or Component Specifications
  Engineering Standards and Procedures
  Action Taken on Suggestions to Reduce
    Defects
  Product/Design Safety Meeting Reports
  Warning Labels and Precautionary
    Statements
  Product Installation and Operating
    Instructions
  Inventory Records

  Equipment History
  Production Identification
  Production Procedures
  Production Reports
  Production Specifications
  Quality Control Procedure Checklists
  Quality Control Manual
  Quality Control Reports
  Product Acceptance and Rejection Reports
  Testing Data—Independent Consultants,
    Independent Laboratories, FMEA, FTA,
    etc.
  Testing Data (Internal Inspection and Test
    Procedure Records)
    Dates conducted
    Identification of units or batches passing
      tests successfully
    Reasons for any rejections
    Action taken to correct any deficiencies
    Identifying data

*Personnel Records*
  Personnel History
  Personnel Testing
  Job Descriptions
  Medical Records

*Purchasing and Stores Records*
  Invoices
  Receiving Reports
  Specifications
  Purchase Requisitions

*Traffic Records*
  Bills of Lading
  Damaga Claims
  Inspection Reports
  Routing Records
  Checklists covering inclusion of instruction
    manuals in shipments

*Legal Records*
  Cases, Files, etc.
  Claims, Evidence, etc.
  Patents
  Information Files
  Regulation Compliance Reports

FIG. 22-6.

cords are being maintained, what they contain, nd for how long they should be retained.

There are several guidelines that should be pplied to the implementation of a PS&LP cordkeeping program. Some of the reasons for eeping records are:

In compliance with those federal regulations hat cover the design, manufacture, and sale of the ompany's products

To demonstrate determination on the part of ompany management to market a quality roduct

To establish the care taken to produce and sell a afe, reliable product

To facilitate the traceability of the product nd/or customer

To establish a sound data base for such parameters as cost of insurance, sources of supply, product recall or field-modification expense equirements, etc.

## ield-information system

Because a company must receive information eedback from the field about the performance of ts products, the PS&LP program auditor must letermine the effectiveness of a company's field-nformation system in relation to the type of roduct involved and the product distributing ystem. What the program auditor must thoroughly evaluate is (a) the company's capability to dentify and trace its product from the raw material through final sales and distribution stages, (b) a company's ability to acquire and use field data complaints, incidents, and accidents), and (c) the company's desire to use these two factors to mplement product field modification or recall action, where appropriate.

**Data collection and analysis of complaints, ncidents, and accidents.** Every company hould have a reporting system that will permit it o acquire and subsequently evaluate product nformation from the "ultimate testing laboraory"—the customer. This information should be orthcoming from a variety of sources both within and without the organization (service personnel, alespeople, repair, distributors, retailers, etc.).

A reasonably detailed report used with a data collection and analysis system should enable a company to accurately evaluate each complaint,

incident, and accident received and realistically assess any problem with a product as it develops.

For maximum effectiveness, data should be directed to one individual in the company, the PS&LP program coordinator.

The program auditor should also be able to verify, through company records, the results of any field data analysis and what corrective action, if any, was taken.

Diversification of manufactured products prohibits the spelling out of a specific data collection and analysis system applicable to all companies. However, every data reporting system must provide the answers to the following questions:

• *Who is the customer?* The customer's name and location, and where the product is being used, must appear on the product complaint form.

An accumulation of complaint records by name of the customer sometimes reveals problems associated with specific products. Further investigation may determine that unusual environmental or customer application problems exist.

A tabulation of complaint records by geographic area can occasionally pinpoint transportation, handling, or storage problems.

• *What kind of product is involved?* A company must be able to specifically determine which product or product line is causing a problem. A company's products should be satisfactorily labeled etc., and the complaint report form being used should be elaborate enough to provide information that will precisely identify the product, thus ensuring that the product was, in fact, manufactured by the program auditor's company. Space should be provided on the complaint report form for recording information such as:

Model name
Serial number
Lot number
Manufacturing date code
Carton sequence number
Contract number.

The purpose in recording this data is (a) to permit tracing the approximate date of manufacture and the responsible operator, (b) to determine the pertinent engineering specifications, and (c) to associate the product with particular batches of raw materials or component parts. If sufficient data is provided, a company, upon

**653**

analysis, can determine what, if any, corrective action (manufacturing, design, etc.) should be taken.

• *What is the problem?* A complete description of the customer's problem must be obtained by a company if meaningful corrective action is to be taken. A company must be capable of determining if a malfunction occurred or if the appearance of the product rendered it unfit for service. A completed complaint report form should include answers to the following questions:

What was the nature of the defect?

Was it possible to install the product properly?

Were the operating and installation instructions easy to understand?

Were all the necessary parts received?

Was the appearance of the product satisfactory when first received?

Was the performance of the product initially satisfactory?

Was the appearance of the product satisfactory after a period of operation?

Did discoloration or other deteriorations in appearance or performance become evident with the lapse of time?

A company should also be interested in obtaining data pertaining to the efficiency of the product packaging, transportation, and handling systems, particularly if the complaint may have resulted from product damage incurred in transit.

• *How is the product being used?* As discussed earlier, a company should take into consideration potential uses for the product when it is being designed. It sometimes happens, however, that a customer subjects the product to conditions that were not anticipated by the designers. It is important, therefore, that as much detail as is practical be reported on the customer's use of the product. The complaint report should provide answers to questions such as:

Is the product being used in the manner for which it was intended?

How is it mounted or installed?

What environmental conditions has the product been subjected to?

Has the product been altered or modified in any manner by the customer?

When a few important questions are directed

to a customer having a product problem by th service, sales, and repair personnel, and the di tributor or retailer, information may be foun that will augment a company's test program an provide the basis for corrective action and pro uct design improvements. This informatic should be reviewed by the designated individu within a company's organization (PS&LP pr gram coordinator).

In many cases, a preliminary screening customer complaints, accidents, or "near miss incidents (occurrences not involving propert damage or bodily injury but having the potenti to do so) will indicate potential product hazard

When it is determined that a potential hazar exists, a company should be prepared to instigat field investigations promptly, in order to dete mine its source (design, manufacturing, qualit control, etc.).

The causes, as determined by the field invest gation, should then be analyzed to determine if trend is developing or if the product problems ar unrelated. This information should be provided t the PS&LP program coodinator, to decid whether to recommend that further action b taken.

A company must be prepared to act upo appropriate recommendations. This is the funda mental goal of a data collection and analysi system and the underlying reason for using centralized complaint report evaluation syster leading to product field investigations.

The PS&LP program auditor must be pre pared to evaluate the company's effectiveness i taking action based upon the informatio received through its data collection and analysi system. The type of action taken might includ changes in design, manufacturing, quality con trol, or advertising procedures, or the implemen tation of a product field-modification or recal program. If *no* action is taken by a company, the the overall system is basically of no value in th manufacture of safe, reliable products.

The surest means available to the progran auditor to evaluate a company's data collectio and analysis system is to request a review of th company's complaint, loss, field data, and simila files.

If the company does not have any, or if they ar poorly coordinated, then it may be safely assume that the company does not significantly use th source of information to help it manufacture saf products.

**Product traceability.** The need for product call or field modification can become a reality r the manufacturer of almost any product and n also involve those who supply component irts, materials, and services for those products. herefore, the PS&LP program auditor must be epared to evaluate the company to determine hether it is capable of implementing a success- l product recall or field-modification program iould one become necessary because of informa- on developed by the company's data collection id analysis system.

In the event that substantial performance or fety defects are determined to exist in some or l of a company's products that have already en shipped, it is incumbent upon the company recall or field-modify these products.

The identification of the specific lots, batches, iantities, or units of the product to be recalled or odified in the field can be a difficult procedure iless a system of adequate traceability has been tablished by a company during the product lanning and manufacturing stages, as discussed irlier in this chapter. Every company's record- eping system should be extensive enough to rovide adequate product traceability from esign, through production, and delivery of the roduct to the customer. In addition, recall or iodification should be considered in those cases here the company is aware of or has itself eveloped an "improvement" to its product (for cample, a guard, shield, etc.). If the improve- ent has been developed subsequent to the sale of irlier product models, a company must be pre- ared to advise its customers of the available roduct improvement, the hazard it eliminates, id what they must do to incorporate it into their roduct models.

If a product recall or field-modification pro- ram does become necessary, the quantity of roduct that must be recalled or modified by a ompany and the cost to do so can be minimized if ie exact number of defective products, parts, or omponents can be pinpointed.

Where practical, a company's products should e identifiable, even though the means of marking product so that the identification survives use is ometimes difficult, and sometimes impossible. his difficulty notwithstanding, no code, date, rial number, or other marking will be useful iless it can be used to identify which batches, iaterials, components, processes, etc. were esponsible for the suspect products. Therefore, a

company must use and maintain a continuous log of all batches, materials, processes, and product changes. This log must be sufficiently detailed to enable a company to correlate it with its product marking or identification system.

The advantage to a company of having a good product information retrieval system is, gener- ally, reduced product recall or field modification. Other advantages include the greater ease with which replacement parts can be furnished to customers and service centers and the opportu- nity that traceability provides for correlating product returns, complaints, and field experience records with changes in product design, produc- tion, and quality control procedures. In addition, pronouncements by the Consumer Product Safety Commission clearly indicate that if a company's records to not enable it to recall or modify its products effectively, the CPSC may resort to a public notice advising the news media of the potential hazard. Thus there are obvious PS&LP and economic advantages to be realized by a company implementing a system permitting the expeditious recall or field modification of its products.

## Field-modification program plan

The following product recall or field modifica- tion program plan presents the general proce- dures to be considered by a company in the implementation of such a program. Each com- pany's needs will, of course, be different and must be defined by the PS&LP program auditor after evaluating the company's recordkeeping pro- gram and product traceability systems capability.

Based on information acquired from com- plaints, incidents, and accident reports from cus- tomers, distributors or dealers, and state (or provincial) or federal agencies, a company must be capable of determining immediately if a sub- stantial hazard exists. Techniques for making this determination include: on-site investigation of the complaint, incident or accident; hazard and/or failure analyses of the unit involved in the complaint, incident or accident by the company or an independent laboratory; analyses of other units of the same product batch; evaluation of in- house test, or other, records.

If a company finds that a substantial product hazard does exist, the following steps should be taken, as appropriate:

• Cease production and distribution of the hazardous product.

- Involve legal counsel in planning and conducting a product recall or field-modification program.

- Determine the number and identity of the defective products from the design, production, and quality control records.

- Determine from sales and distribution records, the geographical areas and, if possible, customers who purchased the defective products.

- Assign responsibility for estimating the cost of the proposed product recall/field-modification to an appropriate individual/department.

- Supply the individual(s) responsible for actually making the decision to recall or field-modify the product with reports on the seriousness of the hazard, the number of units involved, and the estimated cost to recall or modify.

- Have the above individual(s) notify the Consumer Product Safety Commission of a substantial hazard if the product comes under the Consumer Product Safety Act and have them coordinate all subsequent product recall or field-modification activities with the Consumer Product Safety Commission. (For products coming under the jurisdiction of other federal government agencies, i.e., drugs, foods, automobiles, etc., the product defect or hazard should be reported to the appropriate agency and the recall or field modification coordinated with them.)

- Notify dealers and/or distributors of the safety problem and advise them that the product recall or modification program will commence on a certain date. Dealers and distributors must be provided with the procedures to be taken when the program commences (replacements of defective products, modification of defective products, etc.). The reimbursement steps enabling dealers to recover their cost for time, labor, etc., must also be outlined.

- Initiate procedures to provide dealers and/or distributors with replacement products or parts for the recall or field-modification program.

- Telephone major customers and define the problem and product recall or field-modification program steps.

- Follow up with the formulation of a produ hazard letter to be sent to all customers. Th letter must clearly spell out the product haza and its estimated severity. The company shou notify customers by telegram or by certified m if the product hazard is estimated to be seriot The action steps the customer should take mu be clearly stated: e.g., discontinue use immed ately, take product to nearest dealer or distribut for refund, replacement, repair, or whatever.

- Formulate press releases for newspapers, radi and/or television presenting the compan action in the best possible light.

- Send letters or telegrams to customers, distri utors, and dealers announcing the product rec or field-modification program. Place formulat advertisements in major newspapers and on maj radio and television stations announcing th recall or field-modification program.

- Develop and retain records defining the effe tiveness of the product recall or field-modific tion program as a function of dealer or distribut and by city and geographical area. The compar must follow-up in those instances where r response has been forthcoming from customer

- Report results, as appropriate, to the Consum Products Safety Commission and other feder regulatory agencies.

Note that when a company's customer record are incomplete or nonexistent, recommende procedures are to:

1. Determine the geographical areas where th defective products were sold.

2. Formulate newspaper, radio, and televisic station advertisements for use in the appropr ate geographical sales areas. (The purpose these advertisements is to announce the prod uct hazard and the planned product recall field-modification program. Action steps t take in complying with the program should b given.)

### Independent testing

As an integral part of the PS&LP program, company should either have adequate intern product testing facilities or have an affiliatio with an independent testing laboratory that ca provide whatever testing is required.

In certain instances, companies maintaining bona fide laboratory or adequate testing facilities could be encouraged to certify on their own authority and reputation that their products comply with existing standards, or in those instances where no standards exist, that their products comply with an appropriate standard that the company has developed.

**Types of product testing** that a company might seek to have performed by an independent testing laboratory could include:

The determination of physical characteristics, such as tensile strength, abrasion resistance, or weathering

The testing of mechanical and electrical parameters for certain product classes

Chemical analyses

Nondestructive testing including X ray, ultrasonic, and magnetic particle examination

The testing of thermal and flammability characteristics

Nuclear and radiological testing

Human factors (preference testing).

Some of the reasons why a company should use the services of an independent testing laboratory are as follows:

Such use may be mandated by code, specification, or the rules of a regulatory agency.

The independent laboratory may play an important role in a voluntary trade association program for certification and labeling.

The company may be overloaded in its own laboratory.

The company may lack general or specialized test facilities.

The independent laboratory may be needed to conduct tests required in litigation and/or to have its technical personnel serve as expert witnesses.

The independent laboratory may be used to conduct programs used in advertising claim-substantiation programs.

In the buyer-seller relationship, the laboratory's test report may serve to indicate compliance on the part of the supplier with the company's purchase specification.

• To verify product, component, and packaging compliance with existing standards or, in the absence of such standard, with an appropriate standard developed by the independent laboratory.

**Selecting a testing laboratory.** The following criteria may be useful in the selection of a good independent testing laboratory.

A *competent laboratory* should be sought, that is, one that has either had direct experience in the disciplines required or has shown that it has conducted programs in similar fields and is willing to staff and equip for a company's particular needs.

*Complete objectivity* is a very important attribute for a laboratory performing tests as a product evaluation tool. A good laboratory will "call it as it sees it" *every* time. Laboratory personnel are not product experts, they are testing experts and a good laboratory should have some staff members that have spent a significant part of their working lives performing objective evaluations for others.

*Equipment is important.* It should meet any pertinent specification requirements, be in a good state of repair, and be calibrated on a prescribed scheduled basis. Records of calibration should be maintained properly.

*Interest.* A subjective but important measurement of an independent testing laboratory is the degree of interest shown by the laboratory staff in a company's problem.

*Representation.* Is the laboratory staff willing to have a company representative witness the testing? Will they phone the company about important developments? Will a testing schedule be maintained? Are training seminars conducted by the laboratory's senior and more experienced staff members to ensure that new personnel are properly indoctrinated?

*Continuity* is another important factor. A good laboratory plans to be around for the next year, decade, century. It should not experience a high turnover in its staff. It should have a good financial base and not be subject to minor setbacks.

## PS&LP Program Audit Report

A great deal of general information on PS&LP program evaluation has been provided in the preceding pages of this chapter. This general information covers all the facets of a company's PS&LP program activities that a program auditor must consider. In addition, the program auditor will generate a sizable body of information pertaining to a company's PS&LP program. This information must be assembled, organized, and presented to top management in a coherent format.

There are a few important PS&LP program audit report preparation ground rules that must be complied with if the program auditor is to prepare consistently high quality reports that are of the greatest use to management.

The overall PS&LP audit program report should be timely, succinct, understandable (clarity is essential), well organized, and complete. It should represent the program auditor's opinion of the company's PS&LP program and no one else's. The program auditor must not permit his opinion of the company's program to be coerced by an external influence from any source.

The audit report should have a summary of findings as its initial section for management's benefit during review. This summary section must clearly express the program auditor's opin-ion of the company's overall PS&LP program and whether or not he has found it necessary to prepare recommendations to correct deficiencies detected during the audit. If recommendations are made, they must be adequately supported in the body of the report, practical, and simple to comply with, if possible. In other words, recommendations, whenever possible, should attempt to use the company's already existing systems and procedures. Recommendations must be directed toward correcting specific problems. Top management must be clearly advised as to the degree of importance of each recommendation and the possible consequences if the company fails to comply.

The program auditor should estimate a realistic time frame for recommendation compliance. For example, how long should it reasonably take the company to implement each recommendation on a day-in and day-out basis. This estimate is extremely useful in conjunction with the program auditor's evaluation of the degree of importance of each recommendation.

It must be clear to top management why the program auditor has formulated an opinion about the company's PS&LP program. Otherwise, the value and impact of the program auditor's efforts to qualitatively evaluate and materially improve an existing PS&LP program or control system will be seriously mitigated.

## References

American National Standards Institute, 1430 Broadway, New York, N.Y. 10018. "Catalog of American National Standards" (issued annually).

Brown, D.B. *Systems Analysis and Design for Safety.* Englewood Cliffs, N.J., Prentice-Hall, Inc., 1976.

Consumer Products Safety Commission, Washington, D.C. *Handbook and Standard for Manufacturing Safer Consumer Products,* 1975.

Dallas, D.B., *ed. Tool and Manufacturing Engineers Handbook,* 3d ed. Dearborn, Mich., Society of Manufacturing Engineers.

Gray, I., *et al., Product Liability—A Management Response.* New York, N.Y., AMACOM, 1975.

Hammer, W. *Product Safety Management and Engineering,* Englewood Cliffs, N.J., Prentice-Hall, Inc., 1980.

Kolb, J. and Ross, Steven. *Product Safety and Liability,* New York, N.Y., McGraw-Hill Book Company, 1980.

Malasky, S.W. *System Safety,* Rochelle Park, N.J., Hayden Book Co., Inc., 1974.

National Bureau of Standards, Washington, D.C. 20234.
   *An Index of U.S. Voluntary Engineering Standards,* Spec. Pub. No. 329. Standards Information Service.

National Safety Council, 444 N. Michigan Ave., Chicago, Ill. 60611.
   Industrial Data Sheets (listing available).
   "Product Safety and Loss Prevention: Guidelines for Retailers, Wholesalers, and Importers," 1978.

"Product Safety and Product Loss Prevention: Guidelines for Management," 1976.
*"Product Safety Up-to-Date* (bimonthly newsletter).

Poust, J.G., and Ross, K., *eds. Products Liability of Manufacturers: Prevention and Defense.* New York, N.Y., Practicing Law Institute, 1977.

Product Safety and Liability Prevention Committee (ASQC), Milwaukee, Wis. *Product Recall Planning Guide.*

*Quality Assurance Program Evaulation.* West Covina, Calif., L. Marvin Johnson & Associates.

*Restatement of Torts*, Second Series. Philadelphia, Pa., American Law Institute, 1965.

Thorpe, J.F. *What Every Engineer Should Know About Product Liability.* New York, N.Y., Marcel Dekker, Inc., 1979.

Underwriters Laboratories Inc., 333 Pfingston Rd., Northbrook, Ill. 60062. *Standards for Safety Catalog.*

U.S. Consumer Product Safety Commission, Washington, D.C. 20207.
"Catalog of Publications, Radio, Films, Slides, Fact Sheets, TV."
"Handbook and Standard for Manufacturing Safer Consumer Products," 1975.

Weinstein, A.S. *Products Liability and the Reasonably Safe Product.* New York, N.Y., John Wiley and Sons, 1978.

# Motorized Equipment

# Chapter
# 23

# 23—Motorized Equipment

Motorized equipment discussed in this chapter includes trucks, passenger cars, buses, motorcycles, and off-the-road equipment such as bulldozers, cranes, and road-graders. Powered industrial trucks and handtrucks are covered in the *Engineering and Technology* volume, Chapters 3 and 6, "Manual Handling and Material Storage," and "Powered Industrial Trucks," respectively.

Safe operation of vehicles is the result of planning and action, not chance. Often the problem of ensuring their safe operation is given insufficient attention; the reason may be lack of awareness of the problem or the difficulties of organizing an adequate safety program and providing good supervision.

In about 85 or 90 percent of all motor vehicle accidents, unsafe acts of drivers or inadequate or improper maintenance of equipment can be identified as the cause; only 10 to 15 percent are due to mechanical failure of vehicles. Modern vehicle accident prevention effort focuses attention on these two principal accident factors—driver failure and vehicle failure—because both can be controlled.

Experience has shown that driver failure can be controlled by a carefully planned program of driver selection, training, and supervision, and that vehicle failure can be reduced by systematic preventive maintenance. Also the unsupervised fleet will have higher accident losses than the supervised one.

## Cost of Vehicle Accidents

The total cost of a vehicle accident far exceeds the amount recovered from the insurance company. Control of accidents in the large motor transportation fleet is especially desirable because insurance premiums reduce profit. Insurance premiums fluctuate with accident frequency and dollar losses sustained by a fleet.

As discussed in Chapter 7, "Accident Investigation, Analysis, and Costs," the cost of insurance is only one of the costs that are levied against a company as a result of an accident. There are indirect (uninsured) costs, also. As with other work accidents, these may be several times the direct costs. Indirect costs may be listed as follows:

1. Salary paid, and loss of service of, the employee injured in an accident. Loss of a key employee at a critical time is incalculable.

2. Added workers' compensation costs resulting from a disabling injury.

3. Loss of the vehicle while it is being repaired or replaced.

4. Cost of supervisory time spent in investigating, reporting, and in cleaning up after the accident.

5. Cost of repairing the company vehicle.

6. Cost of repairing or replacing other company property.

7. Poor customer and public relations resulting from a company vehicle having been involved in an accident.

8. Cost of replacing and training an injured employee.

9. Time lost by co-workers in discussing the nature of the accident and the extent of the injury.

In addition to appealing to the profit motive, the most telling argument for controlling accidents is the company's moral obligation to the employee and to the public. The employer, through his authority to hire, supervise, discipline, and discharge employees exercises a high degree of control over their driving performance. Motor vehicle collisions are, in fact, wasteful errors traceable to poor management of the fleet operation.

Management can exercise that control by employing the simple and proven techniques of driver safety education and supervision.

## Vehicle Safety Program

A vehicle safety program should provide for the following:

1. A definite safety policy, originated, supported and emphatically enforced by top management, with delegated authority

2. A safety director (full or part time) to advise top management

3. A driver safety program, including driver selection procedure, driver training, and interest-sustaining activities. Proper supervision and instruction are mandatory for success.

4. An efficient system for accident investigation, reporting, analysis for cause, determination of

appropriate corrective action, and followup.

Preventive maintenance procedures.

## esponsibility

The first requirement of a good, driver safety rogram is that management, from the president o the immediate supervisor, must accept responbility for safe operation of company vehicles. As a the case of other desirable qualities of job erformance, management must first demand a afe operation, define standards of acceptable erformance, and then organize means for the valuation and correction of job performance to eet these standards.

Management must evolve and enforce the olicy that practical accident prevention is a equirement of employment.

A safety professional is usually responsible for apervising the company's program for the safe peration of all automotive equipment. In a small adustrial concern, this may be a part-time assignent. Some of the duties of the safety professional re:

. Advise management on accident prevention and safety.

. Develop and promote safety activities and work injury prevention measures throughout the fleet.

. Study and recommend fleet safety policy in relation to equipment and facilities, personnel selection and training, and other phases of fleet operation.

. Evaluate driver performance.

. Conduct and arrange for effective safety training.

. Review accidents for determination of cause. Compile and distribute statistics on accident-cause analysis and experience. Identify problem persons, operations, and locations.

. Maintain individual driver-safety records, and administer the Safe-Driver Award incentive program.

. Procure (or prepare) and disseminate safety educational material.

## river safety program

A driver-safety program for a fleet should nclude the following five basic accident preven-

tion procedures.

1. Set up an in-service driver training program.

2. Discuss preventability of each accident with persons concerned.

3. Require immediate reporting of every accident.

4. Compute and publicize the fleet accident record.

5. Maintain an accident-record card for each driver.

The planning and administration of a safety program for motor transportation fleets are described in greater detail in the National Safety Council's *Motor Fleet Safety Manual* and in the *Small Fleet Guide.*

An accident is defined as "any incident in which the company vehicle comes in contact with another vehicle, person, object, or animal, which results in death, personal injury, or property damage, regardless of who was injured, what property was damaged or to what extent, where it occurred, or who was responsible." (Another definition appears in the Preface to this volume.)

This definition includes even minor accidents involving little more than a fender scratch. All vehicle accidents, major and minor, are of importance to the safety supervisor since he is primarily concerned with the eradication of faulty driving habits or attitudes. Minor accidents, just as much as the more spectacular ones, provide clues to such faults.

## Accident reporting procedure

Each driver should be required to make out a complete accident report on a standard accident report form for every accident in which his vehicle is involved. If possible, this report should be turned in to the supervisor on the day the accident occurs. National Safety Council "Form Vehicle 1" is a good example of an accident report form. (See the Council's *Motor Fleet Safety Manual* for illustrations of forms.)

Drivers should be told how to fill out the accident report form accurately and intelligently. Failure to report an accident, no matter how slight, or falsification of data on an accident report should be made cause for disciplinary action against the driver.

Drivers should be required to complete the report at the scene of the accident, if possible, and

**663**

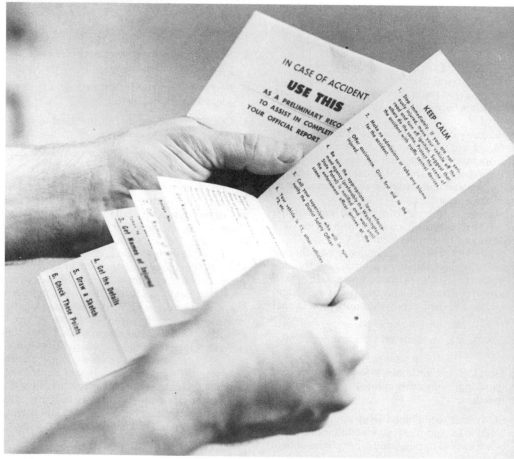

FIG. 23–1.—Accident report packet can be carried in the glove compartment. Instructions and checklist forms are give

then send it promptly to their supervisor.

The number of failures to report an accident can be controlled by a vehicle inspection before and after each trip, noting any changes in the condition of the vehicle.

An accident report packet that can be carried in a glove compartment will be found very useful. This packet (Fig. 23–1) should provide for a memorandum report of the accident. In addition to serving as a checklist, it should contain a pencil, plain paper, courtesy cards, and a list of telephone numbers of company officials and of insurance representatives. The necessary note-taking material will thus be available at the scene of an accident.

Specially printed courtesy cards will save time

and will help the driver get names and addresses key witnesses (Fig. 23–2). Drivers should impressed with the importance of identifying many witnesses as possible.

In the case of serious accidents, especial those resulting in a fatality or personal injury, representative of the company—the manage safety director, or claim agent—should make personal investigation at the scene of the accide as quickly as possible.

The purpose of such an investigation is verify the accuracy of information submitted the driver on the accident report form and obtain other data which might prove valuable for accident prevention work or for defense again unjust claims.

**664**

FIG. 23-2.—When distributed, filled in, and collected, courtesy cards help determine who saw the accident in case witnesses are needed later.

✚ **National Safety Council**
**MOTOR  TRANSPORTATION**
**AWARD  AND  ACCIDENT  RECORD**

| JAN | FEB | MAR | X APR | MAY | JUN | JUL | AUG | SEP | OCT | NOV | DEC |
|-----|-----|-----|-------|-----|-----|-----|-----|-----|-----|-----|-----|

Name    Smith,          Bill          E.
        *Last*          *First*       *Middle*

Location    Midwest Division

Company    Highway Express

Address    123    Home St.,    Any Town
           *Number*   *Street*

Badge Number    123    Date Employed    Feb.    1    19--   Age 29
                                        *Month*  *Day* *Year*   *At Emp.*

### SAFE  DRIVER  AWARD  RECORD

Earned    2    Year N.S.C.   Award during period
from    3-2-19--    to    3-2-19--    with
Company    Overnight Freight, Inc.
Certified by    F. J. O'Connell, Supt.

DRIVING  TESTS

| Date | Score | Remarks |
|------|-------|---------|
| 2-4-19-- | 90 | Slow reaction time |
|  |  |  |

| Award earned | Certificate Number | Date Award earned | Preventable Accidents | | Non-Driving Time | |
|---|---|---|---|---|---|---|
| | | | File No | Date | From | To |
| 3 | 468950 | 3/2/19-- | 1016 | 4/10.19-- | 12/1/19-- | 1/1/19-- |
| 4 | 501850 | 3/2/19-- | | | | |
| 5 | 600100 | 4/2/19-- | | | | |
| | | | | | | |
| | | | | | | |
| | | | | | | |
| | | | | | | |

REMARKS:    12-1-19--  took on month leave of absence.

Form Vehicle 6          PRINTED IN U.S.A.          STOCK No. 229.36

FIG. 23-3.—Award and accident record should be kept as part of each driver's personnel record. Form is useful in administering a company award plan and in counseling accident repeaters.

### Corrective interviewing

As soon as possible after an accident, the company driver involved should be interviewed by the safety professional to determine whether or not the driver might have prevented it. If, after reading the report and discussing the matter with the driver, the safety professional feels that the driver could have helped prevent the accident, it should be classified "Preventable."

In this case, the safety professional must explain to the driver what he did or failed to do that contributed to the accident. He must also make sure that the driver understands what he must do to prevent similar accidents in the future.

If, in the safety professional's opinion, the driver did everything he reasonably could to prevent the accident, it should be classified "Nonpreventable."

It might be pointed out here that responsibility for the prevention of accidents includes more than careful observance of traffic rules and regulations. Drivers must drive in such a manner as to prevent accidents, regardless of faulty driving or nonobservance of traffic laws on the part of other drivers.

### Driver record cards

A record card should be maintained for each employee who drives a company vehicle. This card furnishes not only a record of accidents, but also the information needed for safe driver award plans or other forms of recognition (Fig. 23–3). The date of each accident and the accident category (preventable or nonpreventable) should be entered on this card. The safety professional should review the cards at least every six months and note those drivers who have had an accident.

When a driver becomes an accident repeater, management should make every effort to rehabilitate him through counseling, retraining, closer supervision or reassignment.

If all efforts fail to curb preventable accidents for a driver, discharge or assignment to nondriving duties will be in the best interests of both the firm and the employee.

### Fleet accident frequency

A useful accident control tool is the practice of computing the accident frequency rate of the fleet each month or quarter, in terms of number of accidents per 1,000,000 vehicle miles. Vehicle miles should be computed from odometer read-

ings of all vehicles and not left to rough guesses based on route mileages unless the operations of the fleet are stable from day to day. The standard formula for figuring a fleet accident rate is:

$$\text{Fleet accident frequency rate} = \frac{\text{No. of accidents} \times 1,000,000}{\text{miles driven}}$$

By keeping a monthly record of frequency rates, the safety professional can:

1. Tell whether group safety performance is improving or getting worse

2. Compare the record with like periods to evaluate seasonal trends

3. Compare the status of the fleet with that of other fleets having similar operations.

He can then plan a program accordingly. Accident frequency rates are also of interest to management since they show the effectiveness of the safety program.

(The National Fleet Safety Contest, conducted annually by the National Safety Council, issues a monthly bulletin that gives the accident frequency rates of all participating fleets and thus provides a means for comparison of a company's experience with that of similar fleets.)

### Selection of drivers

For some jobs that require vehicle driving, such as that of a sales representative or technician, other qualifications unfortunately often outweigh a safe driving record, so that the prospective employee's competence as a driver is sometimes investigated in an incomplete fashion or not at all.

However, when a person is to be hired for a job in which driving is the primary function, every effort must be made to select an individual who can be expected to drive safely. In making that selection, the following factors should be considered.

Age. Males under 25 years of age, especially those under 21 (who lack formal driver training) are not considered good accident risks by insurance companies. The personnel officer should take special pains to analyze the qualifications of applicants under 25, and should assign to driving only those who evidence mature, stable personalities (preferably those who have successfully completed driver training courses).

**Experience.** Individuals who have a record of frequent involvement in vehicle accidents should not be assigned to drive company vehicles. An individual's safety record should be investigated (a) in a personal interview, (b) by consulting with former employers, and (c) by checking the state motor vehicle department for accident reports, and (through them) the national driver register service for out-of-state or two license revocations. The National Highway Traffic Safety Administration, Washington, D.C. 20591, maintains a central national register of motor vehicle operators' permits or licenses revoked or suspended for highway safety code violations. Service is only to state officials, so query your Secretary of State for this information.

**Attitude.** Dissatisfied, timid, cocky, troublesome, or otherwise temperamental or unstable individuals often do not make good drivers.

**Personal traits.** A close relationship has been noted between the ability to drive safely and such personal traits as dependability, courtesy, pleasant personality, and the ability to get along harmoniously with other people.

Conversely, persons who tend to be antisocial, argumentative, and impulsive are suspect as drivers.

Individuals differ in their ability to act safely. The fleet safety program must therefore begin at the employment office.

In determining standards of selection, a careful analysis of the job and of the qualifications a driver should have in order to perform it satisfactorily should be made. Results of the job analysis are embodied in a job description in which the separate tasks involved in the job are completely and accurately described.

After the job has been analyzed, the next step is to decide what qualifications the applicant must have to perform the job satisfactorily. There should be a sound reason for each qualification finally imposed. It may be helpful to study the qualifications of those employees who are performing the job in an average or better than average manner. Their qualifications should indicate the requirements expected in new employees. Interstate carriers must comply with driver qualification regulations of the U.S. Department of Transportation.

Safe driving should always be paramount.

Otherwise, accident losses might completely offset any advantages gained through a driver's other special abilities.

## Information-gathering techniques

After job essentials and qualifications have been determined the next step is to develop methods for gathering and sifting employment data about each applicant. Standard employment procedure includes:

Application form
Personal references
Interview
Psychological tests
Driving tests
Physical examination

Illustrations of the forms and more descriptive detail will be found in the Council's *Small Fleet Guide*; see References.

The **application form** is a printed or duplicated form on which the applicant submits details of past employment and other personal data. What a person has done in the past is a good indication of what he can be expected to do in the future. The completed form also saves time during the interview, since essential data are made available to the interviewer at a glance.

Questions on the form should bear directly on the basic qualifications for the job, and should be arranged in logical sequence. Specifically, questions on driving experience should include mileage and years spent as a driver and types of vehicles operated, seasons of the year and geographical areas in which vehicles were operated, preventable and nonpreventable accidents experienced, number of convictions for traffic and other violations, number and type of driver's licenses held, and safe driver awards received.

**Personal references.** The applicant should furnish the names and addresses of previous employers in the space provided on the application form, and these references should be checked. Additional reference sources are the local credit bureau, police department, and state motor vehicle department, as mentioned before.

A properly conducted interview should reveal additional facts about the applicant's employment experience, knowledge of traffic regulations, attitude, personality, appearance, family

**667**

life, and general background.

The interview should be conducted in private, and the applicant should be seated and put completely at ease. The interviewer should keep in mind at all times the inventory of basic qualifications. A checklist of these may be made up to serve as a guide. After the interview, the applicant can be rated on each of the qualifications listed.

**Psychological tests** are devices for obtaining samples of behavior under controlled conditions. They can be useful in the selection process if the behavior traits sampled are known to be related to job success and if interpretation of the results is made by a qualified person. However, since available tests are not reliable instruments of prediction, tests alone should not be the basis for selection. The personnel officer should never use tests as a substitute for other ways of securing employment information. Until tests can be developed which will correlate very highly with our accident criterion, it is not practical to rely on them only.

Many of the large trade associations have had personnel specialists develop standardized personnel selection procedures for their member organizations. These procedures usually include psychological tests that have been found applicable to driver selection.

Small fleets that are not members of an association providing this service should be able to retain, for a reasonable fee, a qualified personnel psychologist for advice on this matter. The psychology departments of some state universities give valuable advice on this problem through their extension services.

**Driving tests.** Each applicant should undergo an actual driving test or a perceptual-motor test as part of selection procedure. Some firms rely on a perceptual-motor test for indication of driving ability and on an extensive driver training course following employment for developing that ability.

Driving tests are of two kinds, the driving range type and the in-traffic type. The requirements of a good driving test in traffic can be listed as follows:

1. The road test should be long enough to sample fairly a number of typical driving situations. Certainly 20 minutes should be considered minimum.

2. The test should include typical maneuvers i heavy traffic as well as on freeways, in order t really test a driver's ability. Almost anyone ca successfully "drive around the block."

3. A standard scoring procedure and predeter mined test route should be used so that the tes will be the same for all drivers examined.

4. The examiner should check definite item concerning the driver's performance (in orde to reduce subjective judgment) and point ou driving faults that may be corrected by prope training.

The applicant's test performance will indicat if driver training is needed, and will indicat weaknesses that can be corrected during th training period. Tests for interstate drivers mus meet the requirements of the U.S. Dept. o Transportation.

**Physical examination.** Applicants should b examined by a qualified physician before bein hired. For firms engaged in interstate commerce physical examination of all new drivers i mandatory and drivers must be reexamined ever two years. The regulations prescribed by the U.S Department of Transportation, National High way Traffic Safety Administration, for bus an truck operators coming under its jurisdiction (se References) require physical examinations for al drivers and provide that motor carriers must hav on file for each driver a certificate showing him t be physically qualified.

Most drivers are, in addition, given a series o psycho-physical tests of vision, depth perception and hearing. Substandard findings are submitte to competent medical authority for evaluation Drivers are told of their weaknesses and how bes to compensate for them.

## Driver training

Individual training by a skilled instructor for al employees assigned to drive company moto vehicles is a highly desirable objective. Variou types of courses can be given.

REMEDIAL, for drivers who get into trouble

REFRESHER, for periodic updating of all drivers

SPECIAL, for operators of specialized equipment

A training course must be planned to fit each

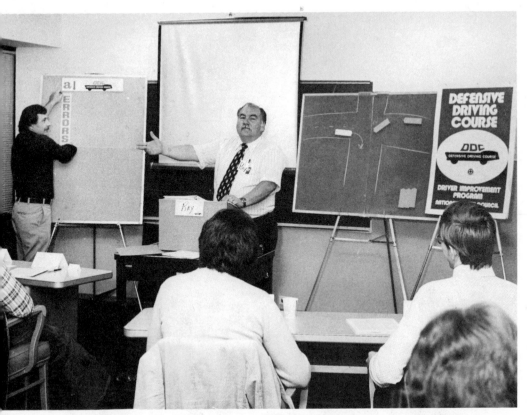

IG. 23–4.—Training session in National Safety Council "Defensive Driving Course" uses many visuals.

ob, training materials assembled, and classroom acilities provided. The objective, however, is well worth the investment. The driver training course should cover the following points.

**State and municipal driving rules.** Most state or provincial) motor vehicle departments publish the rules and regulations of the road for those seeking drivers' licenses. The training course should cover salient points in such booklets.

**Company driving rules.** Each company has rules governing the use of company vehicles: how he vehicles may be obtained, where they may be operated, where parked and under what conditions, speed to be observed, and so on. These rules should be covered thoroughly in the training course.

**What to do in case of an accident.** This topic should include instructions on how to make out company accident report forms, how individual driver records affect the employee, what to do in case of a vehicle accident away from the plant, and similar points. See Fig. 23–1.

• **Defensive driving.** This concept embraces all the commonsense rules of safe and courteous driving. Defensive driving instruction seeks to build in the prospective driver a high sense of responsibility not only for the safety of his own vehicle, but for the safety of other street and highway users who are less skilled and who have had less training and practice (Fig. 23–4) than he has had. At this time, the company's safe driver award or incentive plan should be explained.

### Safe driving incentives

One of the basic assumptions of a safety program is that most drivers believe that they know how to drive much better than they really do. Proceeding on this assumption, then, most safety

**669**

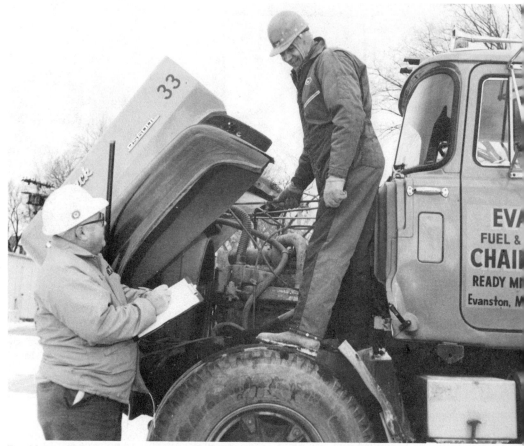

Fig. 23–5.—Although maintenance personnel are responsible for giving the driver a vehicle that is in top mechanical condition, it is the driver who must assure himself at the start of each trip that the vehicle *is* in good condition. Here the safety director goes over the checkpoints.

*Courtesy Evanston (Illinois) Fuel and Material Co.*

professionals regard it as part of their job to provide effective motivation in various ways so that drivers will use more of their driving skill more of the time. To supply this motivation directly or indirectly, the safety professional should:

1. Require a detailed report of every accident

2. Interview the driver after each accident to determine whether or not he could have prevented it

3. Keep a record of each driver's safety performance

4. Recognize safe driving performance. Safe driver awards and cash or merchandise prizes for driving for stated periods without a preventable accident are strong motivations

5. Provide continuous safety instruction and reminders. Use all media: company news letters and bulletins, booklets, posters and bulletin board displays, and meetings and direct personal conversation. ("Talk Topics - Fleet Books 1 and 2," both published by National Safety Council, contain 5-minute safety talks for drivers. Also refer to Chapter 11 and 12 earlier in this volume.)

## Safety devices

Many accidents involving motor vehicles are due to lack of safety devices and particularly to inadequate maintenance. Therefore, fundamental requirements for safe operation are that trucks be equipped with the necessary safety devices and that vital parts, such as tires, brakes and steering mechanisms, and headlights, taillights, and horn be maintained in first-class condition. (See Fig. 23–5).

Safety devices include the following:

Directional signals
Windshield wipers
Windshield defroster
Fire extinguisher
Power steering
Low air-pressure warning system
Rock guards over the drive tires
Adequate outside mirrors
Backup light
Audible backup signal for heavy-duty trucks
Nonslip surfacing on fenders, floors, and steps
Safety belts
High-quality tires
Automatic sander
Anti-jackknife device
Reflective markings

In addition, the following devices are recommended for dump trucks.

A light or indicator to show when the body is in a raised position

A Caution sign on the rear of "packer-loader" trucks

Cab protector or canopy

A built-in body prop

**Loading and unloading of trucks.** To reduce the danger to the driver from falling material while the truck is being loaded, the truck should be spotted so that the load does not swing over the cab or seat. (See Fig. 23–6.) If a truck cannot be so located and does not have a protective canopy over the cab, the driver should dismount and stand clear of the truck.

Certain hazardous materials and cargo require placarding and special precautions especially when loading and unloading. The DOT and EPA regulations must be followed where applicable.

Accidental injuries incurred in the loading and unloading of materials, such as lumber, pipe, equipment, and supplies, are especially numerous, but can be avoided if these precautions are followed:

1. The bulk and weight capacity of the truck should be observed.

2. Loads that may shift should be blocked or lashed. Tiedowns (ropes, chain, boomers) should be tightened on the right side or top of the load.

3. If material extends beyond the end of the tailgate, a red flag (or, at night, a red lamp) should be fastened to the end of the material. No material should extend over the sides.

4. Before loading or unloading a truck, the brakes must be securely set or the wheels blocked to protect the workers both on the truck and on the ground.

5. A truck should not be moved until all workers are either off the truck or properly seated on seats provided and are protected from injury if the load should shift during transit.

6. To avoid falling when unloading a flatbed truck, employees should keep away from the sides of the truck, especially when shoes, floors, and loads are wet or muddy.

7. Be alert for pinch points when loads are being pulled, hauled, or lifted.

8. All safe practices for material handling, such as using mechanical handling equipment, getting sufficient help, and so on, should be observed.

9. Specialized training depending on the classification of the cargo (flammable, corrosive, radioactive, etc.) should be included.

**Detached trailers.** When loading and unloading detached trailers with a lift truck, be sure that the wheels are adequately blocked.

It is important to place the chock properly when trailers are at the dock being loaded and unloaded. Preferred location of chocks is under the rear set of wheels (see Chapter 6 of the *Engineering and Technology* volume, "Powered Industrial Trucks"). If trailer is not blocked properly, the vehicle may move because of an incline or be set in motion by the loading or unloading operation.

The trailer nose can be supported by screw or hydraulic jacks—one on each side of the nose—in order to strengthen the support of the landing

# 23—Motorized Equipment

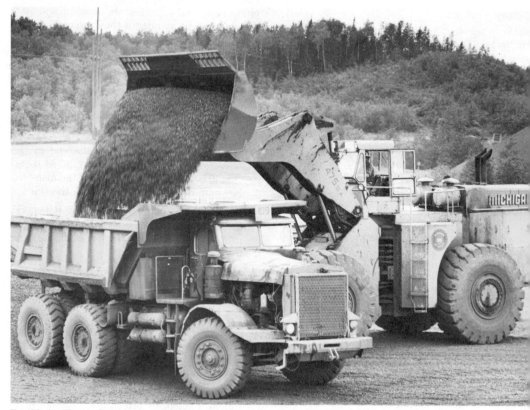

FIG. 23-6.—The truck and loader are properly positioned for safe loading of materials. Loader is approaching the driver's side of the truck, not the blind side, and the driver is in the cab of the truck, not on the ground next to it. (Note the protective canopy over the cab.) The bucket is well positioned to drop the load in the center of the truck bed, reducing spillage. The loader operator has a full view of the truck, the bucket and the material. Note the excellent housekeeping—loose material is leveled around the entire loading operation and the haul road is well maintained.

*Courtesy National Safety Council* Construction Newsletter.

gear assembly. Under a heavy forklift load, landing gears have collapsed from the weight because of dolly metal rust or fatigue, defective struts, or some other cause. (See Fig. 6-17, pages 234—235 of the *Engineering and Technology* volume.)

## Preventive maintenance

Well-managed motorized equipment, both highway and off-the-road, is covered by an extensive and more-or-less complicated preventive maintenance program, the primary considerations of which are safety, economy, and efficiency. Such a program, based on either the mileage or the operating hours of the equipment as recommended by the manufacturer determines

when oil will be changed, tires rotated or replaced, and minor and major overhaul jobs undertaken.

The objectives of such a program are:

1. To prevent accidents and delays

2. To minimize the number of vehicles down for repair

3. To stabilize the work load of the maintenance department

4. To save money by preventing excessive wear and breakdown of equipment

Such a program should, as a matter of course

over all mechanical factors relating to safe operation of all motorized equipment, such as brakes, headlights, rear and stop lights, turn signals, tires, windshield wipers, muffler and exhaust system, steering mechanism, glass, horn, and rearview mirrors. (These are discussed more fully a little later in this chapter.) The manufacturer of the equipment used by the company can help with the specifications.

If at all possible, each driver or operator should be assigned a specific vehicle in order to fix responsibility for reporting defects as well as to encourage drivers and operators to take better care of their vehicles.

Drivers and operators can play an important role in a preventive maintenance program if they are properly instructed and motivated. Because they are most familiar with the vehicle and how it normally operates, they are usually the first to notice when minor (as well as major) mechanical defects develop.

Drivers should check their vehicles before each dispatch. At the end of the workday, they should submit a checklist report of repairs or adjustments needed before the vehicle is used again. It is important that maintenance personnel follow up on these, otherwise the benefit is lost.

A printed checklist (adapted from the outline that follows) should be furnished all drivers and operators for the inspection. On completion, they should give the inspection form to the supervisor. This form acts as a reminder as well as a checklist, and should normally cover the following items:

BRAKES. Brakes should apply evenly to all wheels so that a vehicle does not swerve when the brakes are applied. This even application also gives maximum braking effectiveness.

HEADLIGHTS should function and be properly aimed to avoid blinding other motorists and to give maximum road lighting efficiency. The dimming switch and upper and lower beams should work properly.

CONNECTING CABLES on a combination vehicle should have strong connections that will not be affected by the vibration of the vehicle. All other cables, such as brake and electrical, should be free of defects.

STOP LIGHTS, turn lights, rear lights, and side-marker lights should be checked.

TIRES should be inflated to manufacturer's recommended pressure, and checked regularly for adequacy of tread and for cuts or breaks. Dual tires should be well matched.

WINDSHIELD WIPERS must wipe clean and not streak.

STEERING WHEEL should be free from excessive play. Front wheels should be properly aligned.

GLASS should be free from cracks, discoloration, dirt, or unauthorized stickers which might obscure vision.

HORN should respond to a light touch.

REARVIEW MIRRORS should give the driver a clear view of the rear. So outside rearview mirrors can provide maximum sight advantage, portions can be conventional and convex.

STALLING PROBLEMS should be investigated and corrected immediately.

INSTRUMENTS should be in good working order; they are essential to safe and economical operation.

EXHAUST SYSTEM should be checked for leaks to protect against carbon monoxide gas. The exhaust manifold, pipe connections, and muffler should be inspected periodically, and leaky gaskets replaced.

EMERGENCY EQUIPMENT in every vehicle should include a fire extinguisher, essential tools for road repairs, spare bulbs, flares, reflectors, flags, and such other equipment deemed necessary in case of fire, accident, or road breakdown. These items should be periodically checked to make sure of their availability and usability. Interstate vehicles must be equipped with emergency items prescribed by the U.S. Department of Transportation.

Many states and cities require periodic safety tests and inspections for all vehicles. The maintenance superintendent should know the applicable inspection standards. The preventive maintenance policy of the company should require all vehicles to meet these requirements.

## Repair Shop Safe Practices

The vehicle safety supervisor also should take an active interest in the work habits of automotive repair shop employees to determine their safety attitudes, and should cooperate with the plant safety supervisor. An effective program

**673**

must ensure that all employees engage in safe work practices. Also, that all federal and state (provincial) regulations are followed.

## Servicing and maintaining equipment

Serious injuries occur in servicing and maintaining trucks. Heavy equipment requires mechanical aids for handling heavy parts. Hoists for lifting parts in and out of trucks and for moving parts about the shop not only prevent accidents, but also make work easier and save time. See the discussion in Chapter 3, "Manual Handling and Material Storage," in the *Engineering and Technology* volume.

Serious injuries are likely to occur from unexpected movement of equipment undergoing repair. Brakes should be set and wheels should be blocked. If work must be done under a raised body, the body must be secured or blocked against coming down in case the hoist of jack control levers or pedals are inadvertently struck and the load released.

A jack often is used to raise equipment, which then becomes a support in an unstable position. Because serious injuries occur when a truck falls off a jack, it is important that the jack be set on a firm foundation and be exactly perpendicular to the load. To help prevent the jack from slipping, a thin wood block between the top of the jack and the load is recommended. When the truck has been raised to the desired height, it should be supported by stanchions, blocking, or other secure support.

No work should be done near the engine fan or other exposed moving parts until the engine has been stopped. If the engine must be run to inspect or check on moving parts, keep a safe distance away and do not attempt an adjustment. Jewelry, especially rings, should not be worn.

Close-fitting unfrayed clothing, safety shoes, and goggles are essential for repair people.

Burns are frequent in the servicing of trucks. An employee should use a heavy work glove, "bleed-off" any steam, and then remove the cap. Gasoline or alcohol used near hot engines and spilled on them can cause a serious fire. Suitable funnels and safety containers should be used.

## Tire operations

A particularly serious hazard in inflating truck tires is the possibility that the locking ring may blow off at a high pressure. Use of a tire safety rack will greatly reduce the hazard. All truck tires should be checked to make sure that the valve ha been removed and the tire fully deflated prior t disassembly. Tires must be inflated in ste "cages" that will restrain flying objects should blowout occur. A locking ring must be seate properly and must not be yanked free by bein twisted. A defective locking ring or rim should b replaced with a sound one. Ring and rim sea should be clean.

It is advisable to use inflators that can be prese and have locking attachments so that the worke does not have his hand or arm in the danger are even if the tire is in a cage.

Blowouts may occur because of overinflatio of the tire, improper placement of the tire on th rim or wheel (causing pinching or chafing of th tire or tube), or improper mounting of lock-rinj or rims. Records show that most accidents in th handling of truck tires occur while tires are bein inflated.

Only employees thoroughly familiar with th hazards and safe methods involved in handlin tire equipment should inspect, install, repair, an replace tires and rims.

Other hazards are strains or hernias resultin from lifting heavy tire assemblies. Mechanic lifting and moving devices should be provided s that workers are not required to lift heavy tire

Rubber cement and flammable solvents use for patching inner tubes, and casing compound used for filling tire cuts, should be kept in safet cans.

Electric heating elements used for vulcanizin or branding tires should be inspected regularl Defective wiring should be replaced.

Where power-driven rasps or scrapers are use for casings or inner tubes, the operators must wea eye protection. A local exhaust system should b applied to these machines to keep the fine rubbe dust out of the workroom air.

## Fire protection

Because fire is a hazard in the operation o heavy-duty trucks, they should be equipped wit Type B-C fire extinguishers, listed by the Unde writers Laboratories as suitable for use on burn ing oil, gasoline, grease, and electrical equipmen The extinguisher may be placed in a convenien location in the cab or on the running board, an the driver should be taught how to operate it Monthly inspection of firefighting equipment i advisable.

The repair shop should also have an adequat

number of fire extinguishers of the ABC type and employees who are trained in their use.

If cutting, burning, or welding must be done near fuel oil tanks, an extinguisher should be at hand. A tarpaulin should be used to cover fuel, oil tanks, or combustible materials to protect them against sparks and excessive heat. Such work should not be performed on a fuel tank or other container until it has been drained and thoroughly purged of vapors.

Fueling requires certain precautions to avoid fires. The engine should be stopped. Smoking should be prohibited. Safety containers and a grounded fuel hose should be used for fueling. When the tank is being filled, the metal spout of the hose should firmly contact the tank to ensure grounding and to neutralize static charges sufficient to ignite fuel vapors and cause an explosion or fire.

Fires occur in shops each year because gasoline and similar flammable solvents are used for cleaning parts. Safe, nontoxic cleaning liquids that are nonflammable and do not injure the skin are available and should be used.

The likelihood of a fire in a shop also can be reduced by good housekeeping, especially the disposal of oily waste and similar materials in covered metal containers.

Fire prevention procedures apply to all motorized equipment, such as, power cranes, shovels, bulldozers, as well as trucks.

Details are covered in the *Engineering and Technology* volume, Chapters 16, "Flammable and Combustible Liquids," and 17, "Fire Protection."

## Grease rack operations

In greasing operations, a person may slip and fall because of accumulated grease and oil on the floor, injure his hands on sharp or rough edges on the vehicle, incur strains in trying to rock the vehicle to make grease penetrate into stiff bearings or springs, inhale sprayed or atomized oils used for spring lubrication, or suffer hand and head injuries from high-pressure guns.

Floors should be kept free of grease and oil to prevent slips and falls. Spills which occur during the working day should be immediately cleaned up or covered with an oil-absorbent compound.

Remind workers to keep their hands away from sharp or rough edges and to obtain immediate first aid treatment for all cuts and scratches.

Warn workers against putting their hands in front of the grease gun nozzle when the handle is pulled. Instances have been reported in which quantities of grease have been forced under the skin of workers by high-pressure grease guns.

Tops of grease cylinders should be securely fastened into place; otherwise, covers may blow off and seriously injure anyone who may be nearby.

All equipment should be inspected weekly and repairs should be made when needed.

Workers should be warned of the danger of inhaling sprayed or atomized oils while lubricating springs. They should stand clear of the lubricant spray, which settles quickly, and must not direct the spray at other employees.

## Wash rack operations

When washing vehicles, a person can slip and fall on wet floors, incur cuts or abrasions from the sharp or rough edges of the vehicle, or suffer burns from careless use of hot water or steam.

The concrete floor of the wash rack should be rough troweled to produce a nonslip surface. While washing cars, employees should wear safety toe rubber boots, preferably with nonslip soles and heels, and a rubber coat or apron.

Workers should never point the high velocity steams of hot or cold water at another person because injury may result.

Workers should direct the hose, particularly under the vehicle, in such a way as to avoid being struck by a backlashing stream of water and dirt.

Where a hot water hose is used, cover the metal parts to avoid skin contact and consequently prevent burns. Heavy-duty gloves and face shields should be used when necessary. A portable fan may be needed to blow steam away, so that the operator can see the work. Washers should be alert for sharp and rough edges on the vehicle which might cause cuts and abrasions. A periodic scheduled cleanup of the entire wash rack and associated equipment is recommended.

## Battery charging

The principal hazards of battery charging operations are acid burns during filling, back strains from lifting, electric shocks, slips, falls, and explosions.

Employees should wear safety apparel suitable for battery shops; this includes splash-proof goggles, and acid-proof gloves, aprons, and boots with nonslip soles. (Rubber boots and aprons must be worn when batteries are being filled. Goggles should be worn when working around batteries to prevent acid burns to the eyes.)

A wood-slat floor should be used and kept in good condition, to prevent slips and falls and to protect against electric shocks from batteries being charged.

Fire doors should be installed between charging rooms and other areas where flammable liquids are handled and stored.

The manufacturer's recommendations as to the charging rate for batteries of various sizes should be closely followed in order to prevent rapid generation of hydrogen. Potentially explosive quantities of oxygen and hydrogen are developed in cells of batteries. This is particularly true if the battery is defective or if a heavy charge has been or is being applied. The lower the water in the battery, the greater the cavity for the accumulation of gas.

Care should be taken to prevent arcing while batteries are being charged, tested, or handled. Tools and loose metal (and even lifting hoist chains) should not be in such a position that they may fall on batteries and cause a short circuit, which in turn can result in serious burns or an explosion.

When manual lifting is necessary, sufficient help should be provided to prevent strains, sprains, or hernias. Hand carts for transporting batteries are commercially available or can be made in a company shop.

Acid carboys should be handled with special care to prevent breakage and possible injury due to splashing of acid. Acid carboys should never be moved without their protecting boxes. They should not be stored in excessively warm locations or in the direct rays of the sun. Carboy tilters can be used. (See Chapter 3 of the *Engineering and Technology* volume, "Manual Handling and Material Storage.")

A summary of recommendations for changing and charging batteries is given in Chapter 6 of the *Engineering and Technology* volume, "Powered Industrial Trucks."

• **First aid for chemical burns.** Many batteries contain an acid electrolyte; some, such as the nickel-iron battery, contain an alkali solution. Whether it be acidic or alkaline, if electrolyte gets on a person's skin, it must be washed off immediately with large quantities of running water. Neutralizing agents are so often mishandled, they can often do more harm than

good—only use them if first aid directions are available on labels or through company or plant directions. Get medical aid at once.

• **First aid for burns of the eye.** Irrigate the eye thoroughly with large amounts of clean water. Place a sterile dressing over the eye to immobilize the lid and get medical aid at once. Well-marked supplies of appropriate neutralizing agents can be kept close at hand for immediate use. Check with company physician. A safety shower and eyewash fountain are required by OSHA wherever acids or caustics are used. See Chapter 19, "Occupational Health Services."

## Gasoline handling

The handling and storing of gasoline should comply with the provisions of the National Fire Protection Association *Flammable and Combustible Liquids Code*, NFPA 30, which is discussed in Chapter 16 of the *Engineering and Technology* volume, "Flammable and Combustible Liquids."

Use of gasoline must be prohibited for all cleaning. Solvents with higher flash points are available and are equally effective and much safer. Even when higher flash point solvents are used, if carburetor or gas line parts are cleaned, the solution should be changed regularly since the admixture of small quantities of gasoline will tend to lower the flash point, and increase the danger of fire and explosion.

Grease, oil, and dirt may be removed from metal parts by nonflammable solutions, or by high-flash point solvents in special degreasing tanks with adequate ventilating facilities.

Use of gasoline to remove oil and grease from garage floors must be prohibited. Nonflammable cleaning compounds are commercially available and should be used.

Gasoline should not be used for removing oil and grease from hands. Soaps are available that will effectively remove greasy dirt from the skin without danger of injury. There are also protective creams and ointments which, if applied before starting work, will protect the skin from dirt and grease.

In some shops, employees use gasoline to clean work clothes. This unsafe practice must be prohibited.

If gasoline is spilled, it should be taken up immediately. If gasoline in quantity gets into the sewage system, the fire department should be notified so that the sewers can be flushed. Because gasoline vapor is heavier than air, it collects in low spots, such as basements, elevator pits, and sumps. These places should be kept ventilated whenever gasoline vapors are present.

## Other safe practices

**Using jacks and chain hoists.** Vehicles jacked up or hung on chain hoists should always be blocked with stanchions, pyramid jacks, or wood blocks (which have first been carefully inspected). The best jack for general garage use is the hydraulic-over-air type—if one system fails, the other prevails. Ordinary pedestal jacks are not to be used, especially the type supplied for passenger cars, as the vehicle may be tipped or jarred off the jacks and cause injury.

When a person is working under a vehicle that is blocked up, other employees should not work on the car in such a manner that the car may be knocked from its blocks.

Employees who work under vehicles should be safeguarded from danger when their legs protrude into passageways. Barricades should be used for protection, or else the worker's entire body should be under the vehicle.

A frequent cause of injury to employees who work under vehicles is dirt and metal chips falling into the eyes. To protect the eyes, employees working under these conditions, should wear suitable eye protection—goggles or plastic eye shields. However, because they sometimes fog, the fog-resistant type should be used, if necessary.

**Removing exhaust gases.** Repair shop employees should use local exhaust and ventilating facilities to prevent accumulation of vehicle exhaust gases within the shop.

**Repairing radiators.** Where radiators are boiled out or tested for leaks, the operator should be provided with both chemical goggles and a face shield of clear plastic. The entire face needs protection.

**Cleaning spark plugs.** All mechanics using sandblast spark plug cleaners should wear goggles or face shields.

**Replacing brakes.** When cleaning around brake drums and backing plates, in the process of replacing brakes, the use of air pressure can send asbestos filings from the brake area into the breathable air and cause respiratory problems.

Rather than use compressed air to clean, vacuums, chemical wash solutions, or steam cleaners should be used.

**Controlling traffic.** Movement of vehicles inside shops and garages should be regulated by rigidly enforced traffic rules. Traffic lanes and parking spaces should be painted on the floors and the direction of traffic flow indicated. Vehicles with air brakes should not be moved until sufficient air pressure has been built up.

Every driver should stop his vehicle, then sound the horn before passing through the entrance or exit door. Signs requiring this procedure should be posted in conspicuous places. Mirrors should be installed at blind corners.

Vehicles should be moved in low gear and at low speed inside shop areas, especially up and down ramps.

**Other sources of injury** are jumping across open inspection pits, falling off ladders, hurting backs while trying to move supplies and equipment, and using hand tools improperly. Prevention of all work injuries requires proper selection and training of employees, careful supervision of their work habits, review of all injury causes, and the creation of safety-mindedness in all employees.

## Training repair shop personnel

Apprentices and new employees should be trained to do each job in the most efficient manner. Job instruction should include the safety rules and regulations pertaining to each job and the reason for such rules. The new mechanic should be thoroughly indoctrinated concerning the company's policy toward safety. He should understand the organization of the safety program and the part he is expected to play in it.

Having been indoctrinated and trained to work safely, the new employee must be kept actively interested in observing accepted safe practices in the conduct of his job. There are many devices available to the safety director to accomplish this end, including safety supervision, safety contests, safety meetings, posters, safety bulletins, and pamphlets. See Chapter 9, "Safety Training."

More details on mechanical and chemical safety can be found in the *Engineering and Technology* volume and in *Fundamentals of Industrial Hygiene,* respectively.

# 23—Motorized Equipment

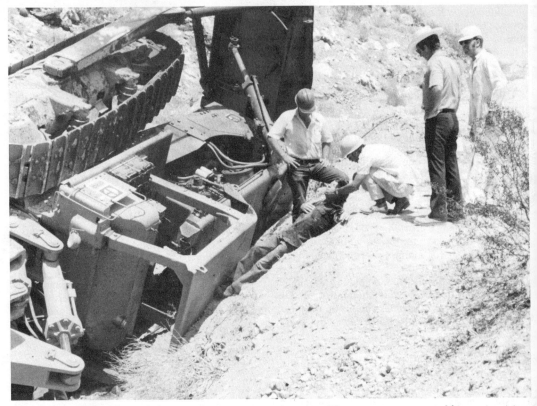

FIG. 23–7.—This is only a simulation, but it illustrates a very real situation. The operator was protected from serious injury by his safety belt and the ROPS canopy; however, this accident would not have occurred had the operator followed the rules of safe operation.

*Courtesy National Safety Council* Construction Newsletter.

## Off-the-Road Motorized Equipment

Heavy-duty trucks are mentioned again here because they are used extensively for special off-the-road operations in such industries as quarrying, mining, and construction. When on the road, they are, of course, governed by the same safe-driving practices as other types of automotive equipment.

The use of heavy-duty trucks, mobile cranes, tractors, bulldozers, and other motorized equipment in quarrying, mining, and construction presents the possibility of accidents. Workers near equipment can be struck, run over, and killed; equipment sometimes slips over embankments, injuring people (Fig. 23–7). Even personnel who are involved in servicing and maintaining equip-

ment can find it hazardous. (See Fig. 23–8.)

Many accidents, even those that do not injure anyone, result in costly damage to equipment, loss of efficiency and production, and high maintenance costs.

In general, prevention of accidents to heavy equipment requires:

1. Safety features on equipment

2. Systematic maintenance and repair

3. Trained operators, and

4. Trained repair personnel.

Safe and proper operation of equipment will be found in the manufacturer's manuals. Many driving practices are the same as those necessary

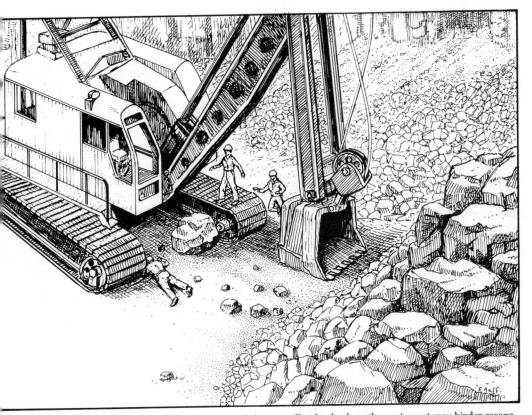

FIG. 23–8.—Workers must not go between equipment and the pit wall or bank where the equipment may hinder escape from falls or sides of the bank. In the situation shown here, a lubrication man was fatally injured when he was crushed between a track pad of an electric power shovel and a boulder that had rolled down a 50-ft-high pile.

*Courtesy Mine Safety and Health Administration.*

or the safe operation of highway vehicles. Off-the-road driving, however, involves special hazards and requires special training and safety measures.

### Haul-roads

Roadway improvements pay for themselves because they reduce accidents and lower maintenance costs.

Both temporary and permanent roads often are too narrow for heavy equipment and for two-way traffic, especially at curves and fills. Enough space must be provided at curves so that large trucks need not cross the centerline of the road. Curves should be banked toward the outside.

Both temporary and permanent roadways require regular patrolling and maintenance. Too often, serious accidents, breakdowns, delays, and unnecessary maintenance expense can be traced to neglected roadways. Road patrols should be provided with protective equipment, such as barricades, warning signs, red flags, flagmen, and flares.

Seasonal conditions create road hazards that require prompt attention. Some companies provide sprinkler trucks to protect their employees against harmful dusts, discomfort, and the possibility of accidents during dry and windy periods. Others keep dust down by spraying oil with an asphalt base, on the road surface.

Skidding on snow and ice is a serious hazard during the winter. Snow and ice should be

**679**

removed by means of snowplows or blade graders as promptly and as completely as possible.

When roadways are built close to high banks, the slopes of the banks should be inspected for loose rocks, especially after rain and freezing or thawing weather. Loose rock should be barred down, that is, pried out with a steel bar.

Where trucks enter public highways, signs should be installed warning the highway traffic. Design, color, and placement of the signs should be in accordance with U.S. Department of Transportation, Federal Highway Administration, Washington, D.C., *Manual on Uniform Traffic Control Devices for Streets and Highways*, also published as American National Standard D6.1 (see References). If operations are conducted at night, these signs should be made of a light-reflecting material or lighted directly.

## Driver qualifications and training

The modern heavy-duty vehicle or other off-the-road equipment is a carefully engineered and expensive piece of equipment and warrants operation only by drivers who are qualified physically, mentally, and by training and experience. The physical and mental qualifications for an efficient and safe operator of heavy over-the-road equipment (discussed earlier in this chapter) apply also to drivers of off-the-road vehicles.

No driver should be allowed to work until his knowledge, experience, and abilities have been determined. The amount of time varies for a prospective driver or operator to become thoroughly acquainted with the mechanical features of the truck or piece of equipment, safety rules, driver reports, and emergency conditions. Even an experienced operator should not be permitted to operate equipment until the instructor or supervisor is satisfied with his abilities.

Because accidents caused by unsafe practices outnumber those resulting from unsafe condition of equipment and roadways, the time required for thorough checking and training is well warranted. After an employee has been trained, continuing supervision is required to make sure that he continues to operate in the way in which he was instructed.

## Operating vehicles near workers

Workers are exposed to the danger of being struck or run over by vehicles, particularly around power shovels, concrete mixers, and other equipment, in garages, shops, dumps, and construction areas.

**Backing.** The most dangerous movement i backing, especially for packer-loader trucks (Fig 23–9), used by municipalities and private cor tractors for refuse collection.

Some construction companies require driver to blow three blasts of the horn for a back-u signal.

An automatic audible signaling device to wari workers of a vehicle backing up is required b OSHA regulations.

Where a number of employees are working the driver should call upon another employee t signal whether or not the path is clear befor backing or making any other movement. Th person, giving the signals, should always take position within sight of the driver. Also, a stan dard set of signals should be devised to ensur proper communication.

**Moving forward.** Serious accidents also occu during forward movements. The hazard to work ers increases with the greater height and capacity of trucks. A driver often fails to see worker crossing from the right immediately ahead of th truck. Thus, drivers often are required to blow two blasts on the horn before starting forward

## Procedures for dumping

Vehicle operations on dumps and banks involve the danger of the vehicle going over the crest while dumping a load. A person trained in proper dumping procedures is probably the best insurance against loss of life and damage to equipment. Drivers are required to follow his instructions and signals, especially in backing to dump. Prearranged signals must be used at all times.

The person responsible for dumping must know how close to the edge a vehicle can approach safely under various weather conditions. He positions himself on the driver's side of the vehicle (a) so that the signals can be easily seen and (b) so the driver will have him in sight, and there will be less danger of his being run over. To protect him further, the driver should turn from his left when backing, so that he will have a maximum view of the area into which the rear of the truck is moving. Also, the signaller must stay clear to avoid being struck by falling material.

Left-hand driving also reduces the danger of going over the crest, especially in the operation of

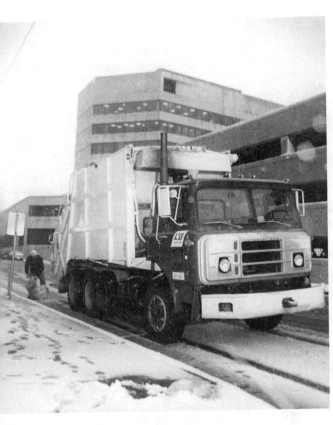

FIG. 23–9.—Enclosed, compactor-type refuse collection truck. Backing is a most dangerous operation because of poor visibility.

*Courtesy International Harvester Co.*

ide dump trucks, since the driver is on the crest ide.

To avoid hitting overhead lines or other low learances, the dump box should be lowered as oon as the load is dumped.

To help prevent the crest from caving in, tockpiles and dumps frequently are graded oward the crest so that vehicles back up the lope. Loads also may be dumped a safe distance rom the crest and then leveled by a grader or ulldozer (Fig. 23–10).

Strongly built cabs and cab protectors on anopies and especially safety belts are effective n preventing injuries if vehicles overturn. The nclination to jump clear of a vehicle that is eginning to roll or slide over an embankment is ll advised. It is far safer to remain in the cab.

Holes, ruts, and similar rough places on umps, and roadways may cause the front wheels f a truck to cramp so that the steering wheel pins, injuring fingers, arms, and ribs, particularly

if the truck is not provided with power steering. Gripping the wheel on the outside and not by the spokes, driving at reduced speed, and observing the ground ahead for rough places will help the driver avoid such injuries.

Floodlighting during night operations helps to prevent accidents.

### Protective frames for heavy equipment

All bulldozers, tractors, and similar equipment used in clearing operations must be equipped with substantial guards, shields, canopies, and grilles to protect the operator from falling and flying objects (Fig. 23–7, –10, and –11).

Crawlers and rubber-tired vehicles, self-propelled pneumatic-tired earth movers, water tank trucks, and similar equipment must be equipped with steel canopies and safety belts in order to protect operators from the hazards of rollover (Figs. 23–6 and –17). Drivers should be trained and required to wear the safety belt.

**681**

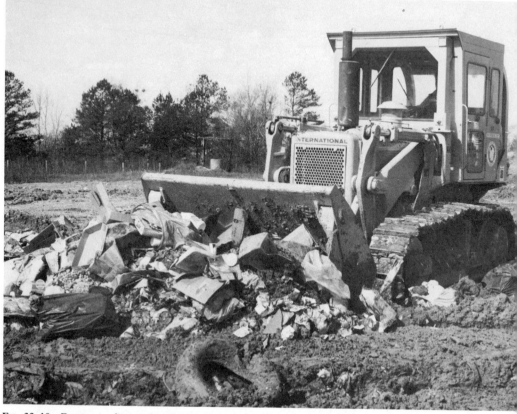

FIG. 23–10.—Dumps are frequently graded uphill toward the crest. Steel canopy protects the operator. *Courtesy International Harvester Company.*

A canopy and its support should be designed and made to be able to support not less than two times the weight of the prime mover. This calculation is to be based on the ultimate strength of the metal and integrated loading of support members, with the resultant load applied at the point of impact. In addition, there should be a vertical clearance of 52 in. (132 cm) from the deck to the canopy where the operator enters or leaves the seat.

For more details, see National Safety Council Industrial Data Sheet 622, *Tractor Operation and Roll-over Protective Structures.*

### Transportation of workers

Some jobs—for various reasons—require that workers be transported to and from the work site. However, transporting employees to and from

work can involve special risks and consequentl special precautions must be taken. Where suc transportation is a regular occurrence, a bus c other vehicle designed to transport passenger can avoid many of the particular risks.

Hazards are more likely to exist when tran portation of workers is performed on an irregula basis. Often, under these conditions, an ope cargo truck of some kind is used as the transport ing vehicle. If so, workers should be advised of th following safety procedures:

● Getting on. Look before and where you step Use every handhold available, even a helpin hand from someone already on the truck. Ste squarely; never at an angle. No one should eve attempt to board a moving vehicle—regardless o how slow it may be traveling.

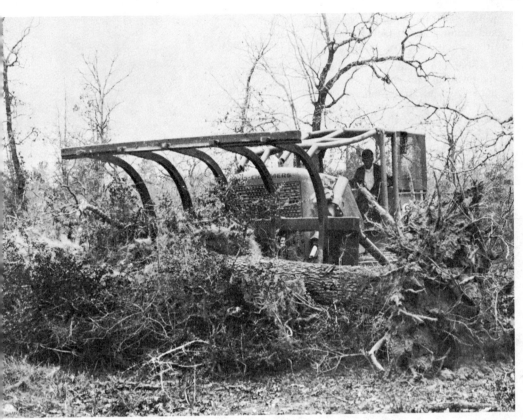

FIG. 23–11.—Crawler tractor equipped for site clearance has protective frame and screens to protect operator from falling and flying objects.

*Courtesy Spade Plow Inc.*

If possible, benches should be provided. In no case, however, should the passengers remain standing while the vehicle is in motion. If necessary, they should sit on the truck bed.

Avoiding horseplay. Of all the many negative actions that a group of people may take, this is one of the most stupid and dangerous. Some companies will go as far as firing anyone caught indulging in this type of activity. Horseplay is inherently dangerous, and in a moving vehicle, it may be fatally so.

Getting off. Workers should again look before they step, then get off slowly and easily, using every possible handhold. Under no circumstance should anyone attempt to jump off a moving vehicle. Many injuries occur as a result of jumping off a vehicle, whether it is moving or not.

## Towing

Towing is a hazardous operation, especially when coupling or uncoupling the equipment. Workers can be crushed when a truck or other piece of equipment moves unexpectedly while they are between the two pieces of equipment.

The following safe practices are essential to prevent accidents in the coupling or uncoupling of motorized equipment:

1. No one should go between the vehicles while either one is in motion.

2. Vehicles must be secured against movements by having the brakes set, the wheels blocked, or both.

3. A driver should not move his vehicle while someone is between it and another vehicle, a

**683**

wall, or anything else that is reasonably solid and immovable. In fact, before moving, the driver should receive an all-clear signal.

4. Tow bars are usually safer than towing ropes. If ropes, which may be more convenient to use under certain circumstances, are employed, they must be in good condition and of sufficient size and length for the towing job.

5. Equipment towed on trailers should be secured to the trailer.

## Power shovels, cranes, and similar equipment

Safe operation of power shovels, draglines, and similar equipment begins with purchase of the machines. A good policy is to spell out in the equipment specifications that guards must cover gears, and that safe oiling devices, handholds, and other safeguards be provided. In any case, before equipment is put into operation, it should be thoroughly inspected and necessary safety devices should be installed.

To keep workers from being injured when caught between truck frames, crawler tracks,

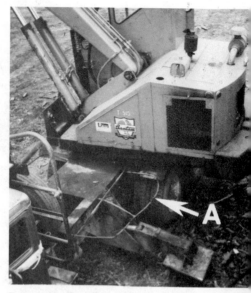

FIG. 23–12a.—A 7/8 in. wire rope is used to provide warning barricade across the pinch point of a hydraul loader. Rope is flexible enough so it does not crea another pinch point between the cab and the rope.

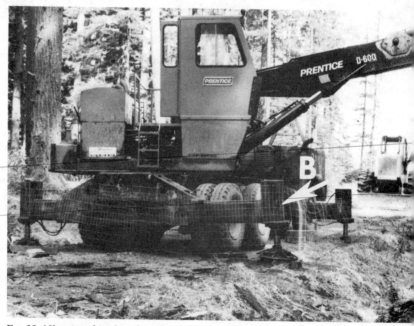

FIG. 23–12b.—Attaching lengths of fencing around the outriggers of this loader creates a clearl visible warning barricade.

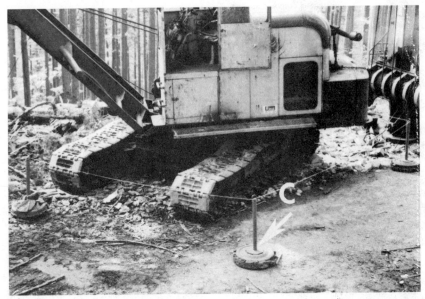

FIG. 23-12c.—Rope and brightly painted metal stands (with heavy bases) form an effective barricade around this crane in a woods operation.

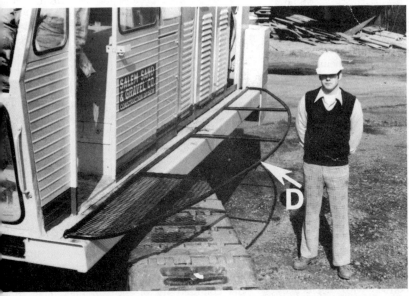

FIG. 23-12d.—Lightweight metal frame can be pulled up and out of the area. Barricade is not covered with screen to prevent it from being used to store tools and materials.

*Courtesy State of Oregon, Accident Prevention Division.*

**685**

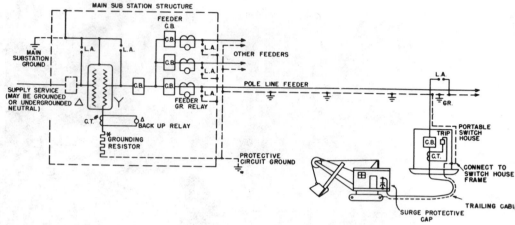

FIG. 23–13.—A grounded safety neutral system for electric-powered units.

*Courtesy General Electric Co.*

cabs, and counterweights of cranes and shovels, a barricade can be used to warn employees who are working near operating equipment that they are close to a hazardous area. Signs, flashing lights, and other warning devices can also be used to alert people to the hazards. Examples are shown in Fig. 23–12. Barricades are easily moved when equipment is moved.

Both operators and maintenance personnel, whether experienced or not, should be instructed in the recommendations of the manufacturer pertaining to lubrication, adjustments, repairs, and operating practices, and should be required to observe them. A preventive maintenance program for shovels and other equipment is essential for safety and efficiency. Frequent and regular inspections and prompt repairs are the bases for effective preventive maintenance.

Generally, the operator is responsible for inspecting the mechanical condition of such items as holddown bolts, brakes, clutches, clamps, hooks, and similar vital parts.

Wire ropes should be kept lubricated in accordance with the manufacturers' instruction, and should be inspected daily since rope failures can cause serious accidents. Ropes are particularly likely to develop weakness at the fastenings, at crossover points on drums, and in the sections that are in frequent contact with the sheaves.

**Grounding systems.** In order to prevent electrical shock, electrically powered equipment requires a good earth grounding system to protect workers from electrical faults in trailing cables at the machine. Though the cable may make close physical contact with the surface of the ground, the resistance to the flow of current from the frame of the equipment and cable to the earth usually is high because of wire insulation. A machine-to-ground fault resistance of 100 ohms and a current of 10 amperes means an electric shock hazard of about 1000 volts. A leakage fault current of 1/50 ampere is very painful and can result in the loss of muscular control. As little electric current as 1/10 ampere through the body may result in death. (See Table 15-A in Chapter 15, "Electrical Hazards," in the *Engineering and Technology* volume.) Since these low leakage currents can be forced through wet skin by commercial 120 volts AC, no employee should be exposed even momentarily to this electrical hazard. Fig. 23–13 shows a grounded safety neutral system.

A good earthground system may be made by driving copper-clad steel rods, or electrodes, into suitable soil for a distance of at least 8 feet (2.4 m). Rods, which are available commercially for this purpose, lower the earth resistance and provide better ground. Since the number of rods and their spacing depend considerably on soil conditions, the conductivity of the soil may have to be increased by treatment with common salt, sodium nitrate, copper sulfate, or similar chemicals which are carried into the soil by rain. A ground

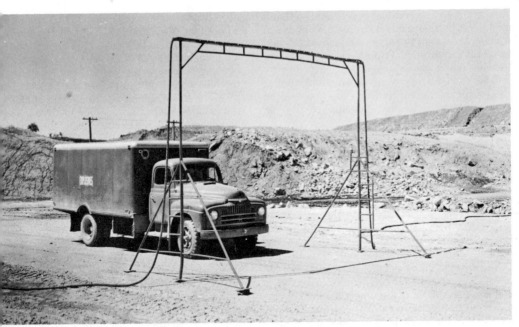

FIG. 23-14.—To minimize wear, a structure can be used to elevate trailing cables when they cross over roads.

g system having a total resistance of 1 ohm, including the cable, can be obtained in many areas by proper design and construction. (Chapter 15, "Electrical Hazards," in the *Engineering and Technology* volume, for a thorough discussion of grounding.)

The pole line ground wire should have at least the same wire gage size as the power wires. Wherever power is tapped from the power line, a connection is made from the pole ground wire to a ground wire in the cable. A good cable has metal shielding outside the insulating material around each conductor, and the ground conductor is in full electrical contact with the shielding. The shielding should have electrical continuity, and, if broken, it should be bridged.

The ground wire in the cable is connected to the frame of the equipment where there should be good metal-to-metal contact. If necessary, paint or other covering should be scraped off to achieve good contact. A resistor between the pole line ground wire and the transformer neutral limits the amount of current to not more than 50 amperes, eliminating dangerous voltages at the shovel and permitting sufficient current to open the circuit breakers.

The neutral ground system permits the opera-tion of all equipment except the machine where the fault occurs. The machine is segregated from the rest of the system by the immediate operation of a circuit breaker actuated by the fault. Suitable switching equipment in the neutral grounded system eliminates the danger from several faults existing at the same time in different phases at different locations, except for the interval required for the circuit breakers to open.

The equipment ground should not be con-nected to the substation ground in any way, to avoid energizing the equipment by a fault in the power supply system.

Circuit breakers and other devices in the grounding system should be inspected monthly. The resistance of the ground rods or system also should be checked regularly. A megohmmeter test of the cable insulation is a recommended part of cable inspection. Defective cable insulation should not be taped—the cable should be replaced.

Workers should be provided with rubber gloves and insulated tongs or hooks for handling trailing power cables.

Minimum wear and damage to trailing cables is important for safety. They should be protected from blasting operations as much as possible but kept as close to operations as practical so that a minimum length of cable is required. Tripods and wooden construction horses can be used to keep cable off the ground. Tripods are preferable to trenches where cables cross roads. (Fig. 23–14).

The electrical parts of shovels and similar equipment, including trailing cables, should be inspected regularly and maintained by an electrician.

**Maintenance practices.** If a shovel is operating in a deep excavation, repairs or adjustments should be made with the shovel in a safe position where it will not be endangered by falling or sliding rock or earth.

When repairs are to be made, the operator is responsible for setting the brakes, securing the boom, lowering the dipper or bucket to the ground, taking the machine out of gear, and before leaving the machine, exercising similar precautions to prevent accidental movement.

Before starting any job, maintenance personnel should notify the operator about its nature and location. If the work is to be done on or near moving parts, the controls should be locked out and tagged, and the lock and tag should be removed only by authorized persons. This precaution is essential to prevent the operator from starting the equipment inadvertently.

Parts that must be in motion while workers are working on them should be turned slowly, by hand if possible, in response to guidance or on signal if two or more persons must be involved. This precaution applies particularly to those who work around gears, sheaves, and drums. Workers who grasp ropes just ahead of the sheaves risk having their hands jerked into the sheaves. To prevent hand injuries, a rope being wound on a drum should be guided with a bar.

If guards must be removed for convenience in making repairs, the job cannot be considered complete until the guards, plates, and other safety devices have been replaced.

Repair personnel should wear snug-fitting clothing, eye protection, and safety shoes. Gloves should not be worn when working on or near any moving parts of the machines.

**Operating practices.** Slides of rock and material from high faces and banks result in some of the worst accidents in the operation of power shovels. In some instances, the shovel and operator have been buried, and in other cases, workers have

been struck and injured while working around t equipment (Fig. 23–8).

Some quarries that have high faces limit t height of banks to 25 ft (7.6 m) by benching and blasting procedure that forces the rock out fr the face sufficiently to reduce the height of t pile. The shovel operator is thus able to maint the back at a safe slope. When loading unde high face, the operator should swing the shovel the sight side and away from the face, there providing a better view and reducing the ex sure to injury.

Undercutting banks of earth, sand, gravel, a similar materials is dangerous, especially dur winter and spring months. Freezing and thaw may result in a collapse of the overhang material. To maintain a safe slope, the overhar ing material may be blasted.

The shovel operator has responsibility for t safety of other employees whose duties take the into the vicinity of the shovel. These workers m be struck by falling rock, squeezed betwe shovel and the bank or similar pinch points, struck by the dipper. No worker should enter dangerous location without first notifying t operator who, in turn, should not move t equipment.

Dippers should be filled to capacity but n overflowing, to prevent falling material fr endangering workers and to eliminate excessi spillage. Insofar as possible, loading should done from the blind side. The operator should n swing a load over a vehicle nor load a truck un its driver has dismounted and is in the clear, unle the truck is provided with a canopy designed the protection of the driver. Rail cars and mot trucks should be loaded evenly so that earth rocks do not overhang the sides.

Housekeeping on and around the shov should be stressed. The operator should ke tools in a definite place and keep the cab floor fr of grease and oil. Ice and snow should be remov promptly, and a bulldozer should keep the ar around the shovel free of rocks and ruts.

One should get on or off a shovel or dragli only after having notified the operator, who, turn, should swing the platform so that the han hold can be grasped and the steps or tread use No one should get on or off by jumping onto t tread, either while the operator is making a swi or while the equipment is stationary.

No unauthorized person should be permitte on a shovel or dragline.

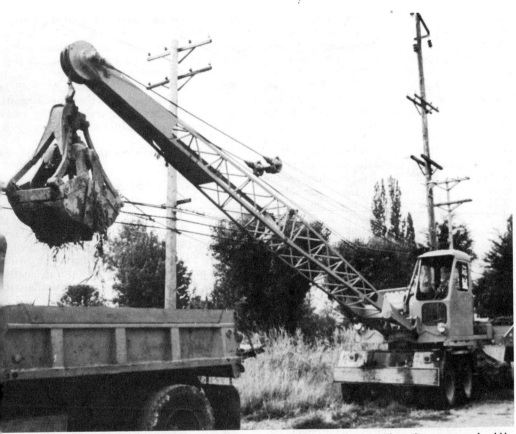

FIG. 23–15.—When mobile cranes must be operated in the vicinity of electric power lines, the utility company should be consulted first to determine whether the lines should be deenergized. OSHA and many state regulations require that booms and wire ropes be kept a minimum of 10 ft (3 m) away from power lines.

*Courtesy Washington State Department of Transportation.*

**Mobile cranes.** The outstanding characteristic of accidents involving crawler and similar types of cranes is the severity of the injuries. Although these accidents occur with relative infrequency, the injuries are about twice as serious as those resulting from accidents involving other types of heavy equipment. For this reason, a crane operator particularly should be selected for his intelligence, stability, and willingness to follow instructions.

The operator is largely responsible for the safe condition of the crane and should make regular inspections of brakes, ropes and their fastenings, and other vital parts, and promptly report worn, broken, and defective parts. Like other equip-

ment, mobile cranes should be maintained on a regular schedule.

The operator is responsible for the safety of the oiler an also has a large measure of responsibility for preventing injuries to hookers or riggers and others working around the equipment. However, anyone working in the vicinity of a crane has the responsibility to stay clear of the boom. In no case should anyone work or cross under the boom.

Some of the worst accidents result from overloading cranes. In no case should the load limits specified for various positions of the boom by the manufacturer be exceeded. These load limits should be conspicuously posted in the crane cab. If there is doubt about the weight of a load, the

**689**

capacity of the crane to handle the load safely should be tested by first lifting the load slightly off the ground. Operating a crane on soft or sloping ground is dangerous. The crane should always be level before it is put into operation. Outriggers give reliable stability only when used on solid ground. The use of makeshift methods to increase the capacity of a crane, such as timbers with blocking, is too dangerous to be permitted.

Boom stops limit the travel of the boom beyond the angle of 80 degrees above the horizontal plane and prevent the boom from being pulled backwards over the top of the machine by the boom-hoisting mechanism or the sudden release of a heavy load suspended at a short radius. Either of these occurrences usually result in serious damage to the equipment and injuries to the operator or other workers.

Accidents usually occur when the operator is performing more than one operation and becomes confused or distracted and excited. Also, clutch linings may swell during wet weather, and the master clutch or the boom clutch, or both, may "drag" and cause the boom to be pulled over backwards. Clutches should be tested before starting work on rainy days and the clearances adjusted if necessary. Another accident cause is the sudden release of a load when the boom angle is high, for example, from the parting of a sling.

Boom stops are best suited to medium-size cranes (the 5- to 60-ton range). Boom stops should disengage the master clutch or kill the engine and stop the boom before it reaches the maximum permissible angle. One type of stop that meets these requirements has a piston and cylinder; it is spring or pneumatically actuated, and is mounted on the A-frame to intercept the boom as high above the boom hinges as possible. By positive displacement of an actuator mounted on the A-frame, the boom action disengages the master clutch (or ignition breaker or compression release) by means of light rope reeved over a few small sheaves.

When a mobile crane must be operated near electric power lines, the power company should be consulted to determine whether the line can be deenergized. Most fatalities have resulted from contact with power lines, and often the power company's service is seriously disrupted. Various states and OSHA have enacted legislation specifying distances which booms and wire ropes must be kept from power lines. A minimum of 10 ft (3 m) is often specified; however, the recommendations

of the power company and legal requirements should be observed. (See Fig. 23–15.)

An experienced operator working with a untrained or relatively inexperienced hooker or rigger should direct the details of lifts, such as the type of sling and hitch to be used. Although the operator usually can rely on the knowledge of a experienced rigger, the operator has the right to question the safety of a lift and have his supervisor make a decision.

The following safe practices are essential when handling loads.

1. The hook must be centered over the load to keep it from swinging when lifted.

2. Employees should keep their hands out of the pinch point when holding the hook or slings in place while the slack is taken up. A hook, or even a small piece of board, may be used for the purpose. If a worker must use his hand, the sling should be held in place with the flat of the hand.

3. The hooker, rigger, and all other people must be in the clear before a load is lifted.

4. Tag lines should be used for guiding loads.

5. Hookers, riggers, and others working around cranes also must keep clear of the swing of the boom and cab.

6. No load may be lifted or moved without a signal. Where the entire movement of a load cannot be seen by the operator, as in lowering a load into a pit, someone should be posted to guide him. To avoid confusion in signals, only standard hand signals should be used. (See Chapter 4, in the *Engineering and Technology* volume, "Hoisting Apparatus and Conveyors.")

## Graders, bulldozers, and scrapers

Many of the basic safety measures recommended for trucks also apply to graders and other types of earth-moving equipment. All machines should be inspected regularly by the operator who also should promptly report any defects and malfunctioning systems or parts. The safety and efficiency of the equipment are increased by scheduled maintenance.

Only physically and mentally qualified individuals should be selected as operators and trained in correct operating practice, as specified in the manufacturer's manual and by company

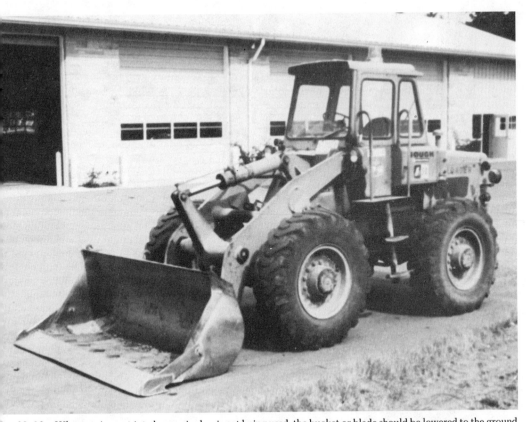

FIG. 23–16.—When equipment is to be repaired or is not being used, the bucket or blade should be lowered to the ground and the engine turned off.

*Courtesy Washington State Department of Transportation.*

requirements. Prevention of injury in the servicing and repairing of machines requires special precautions in addition to the observance of general safe procedures applying to other types of motorized equipment.

**Maintenance.** Brakes, controls, engine, motors, chassis, blades, blade holders, tracks, drives, hydraulic mechanisms, transmission, and other vital parts require regular inspection. Wheel and engine-mount bolts likewise require frequent checking for tightness.

Making adjustments and repairs with the engine running is a dangerous practice, particularly when work is being done near the fan of the engine or when a clutch of a tractor is being adjusted. Refueling should be done only with the engine stopped.

The danger from a locking ring blowing off when the tire of a truck is being inflated applies equally to a tractor tire. (See details under Tire Operations, earlier in this chapter.)

When cutting edges are to be replaced, the scraper bowl or dozer blade should always be blocked up. After the scraper has been lifted to the desired height, blocks are placed under the bottom near the ground plates. Apron arms are raised to the extreme height and a block is placed under each arm, so that the apron can drop enough to wedge each block firmly in place.

Before receiving wire rope on a drum or through sheaves, the operator should disengage the master clutch, idle the engine, and lock the brakes. The engine should be at a complete stop

**691**

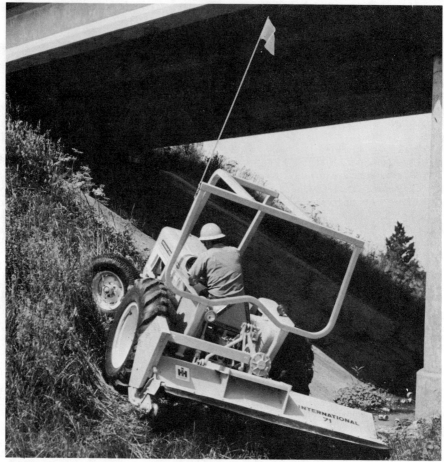

FIG. 23–17.—Mowers should have roll-over protective structures (ROPS), slow-moving vehicle (SMV) emblem, and an orange flag mounted about 10 feet (3 m) high.

*Courtesy International Harvester Company.*

before working with the rope on a front-mounted drum.

If an operator is assisting a repair worker and working behind the scraper with the tail gate in the forward position, a block should be placed behind the tail gate so that it cannot fall. This precaution is necessary in case someone should release the power control unit brake permitting the tail gate to come back.

When ropes are to be replaced on scrapers, the tail gate should be back at the end of its travel.

**General operating practices.** The operator must look to the front, sides, and rear before moving his machine and be constantly alert for employees on foot when operating near other equipment, offices, tool and supply buildings, and similar places.

Speeds are largely governed by conditions. Slow speeds are essential in driving (*a*) off the road and beyond the shoulder, on steep grades, and at rough places to avoid violent tilting which may throw the driver off the machine or against levers and cause serious injury, (*b*) in congested areas, and (*c*) under icy and other slippery conditions. No one other than the operator should be permit-d on the vehicle at the same time.

Jumping from a standing machine can result in sprained ankles and other injuries. The safe practice is to step down after looking to make sure that the footing is secure and there is no danger from other vehicles. Ice, mud, round stones, holes, and similar conditions cause many falls. For the same reason, deck plates and steps on equipment should be free of grease and other slipping hazards.

An operator should not drive the equipment into a haul road without first stopping and looking both ways, regardless of whether or not the place of entry is marked with a stop sign. Generally, loaded equipment is given the right of way on job or haul roads.

Before an operator leaves his equipment, even for a short time, the bucket or blade should be lowered to the ground and the engine stopped (see Fig. 23–16). A safe parking location is on level ground, off a roadway, and out of the way of other equipment.

The operator should never leave his equipment on the inclined surface or on loose material with the engine running—the vibration may put the equipment in motion.

**Procedures on roadways.** When graders, scrapers, and other earth-moving equipment are in operation along a section of a road, the precautions discussed next will help prevent accidents to the public, employees, and equipment.

Traffic must be warned, by barrier signs at both ends of the road section undergoing construction, that there is danger ahead. Primary warning signs, such as ROAD UNDER CONSTRUCTION or BARRICADE AHEAD, should be placed 1500 ft (460 m) from the end point of operation.

Orange flags or markers at the ends of blades, which may project beyond the tread of a machine, serve to warn persons and other equipment operators.

An orange flag on a staff that will project the flag at least 6 ft (1.8 m) above the rear wheel of a blade grader is recommended for operation in hilly country. (See Fig. 23–17.)

Operators of motor graders should keep to the right side of a roadway. When blading against traffic is necessary, flags and barricades should be used to warn traffic. Warning signs must be placed at a considerable distance from the work area. This distance increases as the "speed" of the highway increases. Suggestions are given in

National Safety Council's Data Sheet 614, *Surface Surveying*, and DOT *Manual on Uniform Traffic Control Devices for Streets and Highways*, ANSI D6.1. Most states use the latter standard (DOT) as minimum requirements, with additional traffic control where conditions dictate.

Where operations are extensive, flagmen should be placed at each end of the working area so that they are visible to oncoming traffic for at least 500 ft (152.5 m).

Where earth-moving equipment is stopping, turning, or backing at curves, crests of hills, and similar dangerous locations, flagmen must be stationed. Such movements generally require a clear view of approaching traffic for a distance of about 1000 ft (305 m) for safety.

Flagmen must also be used where the working area is congested by other equipment, workers, building, excavation, and similar hazards. See Fig. 23–18 for hand signaling procedures.

**Coupling and towing equipment.** An operator should not back up to couple a tractor to a scraper, sheepsfoot roller, or other equipment without having first checked to make sure that everyone is in the clear. If the operator is assisted by a person on the ground, he should not move the equipment until signaled.

Before an employee is allowed to couple the trailing equipment, the tractor should be stopped, the shift lever put in neutral, and the brakes set. The wheels of the equipment to be coupled should be blocked.

All equipment being towed should be secured by a safety chain attached to the pulling unit, in addition to the regular hitch or drawbar, since a drawbar failure can result in a serious accident.

When a scraper is towed from one job to another, the operator should use a scraper bowl safety latch, or place a safety bolt in the beam to give maximum clearance for road projections such as crossing. This precaution prevents the bowl from striking the ground or pavement and injuring persons or damaging equipment.

**Clearing work.** Work requiring exposure to low limbs of trees or to high brush involves serious hazards which can be readily overcome by suitable protective measures and safe practices. (See Fig. 23–11.)

When using a bulldozer, it is best to equip it with a heavy, well supported, arched steel mesh canopy to protect the operator. See section on

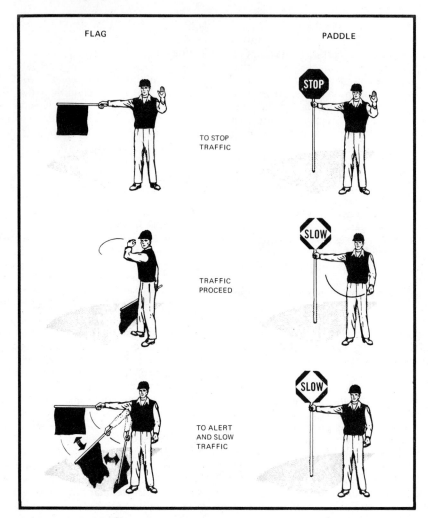

FLAG                                PADDLE

TO STOP
TRAFFIC

TRAFFIC
PROCEED

TO ALERT
AND SLOW
TRAFFIC

FIG. 23–18.—Hand signaling devices used by flagmen. Flag and background of STOP sign are bright red. Diamond of SLOW sign is orange.

*From American National Standard D6.1-1978.*

Protective Frames for Heavy Equipment, earlier.

Goggles should be worn to protect the eyes from whipping branches.

Head protection provides protection from falling dead branches. When a bulldozer shoves hard against the butt of a large dead tree, the tree may crack in the middle or limbs may fall onto the machine. Dead branches or tops also may drop from live trees. A safe procedure to eliminate the danger is to cut the roots on three sides and then apply the power to the fourth side. A long rope may be used to pull over large trees, but it must be determined in advance that the tractor and operator will be in the clear when the tree falls.

Operators have the responsibility of seeing that all workers in the area are in the clear before pushing over any trees, bulldozing rock, and rolling logs.

**Special hazards.** Fatalities can easily occur

hile equipment is operated on dumps and fills, ar excavations, and on steep slopes.

The bulldozer blade should be kept close to the ound for balance when the machine is traveling a steep slope.

When a tractor-dozer is to be driven down a ope, three or four loads of dirt should be dozed the edge of the slope and kept in front of the ade.

If the dirt is lost on the way down, the operator ould not lower the blade to regain the load cause of the danger of overturning. Using the ade as a brake on a steep slope should only be done in cases of extreme emergency.

How close to an excavation or the crest of a dump a machine can be safely operated depends on ground condition. Wet weather requires equipment to operate a greater distance from the edge or crest. Someone to signal the driver is especially essential when the ground is treacherous.

Sometimes employees, the public, livestock, and property are endangered when material is pushed over the edge in side hill work. In such cases, sufficient clearance below must be provided before the work begins.

## References

American Automobile Association, 1712 G St. NW., Washington, D.C. 20006.
   "Driver Training Equipment" (catalog).
   *Sportsmanlike Driving* (a textbook).

American Trucking Associations, Inc., 1616 P St. NW., Washington D.C. 20036. *Federal Motor Carrier Safety Regulations, U.S. Dept. of Transportation Federal Highway Administration, Parts 390-397, Issued January 1977.* (Pocketsize edition for issuing to drivers.)

American Insurers Highway Safety Alliance, 20 N. Wacker Drive, Chicago, Ill. 60606. *Code of the Road.*

The Associated General Contractors of America, Inc., 1957 E St. NW., Washington, D.C. 20006. *Manual of Accident Prevention in Construction.*

Association of Casualty and Surety Companies, 110 William St., New York, N.Y. 10038.
   *Guide Book, Commercial Vehicle Drivers*
   *Truck and Bus Drivers Rule Book*

National Fire Protection Association, 470 Atlantic Ave., Boston, Mass. 02210. *Flammable and Combustible Liquids Code, NFPA 30.*

National Safety Council, 444 N. Michigan Ave., Chicago, Ill. 60611.
   *Accident Investigation Manual (Motor Vehicle)*
   *Alcohol and the Impaired Driver.*
   *Aviation Ground Operators Safety Handbook.*
   Defensive Driving Program Materials.
   *Fundamentals of Industrial Hygiene.*
   Industrial Data Sheets
       *Airport Vehicular Traffic,* 539.
       *Barricades and Warning Devices for Highway Construction Work,* 239
       *Berms in Pits and Quarries,* 680.
       *Diving in Construction Operations,* 332.
       *Falling or Sliding Rock in Quarries,* 332.
       *General Excavation,* 482.
       *Grouding Electric Shovels, Cranes, and Other Mobile Equipment,* 287.
       *Lead-acid Storage Batteries,* 635.
       *Liquefied Petroleum Gases for Industrial Trucks,* 479.
       *Motor Graders, Bulldozers, and Scrapers,* 256.
       *Motor Trucks for Mines, Quarries, and Construction,* 330.
       *Mounting Heavy Duty Tires and Rims,* 411.
       *Operation of Power Shovels, Draglines, and Similar Equipment,* 271.
       *Ready-Mix Concrete Trucks,* 617.
       *Snow Removal and Ice Control,* 638.
       *Surface Surveying,* 614.
       *Tractor Operation and Roll-over Protective Structures,* 622.

*Motor Fleet Safety Manual.*
*Small Fleet Guide.*
*Public Employee Safety Guides—Streets, and Highway Maintenance.*
*Talk Topics—Motor Fleet, Book 2.*
*Vehicular Equipment Management.*
*Vehicle Damage Scale for Traffic Accident Investigators.*

New York University Center for Safety Education, Washington Square, New York, N.Y. 10003. Publications list.

North American Association of Alcoholism Programs, 1611 Deveonshire Drive, Columbia, S.C. 29204.

U.S. Department of Defense, Department of the Army, Washington, D.C. 20310.
*Driver Selection and Training, TM 21-300.*
*Drivers' Manual, TM 21-305.*
*General Safety Requirements, EM 385-1-1,* U.S. Army Corps of Engineers
"Methods of Teaching."
*Motor Transportation, Operation, FM 25-10.*

U.S. Department of the Interior, Bureau of Mines, Washington, D.C. 20240.
*Minerals Yearbook.*
Also various handbooks, miners' circulars, and other publications.

U.S. Department of Transportation, Federal Highway Administration, 8th and D Sts SW., Washington, D.C. 20591.
*Manual on Uniform Traffic Control Devices for Streets and Highways.* (Also identified as American National Standard D6.1.)
Title 49, *Code of Federal Regulations, Parts 390-397, Motor Carrier Safety Regulations.*

# Sources of Help

# Chapter
# 24

The safety professional frequently needs highly specialized or up-to-the minute, unpublished information. The sources for obtaining this information are numerous. Professional societies and trade associations are excellent sources of help; however, their charters of responsibility are varied. As an aid in the safety professional's search for information, this chapter selects some sources and defines their functions.

On a particularly difficult problem, it may be necessary to contact a number of sources before an effective solution can be obtained. Governmental authorities and specific organizations can furnish the minimum requirements under the law or applicable standards. Insurance companies or their associations may offer assistance through their knowledge of a similar problem. The trade association in the industry may have developed materials and aids in solving the problems.

The National Safety Council, through its resources and membership, can usually provide added input to the development of an effective countermeasure.

## Service Organizations

### National Safety Council
444 North Michigan Ave., Chicago, Ill. 60611

The National Safety Council is the largest organization in the world devoting its entire effort to the prevention of accidents. It is nonprofit and nonpolitical. Its staff members work as a team with more than 2000 volunteer officers, directors, and members of various divisions and committees to develop and maintain accident prevention material and programs in specific areas of safety. These areas include industrial, traffic, home, recreational, and public. Volunteer-staff teams are also organized in such areas as public information, publications, membership extension, and field organization. Council headquarters facilities include the largest safety library in the world.

At the Chicago headquarters, a staff of more than 350, about half of whom are engineers, editors, statisticians, writers, educators, librarians, and other specialists, carry out the major activities. In addition to its main office in Chicago, the Council has a regional office at 1705 DeSales St. NW., Washington, D.C. 20036.

Recognizing that industry's safety problems often require specialized treatment, the Council has divided its industrial effort into sections guided by the Industrial Division. Each section is administered by its own executive committee, nominated and elected from the membership within that industry. Each executive committee consists of a general chairman, a vice-chairman, secretary, a newsletter editor, subcommittee chairmen, and others elected at the annual meeting held at the National Safety Congress.

The industrial membership of the Council is organized according to the following industries. These sections are designed to provide special help for all facets of the industrial section, as shown below.

AEROSPACE
Missile and aircraft manufacture, related components

AIR TRANSPORT
Ground safety; personnel and equipment

AUTOMOTIVE, TOOLING, METALWORKING, AND ASSOCIATED INDUSTRIES
Machining, fabrication, assembly, general manufacturing

CEMENT, QUARRY AND MINERAL AGGREGATES
Quarrying, processing, manufacturing, production

CHEMICAL
Manufacturing compounds and substances

COAL MINING
Underground and open pit

CONSTRUCTION
Highway, buildings, heavy, home, specialty

ELECTRONIC AND ELECTRICAL EQUIPMENT
Manufacturing and assembly

FERTILIZER
Manufacturing, storage, transportation, retailing

FOOD AND BEVERAGE
Process foods, dairies, brewers, confectioners, distillers, canners and freezers, grain handling and processing, restaurants and fast food

FOREST INDUSTRIES
Logging, manufacturing, converting, pulp and paper, plywood, furniture, and related products

GLASS AND CERAMICS
Manufacturing; flat, containers, miscellaneous products, fiber, refractories, molds

HEALTH CARE
Hospital, patient, employee, visitor safety, security, emergency operations

MARINE
Deep water and inland waterway; crew, passenger, vessel safety, stevedoring, shipbuilding, repair, cargo

MEAT AND LEATHER INDUSTRIES
Meat packing, processing; tanneries and leather products

METALS
Foundries, manufacturing ferrous and nonferrous, fabricating, steel service centers

MINING
Metals and minerals

PETROLEUM
Exploration, drilling, production, pipeline, marketing, retail

POWER PRESS AND FORGING
Metal stamping and forming, forging

PRINTING AND PUBLISHING
Letterpress, offset, newspaper, bindery

PUBLIC EMPLOYEE
City, county, state, federal (employees and governments)

PUBLIC UTILITIES
Communications, electric, gas, water, construction

RAILROAD
Employee, passenger, public safety, freight

RESEARCH AND DEVELOPMENT
Safety; laboratory, physical, fire, health

RUBBER AND PLASTICS
Tires, molded products, belts, footwear, synthetics

TEXTILE
Manufacturing and fabrication, natural and synthetic fibers, ginning

TRADES AND SERVICES
Food service and retailers, other retailers, hotels, motels, mercantile and automotive, financial institutions, warehouses, offices, recreational facilities

The Council assigns a staff professional to each section to assist with programs, membership, organization, and the preparation of informational materials. In this way, each major industry group is assured of representation in the affairs of the Council and has the means to develop material and services to meet its needs.

Section executive committees meet several times a year. Improvement of Council services through new technical materials and visual aids takes a major portion of each committee's meeting time. Since increased membership can improve these services, membership solicitation is an ongoing program. Planning of National Safety Congress programs is given careful consideration. Special committees are often assigned to work on problems unique to an industry and on which there are no ready program materials.

To coordinate the entire Council industrial program, a committee representing all industries, the Industrial Division, meets two times a year. The function of this Division is to review current industrial safety and health problems and to determine on a national scale the best procedures to follow in providing increasingly beneficial programs to industry.

The Industrial Division is made up primarily of industrial members of the Council. It comprises 27 section general chairmen, 27 vice-general chairmen, and other members at large, drawn from business and industry member organizations, governmental agencies, insurance organizations, professional and trade associations, and other groups.

The Industrial Division is divided into 12 standing subcommittees that cover various segments of the occupational safety and health area to assist the 27 Industrial Sections and the Industrial Department in carrying out its responsibilities for occupational safety and health business and industry. The Council's Industrial Department manager is assigned as the staff representative to assist the Industrial Division members in their activities.

**Program materials.** The following Council publications have proven to be particularly useful for industrial and off-the-job safety programs. (Unless otherwise stated, they are published monthly.)

*Family Safety* (quarterly)
*Industrial Supervisor*
*National Safety News*
"OSHA Up-to-Date"
"Product Safety Up-to-Date"

**699**

Section "Newsletters" (one for each of the 27 sections—six issues a year)
*Safe Driver* (issued in three editions—Truck, Passenger Car, and Bus)
*Safe Worker*
*Traffic Safety* (six issues a year)

In addition, the following statistical materials are also available from the Council:

*Accident Facts* (annually)
Section Contest Bulletins (monthly)
"Work Injury and Illness Rates" (annually)

**Technical materials** (see current Council "General Materials Catalog" for a complete listing):
*Accident Prevention Manual for Industrial Operations* (this book)
   *Administration and Programs* volume
   *Engineering and Technology* volume
*Alcohol and the Impaired Driver*
*Aviation Ground Operations Handbook*
*Communications for the Safety Professional*
*Fundamentals of Industrial Hygiene*
*Guards Illustrated*
"Guide to Occupational Safety Literature"
*Handbook of Occupational Safety and Health*
"Industrial Data Sheets" (a series; listing available)
*Industrial Noise and Hearing Conservation*
*Meat Industry Guidelines*
*Motor Fleet Safety Manual*
"National Directory of Safety Films"
*Personnel Safety in Chemical and Allied Industries*
"Power Press Safety Manual"
"Public Employee Safety Guides"
*Safety Guide for Health Care Institutions*
"Safety Handbook for Office Supervisors"
*Safety Manual for the Graphic Arts Industry*
"Safety Reprints" (a series)
"School Transportation: A Guide for Supervisors"
"Small Fleet Guide"
"Successful Supervision"
*Supervisors Guide to Human Relations*
*Supervisors Safety Manual*

**Training and motivational materials:**
Banners
Booklets
Calendars
Films
Posters
Safety slides
Supervisory training pamphlets
Video tapes

**Meetings.** The National Safety Council sponsors the National Safety Congress and Expositio one of the largest conventions held anywher Nearly 200 general or specialized sessions, wor shops, and clinics are held covering the full rang of safety and occupational health topics.

The annual meetings or special business mee ings of a dozen of allied organizations and associ tions are also held concurrent with the Congres greatly enhancing the exchange of views ar information in safety and occupational health

Regional Congresses are held in the spring (th first one was held in Washington, D.C., in 1980) an effort to extend the expertise that is assemble at the annual Congress to a wider audience on th local level. The regional Congress provides a unusual opportunity to hear from leaders ar preeminent speakers representing regional inte ests in business, organized labor, and governmen

**Special services.** Special services availab through the Council to support industrial safet programs include:

*Library.* A computerized data base and th Safety Research Information Service form th bulk of the Council's vast library holdings. Mor than 7000 books and 600,000 reports and pam phlets make it the largest and most compreher sive safety resource of its kind in the world.

*Statistical.* The Council's statisticians provid a highly refined statistical capability. They are recognized source of reliable, accurate, an authoritative data within the safety communit Equipped with data processing and researc tools, they study various types of accident data i the continuing search for clues on the causes c accidents.

*Consulting.* In 1980, the Council introduced loss control management consulting servic aimed at the small to medium-sized manufactu ing company. It is specifically designed to mee the specialized needs voiced by executives c these smaller companies who seek a totally inte grated, yet reduced scale, effort of loss control i safety and occupational health.

**Safety training.** The National Safety Council's Safety Training Institute conducts the following training courses:

Fundamentals of Occupational Safety

Safety Training Methods

Safety Management Techniques

Practical Aspects of Industrial Hygiene

Fundamentals of Hospital Safety

Safety in Chemical Operations

Laboratory Safety

Fundamentals of Accident Prevention for Public Utilities

Motor Fleet Investigation Workshops

See the annual "Safety Training Institute Course Schedule" for dates of presentation and course content.

The Institute also offers two Home Study Courses in "Supervising for Safety" and "Human Relations for Supervisors." These courses are recognized by the National Home Study Council.

Three supervisor training courses are also available for purchase from the Safety Training Institute and have been designed for presentation by in-house training personnel. These programs include the "You Are Mangement" program, which is oriented to the new supervisor; "Supervisor's Development Program" for individuals with six or more months' experience; and the "Human Relations Course for Supervisors," directed toward the more experienced supervisor. (Complete information on these and other courses can be found in the National Safety Council's "General Materials Catalogue.")

The "Forklift Truck Operators Training Course" is an eight-hour program designed to help a company comply with training regulations. The course can be presented in the standard form or can be tailored to fit an individual company's facilities and needs.

Several of the courses offered by the Safety Training Institute are also presented by local safety councils.

The Safety Training Institute can tailor courses and seminars to customer needs and present them at customer locations. Information on costs, scheduling, and specifics is available from the Safety Training Institute.

Safety courses are also sponsored by other educational institutions. See the current "College and University Safety Courses" pamphlet, which is published by the Council. See also the discussion under Educational Institutions at the end of this chapter.

**The Labor Division.** Members of the Council's Labor Division represent unions and governmental labor agencies. This division and its members represent labor and its safety and health viewpoints in many of the Council's areas of work, such as construction, public utilities, coal mining, legislation, defensive driving, and vocational education.

Specific problems requiring labor's review or consensus input may be referred to one of the following committees of the division, subject to approval of the Executive Committee:

Awards
Fire Protection and Public Safety
Government, Labor Agencies, and Standards
Membership
Nominating
Occupational and Environmental Health
Occupational Safety
Off-the-Job and Driver Improvement
Program Planning
Promotion of Safety Training and Education

These committees may refer to the resources of the labor organizations affiliated with the Council.

## Community safety councils

Seventy-seven community and state safety councils located throughout the United States and Canada have been chartered by the National Safety Council. These councils work under the leadership of public-spirited citizens, commercial and industrial interests, responsible official agencies, and other important groups. They are nonprofit, self-supporting organizations whose purpose is to reduce accidents.

Accredited community councils operate under the guidance of a full-time manager and staff and receive continuous service from the National Safety Council. (A list of accredited councils can be obtained from the Council's State and Local Safety Council Relations Department.)

These organizations give assistance to local safety engineers and others concerned with occupational safety. Safety professionals, in turn, render substantial service through participation in the local council's work.

Many of the local councils offer the following services:

• Act as a clearinghouse of information on occupational safety problems, and maintain a library of films and other aids;

• Provide a forum for exchange of experience through regularly scheduled meetings of supervisory personnel;

• Sponsor courses of safety instruction, in some cases with the aid of educational institutions (many now present approved National Safety Council training courses);

• Conduct annual, area-wide occupational safety conferences;

• On request, give advice on safety problems and programs;

• Stimulate and assist in the development of accident prevention programs for all employers;

• Conduct safety contests with awards for outstanding safety records.

The scope and extent of activities of each group depend, of course, upon local conditions and available resources.

## American National Red Cross
17th and "D" Sts. NW., Washington, D.C. 20006

The American National Red Cross, through its more than 3100 chapters, offers free courses in first aid, cardiopulmonary resuscitation (CPR), swimming, lifesaving, and small craft handling.

Experience in industry shows that first aid and safety training contributes to the reduction of accidents—both on and off the job—by creating an understanding of accident causes and effects and by improving attitudes toward safety. In addition, this training prepares individuals to give proper emergency care to accident victims. In some situations, immediate action may mean the difference between life and death.

Arrangements for first aid training can be made through local Red Cross chapters. Most industries prefer to select key personnel to receive training as volunteer instructors who, in turn, can conduct classes for fellow employees. Others may wish to arrange for employee training

by instructors provided through a local chapte[r]

Texts, instructor's manuals, charts, and oth[er] teaching materials and visual aids, such as fil[m] and posters, are available through local chapte[rs]

## Industrial Health Foundation, Inc.
5231 Centre Avenue, Pittsburgh, Pa. 15232

The foundation, a nonprofit research associ[a]tion of industries, advocates industrial heal[th] programs, improved working conditions, and be[t]ter human relations.

The foundation maintains a staff of physician[s,] chemists, engineers, biochemists, and medic[al] technicians.

Activities fall into three major categories:

• To give direct professional assistance to me[m]ber companies in the study of industrial heal[th] hazards and their control.

• To assist companies in the development [of] health programs as an essential part of industri[al] organization.

• To contribute to the technical advancement [of] industrial medicine and hygiene by education[al] programs and publications.

Activities are classified as follows:

*Medical:*
Organization and administrative practices.
Opinions on doubtful X-rays.
Surveys of health problems.
Specific industrial medical problems.
Epidemiology studies.

*Chemistry, toxicology, industrial hygiene:*
Field studies—plant or industry basis.
Toxicity of chemicals, physical agents, processes.
Sampling and analytical procedures.

*Engineering:*
Ventilating systems.
Exhaust hoods.

*Education:*
Training courses in occupational health a[nd] safety for:
    Physicians
    Nurses
    Industrial hygienists and engineers.
Symposia on special subjects of current interest [in] these fields.

The foundation holds an annual meeting of members, conferences of member company specialists, and special conferences on problems common in a particular industry.

The following publications are issued:

*Industrial Hygiene Digest,* monthly (abstracts). Bibliographies on current interest subjects. Technical bulletins. Proceedings of symposia.

## National Society to Prevent Blindness
79 Madison Avenue, New York, N.Y. 10016

The NSPB is the oldest voluntary health agency nationally engaged in the prevention of blindness through a comprehensive program of community services, public and professional education, and research. The Society's industrial service program is guided by its Advisory Committee on Industrial Eye Health and Safety, comprised of experts in the fields of industry, education, medicine, nursing, and accident prevention.

Activities and programs of the department are:

• Promotes and administers the Wise Owl Club of America, eye-safety incentive program, among industrial, military, municipal and educational organizations. Membership in the Club is restricted to those who save their vision from being damaged or destroyed by wearing proper eye-protection both on and off-the-job. Junior Wise Owl Club membership recognizes sight saved by children and teenagers through wearing safety glasses or other forms of protectors.

• Promotes state-wide eye safety for all school and college laboratory and shop students, and their teachers and visitors. Both voluntary and legislative means are used. Provides counseling to school administrators and teachers in establishing and implementing eye safety programs. Encourages amendments to state school eye safety laws which presently exclude compliance by private schools.

• Provides secretarial, counseling, and liaison services for the American National Standards Institute Z87 Committee, engages in upgrading current eye and face protector code Z2.1. Participates as member of other American National Standards Institute studies dealing with topics related to illumination, vision, and eye protection.

• Promotes universal usage of nonflammable prescription and plano safety eyeglasses and sunglasses by the general public through voluntary and legislative means, and encourages cooperation by the eye care professions and the ophthalmic industry.

• Promotes periodic vision testing in industry and technical schools to determine visual defects and their relationship to visual requirements for various tasks and occupations. Provides counsel on improvement of visual working conditions through proper use of illumination and color.

• Provides exhibits on eye health and safety topics at industrial and educational meetings. Distributes literature and films on eye safety.

• Stimulates relationships with organizations, groups, and individuals with a related interest in sight conservation. Addresses industry, safety and educational meetings to project NSPB recommendations and program aims.

## Standards and Specifications Groups

### American National Standards Institute
1430 Broadway, New York, N.Y. 10018

The American National Standards Institute coordinates and administers the federated voluntary standardization system in the United States, which provides all segments of the economy with national consensus standards required for their operations and for protection of the consumer and industrial worker. It also represents the nation in international standardization efforts through the International Organization for Standardization (ISO), the International Electrotechnical Commission (IEC), and the Pacific Area Standards Congress (PASC).

ANSI is a federation of some 1200 national trade, technical, professional, labor, and consumer organizations, government agencies, and individual companies. It coordinates the standards development efforts of these groups and approves the standards they produce as American National Standards when its Board of Standards Review determines that a national consensus exists in their favor.

Many American National Standards, as well as other national consensus standards, have taken on additional importance since the passage of the Williams-Steiger Occupational Safety and Health Act of 1970. In promulgating standards under the act, the Occupational Safety and Health

Administration has stated a definite preference for basing its regulations on consensus standards that have proved their value and practicality by use.

Under ANSI procedures, the responsibility for the management of specific standards projects is divided according to subject matter and assigned to an ANSI Standards Management Board. Standards dealing with safety fall under the jurisdiction of the Standards Management Board. Many American National Standards on safety and health are developed by American National Standards Committees formed under ANSI procedures.

### American Society for Testing and Materials
1916 Race Street, Philadelphia, Pa. 19103

ASTM is the worlds largest source of voluntary consensus standards for materials, products, systems, and services. There are currently more than 6000 ASTM standards.

ASTM membership is drawn from a broad spectrum of individuals, agencies, and industries concerned with materials, products, and systems. The 28,500 members include engineers, scientists, researchers, educators, testing experts, companies, associations and research institutes, governmental agencies, and departments (federal, state, and municipal), educational institutions, consumers, and libraries.

ASTM standards are published for such categories as:

Nonferrous metals
Ferrous metals
Cementitious, ceramic, and masonry materials
Medical devices
Security systems
Energy
Construction
Chemicals and products
Environmental effects
Occupational safety and health
Protective equipment for sports
Electronics
Transportation systems
Business supplies

ASTM recently formed committees on geothermal resources and energy, quality control, food service equipment, and protective coatings for power generation facililties. The committee on consumer product safety has helped develop standards that will assist in protecting the public by reducing the risk of injury associated with the use of consumer products such as cigarette lighters, bathtubs, and shower structures, children's furniture, trampolines, and nonpowered guns.

ASTM standards are of interest to the safety professional since they identify areas of hazard and establish guidelines for safe performance. The society also publishes standards for atmospheric sampling and analysis, fire tests of materials and construction, methods of testing building construction, nondestructive testing, fatigue testing, radiation effects, pavement skid resistance, protective equipment for electrical workers, and others.

These constitute basic reference materials for safety professionals who will frequently be confronted with ASTM standards in processes, a with power plant installations in which vessels, piping, valves, and other component parts are designed and fabricated according to these standards. ASTM standards may also be factors in the raw materials used in protective equipment or other devices.

### Canadian Standards Association
178 Rexdale Boulevard, Rexdale,
Ontario M9W 1R3, Canada

The CSA was chartered in 1919. Until 1944, it was known as the Canadian Engineering Standards Committee. It is a private, not-for-profit organization serving as a standards developer and certifier. It publishes some 1200 standards, including the *Canadian Electrical Code*.

There is a Standards Steering Committee in each of the 38 broad areas of standardization.

### Other standards groups

In addition to the American National Standards Institute, many governmental and other agencies have established specifications used by safety professionals. Many industries through their trade associations have also established either (a) codes covering operations in their own plants or (b) safe practices to be followed in the use of their products. Some of these groups are:

AMERICAN SOCIETY OF MECHANICAL ENGINEERS
AMERICAN WELDING SOCIETY
COMPRESSED GAS ASSOCIATION
DEPARTMENT OF TRANSPORTATION
GENERAL SERVICES ADMINISTRATION
INDUSTRIAL SAFETY EQUIPMENT ASSOCIATION

INTERSTATE COMMERCE COMMISSION

NATIONAL ASSOCIATION OF PLUMBING AND MECHANICAL OFFICIALS

NATIONAL BOARD OF BOILER AND PRESSURE VESSEL INSPECTORS

NATIONAL BUREAU OF STANDARDS

NATIONAL FIRE PROTECTION ASSOCIATION

OCCUPATIONAL SAFETY AND HEALTH ADMINISTRATION

U.S. BUREAU OF MINES

## Fire Protection Organizations

Many safety professionals are also responsible for fire prevention and extinguishmsnt in addition to other aspects of safety.

The following organizations offer help in this field; also see Insurance Associations, later in this chapter.

### Factory Mutual System
### 1151 Boston-Providence Turnpike,
### Norwood, Mass. 02062

The Factory Mutual System is the world's largest mutual industrial insurance group and a world leader in loss control engineering and research. The System is an outgrowth of the philosophy of positive protection instead of just sharing the risk. In other words, recognition of the good risk through rate (premium) reduction is considered preferable to merely allowing the good risks to help pay for the bad.

The System consists of the following companies: Allendale Mutual Insurance (Johnston, R.I.), Arkwright-Boston Manufacturers Mutual Insurance (Waltham, Mass.), Philadelphia Manufacturers Mutual Insurance (Valley Forge, Pa.), Protection Mutual Insurance (Park Ridge, Ill.), Factory Mutual International (London, England), and Factory Mutual Engineering and Research (Norwood, Mass.).

Factory Mutual Engineering and Research provides loss prevention services for policyholders. Its aim is to make properties and production facilities safe from fire, explosion, wind, water, and many other perils for which coverage is provided, including damage to boilers, pressure vessels, and machinery. Engineering services include evaluation of hazards and protection through property inspections by Factory Mutual consultants located in major industrial centers. Research services involve the evaluation of fire protection devices and equipment for approval

and the development of recommendations based on tests and loss experience for the prevention of loss. The Test Center in Rhode Island provides full-scale fire testing, simulating industrial conditions with regards to height, weight, and protection of major industrial storage occupancies.

Loss control training services are available to policyholders, and assistance is given to special technical problems relating to loss prevention as well as the human element aspect. The source of these services is the Factory Mutual Training Resource Center.

Training courses include Practicing Property Conversion, Boiler and Machinery Preventive Maintenance (both developed specifically for insureds), and Designing for Firesafety and Hazard Control (open to all architects and design professionals). These courses are taught by Factory Mutual engineers, research scientists, and training experts.

Factory Mutual's publications include the *Record, Approval Guide, Handbook of Property Conservation, Loss Prevention Data Books,* and *Factory Mutual Resources—A User's Catalogue.* The *Record* is an internationally recognized bimonthly management magazine dealing with property conservation. The *Approval Guide* is a manual which lists industrial fire protection equipment that has been tested and approved by Factory Mutual laboratories. The *Handbook of Property Conservation* and the *Loss Prevention Data Books* cover recommended practices for protection against fire and related hazards. The *Factory Mutual Resources—A User's Catalogue* lists all available FM publications, films, training aids, and workshop kits.

### Industrial Risk Insurers
### 85 Woodland St., Hartford, Conn. 06102

The IRI is an association of forty-five insurance companies that provides underwriting and advisory loss-control engineering services to industry. It maintains a staff of engineers with representation in key industrial centers.

The fire safety laboratory in Hartford contains many types of fire protection equipment for examination and demonstration under working conditions. This laboratory is used for the basic and advanced training of IRI field engineers and for training plant protection personnel of IRI policyholders and of other insurance organizations who are given short courses in the proper use of fire protection devices.

### National Fire Protection Association
470 Atlantic Ave., Boston, Mass. 02210

The National Fire Protection Association is the clearinghouse for information on the subject of fire protection, fire prevention and firefighting. It is a nonprofit technical and educational organization with a membership of some 32,000 companies and individuals.

The technical standards issued as a result of NFPA committee work are widely accepted by federal, state, and municipal governments as the basis of legislation, and widely used as the basis of good practice. More than 50 are used as OSHA regulations. Constantly revised and updated, 240 standards are currently issued by NFPA, which are available in separate booklets.

Many of them supply authoritative guidance to safety engineers. Representative subjects include:

Industrial Fire Loss Prevention
Portable Fire Extinguishers
Sprinkler Systems Organization and Training of Private Fire Brigades
Flammable and Combustible Liquids Code
Hazardous Chemicals Data
Cutting and Welding Processes
Storage and Handling of Liquefied Petroleum Gases
Prevention of Dust Explosions in Industrial Plants
National Electrical Code
Lightning Protection Code
Air Conditioning and Ventilating Systems
Life Safety Code
Safeguarding Building Construction Operations
Protection of Records
Truck Fire Protection
Powered Industrial Trucks

The standards are also published as the "National Fire Codes" in 16 volumes totaling 12,800 pages.

Other publications of interest, such as the employee training course Introduction to Fire Protection, many items on fire safety in health care facilities, and the NFPA Inspection Manual, are available to safety professionals from the association.

The Fire Protection Handbook is also published by NFPA. An authoritative encyclopedia on fire and its control, the 1300-page handbook is divided into 18 sections and 131 chapters.

The current NFPA "Catalog of Publications and Visual Aids" is available from the NFPA Publications Sales Division.

### Underwriters Laboratories Inc.
333 Pfingston Road, Northbrook, Ill. 60062

The Underwriters Laboratories, a not-for-profit organization, maintains laboratories for the examination and testing of devices, systems, and materials, to determine their safety.

The laboratories publish annual directories of manufacturers whose products have proven acceptable under appropriate standards and which continue to pass their followup checking service.

These directories are:

"Automotive, Burglary Protection and Mechanical Equipment"
"Building Materials"
"Electrical Appliance and Utilization Equipment"
"Electrical Construction Materials"
"Fire Protection Equipment"
"Fire Resistance Index"
"Gas and Oil Equipment"
"Hazardous Location Equipment"
"Marine Products"

The Laboratories follow up on listed material at annual or more frequent intervals.

Safety professionals have come to regard the Underwriters' label as a requisite when they purchase fire, electrical, and other equipment which falls in categories tested in the laboratories.

Engineers should be aware, however, that UL listings apply only within the scope of the test made, and may have no bearing on performance or other factors not involved in the examination procedure. If the function of the device or material tested and listed is a safety professional what he wants to know. UL tests are made under conditions of installation and use which conform to the appropriate standards of the NFPA or other applicable codes. Any departure from these standards by the user himself may affect the performance qualifications found by the Underwriters Laboratories.

### Insurance Associations

In addition to the insurance associations listed under Fire Protection Organizations, there are a number of insurance federations with accident prevention departments that produce technical information available to safety people.

## Alliance of American Insurers
## 20 North Wacker Drive, Chicago, Ill. 60606

The Alliance of American Insurers is a national organization of leading property-casualty insurance companies. Its membership includes more than 150 companies that safeguard the value of lives and property by providing protection against mishaps in workplaces and losses from fires, traffic accidents, and other perils. Alliance member companies have a tradition of loss prevention which dates from the organization of the first American mutual insurance company in 1752.

Through its Loss Control Department, the Alliance makes a concerted effort to reduce accidents, fires, and other loss-producing incidents. Under the guidance of its loss control advisory committee, sound safety engineering, industrial hygiene, fire protection engineering, and other loss prevention principles are promoted. Major activities include the dissemination of information on safety subjects, conduct of specialized training courses for member company personnel, sponsorship of research, cooperation in the development of safety standards, development of visual aids, and the publication of technical and promotional safety literature. A catalog of safety materials is available without charge.

Notable among the publications issued by the Alliance are:

*Safe Openings for Some Point-of-Operation Guards*
*Wood Working Circular Saws, Protection for Variety and Universal Types*
*Spreaders for Variety and Universal Saws*
*Nip Hazards on Paper Machines*
*Material Handling Manual*
*Handbook of Organic Industrial Solvents*
*Judging the Fire Risk*
*Tested Activities for Fire Prevention Committees*
*Exit Drills in the Home*
*Handbook of Hazardous Material*
*Safety Memos for Fleet Supervisors*

Other Alliance departments also regularly issue a variety of bulletins, reports, research reports and similar materials that often may relate to and support work safety and accident prevention. The communications department, for example, publishes the general-interest magazine, *Journal of American Insurance*, as well as leaflets, brochures, and other informational and educational materials. Inquiry is invited.

The Alliance cooperates extensively with trade associations, professional societies, and other organizations with similar interests, such as the National Safety Council, the National Fire Protection Association, the American National Standards Institute, Inc., the American Society of Safety Engineers, and the American Industrial Hygiene Association.

## American Insurance Association
## 85 John Street, New York, NY 10038

The American Insurance Association, organized January 1, 1965, is an advisory organization serving a large number of companies in the property-liability insurance field. It is a multi-line organization designed to help its member and subscriber companies meet many of the diverse problems confronting the insurance business today. Embodied in the Association are the traditions, experience, and accomplishments of the National Board of Fire Underwriters, the Association of Casualty and Surety Companies, and the former American Insurance Association.

The Association, through its Engineering and Safety Service staff and subscriber representatives, has working representation on more than 175 committees of the National Safety Council, American National Standards Institute, and the National Fire Protection Association. In addition, the Association has worked closely with other trade, industry, and professional groups with similar interests.

The Engineering and Safety Service develops and publishes a wide variety of safety-related materials which it makes available to the public, in addition to those it produces for its subscriber companies.

Typical of the publications issued for the public are the following:

**Accident Prevention:**

Commercial and industrial
*An Emergency First Aid Guide*
*Safe Use and Care of Hand Tools*
*Your Guide to Safety as a Restaurant Employee*
*Your Guide to Safety in the Machine Shop*
*General Safety Instructions*
*Supervisor's Safety Guide Book*

Commercial vehicle fleets
*A Control Program for Motor Vehicle Fleets*
*Driver Selection*

**707**

Construction
  *Your Guide to Safety in Demolition-Wrecking
  Operations*
  *Your Guide to Safety on Construction
  Projects*

Home, traffic, and off-the-job
  *Boating Safety*
  *Family Safety Off the Job*

Public and semi-public
  *Safe Hospitals*
  *Safe Schools*
  *Your Guide to Safety as a Hospital
  Employee*

**Fire and natural hazards:**

Codes (suggested)
  *Fire Prevention Code*

Fire resistance ratings
  *Fire Resistance Ratings*

Fire prevention education
  "Self-Inspection Blanks" (camps, churches,
  farms, hospitals, hotels, industrial plants,
  mercantiles, places of assembly, and schools)
  "Sleep Easier with a Smoke Detector"
  "Family Home Safety Check List"
  "Apartment Dweller's Safety Check List"

Standards and recommended safeguards
  *Safe Handling and Use of LP-Gas*

Research publications
  *Fire, Explosion, and Health Hazards of
  Organic Peroxides*

**Special-interest bulletins:**

The Association has more than 250 special-interest bulletins, covering subjects like salamanders, fire-flow tests, small hose, and other items that do not require the full treatment given a standard. They contain information of special interest to firefighting services, municipal building inspectors, and fire protection people generally. An index to the bulletins is available on request.

**Highway emergency bulletins—police and fire:**

These bulletins promote public safety in the highway transportation of extra-hazardous commodities and furnish fire and police officials with educational and training material.

Technical surveys
  *Hazard Survey of the Chemical and Allied
  Industries*

A complete list of publications may be obtained by writing to the American Insurance Association.

## Professional Societies

### American Society of Safety Engineers
850 Busse Highway, Park Ridge, Ill., 60068

The American Society of Safety Engineers is the only organization of individual safety professionals dedicated to the advancement of the safety profession and to foster the well-being and professional development of its members.

In fulfilling its purpose, the Society has the following objectives:

Promote the growth and development of the profession

Establish and maintain standards for the profession

Develop and disseminate material which will carry out the purpose of the Society

Promote and develop educational programs for obtaining the knowledge required to perform the functions of a safety professional

Promote and conduct research in areas which further the purpose and objectives of the Society

Provide forums for the interchange of professional knowledge among its members

Provide for liaison with related disciplines

An annual professional development conference is conducted for members.

The Society is actively pursuing its Professional Development Programs including the development of curricula for safety professionals, accreditation of degree programs, member education courses, additional publications, and defining research needs and communications to keep safety practitioners current. In addition, the Society has increased its participation and activity in national government affairs.

The Society has established a separate research corporation, the American Society for Safety Research, because of its concern for the need for greater research efforts in the prevention of accidents and injuries. The Society believes that increased research will improve accident and injury control techniques, thus will serve the terests of its members as well as contributing to the economy of our nation and to the health and welfare of all persons.

The Society was also instrumental in establishing a separate corporation to develop a certification program for safety professionals. This corporation is known as Board of Certified Safety Professionals of America. (See BCSP later in this chapter.)

The members of the Society receive the monthly *Professional Safety* as part of their membership. (Nonmembers may also subscribe.) Articles on new developments in the technology of accident prevention are included, as well as information on the activities of the Society, its chapters and members. The Society also publishes other technical or specialized information, such as "A Selected Bibliography of Reference Materials in Safety Engineering and Related Fields," a glossary of terms used in the safety profession, and a series of Monographs.

Founded in 1911 as the United Association of Casualty Inspectors, it grew from the original enrollment of 35 to more than 15,000 members internationally in 1980.

Chapters engage in a number of activities designed to enhance the professional competence of their members. Most hold monthly meetings featuring speakers, demonstrations, workshops and discussions designed to help members keep abreast of developments in their professional field. A list of chapters grouped by states and listed by name and by location can be obtained from the national office.

## American Association of Occupational Health Nurses, Inc.
575 Lexington Ave., New York, N.Y. 10022

As the national professional organization for the registered nurse working in industry, the association strives to raise the qualifications for industrial nurses, improve nursing services and standards, and provide educational programs for nurses in this special field. *Occupational Health Nursing* is published monthly.

The annual meeting is held in conjunction with that of the American Occupational Health Conference of the American Occupational Medical Association.

## American Board of Industrial Hygiene
475 Wolf Ledges Parkway,
Akron, Ohio 44311

This specialty board is authorized to certify properly qualified industrial hygienists. The overall objectives are to encourage the study, improve the practice, elevate the standards, and issue certificates to qualified applicants.

## American Chemical Society
1155 16th St. NW., Washington, D.C. 20036

This society is devoted to the science of chemistry in all its branches, the promotion of research, the improvement of the qualifications and usefulness of chemists, and the distribution of chemical knowledge.

Articles on safety appear in the monthly publication *Industrial and Engineering Chemistry,* the weekly publication *Chemical and Engineering News,* and in the *Journal of Chemical Education.* Digests of papers dealing with aspects of industrial hygiene appear monthly in *Chemical Abstracts.* The environment is discussed in *Environmental Science and Technology.*

The society has a Committee on Chemical Safety and a Division of Chemical Health and Safety. It also has inaugurated a Chemical Health and Safety Referral Service which is accessible by telephone at 202/872-4511.

## American College of Surgeons
40 E. Erie St., Chicago, Ill. 60611

The American College of Surgeons, in addition to its role in the Joint Action Program with the National Safety Council and the American Association for the Surgery of Trauma, is launching a series of Advanced Trauma Life Support courses for physicians given through the auspices of the College's Committee on Trauma. The object, as always, is improved care for the injured patient.

## American Conference of Governmental Industrial Hygienists
2205 South Road, Cincinnati, Ohio 45238

A professional association composed of industrial hygiene personnel in government (federal, state, county, or municipal government), or working under a government grant. ACGIH was organized in 1938 by a group of governmental industrial hygienists as a medium for the exchange of ideas, experiences, and the promotion of standards and techniques in occupational health.

ACGIH's wide scope of activities are accomplished through the work of its 15 standing committees.

Particularly valuable to safety professionals is *Industrial Ventilation—A Manual of Recommended Practice,* by the Committee on Industrial Ventilation. ACGIH annually publishes a table of recommended threshold limits for chemical substances and physical agents.

A list of publications will be sent on request to ACGIH.

### American Industrial Hygiene Association
475 Wolf Ledges Parkway,
Akron, Ohio 44311

The AIHA is a professional association composed of industrial hygiene personnel. Established in 1939 by leading industrial hygienists as a result of a need for an association devoted exclusively to industrial hygiene, its purpose is to disseminate knowledge of the field and to promote the study and control of environmental factors effecting the health of industrial workers. Requirements for membership are a college degree and three years of industrial hygiene experience.

AIHA publishes "Hygienic Guides" (summarizing current information on physiological effects of specific chemicals, and methods of control), the *American Industrial Hygiene Association Journal,* the *Air Pollution Manual* and the *Industrial Noise Manual,* and reports and monographs. A list of publications will be sent on request to AIHA.

The AIHA, in cooperation with the American Conference of Governmental Industrial Hygienists, sponsors the annual American Industrial Hygiene Conference, the largest national assembly for the presentation and exchange of industrial hygiene information.

### American Institute of Mining, Metallurgical, and Petroleum Engineers
345 East 47th St., New York, N.Y. 10017

The AIME promotes the advancement of knowledge of the arts and sciences involved in the production and use of useful minerals, metals, energy sources, and materials and to record and disseminate developments in these areas of technology for the benefit of mankind.

Publications are *Mining Engineering, Journal of Metals, Journal of Petroleum Technology, Iron and Steelmaker,* all issued monthly and *Transac-*

*tions of the Society of Mining Engineers* (quarterly), *Transactions of the Metallurgical Society* (bimonthly), and *Transactions of the Society of Petroleum Engineers of AIME* and *Society of Petroleum Engineers Journal* (quarterly).

### The American Medical Association
535 No. Dearborn St., Chicago, Ill. 60610

The American Medical Association, with current membership of about 200,000 physicians, has a long record of involvement in public health.

The Department of Environmental, Public and Occupational Health (DEPOH) was organized in 1970 as a combination of AMA's Departments of Occupational Health and Environmental Health. In general terms, it is concerned with the well-being of all population groups whether they be in the work place or in the community. Thus the expertise of the staff covers the health effects of air, water, chemical, and physical stresses; communicable diseases; population growth; injuries; epidemiology; preventive medicine; sports medicine; and problems of the aged and the handicapped.

The department is principally an authoritative source of information for inquiries about environmental, public, and occupational health. In addition, it plans appropriate conferences and courses, prepares authoritative publications for physicians and the public, carries out special assignments and studies, and acts as the AMA liaison in federal health programs and legislation.

Since 1939, AMA has sponsored and organized annual congresses on occupational health. Intended especially to benefit the part-time occupational health practitioner, these congresses have addressed such topical subjects as: the reproductive disorders of workers, mental health in industry, group practice in occupational health, occupational pulmonary diseases, diseases and injuries of the back, and toxic chemicals in the community.

National conferences on the medical aspects of sports, which focus on the prevention and treatment of athletic injuries, are intended for team physicians, coaches, trainers, and administrators. Proceedings of the conferences are published.

The AMA continues to have an active voice in the regulatory process: for example, identifying to the National Institute of Occupational Safety and Health (NIOSH) those AMA physicians who have the expertise to review NIOSH Criteria

Documents. And when the Occupational Safety and Health Administration (OSHA) proposed a rule (in July 1978) to give OSHA and NIOSH complete access to employees' medical records, department staff protested in the public hearings.

The *Journal of the American Medical Association* (JAMA) is published weekly and frequently contains articles on some aspect of occupational health.

## American Nurses' Association, Inc.
2420 Pershing Road,
Kansas City, Mo. 64108

The American Nurses' Association is the voluntary membership organization for all registered nurses. The Division on Community Health Nursing Practice is the component of the ANA which provides authoritative information about the practices of occupational health nursing. The objectives of the division are to improve community health nursing practice including occupational health nursing practice for better employee health care.

Publications of interest are: "Standards of Community Health Nursing Practice," "Concepts of Community Health Nursing," and "A Statement on Certification of Occupational Health Nurses." Titles of other brochures, pamphlets, guides, and articles are included in the association's publications list which will be sent on request. (It should be noted that these other publications do not deal specifically with Community Health Nursing Practice.)

## American Occupational Medical Association
150 N. Wacker Drive, Chicago Ill. 60606

The American Occupational Medical Association fosters the study and discussion of problems peculiar to the practice of industrial medicine and surgery, encourages the development of methods adapted to the conservation and improvement of health among workers, and promotes a more general understanding of the purpose and results of employee medical care.

Some of the association committees are:

Alcoholism and Drug Abuse
American National Standards Institute Liaison
  Representatives
Annual Scientific Meeting
Energy Technology
Ethical Practice in Occupational Medicine
Education Council

Health Achievement in Industry Award
Health Education
Labor Liaison
Medical Center Occupational Health Services
Medical Information Systems
Medical Practice in Small Industries
Noise and Hearing Conservation
Nutrition
Occupational Medical Practice
Psychiatry and Occupational Mental Health
Trauma

The official publication of the association is the monthly *Journal of Occupational Medicine*.

An annual American Occupational Health Conference is held, usually in April, in collaboration with the American Association of Occupational Health Nurses.

## American Psychiatric Association
1700 18th St. NW., Washington, D.C. 20009

This association is concerned with research in all phases of mental disorders, standards of psychiatric education, and the medico-legal aspects of psychiatric practice. It publishes the *American Journal of Psychiatry* bimonthly.

## American Public Health Association
1015 Fifteenth Street, N.W.,
Washington, D.C. 20005

The American Public Health Association is a multidisciplinary, professional association of health workers. Through its two monthly periodicals, *The American Journal of Public Health* and *The Nation's Health* and other publications, APHA disseminates health and safety information to those responsible for state and community health-service programs. Program area Sections are devoted to injury control and emergency health services, and to occupational health and safety.

## American Society for Industrial Security
2000 K St., NW., Washington, D.C. 20006

The American Society for Industrial Security, a professional society of more than 14,000 industrial security executives in both the private and public sector, has 124 chapters in 17 regions worldwide. Committee activities that would be of interest to the safety professional are safeguarding proprietary information, physical security, terrorist activities, disaster management, fire prevention and safety, and investigations.

The Society publishes the magazine *Security Management* monthly and issues a newsletter to its members bimonthly.

The Society certifies security professionals through its Certified Protection Professional (CPP) program.

### American Society of Mechanical Engineers
345 East 47th St., New York, N.Y. 10017

This society, the professional mechanical engineers' organization, encourages research, prepares papers and publications, sponsors meetings for the dissemination of information, and develops standards and codes under the supervision of the Policy Board.

The society developed the following safety codes under the procedures meeting the criteria of American National Standards Institute:

*Safety Code for Elevators*
*Safety Code for Mechanical Power-Transmission Apparatus*
*Safety Code for Conveyors, Cableways, and Related Equipment*
*Safety Code for Cranes, Derricks, and Hoists*
*Safety Code for Manlifts*
*Safety Code for Powered Industrial Trucks*
*Safety Code for Aerial Passenger Tramways*
*Safety Code for Mechanical Packing*
*Safety Code for Garage Equipment*
*Safety Code for Pressure Piping*
*Safety Standards for Compressor Systems*

The ASME Boiler and Pressure Vessel Committee is responsible for the formation and revision of the ASME *Boiler and Pressure Vessel Code.*

The society publishes the *Transactions of the American Society of Mechanical Engineers* and the monthly publications Mechanical Engineering and *Applied Mechanics Review.*

### American Society for Training and Development
P.O. Box 5307, Madison, Wis. 53705

Professional society of persons engaged in the training and development of business, industrial, and government personnel.

### Board of Certified Safety Professionals
Suite 101, 501 S. 6th St.,
Champaign, Ill. 61820

The Board of Certified Safety Professional (BCSP) was organized as a peer certification board in 1969 with the purpose of certifying practitioners in the safety profession. The specific functions of the Board, as outlined in its charter, are to evaluate the academic and professional experience qualifications of safety professionals, to administer examinations, and to issue certificates of qualification to those professionals who meet the Board's criteria and successfully pass its examinations. Contact the BCSP for details on the requirements for certification.

### The Chlorine Institute
342 Madison Ave., New York, N.Y. 10017

Founded in 1924, the institute provides "a means for chlorine producers and firms with related interests to deal constructively with common industry problems—especially in safety, transportation, regulations and legislation, and community relations."

Results of committee deliberations are distributed worldwide to chlorine producers, consumers, and other interested groups and persons. In addition to the *Chlorine Manual* and audiovisual programs, some 70 engineering and design recommendations, specifications, and drawings are available.

### Flight Safety Foundation
5510 Columbia Pike, Arlington, Va. 22204

The Flight Safety Foundation works to improve standards and techniques in all aircraft operations. Its specific objectives are to promote research, to provide a forum where controversial safety issues may be resolved, to disseminate accident prevention information (through such means as articles, bulletins, reports, books, and lectures), to encourage the adoption of proven safety devices or procedures, and to try to foresee hazards and to press for corrective action.

To further these objectives, the foundation acts as a clearinghouse for the collection, analysis, and dissemination of safety information. Its personnel participate in safety discussions and safety studies and conduct safety seminars for aviation personnel. It presents awards and otherwise encourages the growth of safety programs. It acts as a catalytic agent in drawing attention to needed improvements and changes in safety techniques. Its publications include:

*Accident Prevention Bulletin* (monthly)

*rport Operators Safety Bulletin* (monthly)
*r-Taxi Commuter Safety Bulletin* (bimonthly)
*iation Mechanics Bulletin* (bimonthly)
*siness Pilots Safety Bulletin* (monthly)
*bin Crew Safety Exchange* (bimonthly)
*ght Safety Facts and Reports* (monthly)
*licopter Safety Bulletin* (bimonthly)
*man Factor Bulletin* (bimonthly)
*ots Safety Exchange Bulletin* (monthly)

Among the foundation's reports and special
idies are:

*cident Reports and Accident Prevention*
*rcraft Fueling*
*llision Prevention*
*oblem of Bogus Parts*
*mp Service*

## ealth Physics Society
lite 506, 4720 Montgomery Lane,
thesda, Md. 20014

Organized in 1955 and incorporated in 1961,
e HPS has as its objectives: (*a*) to aid and
vance health physics research and applied
tivities, (*b*) to encourage dissemination of infor-
ation between individuals in this and related
lds, (*c*) to improve public understanding of the
oblems and needs in radiation protection, (*d*) to
itiate and develop programs for training of
alth physicists, and (*e*) to promote the health
ysics profession.
*Health Physics* is the official journal of the
ciety.

## uman Factors Society
O. Box 1369, Santa Monica, Calif. 90406

HFS is a society of psychologists, engineers,
ysiologists, and other related scientists who are
ncerned with the use of human factors in the
velopment of systems and devices of all kinds.
*uman Factors* is the official journal.

## uminating Engineering Society of North
America
45 East 47th St., New York, N.Y. 10017

The society is the scientific and engineering
imulus in the field of lighting. The work of the
dustrial Lighting Committee and its numerous
bcommittees for various specific industries
ould be of particular interest to industrial safety
rofessionals. Many other projects, such as street
d highway, aviation, and office lighting, may

also be of interest.

Through the society, safety personnel can
obtain reference material on all phases of lighting,
including authoritative treatise on nomenclature,
testing, and measurement procedures.

The society publishes a monthly magazine,
*Lighting Design and Application*; a quarterly,
*Journal of the Illuminating Engineering Society*;
and the *IES Lighting Handbook*, a reference
guide. In addition, the society publishes approximately 50 other publications on specific lighting
areas such as mining, roadway, office, and emergency lighting.

## International Hazard Control Manager
Certification Board
P.O. Box 50101, Washington, D.C. 20004

Founded in 1976, the Board evaluates and
certifies the capabilities of practitioners engaged
primarily in the administration of safety and
health programs. Levels of certification are senior
and master, with master being the highest attainable status indicating that the individual possesses
the skill and knowledge necessary to effectively
manage comprehensive safety and health programs. The Board offers advice and assistance to
those who wish to improve their status in the
profession by acquiring skills in administration
and combining them with technical safety abilities. Establishes curricula in conjunction with
colleges, universities and other training institutions to better prepare hazard control managers
for their duties. Publications are the *Hazard
Control Manager* (quarterly) and the *Directory*
(annual).

## International Healthcare Safety Professional
Certification Board
9413 Jones Place, Seabrook, Md. 20801

A program to certify health-care safety professionals has been established by the International
Healthcare Safety Professional (HSP) Certification Board. The HSP program is designed to raise
the competence, status, and recognition of health
care safety professionals and assist in the transfer
of technology and the exchange of ideas for
improving safety in health-care activities.

The Healthcare Safety Professional (HSP) certification program has the following objectives:

• Evaluating the qualifications of persons
engaged in hazard control activities in hospi-
tal/health-care facilities.

**713**

• Certifying as proficient individuals who meet the level of competency for this recognition.

• Increasing the competence and stimulating professional development of practitioners.

• Providing recognition and status for those individuals who by education, experience, and achievement are considered qualified.

• Facilitating the exchange of ideas and technology that will improve performance.

The HSP program grew out of professional contacts of health-care practitioners with the founders of the Certified Hazard Control Manager program (CHCM). The relationship spread over several years and resulted in CHCM and a number of National Safety Council Health Care Section members working cooperatively to establish the HSP program.

The National Safety Council's Health Care Section members believed that the health-care field had a significantly large number of safety practitioners with the common interests, skills and experience to justify a certification program. The final version resulted from changes they suggested during the 1979 National Safety Congress in Chicago.

There are three levels of certification: the Executive, requiring five years experience and a baccalaureate degree; the Associate, requiring three years experience and an associate of arts degree; and the Affiliate, which requires assignment as a safety officer, completion of high school or equivalent, plus specified safety courses over a period of two years.

### National Association of Suggestion Systems
435 N. Michigan Ave., Chicago, Ill. 60611

The National Association of Suggestion Systems, incorporated as a nonprofit organization, encourages suggestion system activity in industry, commerce, finance, and government. Specific objectives are:

• To increase appreciation of the usefulness of employee suggestion systems.

• To encourage study of the elements necessary to successful use of employee thinking.

• To provide an opportunity for the personal development of those who represent member institutions.

• To gather and disseminate useful information

through meetings, publications, factual surve and the like.

• To promote personal contacts between sugg tion system administrators and the leaders various industries.

### National Safety Management Society
6060 Duke St., Alexandria, Va. 22302

The National Safety Management Socie founded in 1966, is a nonprofit corporation t seeks to expand and promote the role of safe management as an integral component of to management by developing and perfecting eff tive methods of improving control of accide losses, be they personnel, property, or financi Membership is open to those having manageme responsibilities related to loss control.

### SAFE Association
P.O. Box 631, Canoga Park, Calif. 91303

The SAFE Association is dedicated to advar ing the science and art of space and flight equi ment as they apply to personal safety and surviv systems. Members are designers, engineers, ma ufacturers, and users of safety and surviv equipment.

### System Safety Society
P.O. Box A, Newport Beach, Calif. 92663

The System Safety Society is a nonprofit orga ization of professionals dedicated to safety products and activities by the effective impl mentation of the system safety concept. Th concept is, basically, the application of appropr ate technical and managerial skills to assure that systematic forward-looking hazard identificatic and control function is made an integral part of project, program, or activity at the conceptu planning phase, continuing through design, pr duction, testing, use, and disposal phases. Th objectives include:

To advance the state-of-the-art of system safet

To contribute to a meaningful management a technological understanding of system safet

To disseminate newly developed knowledge to a interested groups and individuals.

To further the development of the professiona engaged in system safety.

Through its local chapters, committees, exec

ive council, publications, and meetings, the society provides many opportunities for interested members to participate in a variety of activities compatible with society objectives. In addition to its operating committees, society activities include publication of *Hazard Prevention*, the official society journal. Published five times a year, it keeps members informed of the latest developments in the field of system safety.

International System Safety Conferences are sponsored biennially.

## Veterans of Safety
4721 Briarbend Dr., Houston, Texas 77035

Membership numbers 1700 safety engineers with 15 or more years of professional safety experience. Founded in 1941, the objective of Veterans of Safety is to promote safety in all fields. Activities include: (*a*) Safety Town USA, to educate preschool and elementary school children in pedestrian safety; (*b*) Most Precious Cargo Program, to improve school bus safety; and (*c*) Unified Emergency Telephone Numbers Program, to establish nationwide uniformity in emergency telephone numbers to contact fire, police and medical aid. Gives annual awards for best technical safety papers published. Maintains placement service.

## Trade Associations

## American Foundrymen's Society
Golf and Wolf Rds.,
Des Plaines, Ill. 60016

The American Foundrymen's Society is the only technical society that serves the interest of the foundry industry. It disseminates information on all phases of foundry operations, including safety, hygiene, and air pollution control.

The following publications are available through the society and should be of interest to the safety professional:

American National Standard Series Z241 for sand preparation, molding and coremaking, melting and pouring, and cleaning and finishing of castings.
*Control of the Internal Foundry Environment*
*Control of the External Foundry Environment*
"Foundry Health and Safety" Series
*Foundry Landfill*
*State-of-the-Art Noise Control for Foundries*
*Solid Waste Disposal*

## American Gas Association
1515 Wilson Blvd., Arlington, Va. 22209

The association, through its Accident Prevention Committee, serves as a clearinghouse and in an advisory capacity to persons responsible for employee safety and to safety departments of its member companies. Its purposes are to study accident causes, recommend corrective measures, prepare manuals, and disseminate information to the gas industry that will help reduce employee injuries, motor vehicle accidents, and accidents involving the public. The committee meets several times a year and conducts an Occupational Safety and Health Symposium each year. It also provides speakers for regional gas association and other gas industry meetings.

The committee has task committees on each of the following aspects of employee safety: awards and statistics, distribution and utilization, education, motor vehicles, posters, publications, gas transmission, and promotional and advisory.

Published material includes suggested safe practices manuals, quarterly and annual reports on the industry's accident experience, posters, and an analysis of disabling injuries occurring to employees of more than 100 gas companies. Sound-slide programs are also produced.

The association also maintains laboratories in Cleveland and Los Angeles, where gas appliances are tested and design certified.

## American Iron and Steel Institute
1000 16th St. NW., Washington, D.C. 20036

AISI represents companies accounting for more than 90 percent of raw steel production in the U.S. Special committees on Safety, Industrial Health, and Industrial Hygiene meet quarterly. Regional Safety Committees meet quarterly to provide informational forums for steel plant safety personnel.

The committees sponsor research, develop safety and health management programs for the steel industry, and plan and conduct seminars for management and professional personnel of the industry on specific topics relating to safety and health.

## American Mining Congress
1920 N. St. NW., Washington, D.C. 20036

Congress membership is from coal, metal, and nonmetal mining companies. This association has a Coal Mine Safety Committee, a Noncoal Mine

Safety Committee, and an Occupational Health Committee.

The monthly *Mining Congress Journal* regularly carries articles and news about safety and health.

## American Paper Institute, Inc.
260 Madison Avenue,
New York, N.Y. 10016

The American Paper Institute, through the Safety and Health Subcommittee of its Employee Relations Committee, conducts a broad safety and health education and information service for the paper industry. The Subcommittee sponsors workshops and seminars on various safety and health subjects. Ad hoc task forces are also established to deal with specific problems requiring rapid response, specialized knowledge, or concentrated effort.

In addition, the institute's Employee Relations Department issues a quarterly "Safety and Health Report," which covers the latest developments in OSHA, NIOSH, paper industry safety issues, notices of upcoming safety and health conferences, and other items of current interest. This report includes detailed summaries of selected fatalities and disabilities which have occurred during the period, outlining a brief description of the accident; the department in which it occurred; the machine, tool or other agency involved; and corrective action taken by the particular mill reporting the accident.

The institute, through its Employee Relations Department, compiles an annual "Summary of Occupational Injuries and Illnesses." It also has an industry-wide Safety Award program, which honors individual mills that have outstanding safety records.

## American Petroleum Institute
2101 L St. NW., Washington, D.C. 20037

The objective of the Committee on Safety and Fire Protection of the American Petroleum Institute is to reduce the incidence of accidental occurrences, such as injuries to employees and the public, damage to property, motor vehicle accidents, and fires. To attain this objective, the Committee on Safety and Fire Protection:

• Provides statistical reports, pamphlets, data sheets, and other publications to assist the industry in the prevention of accidents and the prevention, control, and extinguishment of fires.

• Provides a means for the development an exchange of information on accident preventic and fire protection to be used for education ar training in the industry.

• Provides a forum for discussion and exchang of information concerning safe practices and th science and technology of fire protection an safety engineering.

• Promotes research and development in th fields of accident prevention and fire protectio for the benefit of the petroleum industry as whole.

Safety and fire protection manuals have bee published on such subjects as:

*Driver's Handbook*
*Protection Against Ignitions Arising Out of Stati Lightning and Stray Currents*
*Safe Operation of Inland Bulk Plants*
*Safe Practices in Gas and Electric Cutting an Welding in Refineries, Gasoline Plants, Cyclin Plants, and Petrochemical Plants*
*Cleaning Mobile Tanks in Flammable or Combus tible Liquid Service*
*Cleaning Petroleum Storage Tanks*
*A Guide for Controlling the Lead Hazard Assoc ated with Tank Entry and Cleaning*
*First Aid Training Guide*
*Driver Improvement Course*
*Guides for Fighting Fires in and Around Petro leum Storage Tanks*
*Fire Hazards of Oil Spills on Waterways*
*Guide for Safe Storage and Handling of Heate Petroleum-Derived Asphalt Products and Crud Oil Residue*
*Emergency Planning and Mutual Aid for Product Terminals and Bulk Plants*
*Repairs to Crude Oil, Liquefied Petroleum Gas and Products Pipelines*
*Procedures for Welding or Hot Tapping on Equip ment Containing Flammables*
*Dismantling and Disposing of Steel from Tank Which Have Contained Leaded Gasoline*
*Fueling Fixed, Portable, and Self-Propelle Engine-Driven Equipment*
*Identification of Compressed Gases in Cylinder*
*Preparing Tank Bottoms for Hot Work*
*Pipe-Plugging Practices*
*Flame Arresters for Tank Vents*
*Precautions While Working in Reactors Havin an Inert Atmosphere*

## American Pulpwood Association
### 1619 Massachusetts Ave. NW.,
### Washington, D.C. 20036

This association fosters study, discussion and action programs to guide and help the pulpwood industry in growing and harvesting pulpwood raw material for the pulp and paper industry. The safety and training program of the Association is served through six regional Technical Divisions, each one of which has a safety and training committee.

Available literature includes training guides, notebooks, and technical releases that describe items of personal protective equipment, safe working procedures, and other pertinent accident control items.

## American Road and Transportation Builders
### 525 School St. SW.,
### Washington, D.C. 20024

Accident prevention in the construction of highways is the objective of a three-phase program:

A continuing promotional program,

Development of statistical data on accident frequency and severity in the industry,

Development and utilization of safety standards in the industry.

The program is carried on cooperatively with private and governmental agencies concerned.

Information is disseminated to members through special bulletins, newsletters, and the *American Transportation Builder* (bi-monthly magazine).

The organization is also interested in highway design, signing, lighting, and other factors relating to highway safety.

## American Trucking Associations, Inc.
### 1616 P St. NW., Washington, D.C. 20036

American Trucking Associations is the national federation representing the trucking industry. Through its 3000-member Council of Safety Supervisors, standards for the selection, training, and supervision of truck fleet personnel have been developed—these form the foundation for the ATA Safety Service, a basic safety program for truck fleets.

Guidebooks, forms, and a driver safety program are available through the ATA Department of Safety as are monthly mailings of safety bulletins, driver letters and safety posters. In addition to providing these services and materials, and acting as secretariat for the Council of Safety Supervisors, the Department of Safety Security is the trucking industry's liaison with federal agencies and national organizations concerned with safety of highway truck operations.

Membership in the Council of Safety Supervisors is available to any person concerned with truck safety. In addition to regional and national meetings, committees work on such problems as employee selection, training and supervision, accident investigation and reporting, transportation of hazardous materials, physical qualifications, and injury control.

There are 47 state councils of safety supervisors and eight councils concerned with safety of tank truck operations and of automobile transporters. Such councils conduct monthly and quarterly meetings, and engage in safety engineering activities that relate to their particular interests according to geographic location or type of operation.

## The American Waterways Operators, Inc.
### Suite 1101, 1600 Wilson Blvd.,
### Arlington, Va. 22209

The American Waterways Operators, Inc., is a trade association representing the national interests of operators of towboats, tugboats, and barges engaged in domestic trade primarily on the inland and coastal waters of the United States, as well as those of the shipyards that build and repair these vessels.

AWO has a safety committee that pursues three primary objectives:

• Promotion of individual member company's safety programs,

• More participation by members in the Barge and Towing Vessel Industry Safety Contest, which the association co-sponsors with the National Safety Council, and

• Preparation and distribution of AWO safety posters, which the association issues to its members each month.

The association's manual, *Basic Safety Program for the Barge and Towing Vessel Industry*, is designed either (a) to be adopted as a complete company program, or (b) be used as a guide to develop or supplement an individual company's program. The manual covers methods and techniques for accident prevention, and contains valuable guidelines on all aspects of personnel safety in the barge and towing vessel industry.

### American Water Works Association
6666 W. Quincy Ave., Denver, Colo. 80235

The AWWA Accident Prevention Committee has as its scope the development and continued expansion of safety programs for the water utility industry. Programs presently available include (a) collecting, analyzing, and compiling annual statistics on both employee and motor vehicle accidents and their causes, (b) a safety award program, (c) an audiovisual library, (d) one-and two-day safety seminars for supervisors, (e) a safety audit program, (f) a safety poster program, and (g) a first aid kit program. Publications include a *Safety Practices Manual* and *Safety Talks for Foremen*.

### American Welding Society
2501 NW. 7th St., Miami, Fla. 33125

The society is devoted to the proper and safe use of welding by industry. Through its Safety and Health Committee, the society coordinates safe practices in welding by promoting new and revising existing standards.

"Safe Practices for Welding and Cutting Containers that Have Held Combustibles" is one booklet produced by this Committee and is available to industry. Some recent reports deal with noise, fumes and gases, and health effects.

The society also sponsors American National Standards Institute Committee Z49, whose publication, *Safety in Welding and Cutting*, is the authoritative standard in this field. It deals with the protection of workers from accidents, occupational diseases, and fires arising out of the installation, operation, and maintenance of electric and gas welding and cutting equipment.

Frequent articles on safety in welding appear in the official publication of the society, the *Welding Journal*.

### Associated General Contractors of America, Inc.
1957 E St. NW., Washington, D.C. 20006

This association of contractors specializes in the building, highway, railroad, and heavy construction fields. All areas of the United States are served by the association's 113 chapters, which carry on their own programs and render assistance

to their members.

The association has had better than 50 years of continuing interest in the activities of its Safety and Health Committee, to which member contractors have freely contributed their time and effort. The committee's *Manual of Accident Prevention in Construction* is revised periodically. Each year, the national organization presents awards to members and chapters for significant achievement in accident prevention.

### Association of American Railroads
1920 L St., NW., Washington, D.C. 20036

All Class I railroads (those with an annual revenue in excess of $50 million) are members of the AAR. The following divisions and committees of the association are concerned with safety:

Communication and Signal Section
Engineering Division
Mechanical Division
Medical Section
Operating Rules Committee
Police and Security Section
Safety Section
State Rail Programs Division

The Safety Section holds annual meetings; it issues a monthly newsletter, produces posters and publishes pamphlets on railroad safety.

The Bureau for the Safe Transportation of Explosives and Other Dangerous Articles is also located at the above address.

### Bituminous Coal Operators' Association
303 World Center Bldg.,
Washington, D.C. 20006

The Bituminous Coal Operators' Association has a Safety Department to furnish health and accident services to its members.

### Chemical Manufacturers Association, Inc.
2501 M Street, NW.,
Washington, D.C. 20037

Formerly known as the Manufacturing Chemists Association, Inc., one of CMA's most important services is dissemination of information on the handling, transportation, and use of chemicals.

The association supports an Occupational Safety and Health Committee composed of safety directors, medical directors, and other health-

ated managers selected from its member com-
nies. This committee meets six times a year in
ernate months and develops chemical safety
d health information for use by member com-
nies, state and federal health organizations, and
e public. The committee holds three open
etings each year for those interested in chemi-
 safety and health.

Other committees of the association that
lude safety in their program are the Environ-
ntal Management Committee and the Distri-
tion Committee.

## mpressed Gas Association, Inc.
0 Fifth Avenue, New York, N.Y. 10036

The major purpose of the Compressed Gas
sociation is to provide, develop, and coordinate
chnical activities in the compressed gas indus-
es, in the interest of safety and efficiency in the
S., Canada, and Mexico.

Most of the work of the association is done by
ore than 40 technical committees, made up of
presentatives of member companies who are
ghly qualified technically in their respective
as:

etylene
mmonia
mospheric gases: nitrogen, oxygen, argon and
he rare gases.
rbon dioxide
lorine
yogenic and low-temperature gases
hylene
s specification
logenated hydrocarbons: propane, butane, etc.
ydrogen
ydrogen sulfide
edical gases: nitrous oxide, cyclopropane,
ethylene
ethyl chloride
atural gas
troleum hydrocarbon gases
  Refrigerants: ammonia, flurocarbons
  Aerosol propellants
  Poisonous gases: hydrogen cyanide, phosgene,
    etc.
  Other gases: anhydrous ammonia, chlorine,
    methylamines, sulfur dioxide, carbon mon-
      oxide, fluorine
fety device
eciality gases
lfur dioxide

The association publishes the *Handbook of
Compressed Gases*, which contains complete
descriptions of 49 widely used gases, and gives the
safest recognized methods for handling and storing them. Nearly 80 standards and bulletins are
published with audiovisual training aids. A list is
available on request.

## Edison Electric Institute
1111 19th St., NW.,
Washington, D.C. 20036

The Edison Electric Institute is the association
of the nation's investor-owned electric utilities.
Its members serve 99.6 percent of the customers
serviced by the investor-owned segment of the
industry.

The Safety and Industrial Health Committee is
dedicated to improving working conditions
through development of safe work practices. The
Committee meets twice a year and compiles
reports and publications on subjects of interest to
safety professionals in the utility industry. Also
prepared by the committee are videotape cas-
settes and sound-slide films.

## Graphic Arts Technical Foundation
4615 Forbes Ave., Pittsburgh, Pa. 15213

The Education Council is a coordinating
organization, the membership of which is made
up of large national and various local printing and
allied trade associations. Individual companies
are also members of the council.

In cooperation with the National Safety Council, the Education Council published the *Safety
Manual for the Graphic Arts Industry.*

## Industrial Safety Equipment
  Association, Inc.
1901 N. Moore St., Arlington, Va. 22209

This association has represented manufacturers
of industrial safety equipment since 1934. It is
devoted to the promotion of public interest in
safety and encourages development of efficient
and practical devices and personal protective
equipment for industry.

It is umbrella-like in nature, providing technical improvement through the constant activities
of its 12 separate product groups. Of outstanding
importance is the broad representation of its
members on numerous American National Standards Institute standards committees engaged in
promulgation of industry-wide standards of per-

**719**

formance for specific types of personal protective equipment. Safety professionals can be guided by these codes and can be assured that certified products will conform to published standards.

## Institute of Makers of Explosives
420 Lexington Ave., New York, N.Y. 10017

The institute functions through committees composed of qualified representatives of member companies experienced in the activities assigned to the various groups. A technical committee and a committee on traffic and storage conditions are responsible for the institute's booklets on the safe transportation, handling, and use of explosives. Included among such materials are:

"Typical Storage Magazines"
"American Table of Distances"
"Suggested Code of Regulations"
"Do's and Don'ts"
"Glossary of Industry Terms"
"Safety in the Transportation, Storage, Handling and Use of Explosives"
"Safety Guide for the Prevention of Radio Frequency Radiation Hazards in the Use of Electric Blasting Caps"
"IME Standard for the Safe Transportation of Electric Blasting Caps in the Same Vehicle with Other Explosives"
Blasting cap (dummy) display boards

Blasting cap safety posters are circulated, especially in schools and to youth groups; related material, available for newspaper reproduction, is provided upon request.

## International Association of Drilling Contractors
Suite 505, 211 N. Ervay,
Dallas, Texas 75201

This association works to improve oil well drilling contracting operations as a whole and to increase the value of oil well drilling as an integral part of the petroleum industry.

The association holds an annual safety clinic and has standing and special safety committees of contractor representatives to study current problems.

Safety meetings for tool pushers, drillers, crew members, and safety directors are sponsored by the association; they are conducted throughout the country in locations where these people normally reside.

A Supervisory Accident Prevention Traini Program has been developed to instruct drill and tool pushers in how to establish and maint effective accident prevention programs. Six eight professional safety instructors persona conduct these programs anywhere in the wo where 18 to 25 people wish to enroll. Many otl schools of either two-day or five-day duration a available through the association.

Safety award certificates, cards, safety l decals, and plaques are given to member perse nel and rigs that have completed one or mc years without a disabling injury.

The group has produced safety manuals for t industry, inspection reports, color codes, saf signs, studies on protective clothing, and otl publications. They have produced color filr film strips, and slides on specific drilling rig saf practices. The assocation also produces safe posters keyed to the hazards of the drilli industry.

## International Association of Refrigerated Warehouses
7315 Wisconsin Ave. NW.,
Washington, D.C. 20014

The association's Safety Committee conduct program specifically aimed at reducing accider and injuries in refrigerated warehouses. The p gram includes periodic industry surveys to det mine types of injuries being experienced, th causes, frequency and severity, safety bulleti awards, and information on how to establish a operate a safety program. Members a encouraged to submit problems to the Safe Committee for study and suggested solution

## Iron Castings Society
Cast Metals Federation Building,
20611 Center Ridge Road,
Rocky River, Ohio 44116

The Iron Castings Society is a trade associati that represents gray, malleable, and ductile ir foundries in the United States and Cana Founded in 1975 through a merger of the Gr and Ductile Iron Founders' Society and the Mal able Founders Society, it is a nonprofit, volunta membership organization with administrati headquarters in Cleveland, Ohio. It is govern by an elected board of directors which is assist by eleven standing committees in the formulati of programs and policy to promote the progress s members and the industry.

A booklet developed for the Cast Metals Federation defines safe working conditions in ferrous foundries. Booklets entitled "How You Can Work Safely" are available for foundry employees in either English or Spanish language editions.

## National Association of Manufacturers
### 776 F St. NW., Washington, D.C. 20006

The NAM safety and health activities are carried on under the aegis of its Occupational Safety and Health Committee which has a dual function: (a) promoting sound health and safety policies and programs in industry; and (b) working with the federal government to assure that present regulation of health and safety practices in industry and proposals for new regulations and legislation are realistic from industry's viewpoint.

## National Coal Association
### 130 17th St. NW., Washington, D.C. 20036

The association assists its members in the promotion of safety and accident prevention through the development of coal industry training programs that stress safe operating procedures in the mines. Research in health and safety areas is conducted by NCA's research affiliate, Bituminous Coal Research Inc., located in Monroeville, Pa.

## National Constructors Association
### 101 15th St. NW., Washington, D.C. 20005

NCA is made up of more than 50 national and regional design-construction firms that build large industrial facilities for oil, steel, power, and chemicals. Its Safety and Health Committee carries out many programs to enhance the physical welfare of employees and the public. Other activities include labor and employee relations, government and international affairs, and taxes, insurance, and legal matters.

## National Health Council, Inc.
### 1740 Broadway, New York, N.Y. 10019

For nearly six decades, the National Health Council has provided a national focus for sharing common concerns and evaluating needs and pooling ideas, resources, and leadership services for national organizations in the health field.

Today 86 major organizations, including voluntary health agencies, professional and other membership associations, insurance companies, business corporations, and federal government agencies, are members.

Like its constituents, the Council exists to improve the health of Americans. Its principal functions are (a) to help member agencies work together more effectively in the public interest to identify and promote the solution of national health problems of concern to the public; and (b) to improve further governmental and private health services for the public at the state and local levels.

The tradition of the National Health Council is one of thoughtful exploration of the nation's critical health problems and of taking action on solutions where possible.

## National LP-Gas Association
### 1301 W. 22nd St., Oak Brook, Ill. 60521

Founded in 1931, the association is a nonprofit, cooperative group of producers and distributors of liquefied petroleum gas (LP-gas), manufacturers of LP-gas equipment, and manufacturers and marketers of LP-gas appliances. NLPGA promotes technical information and industry standards in its special field.

Its Safety Committee develops and maintains educational programs to train the public and industry in the safe handling and use of LP-gas and in safe practices for the installation and maintenance of equipment and appliances.

An Educational committee working closely with the Safety committee arranges training school and conferences for dealers and distributors.

The association distributes informational, technical and legislative bulletins and publishes a weekly newsletter for members. It holds an annual meeting and sectional meetings with a definite portion of each program devoted to safety.

The Association publishes a *Safety Handbook*, a training guide, audiovisual training programs, and distributes consumer education leaflets for members to help educate its customers.

## National Petroleum Refiners Association
### 1899 L St. NW., Washington, D.C. 20036

Primarily a service organization for the petroleum refining and petrochemical manufacturing industries, the NPRA also serves as a clearinghouse for new ideas and developments for its membership.

Among the several meetings that are sponsored by NPRA are those of the trade group's ten Fire and Accident Prevention Groups. These are one-day regional meetings that are conducted at different refinery locations and are primarily for first-line supervisors and plant safety and fire protection personnel. These meetings, in ten geographical areas, were established to promote the exchange of information and experiences pertaining to fire and accident prevention in refining and petrochemical operations.

The association also prepares and distributes various safety and fire protection bulletins, information on OSHA and NIOSH activities, and an annual summary of industry data dealing with injury and illness experiences. In an effort to promote safety in plant operations, the NPRA has also established a comprehensive safety awards program.

### National Restaurant Association
Suite 2600, One IBM Plaza,
Chicago, Ill. 60611

The National Restaurant Association, through its Public Health and Safety Department, carries on a program to reduce accidents and hazards that affect the safety of food service employees and patrons.

A major association activity is the preparation and distribution of educational materials to the membership. These included self-inspection guidelines on general safety concerns, OSHA and fire protection, as well as posters and audiovisual programs. This material is also available for purchase through the National Restaurant Association's Educational Materials Center.

The association conducts research to substantiate industry positions on such DOE regulations as Hazardous Occupational Orders and on OSHA. Safety-related information appears in the weekly *Washington Report* and the monthly *NRA News*.

The National Institute for the Foodservice Industry, 20 N. Wacker Dr., Chicago, Ill. 60606, is an educational group affiliated with NRA.

### National Rural Electric Cooperative Association
1800 Massachusetts Ave. NW.,
Washington, D.C. 20036

The association, through its Retirement Safety and Insurance Department, promotes a vigorous and diversified program of accident prevention

among rural electric cooperatives. The followir is a brief resume of safety activities:

**Job Training and Safety Fund.** A fund distributed to state safety committees based c the proportionate amount of premium develope within each state in the casualty dividend poo

**Publications and film.** Safety articles are pul lished each month in the association's magazin *Rural Electrification.* Safety releases are issue several times a year to job training and safet instructors and state safety committees. Safet films have been produced and made available t member systems.

**Meetings.** NRECA publicizes the Nationa Job Training and Safety Conference; staff men bers participate each year.

### National Sanitation Foundation
3475 Plymouth Rd.,
Ann Arbor, Mich. 48106

NSF represents the public health professior business, and industry. It conducts research an educational programs in environmental sanita tion and health through its Council of Publi Health Consultants and Industry Advisor Committee.

Publications include:

*Criteria and Standards* (annually)
"Food Service Equipment" (annual listing)
"Plastics for Potable Water and Drain, Waste and Vent" (annual listing)
"Swimming Pool Equipment" (annual listing)
Standards and educational materials

### National Soft Drink Association
1101 Sixteenth St. NW.,
Washington, D.C. 20036

NSDA's Safety Committee periodicall prepares information bulletins concerning OSH regulations and citations, educational safety pro cedures, and training films.

### New York Shipping Association, Inc.
80 Broad St., New York, N.Y. 10004

New York Shipping Association is composed o American and foreign flag ocean carriers an contracting stevedores, marine terminal opera tors, and other employers of waterfront labo

thin the bi-state Port of New York and New
rsey.

Safety by NYSA is supervised by a director
1o is appointed by the association president.
1e safety director maintains contact with fed-
1l, state, and other agencies involved with
1ustrial safety and health regulations. In this
gard, the safety director disseminates relevant
ta to the member companies of NYSA to assist
em in reducing accidents on piers and at marine
:ilities.

Further, he coordinates industry activity and
1intains liaison with the various stevedoring
d marine terminal companies who operate their
vn company safety and health programs.

## 1rtland Cement Association
120 Old Orchard Rd., Skokie, Ill. 60077

PCA, devoted to research, educational, and
omotional activities to extend and improve the
e of portland cement, is supported by more than
, U.S. and Canadian member companies that
1erate more than 130 cement manufacturing
ants. Occupational safety and health have been
nsidered important by the association since its
rmation in 1916. The Occupational Safety and
ealth Services Department works closely with a
mmittee of member company representatives
provide activities, services and materials that
e responsive to the needs of those companies.

Consultation on technical safety and health
atters is provided and association staff members
sit plants on request to perform safety audits,
fety program evaluations, and health exposure
rveys. Laboratory analysis of substance sam-
es, the use of sampling equipment, and training
r plant personnel in noise and dust monitoring
ocedures also are services available to member
mpanies.

PCA expresses the views and opinions of its
ember companies to governmental organiza-
ons regarding proposed legislation and regula-
ons and other issues affecting the cement
dustry.

To supplement materials used in plant acci-
nt prevention programs, a variety of promo-
onal, informational, and educational items are
epared. Included among these are letters,
emos, pamphlets, manuals, summaries, periodi-
ils, and visual aids. Knowledge and experience
e shared through meetings and conferences.

Outstanding individual and group perform-
ice are recognized through an award program.

Worker awards include the Distinguished Safety
Service award and Silver Honor Roll certificate.
Plant recognition is provided by the PCA Safety
Trophy, Thousand-Day Club, and Certificate of
Merit.

An injury/illness reporting program enables
the association to accumulate data and identify
significant casual and circumstantial factors. This
information is used to define the nature and extent
of cement industry injury/illness experience and
in the preparation of educational and informational materials.

## Printing Industries of America, Inc.
1730 N. Lynn St., Arlington, Va. 22209

Printing Industries of America, an association
of printers' organizations, actively sponsors the
development of safety in the graphic arts through
its affiliated local orgranizations and through its
participation in the Graphic Arts Technical Foundation (described earlier).

## Scaffolding, Shoring, and Forming Institute
1230 Keith Building, Cleveland, Ohio 44115

The institute has a deep interest in safety;
members try to do everything possible to improve
this situation in the construction industry. List-
ings of "Scaffolding Safety Rules," "Steel Frame
Shoring Safety Rules," "Horizontal Shoring Beam
Safety Rules," "Single Post Shore Safety Rules,"
"Suspended Powered Scaffolding Safety Rules,"
"Flying Deck Form Safety Rules," "Rolling Shore
Bracket Safety Rules" are available, as are book-
lets "Recommended Scaffolding Erection Proce-
dure," "Recommended Steel Frame Shoring
Erection Procedure," "Recommended Horizon-
tal Shoring Beam Erection Procedure," "Safety
Requirements for Suspended Powered Scaffolds,"
and "Recommended Safety Requirements for
Shoring Concrete Formwork."

## Steel Plate Fabricators Association, Inc.
2901 Finley Rd., Downers Grove, Ill. 60515

The association has an active safety committee
which prepares publications on safety for member companies and their employees. Some of
these are:

"Supervisor's Accident Prevention Manual for
Field Erection and Construction,"
"Basic Safety Rules for Fabricating Shops," and

"Basic Safety Rules for Field Erection and Construction."

The association conducts a monthly steel plate fabricators safety contest.

## Emergency and Specialized Information

Emergency response systems that can help.

### AVLINE

AVLINE (Audio Visuals on-Line) is a data base maintained by the National Library of Medicine; it contains references to audiovisual instructional materials in the health sciences. All of these materials are professionally reviewed for technical quality, currency, accuracy of subject content, and educational design. AVLINE enables teachers, students, librarians, researchers, practitioners, and other health science professionals to retrieve citations which aid in evaluating audiovisual materials with maximum specificity.

For more information contact:

National Library of Medicine
8600 Rockville Pike
Bethesda, Md. 20014

### CANCERLINE

CANCERLINE (Cancer on-Line) is the National Cancer Institute's on-line data base of approximately 60,000 citations dealing with all aspects of cancer.

For more information contact:

CANCERLINE Information Specialist
National Library of Medicine
8600 Rockville Pike
Bethesda, Md. 20014

### CHEMLINE

CHEMLINE (Chemical Dictionary on-Line) is the National Library of Medicine's on-line, interactive chemical dictionary file created by the Specialized Information Services in collaboration with Chemical Abstracts Service (CAS). It provides a mechanism whereby more than 330,000 chemical substance names, representing nearly 100,000 unique substances, can be searched and retrieved on-line. This file contains CAS Registry Numbers; molecular formulas; preferred chemical index nomenclature; generic and trivial names derived from the CAS Registry Nomenclature

File; and a locator designation which points other files in the NLM system containing information on that particular chemical substance. F a limited number of records in the file, there a Medical Subject Headings (MeSH) terms a Wiswesser Line Notations (WLN). In additic where applicable, each Registry Number reco in CHEMLINE contains ring information inclu ing—number of rings within a ring system, ri sizes, ring elemental composition, and comp nent line formulas.

For more information contact:

Toxicology Information Services
National Library of Medicine
8600 Rockville Pike
Bethesda, Md. 20014

### CHEMTREC

Emergency information about hazardo chemicals involved in transportation acciden can now be obtained 24 hours a day. It is th Chemical Transportation Emergency Cent (CHEMTREC), and it can be reached by a natio wide telephone number—800/424-9300. Tl Area Code 800 WATS line permits the caller dial the station-to-station number withou charge. CHEMTREC will provide the caller wi response/action information for the product products and tell what to do in case of spills, leak fires, and exposures. This informs the caller of tl hazards, if any, and provides sufficient inform tion to take immediate first steps in controllii the emergency. CHEMTREC is strictly an eme gency operation provided for fire, police, ai other emergency services. It is not a source general chemical information of a nonemergen nature.

### ICES

The Information Center for Energy Safel (ICES) was established at Oak Ridge Nation Laboratory (ORNL) by the Energy Research ai Development Administration (ERDA) as national center for collecting, storing, evaluatin and disseminating safety information related the development and use of several forms energy. The Center will analyze current inform tion, prepare state-of-the-art reviews of the safel of the various energy systems, and answer techn cal inquiries. Complete bibliographic data c more than 110,000 documents. Phone number 615/574-0391.

For more information, contact:

formation Center for Energy Safety
ak Ridge National Laboratory
O. Box Y
ak Ridge, Tenn. 37830

## EDLINE

MEDLINE (Medical Literature Analysis and
trieval System on-Line) is a data base main-
ined by the National Library of Medicine; it
ntains references to approximately half a mil-
on citations from 3000 biomedical journals. It is
signed to help health professionals find out
sily and quickly what has been published
cently on any specific biomedical subject. Med-
ie is accessed from a variety of typewriter-like
rminals connected to computers in Bethesda,
d., and Albany, N.Y., via ordinary telephone
es and nationwide communications networks.

For more information, contact:

ational Library of Medicine
800 Rockville Pike
ethesda, Md. 20014

## IOSHTIC

NIOSH's computerized research and reference
rvice, NIOSHTIC is available free of charge to
iy person or organization desiring information
out a subject in the field of occupational safety
id health. NIOSHTIC contains approximately
0,000 documents in 14 different subject areas
cluding toxicology, occupational medicine,
dustrial hygiene and personal protective
quipment.

For more information, contact:

ational Institute of Occupational Safety and
Health
arklawn Building
600 Fishers Lane
ockville, Md. 20857

## oison Control Centers

The Poison Control Division of the FDA pro-
ures information on the ingredients and poten-
al acute toxicity of substances that may cause
ccidental poisonings and on the proper manage-
ient of such poisonings. It assists the approxi-
ately 580 Poison Control Centers through the
.S. These are usually associated with medical
chools or large hospitals and provide treatment

and/or toxicity information to doctors and first
aid instructions to laymen on a 24-hour basis.

For more information, contact:

National Clearinghouse for Poison Control
 Centers
Poison Control Division, Bureau of Drugs
Food and Drug Administration
5401 Westbard Ave.
Bethesda, Md. 20016

## SRIS

The National Safety Council's Safety Research
Information Service (SRIS) includes more than
5000 basic research documents and abstracts.
SRIS is part of the Council's library, which
includes more than 600,000 books and documents
regarding all aspects of safety and health.

For more information, contact:

Safety Research Information Service
National Safety Council
444 N. Michigan Ave.
Chicago, Ill. 60611

## TOXLINE

TOXLINE (Toxicology Information on-Line)
is the National Library of Medicine's extensive
collection of computerized toxicology information containing more than 380,000 references to
published human and animal toxicity studies,
effects of environmental chemicals and pollu-
tants, adverse drug reactions, and analytical
methodology.

For further information, contact:

Toxicology Information Services
National Library of Medicine
8600 Rockville Pike
Bethesda, Md. 20014

## U.S. Government Agencies

There is an overwhelming amount of safety
information available from the federal government concerning all aspects of safety and health,
environmental problems, pollution, statistical
data, and other industry problems.

Because of the constant change in government
agency activities and frequent reorganizations, it
is recommended that the reader consult the
*United States Government Organization Manual*,
published by the Government Printing Office,

**725**

Washington, D.C. 20402. It can be found in most libraries.

Information on the Occupational Safety and Health Administration, the Mine Safety and Health Administration, the National Institute for Occupational Safety and Health, the Environmental Protection Agency, the Public Health Service, and the Environmental Protection Agency can be found elsewhere in this Manual.

## Departments and Bureaus in the States and Possessions

It is important that a safety professional has a good working knowledge of the state agencies responsible for the enforcement of safety and health laws. He should, therefore, contact the proper groups in his specific labor department or other agency and find out how the various boards, divisions, and services function.

Some difficulty can be avoided if the safety professional is familiar with the labor legislation and safety and health codes under which he is working. Codes and laws vary widely in the different states and provinces, and those persons who have safety jurisdiction in plants in a number of places must understand these differences.

In many cases, the standards set up by the code may serve only as a minimum, and the safety professional will want to compare them with American National Standards or other regulations to establish more rigid rules for his own plant. He should also know the jurisdiction rights of the factory inspectors, so that he can better understand the job they have to do and how he can help them in the performance of their duties.

### Labor offices

Labor offices in the several states perform many functions, generally depending on the number and kind of labor problems.

A listing of state and provincial labor offices and the title of the chief executive of each agency or subdivision to whom inquiries should be addressed is given in the U.S. Department of Labor Bulletin 177, "Labor Offices in the United States and Canada." The bulletin, revised periodically, is available from the Bureau of Labor Standards, Washington, D.C. 20210.

### Health and hygiene services

Departments or boards of health and industrial hygiene services are integral parts of the organi-

zation of each of the states, the District of Columbia, and the autonomous territories of the United States.

It is to these organizations that the safety professional must look for his state's specific standards and recommendations on such points occupational health, food and health engineering disease control, water pollution, and other facets of the overall field of industrial hygiene.

Industrial hygiene units usually function full time or, in several states, on a limited basis. In addition to the units that operate under state health departments, a number of other industrial hygiene units are run by municipalities or other local authorities.

In addition to direct industrial hygiene services, these state units are able to bring to industry a more or less complete health program by integrating their work with that of other divisions in the state government, such as sanitation and infectious disease control.

State and local programs coordinate their efforts with the U.S. Department of Health and Human Services, Public Health Service, and the U.S. Department of Labor. They also cooperate with medical societies and nurses' associations. (See descriptions earlier in this chapter.)

The names and addresses of such state, commonwealth, or territorial agencies with which the safety professional may need to communicate, are available in an up-to-date listing of health authorities in Public Health Publication No. 75, "Directory of State, Territorial, and Regional Health Authorities," for sale by the U.S. Government Printing Office. Occupational health personnel are listed in the annual "Directory of Governmental Occupational Health Personnel," available from the Bureau of Occupational Safety and Health, Environmental Control Administration, Consumer Protection and Environmental Health Service, Department of Health and Human Services, 1014 Broadway, Cincinnati, Ohio 45202.

## Canadian Departments, Associations, and Boards

In all provinces of Canada there is a Workmen's Compensation Board or Commission. Some of these handle accident prevention directly. In other provinces there are provisions similar to Section 110 of the Quebec Workmen's Compensation Act, which stipulates "that industries included in any of the classes under Schedule may form themselves into an Association for accident prevention and formulate rules for that purpose. Further, the Workmen's Compensation Commission, if satisfied that an Association so formed sufficiently represents the employers in the industries included in the class, may make a special grant toward the expense of any such association."

It is under these provisions that the various safety associations were organized and are functioning. In some provinces, accident prevention is directly assumed by the board itself by establishing a safety department.

Furthermore, all provinces have legal safety requirements which are administered by the Department of Highways, Department of Labor, and the Department of Mines. These sources can be contacted by writing to the deputy minister of the department located in the capital of each province.

## governmental agencies

**Federal.** Canada Department of Labour, Accident Prevention and Compensation Branch (Director), 340 Laurier Avenue West, Ottawa, Ontario.

This branch is responsible for the implementation and administration of the Canada Labour (Safety) Code, which became effective January 1, 1968. It is also responsible for the development of occupational safety regulations and standards, for the inspection of work places under federal jurisdiction, and for the enforcement of the Safety Code and all regulations prescribed under its authority.

**Provincial.** A listing of provincial labor offices is given in U.S. Department of Labor Bulletin 177, described in the previous section on U.S. Departments and Bureaus in the States and Possessions.

## accident prevention associations

Canada Safety Council, 1765 Blvd. St. Laurent, Ottawa, Ontario K1G 3V4

**Provincial associations.**

Alberta Safety Council, 201-10526 Jasper Ave., Edmonton T5J 1Z7

British Columbia Safety Council, Suite 205, 96 E. Broadway, Vancouver V5T 1V6

New Brunswick Safety Council, Inc., 364 York St., Fredericton E3B 3P7

Nova Scotia Safety Council, 3627 Howe Ave., Halifax B3L 4H8

Quebec Safety League Inc., 5576 Upper Lachine Rd., Montreal H4A 2A7

Saskachawan Safety Council, 348 Victoria Ave., Regina S4N 0P6

Industrial Accident Prevention Association of Ontario, 2 Bloor St. E., Toronto M4W 3C2

Included in this association are ten class associations:

Woodworkers Accident Prevention Assn.
Ceramics & Stone Accident Prevention Assn.
Metal Trades Accident Prevention Assn.
Chemical Industries Accident Prevention Assn.
Grain, Feed & Fertilizer Accident Prevention Assn.
Food Products Accident Prevention Assn.
Leather, Rubber & Tanners Accident Prevention Assn.
Textile & Allied Industries Accident Prevention Assn.
Printing Trades Accident Prevention Assn.
Ontario Retail Accident Prevention Assn.

Quebec Forest Industrials Safety Association, Inc., 580 Grande Allee E., Quebec G1R 2K2

Forest Products Accident Prevention Association, P.O. Box 270, North Bay, Ontario P1B 8H2

Ontario Pulp & Paper Makers Safety Association, 91 Kelfield St., Rexdale M9W 5A4

Ontario Safety League, 409 King St. W., Toronto M5V 1K1

Mines Accident Prevention Association, 199 Bay St., Toronto, Ontario M5J 1L4

Transportation Safety Association of Ontario (Inc.), 2 Bloor St. E., Toronto M4W 3C2

Construction Safety Association of Ontario, 74 Victoria St., Toronto M4W 3C2

Industrial Accident Prevention Association—Quebec, 50 Place Cremazie, Montreal H2P 2T5

Quebec Pulp and Paper Safety Association Inc., 580 Grande Allee E., Quebec G1R 2K2

Quebec Logging Safety Association Inc., 580 Grande Allee E., Quebec G1R 2K2

New Brunswick Industrial Safety Council, P.O. Box 2239, corner Hilyard & Portland Sts., St. John E2L 3V1

Workmen's Compensation Board—Accident Prevention Department, P.O. Box 1150, Halifax, N.S. B3J 2Y2

## International Safety Organizations

### Inter-American Safety Council (Consejo Interamericano de Seguridad)
33 Park Place, Englewood, N.J. 07631

The Inter-American Safety Council was founded and incorporated in 1938, as a noncommercial, nonpolitical, and nonprofit educational association for the prevention of accidents. It is the Spanish and Portuguese language counterpart of the National Safety Council.

The Council is the first and only association of its kind rendering services to all industries and agencies in the Latin American countries and Spain. The objectives are to prevent accidents—to reduce the number and severity of accidents in every activity, both on the job and off the job. The services which the Council provides for its members are paid by membership dues and sales of the Council's monthly publications and other educational materials. All of its work is done from the headquarters in New Jersey.

Membership is open to all industries, organizations, institutions, or other groups with two or more employees, interested in accident prevention in Latin America and Spain. More than 1800 plants or work locations in 22 countries are members or are using the materials and services of the Council. In addition, over 300 universities, technical schools, public libraries, and the like, receive the monthly publications free of charge.

Among the services available to members are: monthly publications, annual contest, special awards, consultation, statistical service, reproduction and translation rights and participation in the election of Council officers. In addition, the Council acts as a clearing house of accident prevention materials available in the United States. A catalog is available from the organization.

The Council's monthly publications include two magazines and safety posters:

Noticias de Seguridad (Safety News)
El Supervisor (The Supervisor)
Safety posters in sizes 8½ by 11 and 17 by 22 inches

In addition, the Council publishes translations

of publications, films, safety slides, training programs and other materials of the National Safety Council and other accident prevention organizations.

### International Association of Industrial Accident Boards and Commissions
P.O. Box 2917, Olympia, Washington 98507

This group, composed of American, Canadian, New Zealand, and Philippine members, is concerned with worker's compensation and safety.

### International Labor Organization
International Labor Office, CH 1211, Geneva 22, Switzerland
1750 New York Ave. NW.,
Washington, D.C. 20006

The International Labor Organization (ILO), a specialized agency associated with the United Nations, was created by the Treaty of Versailles in 1919 as part of the League of Nations. Its purpose is to improve labor conditions, raise living standards, and promote economic and social stability as the foundation for lasting peace throughout the world. To this purpose, one of ILO's functions is "the protection of the worker against sickness, disease, and injury arising out of his employment."

The organization consists of about 140 member countries, including the United States (which joined in 1934). ILO functions through an annual conference of member states, a governing body, advisory committees, and a permanent office, the International Labor Office. ILO is distinctive from all other international agencies in that it is tripartite in character—that is, the conference, the governing body, and some of the committees are composed of representatives of governments, employers, and workers.

In the field of safety and health, the International Labor Office maintains a permanent international staff of medical doctors, engineers, and industrial hygienists. Assistance in specific fields is given by panels of consultants, drawn from all parts of the world to act in an advisory capacity and to discuss problems, draft regulations, or render help in emergencies. The office also maintains an Occupational Safety and Health Information Center (CIS) which analyses and provides abstracts of relevant articles appearing in official publications and journals throughout the world

The United States has several members on the panels and has been represented on all the temporary expert committees and special conferences.

The main tasks of the ILO in the field of occupational safety and health are:

International instruments. These include conventions and recommendations, and also model safety codes and codes of practice.

An *Encyclopedia of Occupational Health and Safety* has been prepared in English and French, to succeed *Occupation and Health*, which was published in 1930. This is designed to provide guidance to a wide range of people concerned with health, safety, and welfare at work. Although problems are reviewed from an international angle, special account is taken of the needs of developing countries.

The compilation of technical studies.

The publication of medical and technical studies.

Direct assistance to governments, by furnishing experts, drafting regulations, supplying information, etc.

Collaboration with other international organizations, the World Health Organization, and the International Organization for Standardization.

Assistance to national safety and health organizations, research centers, employers' associations, trade unions, etc., in different countries.

In general, keeping in touch with the safety and health movement throughout the world and assisting the movement by all the means in its power.

## Pan American Health Organization
### Pan American Sanitary Bureau, 525 23rd St. NW., Washington, D.C. 20037

Originally established as the International Sanitary Bureau in 1902, the Pan American Health Organization serves as the regional office for the World Health Organization for the Americas. The purposes of the PAHO are to promote and coordinate the efforts of the countries of the Western Hemisphere to combat disease, lengthen life, and promote the physical and mental health of the people.

Programs encompass technical collaboration with governments in the field of public health, including such subjects as sanitary engineering

and environmental sanitation, eradication or control of communicable diseases, and maternal and child health.

## World Health Organization
### Avenue Appia, Geneva, Switzerland

The United States became a member of the World Health Organization on June 21, 1948, by joint resolution of Congress. There are over 125 member nations and three associate member nations in WHO.

WHO's objective is the attainment by all peoples of the highest possible level of health—physical, mental, and social. The organization recognizes health as fundamental to the attainment of peace and security, and as being dependent upon the fullest cooperation of individuals and states.

WHO assists countries to strengthen their public health services, including environmental sanitation, mental health, communicable disease control, and health aspects of the peaceful uses of atomic energy. Advisory and demonstration teams are sent to countries requesting assistance.

## Educational Institutions

Many colleges and universities offer formal courses in industrial safety. In a publication "Educational Opportunities in Occupational Safety and Health," compiled by the American Society of Safety Engineers, accredited four-year colleges and universities are grouped by those that offer a degree program with concentration on industrial safety and those that offer one or more credit courses as an elective within engineering or education curricula. About one-half of the 1200 four-year colleges and universities in the U.S. provided catalogues for a recent study in occupational safety and health offered by postsecondary educational institutions.

Four-year and two-year degree programs and credit courses are listed in the ASSE report. Courses in water safety, first aid and safety, firefighting, and driver or traffic education are not listed. The report shows approximately 200 four-year institutions offer one or more courses in the five main occupational categories. Write to the ASSE for a copy of this publication. (Address is listed under Professional Societies earlier in this chapter.)

## 24—Sources of Help

### Bibliography of Safety and Related Periodicals

#### Safety

National Safety Council
444 North Michigan Ave.
Chicago, Ill. 60611

See details of publications in descriptive listing earlier in this chapter.

*Accident Analysis and Prevention* (quarterly)
Pergamon Press Inc.
Fairview Park
Elmsford, N.J. 10523

*Canadian Occupational Safety* (bimonthly)
222 Argyle Ave.
Delhi, Ontario N4B 2Y2, Canada

*Hazard Prevention* (5 times a year)
System Safety Society
P.O. Box A
Newport Beach, Calif. 92663

*Health and Safety at Work* (monthly)
Maclaren Publishing Ltd.
69/77 High St.
Croyden CR9 1QH, England

*Human Factors* (bimonthly)
The Human Factors Society, Inc.
P.O. Box 1369
Santa Monica, Calif. 90406

*Journal of Occupational Accidents* (quarterly)
Elsevier Scientific Publishing Company
52 Vanderbilt Ave.
New York, N.Y. 10017

*Mine Safety and Health* (bimonthly)
Dept. of Labor, Mine Safety and Health Administration
Superintendent of Documents
U.S. Government Printing Office
Washington, D.C. 20402

*Nuclear Safety* (bimonthly)
Nuclear Safety Information Center
Oak Ridge National Laboratories
Oak Ridge, Tenn. 31830

*Occupational Hazards* (monthly)

Industrial Publishing Company
614 Superior Ave., W.
Cleveland, Ohio 44113

*Occupational Safety and Health* (monthly)
Royal Society for the Prevention of Accidents
6 Buckingham Place
London SW1, England

*Professional Safety* (monthly)
American Society of Safety Engineers
850 Busse Highway
Park Ridge, Ill. 60068

*Protection* (monthly)
Institution of Industrial Safety Officers
Great Britain
113 Blackheath Park
London SE3, England

*The Record, The Magazine of Property Conservation* (bimonthly)
Factory Mutual System
1151 Boston-Providence Turnpike
Norwood, Mass. 02062

*Safe Journal* (quarterly)
Safe Association
7252 Remment Ave.
Canoga Park, Calif. 91303

#### Industrial hygiene and medicine

*A.M.A. Archives of Environmental Health* (monthly)

*Journal of the American Medical Association* (weekly)
American Medical Association
535 North Dearborn St.
Chicago, Ill. 60610

*American Industrial Hygiene Association Journal* (monthly)
American Industrial Hygiene Association
475 Wolf Ledges Parkway
Akron, Ohio 44313

*American Journal of Nursing* (monthly)
American Nurses Association
2420 Pershing Rd.
Kansas City, Mo. 64108

*American Journal of Public Health* (monthly)

American Public Health Association
1015 18th St. NW.
Washington, D.C. 20036

*ish Journal of Industrial Medicine* (quarterly)
British Medical Association
Tavistock Square
London WC1, England

*Abstracts* (8 times a year)
International Occupational Safety and Health
  Information Center (CIS)
International Labor Office
1211 Geneva 22, Switzerland

*ustrial Hygiene News Report* (monthly)
Flournoy & Associates
1845 W. Morse Ave.
Chicago, Ill. 60626

*ustrial Hygiene Digest* (monthly)
Industrial Health Foundation
5231 Centre Ave.
Pittsburgh, Pa. 15232

*rnal of Occupational Medicine* (monthly)
Industrial Medical Association
150 N. Wacker Dr.
Chicago, Ill. 60606

*cupational Health Nursing* (monthly)
American Association of Industrial Nurses
79 Madison Ave.
New York, N.Y. 10016

## Fire

*Fire Command!* (monthly)

*Fire Journal* (bimonthly)

*Fire News* (monthly)

*Fire Technology* (quarterly)
National Fire Protection Association
470 Atlantic Ave.
Boston, Mass. 02210

*Fire Engineering* (quarterly)
Dun-Donnelley Publishing Corporation
666 Fifth Ave.
New York, N.Y. 10019

*Fire Prevention* (quarterly)
Fire Prevention Association
Aldermary House
Queen Street
London EC4, England

*Fire Surveyor*
Victor Green Publications Ltd.
106 Hampstead Rd.
London NW1 2LS, England

Many of the state departments of labor and federal agencies publish periodicals which are available upon request. With the exception of the state agencies, most of the others are mentioned under the subject headings in this section.

A number of trade journals have sections devoted to industrial safety. The safety professional should become acquainted with those servicing the industry in which he is primarily interested.

# Index

# Index

American Gas Association, 715
American Medical Association, 710-711
American Mining Congress, 715-716
American National Red Cross, 702
  emergency aid, 470
  first aid, 560-566
American National Standards Institute, 140, 153, 180,
    703-704
  see also Z16
American Nurses' Association, 711
American Occupational Medicine Association, 711
American Paper Institute, 716
American Petroleum Institute, 716
American Psychiatric Association, 711
American Public Health Association, 711
American Pulpwood Association, 717
American Road and Transportation Builders, 717
American Society for Industrial Security, 711-712
American Society of Mechanical Engineers, 712
American Society of Safety Engineers, 16, 82, 331,
    372, 708-709
  accredited schools, 729
American Society for Testing and Materials, 704
American Society for Training and Development, 712
American Trucking Associations, 717
American Water Works Association, 718
American Waterways Operators, 717-718
American Welding Society, 718
Amplifying systems, 398-399, 614
Analytical trees, 95-96
Annual reports, 161, 173, 208, 362, 372
Anthropometry, 284-287
  wheelchair handicapped, 592-594
Antiseptics and dressings, 183
Approach-approach conflict, 311-312
Approach-avoidance conflict, 312
Arm protectors, 530-531
Asbestos clothing, 527
Assistant Secretary for Occupational Safety and
    Health, 25
Associated General Contractors of America, 718
Association of American Railroads, 718
Association of Iron and Steel Electrical Engineers, 6
Attitudes, human, 302-303, 314-317
  changing, 315-317
  complacency, 421
  determination, 315
  in driver selection, 667
  on product safety, 641
  supervisory training, 244-251
Audience, publicity, 373-374
Audio aids, 414-415
Audiovisuals, 385-415
  color use, 394
  commercial vs homemade, 388-391, 413-414
  cost, 387, 388, 413
  effectiveness, 386-391
  features and limitations, 388-389
  mobile, 401

Audiovisuals—Continued
  nonprojected, 398, 402-405
  posters; see Posters
  preparation, 391-398
  projected, 400, 405-411
  rehearsal, 401-402
  relative merits, 388-389
  screens, 399-400
  seating, 400
  selection, 387-389
  slides, 405-406
  sound, 396-397
  videotape, 386, 391, 411-414
Auditory displays, 291-295
"Average person" fallacy, 287, 303-304
AVLINE response system, 724
Avoidance-avoidance conflict, 312
Awards
  "clubs," 477
  contest, 341, 346, 347, 348
  driver, 669-670
  presentations, 349-350
  publicity, 372-376
  suggestion, 363-365

## B

Back injury, 193; see also Injuries
Bacteria in food, 554
Barrier creams, skin, 547
Battery charging, 675-676
Behavior, human, 302-317
Behavioral responses, 292-293
Belts, safety, 516-522
  construction, 519-521
  inspection and testing, 521-522
  lifelines, 516-518, 522
  maintenance, 521
Bicycles, parking of, 601
Bilevel reporting, 179, 180
Biological factors in hazard control, 65
Biological monitoring, 127
Bituminous Coal Operators Association, 718
Board of Certified Safety Professionals, 16, 82, 24?
    372, 712-714
Boards, visual aid
  chalk, 402-403
  flannel, 404
  hook and loop, 404
  magnetic, 404-405
  story, 391-393
Body measurements, 284-287
Bonus, safety, 349
Books
  historical safety, 21-22
  industrial safety, 362, 382
  rule, 260-261, 669

# Index

# Index

# Index

urricanes, 441-442
ygiene approach to motivation, 310

## I

lness records, 159-160, 180-188; *see also* Injuries
luminating Engineering Society of America, 713
lumination
  evaluation, 427
  office, 426-427
lustrations
  for publications, 361, 362, 381, 391-396
  photographic, 396-397
mpairment, work-related, 224-225
mpervious clothing, 531-533
mportance principle, 297
ncentives; *see* Awards
ncidence rate, OSHA, 187-188
ncidents, list of, 67
ndividual differences, 303-306
nductive method, 95
ndustrial Health Foundation, Inc., 702-703
ndustrial hygiene, 127-131
  associations, professional, 702-703, 709-710
  government services, 27, 726, 729
  handicapped workers, 586, 588
  hygienist, 86, 131-132, 550
  periodicals, 730-731
ndustrial Risk Insurers, 705
ndustrial Safety Equipment Association, 719-720
nflation, adjusting for, 214
nformation
  displays, 289-290
  man as processor, 294
  personnel, need of, 667-668
  sources, 698-731
  *see also* Books
nformation Center for Energy Safety (ICES), 724-725
njuries
  disabling, 147, 185-186, 189, 191-193, 196, 197,
      419, 422-424
    definitions, 185, 192
    significance of changes, 140, 188-189
  frequency rate formulas, 191
  investigation of, 154, 200-206
  nonoccupational, 190, 596-597
  off-the-job, 189-190
  office, 419-424
  product-related, 624
  production hindrance, 140
  rates, 11, 24-25, 98, 191
    OSHA incidence rates, 187-188
  recordkeeping, 159-179, 185, 190-197
  reducing exposure to, 139-141
  severity of, 203
  workers' compensation, 223-225
njury rate contests, 339-342

Insect control, 544
Inspection
  conducting, 119-127
  definition, 98
  facilities, 38-39
  follow-up, 125-127, 135-136
  frequency of, 117-119
  measurement and testing, 127-133
  mine, 52-53
  OSHA, 29, 35-39, 103, 117
  philosophy of, 98-99
  planning for, 101-121
  quality control, 644, 645, 646-647
  report, writing of, 123-125
  types of, 99-101
  workplace, 35-39
Institute of Makers of Explosives, 720
Insurance
  associations, 706-708
  compulsory, 20
  costs, 209, 214-215, 239
    administrative, 230-231
  disability, 235-239
  handicapped employees, 584-586
  premium discount, 231-232
  private programs, 237-238
  product liability, 641-642
  rehabilitation, 234
  self, 230, 238-239
  workers' compensation, 220, 229-233, 237-239; *see*
      *also* Workers' Compensation
Intensity, principle of, 320
Inter-American Safety Council, 728
Intergroup contests, 343-344
International Association of Drilling Contractors, 720
International Association of Industrial Accident Boards
    and Commissions, 728
International Association of Refrigerated Warehouses,
    720
International Hazard Control Manager Certification
    Board, 713
International Healthcare Safety Professional Certifica-
    tion Board, 713-714
International Labor Organization, 728-729
Interviewing, 377-379
  accident investigation, 134-135
  personnel, 667-668
Invariance, principle of, 293-294
Invitee, legal definition, 596
Iron Castings Society, 720-721
Isotopes, emergency handling of, 449

## J

Jacks, vehicular, 674, 677
Janitorial service, 551

# Index

# Index

**745**

# Index

# Index

Toxicology, experimental, 470
TOXLINE information network, 725
Trade associations, 715-724
Trailers, truck, loading, 671-672
Training; *see* Education
*Transactions, Safety Congress*, 14
Transfer of training, 321
Transparencies; *see* Slides
Transporation during emergencies, 466
Trucks, motor; *see* Motor vehicles

## U

Ultraviolet rays, 495
Underwriters Laboratories Inc., 153, 706
Uninsured (indirect) costs, 209, 214
United States government agencies, 725-726
Unsafe acts, 63-64, 122, 140-141, 207, 272
Utility control squad, 460

## V

Vacillation, 312
Validity of measurement, 305
Variances, federal standards, 34-35, 51
Vehicles, motor; *see* Motor vehicles
Vending machines, 552
Ventilation, office, 426, 427
Veterans of Safety, 715
Videotape, 386, 391, 411-414
    *see also* Audiovisuals *and* Television
Vietnam Era Veterans' Readjustment Assistance Act of 1974, 580, 581
Violations, OSHA, 39-41, 43
Vision tests, 571
Visual displays, 290-291
Visuals; *see* Audiovisuals
Vocational rehabilitation, 234-235

## W

Wage loss theory, 236
Wages lost, 222
Walkways; *see* Passageways
Walsh-Healey Act, 19, 24, 25
Warden service during emergencies, 465-466
Wash rack, vehicular, 675
Washrooms, 547-548
    for handicapped, 591-593

Wastes
    containers, 434, 435
    disposal, 434
    garbage, 544-545
    material, 98
    sewage, 543-544
Water, potable, 538-543, 545
Water systems, disinfecting, 541-542
Weather
    adverse, 449
    National Service, 442
Wells, water, 541
Wheelchairs, 592-594
Whole *vs.* part learning, 319
Williams-Steiger Occupational Safety and Health Act of 1970; *see* Occupational Safety and Health Act of 1970
Windchill factors, 450
Window belts, 519
Withdrawal behavior reaction, 313
Witnesses, accident, 664, 665
Women
    injuries, 421-422
    protective caps, 477, 480
    protective clothing, 533-535
    security, 468
    shoppers, 608
Wool clothing, 527
Work accidents, definition, 208
Workers' compensation
    administration, 227-229
        Canadian, 727-728
    benefits, 225-227, 230-231, 233
    cost levels, 220, 223, 230-231, 239
    coverage, 223-225, 229-230, 232
    disabilities, 225-226, 235-237
    financing, 229-231
    history, 4-5, 220-221
    insurance services, 234, 237-238
    objectives, 222-223, 228
    rating systems, 232, 239
    rehabilitation, 227, 233-235
    safety efforts, 231-232, 239-240
World Health Organization, 729

## X

X-ray examination, 183
X-rays, medical, 570-571

## Z

Z16 definitions, 140, 180, 190-197, 200, 204-206